Chronic and Recurrent Pain

Special Issue Editors

Lynn S. Walker

Carl L. von Baeyer

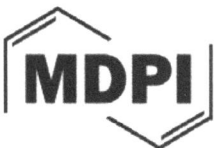

MDPI

Special Issue Editors
Lynn S. Walker
Vanderbilt University School of Medicine
Nashville, USA

Carl L. von Baeyer
Max Rady College of Medicine
University of Manitoba
Winnipeg, Canada

Editorial Office
MDPI AG
St. Alban-Anlage 66
Basel, Switzerland

This edition is a reprint of the Special Issue published online in the open access journal *Children* (ISSN 2227-9067) from 2016–2017 (available at: http://www.mdpi.com/journal/children/special_issues/chronic_pain).

For citation purposes, cite each article independently as indicated on the article page online and as indicated below:

Author 1; Author 2. Article title. *Journal Name.* **Year**, *Article number*, page range.

ISBN 978-3-03842-416-1 (Pbk)
ISBN 978-3-03842-417-8 (PDF)

Table of Contents

Section 4: Assessment and Treatment

About the Special Issue Editors

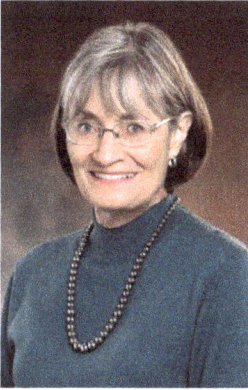

Lynn S. Walker is Professor of Pediatrics at the Monroe Carell Jr. Children's Hospital at Vanderbilt University. She directs a program of research that aims to identify biopsychosocial processes in the development and maintenance of pediatric pain. This work focuses on chronic abdominal pain as a prototypic functional pain condition without significant organic pathology. In a landmark long-term prospective study of several hundred pediatric abdominal pain patients, Dr. Walker's team has identified childhood characteristics that predict persistent pain, disability, and mental health problems in these patients as they reach adulthood. Currently, she is conducting a randomized clinical trial of online cognitive behavior therapy for adolescents with chronic abdominal pain.

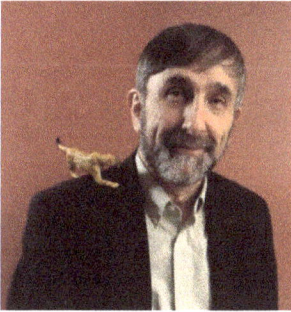

Carl L. von Baeyer, Professor Emeritus, at the University of Saskatchewan, Saskatoon, Canada, now holds appointments in clinical health psychology and pediatrics at the University of Manitoba, Winnipeg, Canada. He has guided the development of a pediatric chronic and complex pain program and has led studies in this field. He is President of the Special Interest Group on Pain in Childhood, International Association for the Study of Pain. He recently received the American Pain Society's 2017 Jeffrey Lawson Award for Advocacy in Children's Pain Relief.

Preface to "Chronic and Recurrent Pain"

For many years people assumed that children did not experience chronic pain. However, recent epidemiological studies show that chronic pain, defined as constant or recurring pain lasting three months or longer, is common in childhood. As many as 40% of schoolchildren aged 5–18, for example, report symptoms frequent and intense enough to meet the criteria for chronic pain, though only around 5% are significantly disabled in their school, family, recreational and social life. Empirical studies have characterized pediatric chronic pain conditions including headaches, abdominal pain, chest pain, and musculoskeletal pains including fibromyalgia. These pain conditions are often associated with school absence, emotional distress, disruption in family activities, and significantly reduced quality of life in both the affected child and their families. For some of these children, chronic pain persists from childhood into adulthood, causing substantial long-term personal and financial costs to the individual, society, and our health care systems.

Despite the prevalence and serious consequences of pediatric chronic pain, it is still under-recognized and under-treated. Too often, chronic pain is treated as a symptom of something else, rather than as a separate condition requiring its own treatment. The goal of this edited volume is to present recent advances in the understanding and treatment of pediatric chronic pain.

This book is grounded in the biopsychosocial approach that has replaced the traditional biomedical approach to chronic pain. Rather than focusing exclusively on the identification of physical pathology and treatment of disease, a biopsychosocial approach investigates biological, psychological, and social factors that contribute to pain and may be a useful focus for treatment. The organization of the book reflects the biopsychosocial approach to chronic pain with sections that address biological factors (Section 1), psychological factors (Section 2), and social factors (Section 3). A final section on assessment and treatment of chronic pain (Section 4) describes clinical approaches that focus on one or more of these factors.

Our aim is to reach all professionals who provide services to children with chronic pain. This includes pediatricians, nurses, guidance counselors, school teachers, social workers, physical and occupational therapists, psychologists, psychiatrists, and others, as well as trainees in these fields. While professionals may be drawn to the section most relevant to their particular discipline, other sections will introduce them to the knowledge base and treatments provided by other disciplines. We hope that the range of topics covered will facilitate communication and multidisciplinary treatment of pediatric chronic pain.

Lynn S. Walker, and Carl L. von Baeyer
Guest Editors

Section 1:
Biological Factors

Review

Beyond Acute Pain: Understanding Chronic Pain in Infancy

Miranda DiLorenzo [1], Rebecca Pillai Riddell [1,2,*] and Liisa Holsti [3,4]

1   Department of Psychology, York University, Toronto, ON M3J 1P3, Canada; mgdilo@yorku.ca
2   Department of Psychiatry, The Hospital for Sick Children and the Department of Psychiatry, University of Toronto, Toronto, ON M5T 1R8, Canada
3   Department of Occupational Science and Occupational Therapy, B.C. Children's Hospital Research, Vancouver, BC V5Z 4H4, Canada; liisa.holsti@ubc.ca
4   Women's Health Research Institute, Vancouver, BC V6H 3N1, Canada
*   Correspondence: rpr@yorku.ca; Tel.: +416-736-2100 (ext. 20177)

Academic Editor: Lynn Walker
Received: 13 September 2016; Accepted: 3 November 2016; Published: 9 November 2016

Abstract: This topical review presents the current challenges in defining chronic pain in infants, summarizes evidence from animal and human infant studies regarding the biological processes necessary for chronic pain signaling, and presents observational/experiential evidence from clinical experts. A literature search of four databases (CINAHL, EMBASE, PsycINFO, and MEDLINE) was conducted, along with hand searches of reference lists. Evidence from animal studies suggest that important neurophysiological mechanisms, such as the availability of key neurotransmitters needed for maintenance of chronic pain, may be immature or absent in the developing neonate. In some cases, human infants may be significantly less likely to develop chronic pain. However, evidence also points to altered pain perception, such as allodynia and hyperalgesia, with significant injury. Moreover, clinicians and parents in pediatric intensive care settings describe groups of infants with altered behavioral responses to repeated or prolonged painful stimuli, yet agreement on a working definition of chronic pain in infancy remains elusive. While our understanding of infant chronic pain is still in the rudimentary stages, a promising avenue for the future assessment of chronic pain in infancy would be to develop a clinical tool that uses both neurophysiological approaches and clinical perceptions already presented in the literature.

Keywords: infant; pain; acute; chronic; NICU; persistent pain

---

1. Introduction

Pain is defined as a negatively-valenced experience with core sensory, social, emotional, and cognitive properties [1]. Unfortunately, due to the sole reliance on self-reporting, infants were initially thought to be incapable of experiencing pain due to their inability to use language to communicate their subjective experience. The seminal work of pioneering scientists [2,3] combined with a public outcry from parents [4], helped end a troubling era of medical practice where scientists and clinicians generally did not acknowledge infant pain [5]. Indeed, research using both animal and human models provides strong evidence to show that infants have the necessary peripheral and central anatomical and neurophysiological systems required for nociceptive transmission, even at very early gestational ages [6–8]. Moreover, in humans, unexpected early pain and stress exposure is associated with long-term changes in brain structure (e.g., reduced white matter microstructure and subcortical grey matter), pain processing (e.g., dorsal horn central desensitization), stress-response system functioning (e.g., high basal cortisol levels), and development (e.g., poorer cognition and motor function), particularly for preterm infants cared for in neonatal intensive care units (NICUs) [9–12].

In response to this growing body of evidence, a plethora of measures have been developed to assess acute infant pain [13,14], and various trials have been conducted that evaluate the effectiveness of pharmacologic [15], behavioral, and physical treatments aimed at mitigating the adverse effects of acute procedural and post-operative pain in infants [16–18].

Most recently, both in the clinical setting and in the research community, more attention has been directed at understanding and investigating pain that persists beyond the acute period in infants [19,20]. Currently, no uniform definition exists for chronic pain of infants that has received widespread endorsement. The International Association for the Study of Pain defined chronic pain in adults as pain that lasts or recurs for more than 3 to 6 months after an injury [21]. However, the applicability of using an arbitrary timeline to define chronic pain for infants who have not lived long enough, yet who have long-lasting (relative to their age) painful conditions, such as osteogenesis imperfecta or epidermis bullosa, appears inappropriate [19]. Thus, it is clear that a specific time criterion cannot be applied specifically to newborn infants. The terms "chronic" or "persistent" pain (these terms are used both interchangeably and differentially in the literature) will both be applied in this paper as used by the original authors or best fitting the context deemed by the current authors. Both these labels (chronic or persistent) have also been defined as pain that has no biological value, pain that persists beyond normal healing time (i.e., 'non-functional', with acute pain being considered 'functional'), or pain that persists when repair has seemingly ended [21]. However, these definitions do not take into account basic physiological mechanisms of this condition, which does not provide clarity regarding treatment and prevention. Instead, a definition is needed with greater focus on models that define infant chronic pain based on the underlying mechanisms of the nervous system. Given that the generalizability of such neurobiological animal models to explain pain in adults has yet to be applied definitively, the application of neonate animal models to the unique context of the developing infant nervous system appears premature.

Thus, for this topical review, the foci will be to: (1) summarize the evidence from animal and human infant studies reporting on the neurophysiological processes that underlie different types of chronic pain in infancy; (2) present evidence gathered from expert researchers and clinicians about infant chronic pain. Our intention is to integrate these lines of evidence, in order to further our understanding of pain beyond acute in infancy, and to inform future research and clinical recommendations.

2. Materials and Methods

The literature search considered peer-reviewed papers included in the following electronic databases: the OVIDSP platform was used to run the search strategy in MEDLINE and EMBASE, ProQuest was used for PsycINFO, and EBSCOHost was used for CINAHL. Articles indexed from inception to 12 November 2012 were included in the initial search and the search was updated in August 2016. Electronic search terms included "infant newborn", "infant premature", "chronic pain", "nociceptive pain", "intractable pain", "ex-prematurity". To be included in this review, papers had to: be written in the English language, have an abstract available online, and involve infant pain that persists beyond the acute period. The search yielded 262 abstracts that were independently assessed against the above pre-specified inclusion criteria. Additional literature was gathered by reviewing the reference lists of the papers obtained from the original search. The literature was sorted into categories relating to neurophysiological processes that focused on pain beyond acute, and clinical studies that highlighted the applied aspects of pain beyond acute in infancy. In total, 58 papers met the criteria for inclusion in the current review.

3. Neurophysiological Developmental Changes in Pain Processing

Compared to temporal or evaluative definitions, current conceptualizations outside of infancy assert that biological mechanisms underlying the pain state are the best way to categorize chronic pain. For example, Woolf [22] proposed a three-pronged classification involving nociceptive pain that provides early signaling of damage, and inflammatory pain which inhibits movement to promote healing. Both nociceptive and inflammatory pain are adaptive and protective. In contrast, "pathological" pain, which can be further divided into neuropathic pain (involving nerve damage) and dysfunctional pain (reflecting abnormal nervous system function) is maladaptive and is considered a "disease of the nervous system". It is clear that a neurophysiological approach to defining chronic pain in infancy is necessary; however, understanding the underlying mechanisms has provided a challenge for researchers because of the immature infant nervous system.

While much of the pain processing system in adults is also functional in infants, the first year of life is marked by significant structural and functional changes in pain pathways, and as a result, pain is processed differently in infants than in adults [23,24]. Animal models, particularly those using rats, tell us a lot about the developmental changes that occur in infant pain pathways, since the changes seen in the two post-natal weeks of rats parallel the neurobiological development in human infancy [25]. This research using animal models has helped to highlight certain developmental changes in somatosensory circuitry that occur over the period of infancy, which have direct relevance to the processing of persistent or chronic pain states in infancy.

Generally, researchers have noted early maturation of nociceptive processing in the periphery of neonate rats; however, their central processing of pain develops more slowly [25]. Early in development, large diameter Aβ primary afferent fibers, which typically relay non-noxious tactile information to the dorsal horn, extend beyond their final resting place in the dorsal horn during infancy [26,27]. The functional implications of the immature Aβ fiber termination is that the low threshold fibers are able to access and activate high-threshold Aδ and C-fibers that usually process noxious information [26]. Consequently, as shown in a study evaluating premature human infants, infants are unable to discriminate between non-noxious and noxious inputs until approximately 35 weeks' gestational age [6]. Further research in neonatal rat models shows that the low threshold tactile afferents (Aβ fibers) retract from the site of high-threshold input until completely segregated after a few weeks of life [28].

In addition to the structural changes of primary afferent innervation of the dorsal horn in early life, key developmental changes also occur in the intrinsic properties of the dorsal horn during infancy. Using rodent models, at birth, the receptive fields in the dorsal horn are large, and decrease in size over the first two postnatal weeks. Stimulation of these "wider" cutaneous receptive fields at early postnatal ages can enhance signaling and evoke long-lasting excitation [29,30]. Furthermore, many neurotransmitters and signaling molecules involved with nociceptive processing are expressed early in development in rodent models, but do not reach adult levels until after infancy [25,31]. Particularly, an imbalance exists between excitatory (e.g., glutamate) and inhibitory (e.g., GABA and glycine) neurotransmitters and their respective receptors that favors excitatory transmission [25]. An increase in excitatory input is observed because both glutamergic receptors, N-methyl-D-aspartate (NMDA) receptor and α-amino-3-hydroxy-5-methyl-4-isoxazolepropionic acid (AMPA) receptor, are highly expressed in the neonatal rat spinal cord before being down-regulated to adult levels [32–34]. Further contributing to this imbalance is the fact that particular inhibitory mechanisms are either weak or absent in early postnatal life. Indeed, glycinergic mini-inhibitory postsynaptic currents are absent within the most superficial laminae of the dorsal horn until the second postnatal week of rodent models, but responses to exogenous glycine can still be evoked [35]. These research findings suggest that during infancy the functional receptors of glycine may be present, but that the glycinergic neurons are absent, resulting in less inhibitory signaling. Additionally, GABA has a reduced inhibitory drive at birth compared to adulthood. A balance of spinal excitability and inhibitory mechanisms is imperative for normal tactile and nociceptive processing [28]; however, stasis is not established between the excitatory and inhibitory drives until later in infancy.

A final key neurodevelopmental change in nociceptive processing includes the delayed maturation of brainstem descending pain pathways that play a major role in the control of pain transmission [36]. Descending pathways from the brainstem to the spinal cord are present in utero in animal models, but functional inhibition of nociceptive signals is not thought to be effective until 2–3 weeks post-delivery [37,38]. Hathway et al. [39] showed that in rats, the rostroventral medulla (RVM), which houses the main output nuclei for brainstem descending control, undergoes drastic maturation after the 21st postnatal day (P21). Lesioning and electrical stimulation of the RVM has revealed that its control over nociceptive circuits is entirely facilitatory before P21 in rats [39,40]. It is only after three postnatal weeks that inhibitory pathways exert an influence. Researchers have argued that the RVM-mediated facilitation of nociception in early life plays a significant role in sustaining pain from neuropathic and inflammatory injury [39,41]. Importantly, the functional development of the descending inhibitory pathways has been shown to be concomitant with the refinement of noxious withdrawal reflexes observed in early human development [42]. Therefore, together, these significant neurobiological developmental changes suggest that infants are more, rather than less, sensitive to pain than older individuals.

4. Types of Chronic Pain in Infancy

Neuropathic pain and inflammatory pain are the two main types of chronic pain [43]. Inflammatory pain manifests as a consequence of tissue damage/inflammation (e.g., surgical injury with resulting tissue inflammation) and neuropathic pain arises from nervous system lesions (e.g., brachial plexus injuries). Neuropathic pain is rare in infants; whereas, persistent inflammatory pain is observed more frequently [31]. The development of inflammatory pain, or the protection against the development of neuropathic pain, can be ascribed to certain pain circuitry immaturities, such as those discussed previously.

4.1. The Development of Persistent Pain Associated with Tissue Injury and Inflammation

The development of an inflammatory pain syndrome in response to tissue injury has been well documented in animal models [24]. Plantar hindpaw incision is a post-operative pain model used widely as it is highly reproducible in both neonatal and in adult rodents [31]. In neonatal rodents, surgical incisions of the plantar hindpaw produce inflammation-induced primary hyperalgesia (decreased pain threshold) from the age of P3 to P17 [44]. Hyperalgesic responses to injury in neonates is not specific to surgical trauma. Inflammogenic molecules, such as mustard oil, can also cause hyperalgesic responses in neonatal rats. Mustard oil is a potent activator of C-fibers (nociceptive cells) and produces primary hyperalgesia and secondary hyperalgesia (pain arising from the tissue surrounding a wound) in both adult and in neonatal rats [45]. However, the pain responses to mustard oil are smaller in neonate rats compared to adult models, which reflects neurodevelopmental immaturities of nociceptive cells within the dorsal horn [46].

More long-term consequences of inflammation associated with hindpaw incisions in neonatal rat models, include significant changes in the resting membrane potential of large diameter sensory neurons that persists beyond the time in which behavioral pain responses are observed [47]. The change in resting membrane potential causes the sensory neurons to be much more excitable. Aforementioned neurobiological immaturities, such as the relative lack of brainstem inhibitory descending controls and the imbalance of inhibitory and excitatory neurotransmitter activity in neonates, are purported to play a role in this biophysical change observed in resting membrane potential [31]. Another example of long-lasting consequences of tissue injury involves changes in microglia, which are cells within the central nervous system that contribute to the manifestation of chronic pain states in animal models [43]. Neonatal skin incision changes the phenotype of microglia, which can alter sensory afferent cells, intrinsic dorsal horn cell responses, and consequently, cause an increase in sensory neuron excitation.

In comparison to rat models, direct evidence of the development of pain associated with inflammation and tissue injury from human infant studies is quite limited. Follow-up studies of infants hospitalized in the NICU, or those who had surgery during the neonatal period, show that they are vulnerable to aspects of altered central pain processing which appear to place them at heightened risk for developing chronic pain. For example, following exposure to heel lance and to surgery with anesthesia, infants had lowered thresholds to tactile stimulation up to the post conceptual age of 35 weeks (sensitization) [48] and decreased thresholds during the first year of life (primary hyperalgesia) [49]. Secondary hyperalgesia was also exhibited in infants, even when the injury was to the contralateral side [50]. In addition to secondary hyperalgesia, infants develop allodynia (pain arising from previously innocuous stimulation) as a result of central sensitization [3,51].

What is not clear is whether or not these changes observed in human infants could be considered "adaptive"; that is, sensitization after minor and major trauma is meant to be protective [52]. As such, the question arises whether evidence of these neonatal changes in pain processing systems are preliminary evidence for chronic pain and thereby considered "maladaptive" [22]. Interestingly, even though the "priming towards excitation" described above suggests that these infants could be at a heightened risk for developing chronic pain because of maladaptive processes, another line of research indicates that infants may be "protected" from some forms of chronic pain [53].

4.2. The Development of Pain Associated with Nerve Injury

Research in rodent models does suggest protection against the development of chronic neuropathic pain in infancy [54–58]. After peripheral nerve injury, persistent mechanical allodynia does not occur until 3 post-natal weeks [54]. In addition, microglia in the dorsal horn involved in the immune response to nerve injury are activated only at very low levels following nerve injury in young animals even up until P16 [55]. This response does not occur because neonatal animals lack innate immune responses, but is more likely a result of absent T-cell activation and infiltration indicating that nerve damage has taken place [56]. Thus, since infant rats are capable of developing clear pain hypersensitivity upon inflammation [44], the lack of neuropathic pain behavior following nerve injury in young animal models has been attributed to immature neuroimmune pathways, rather than a failure of pain processing [57]. In line with this notion, a more recent study by McKelvey et al. offers a novel mechanistic explanation for the absence of pain following nerve damage in infancy. In contrast to adult nerve injury, which triggers a proinflammatory immune response in the dorsal horn, nerve injury in infants triggers an anti-inflammatory immune response with significant increases in IL-4 and IL-10 [58]. Interestingly, the blockade of the anti-inflammatory activity of IL-10 unmasks neuropathic pain behavior suggesting that nerve injury in infancy is not absent, but rather is suppressed by the IL cytokine proteins. Nevertheless, the immature presentation of these factors associated with the development of pain associated with nerve injury have not been studied in human infants and thus provides exciting lines of evidence to pursue.

Similar to the neuropathic pain animal models, under some conditions in which adults and older children would be at risk for developing neuropathic pain, infants appear to be protected. For example, infants who experience complete avulsion of the brachial nerve at delivery, when assessed between 3 and 23 years, do not report chronic pain; and in fact, following surgical repair, they show vastly improved sensory recovery compared to motor recovery, and have normal sensation in other areas of the body [59]. Very few infants with this injury go on to exhibit behaviors which may indicate ongoing chronic pain in childhood [60]. Some postulate that these results occur because nerve conduction velocity in children under the age of two years is 50% lower than in adults [59,61]. In addition, very few children with congenital amputations report phantom pain (<10%) [62]. Yet, in older children (5–19 years) and in adults who undergo amputation, prevalence rates of phantom pain can be as high as 80% [63,64]. Moreover, associations between developing persistent pain after inguinal hernia repair were very low in those operated on in the first 3 months of life [65]. Indeed, Tsai et al. found that infant postoperative chronic pain was minimal and transient after inguinal hernia repair [66]. A similar trend was found for thoracotomy and strenotomy procedures; the prevalence of chronic pain was low in children that underwent these procedures before school entry [67,68].

5. Reconciling Clinical Observations with Pre-Clinical Research

While biologically-based models, particularly rodent models, provide an important foundation for building a conceptualization of the mechanisms of infant persistent pain, actual clinical experience with infants suspected of having ongoing pain provides important complementary information.

To explore the perspectives of infant caregivers on "chronic pain" in infants, based on their observations and caregiving experiences, Pillai Riddell et al. conducted in-depth interviews with a multi-disciplinary sample of highly experienced clinicians (average years of experience was 17 years) from three separate university-affiliated tertiary care centers [19]. While most accepted the idea of chronic pain existing in infants, agreement in regards to a definition was elusive. In contrast to the adult literature where chronic pain is most often cited as pain lasting more than 3 to 6 months [69], a significant proportion of clinicians thought that infants could experience persistent pain after weeks if the context included a clinical presentation of a disease type known to be associated with ongoing pain in infants, such as in epidermolysis bullosa.

Pillai Riddell et al. highlighted another definitional issue on pain beyond acute that was expressed by clinical experts identified as 'iatrogenically prolonged' pain, which is applicable to infants requiring prolonged hospitalization in the NICU [19]. They differentiated infants with unremitting conditions that cause persistent pain, from those undergoing a series of acute or acute-prolonged pain experiences (i.e., pain induced and maintained by repetitive medical procedures) that result in a "chronically pained state". Thus, the acknowledgment was made that these infants may not have a persistent pain state resulting from changes in the nervous system, but rather experience prolonged pain as a result of iatrogenic procedures that are added cumulatively to pain related, earlier procedures that have yet to abate.

Both a sample of clinicians and a follow-up study with parents who had infants currently suspected of having chronic pain (conservatively defined as conditions known to be chronically painful in older populations) independently described two types of infant persistent pain behavioral profiles: the "hyperreactive" and "hyporeactive" infant [19]. The majority of health professionals in these samples suggested that an infant who is "hyporeactive" (exhibits little to no reaction to an acute pain procedure), may be experiencing chronic pain. However, other professionals in the sample suggested the opposite, whereby an infant who is "hyperreactive" (exhibits an exaggerated response to an acute pain procedure), indicates that an infant is experiencing chronic pain. These differing labels further confound the problem of how best to define chronic pain in infants, and consequently, how to integrate the aforementioned findings from pre-clinical and clinical science. The "hyporeactive" infant does not appear to interact with caregivers or even to react to extensive noxious stimulation. Health professionals describe infants as "hyporeactive" if they do not respond behaviorally when a known painful procedure is performed. In contrast, the "hyperreactive" infant exhibits heightened distress even in anticipation of an impending noxious procedure and was described to have behaviorally higher peak distress during painful procedures.

More recently, using a web-based survey technique, van Ganzewinkel et al. invited international neonatal experts and parents to define chronic pain [20]. When responding to the questions relating to what is chronic pain, experts described no known endpoint and they described a concept whereby pain is present, despite the lack of a proximal event or procedure. In addition, consensus by the group indicated that pain would interfere with development and prolong healing times. Not surprisingly, when etiology was discussed, rather than biological mechanisms relating to aberrant pain pathways, painful conditions and situations were listed. However, specifics with regards to diagnostic factors could not be identified.

6. A Need for Chronic Pain Assessment

Both the aforementioned studies working with clinicians suggest that the manifestation of pain beyond acute in infancy is still not well understood. Encouragingly, despite the lack of definitive criteria regarding the mechanisms or the definition of chronic pain in infancy, the belief that it does exist appears to be commonly accepted. Reaching a consensus on both clinical observations and neurobiological mechanisms of chronic pain in infancy is necessary to develop valid assessments. Currently, neither clinicians nor researchers have yet to devise a strategy that can definitively determine whether or not a newborn is experiencing chronic pain, and as a result, chronic pain is difficult to treat effectively [20]. Although a plethora of assessments for acute pain exist, with varying psychometric properties established, most research to date indicates that behavioral and physiological markers of acute pain may not be applicable to chronic pain [70–72]. Researchers have suggested that clinical observations in the NICU (e.g., NEOPAIN trial) [73] and the development of scales, such as the COMFORTneo scale [74] or the EDIN scale [75], show promise in isolating indicators that do not focus on simply peak distress response [74]. Nevertheless, pediatric pain experts have yet to agree on any type of clinical cluster of behaviors or physiological indicators that could form the basis of the tool. The lack of self-reporting in infancy further complicates these problems. Given that infants who have been exposed to prolonged pain have been described as both over and under-responsive, clinicians are unsure of how to determine whether or not the unresponsive infant has stopped responding because of the cessation of pain or has exceeded its capacity to respond to too much pain.

7. Concluding Remarks

Despite decades of research demonstrating that human infants are capable of experiencing pain, the evidence between acute and chronic pain and between animal and human research has developed disproportionately. This has resulted in limited knowledge of how the pre-clinical science on chronic pain relates to the human infant experience, although an understanding of acute behavioral responses to neonatal and infant pain appears generally well-established. However, the potential for infants' capacity for chronic pain is still in need of fundamental research across different pain paradigms (e.g., postsurgical persistent pain syndromes, iatrogenically-prolonged pain exposure). From such a foundation, researchers and clinicians can build a knowledge-base of persistent pain during early human life that reconciles what is known from the collective lines of research. Longitudinal prospective studies tracking infants from birth who are suspected of chronic pain conditions may help to rectify the different clinical pictures seen in chronic pain. The ultimate goal is that a clinical tool is eventually designed that effectively marries both the physiological substantiated mechanisms and clinical perceptions that have been already offered in the literature regarding chronic pain in infancy. This convergence of biological and behavioral/observational evidence could ultimately inform a more accurate assessment, and safe, effective, and ethical treatment of infants who suffer from pain beyond the acute period.

Acknowledgments: This research was funded by infrastructure, operating, and/or salary awards from the Canada Foundation for Innovation, the Canadian Institutes for Health Research, the Ontario Ministry of Research, and the Innovation and York Research Chairs Program awarded to R.P.R. and awards to M.D. from the Social Sciences and Humanities Council of Canada, and the Meighen Weight Graduate Scholarship in Maternal-Child Health. M.D. is also a trainee member of Pain In Child Health (PICH), a strategic research training initiative of the Canadian Institutes of Health Research. L.H. is supported by the Canadian Institute of Health Research Canada Research Chair in Neonatal Health and Development. We would like to gratefully acknowledge Gary Walco and Bonnie Stevens for their input on an earlier version of this manuscript (2012).

Author Contributions: R.P.R. and L.H. conceptualized the manuscript; L.H. completed the initial literature search in 2012, and M.D. updated the search in 2016. All authors contributed to writing the manuscript.

Conflicts of Interest: The authors declare no conflicts of interest.

References

1. De Williams, A.C.; Craig, K. Updating the definition of pain. *Pain* **2016**, *157*, 2420–2423. [CrossRef] [PubMed]
2. Anand, K.J.; Sippell, W.G.; Aynsely-Green, A.A. Randomised trial of fentanyl anaesthesia in preterm babies undergoing surgery: Effects on the stress response. *Lancet* **1987**, *329*, 243–248. [CrossRef]
3. Fitzgerald, M.; Millard, C.; Macintosh, N. Hyperalgesia in premature infants. *Lancet* **1988**, *331*, 292. [CrossRef]

4. Boffey, P. Infants' Sense of Pain is Recognized, Finally. Available online: http://www.nytimes.com/1987/11/24/science/infants-sense-of-pain-isrecognized-finally.html (accessed on 27 August 2016).

5. Rodkey, E.N.; Pillai Riddell, R. The infancy of infant pain research: The experimental origins of infant pain denial. *J. Pain* **2013**, *14*, 338–350. [CrossRef] [PubMed]

6. Fabrizi, L.; Slater, R.; Worley, A.; Meek, J.; Boyd, S.; Olhede, S.; Fitzgerald, M. A shift in sensory processing that enables the developing human brain to discriminate touch from pain. *Curr. Biol.* **2011**, *21*, 1552–1558. [CrossRef] [PubMed]

7. King, T.E.; Barr, G.A. Spinal cord ionotropic glutamate receptors function in formalin-induced nociception in preweaning rats. *Psychopharmacology* **2007**, *192*, 489–498. [CrossRef] [PubMed]

8. Ruda, M.A.; Ling, Q.D.; Hohmann, A.G.; Peng, Y.B.; Tachibana, T. Altered nociceptive neuronal circuits after neonatal peripheral inflammation. *Science* **2000**, *289*, 628–630. [CrossRef] [PubMed]

9. Grunau, R.E.; Holsti, L.; Peters, J.W.B. Long-term consequences of pain in human neonates. *Semin. Fetal Neonatal Med.* **2006**, *11*, 268–275. [CrossRef] [PubMed]

10. Grunau, R.E.; Tu, M.T.; Whitfield, M.F.; Oberlander, T.F.; Weinberg, J.; Yu, W.; Thiessenm, P.; Gosse, G.; Scheifele, D. Cortisol, behavior, and heart rate reactivity to immunization pain at 4 months corrected age in infants born very preterm. *Clin. J. Pain* **2010**, *26*, 698–704. [CrossRef] [PubMed]

11. Brummelte, S.; Grunau, R.E.; Chau, V.; Poskitt, K.J.; Brant, R.; Vinall, J.; Gover, A.; Synnes, A.R.; Miller, S.P. Procedural pain and brain development in premature newborns. *Ann. Neurol.* **2012**, *71*, 385–396. [CrossRef] [PubMed]

12. Grunau, R.E.; Whitfield, M.F.; Petrie-Thomas, J.; Synnes, A.R.; Cepeda, I.L.; Keidar, A.; Rogers, M.; MacKay, M.; Hubber-Richard, P.; Johannesen, D. Neonatal pain, parenting stress and interaction, in relation to cognitive and motor development at 8 and 18 months in preterm infants. *Pain* **2009**, *143*, 138–146. [CrossRef] [PubMed]

13. Ranger, M.; Johnston, C.C.; Anand, K.J.S. Current controversies regarding pain assessment in neonates. *Semin. Perinatol.* **2007**, *31*, 283–288. [CrossRef] [PubMed]

14. Stevens, B.; Lee, G. Neonatal and Infant Pain Measurement. In *Oxford Textbook of Pediatric Pain*; Oxford University Press: Oxford, UK, 2013; pp. 353–359.

15. Anand, K.J.S.; Hall, R.W.; Desai, N.S.; Shephard, B.; Bergqvist, L.L.; Young, T.E.; Boyle, E.M.; Carbajal, R.; Bhutani, V.K.; Moore, M.B.; et al. Effects of morphine analgesia in ventilated preterm neonates: Primary outcomes from the NEOPAIN randomised trial. *Lancet* **2004**, *363*, 1673–1682. [CrossRef]

16. Pillai Riddell, R.R.; Racine, N.M.; Turcotte, K.; Uman, L.S.; Horton, R.E.; Din Osmun, L.; Ahola Kohut, S.; Hillgrove Stuart, J.; Stevens, B.; Gerwitz-Stern, A. Non-pharmacological management of infant and young child procedural pain. *Cochrane Database Syst. Rev.* **2011**. [CrossRef]

17. Shah, P.S.; Aliwalas, L.L.; Shah, V.S. Breastfeeding or breast milk for procedural pain in neonates. *Cochrane Database Syst. Rev.* **2012**. [CrossRef]

18. Stevens, B.; Yamada, J.; Ohlsson, A.; Haliburton, S.; Shorkey, A. Sucrose for analgesia in newborn infants undergoing painful procedures. *Cochrane Database Syst. Rev.* **2016**. [CrossRef]

19. Pillai Riddell, R.R.; Stevens, B.J.; McKeever, P.; Gibbins, S.; Asztalos, L.; Katz, J.; Ahola, S.; Din, L. Chronic pain in hospitalized infants: Health professionals' perspectives. *J. Pain* **2009**, *10*, 1217–1225. [CrossRef] [PubMed]

20. Van Ganzewinkel, C.J.; Anand, K.J.; Kramer, B.W.; Andriessen, P. Chronic pain in the newborn: Toward a definition. *Clin. J. Pain* **2014**, *30*, 970–977. [CrossRef] [PubMed]

21. American Pain Society Task Force on Pediatric Chronic Pain Management. Assessment and Management of Children with Chronic Pain. Available online: http://www.ampainsoc.org/advocacy/downloads/aps12-pcp.pdf (accessed on 9 August 2016).

22. Woolf, C.J. What is this thing called pain? *J. Clin. Investig.* **2010**, *120*, 3742–3744. [CrossRef] [PubMed]

23. Fitzgerald, M. The development of nociceptive circuits. *Nat. Rev. Neurosci.* **2005**, *6*, 507–520. [CrossRef] [PubMed]

24. Fitzgerald, M.; Walker, S.M. Infant pain management: A developmental neurobiological approach. *Nat. Clin. Pract. Neurol.* **2009**, *5*, 35–50. [CrossRef] [PubMed]

25. Beggs, S.; Fitzgerald, M. Development of peripheral and spinal nociceptive systems. In *Pain in Neonates and Infants*, 3rd ed.; Elsevier: New York, NY, USA, 2007; pp. 11–24.

26. Beggs, S.; Torsney, C.; Drew, L.J.; Fitzgerald, M. The postnatal reorganization of primary afferent input and dorsal horn cell receptive fields in the rat spinal cord is an activity-dependent process. *Eur. J. Neurosci.* **2002**, *16*, 1249–1258. [CrossRef] [PubMed]

27. Fitzgerald, M.; Butcher, T.; Shortland, P. Developmental changes in the laminar termination of A fibre cutaneous sensory afferents in the rat spinal cord dorsal horn. *J. Comp. Neurol.* **1994**, *348*, 225–233. [CrossRef] [PubMed]

28. Beggs, S. Long-term consequences of neonatal injury. *Can. J. Psychiatry* **2015**, *60*, 176–180. [PubMed]

29. Jackman, A.; Fitzgerald, M. Development of peripheral hindlimb and central spinal cord innervation by subpopulations of dorsal root ganglion cells in the embryonic rat. *J. Comp. Neurol.* **2000**, *418*, 281–298. [CrossRef]

30. Torsney, C.; Fitzgerald, M. Age-dependent effects of peripheral inflammation on the electrophysiological properties of neonatal rat dorsal horn neurons. *J. Neurophysiol.* **2002**, *87*, 1311–1317. [PubMed]

31. Hathway, G.J. Acute and chronic pain in children. In *Behavioral Neurobiology of Chronic Pain*; Springer: Berlin, Germany, 2014; pp. 349–366.

32. Baba, H.; Doubell, T.P.; Moore, K.A.; Woolf, C.J. Silent NMDA receptor-mediated synapses are developmentally regulated in the dorsal horn of the rat spinal cord. *J. Neurophysiol.* **2000**, *83*, 955–962. [PubMed]

33. Bardoni, R.; Magherini, P.C.; MacDermott, A.B. Activation of NMDA receptors drives action potentials in superficial dorsal horn from neonatal rats. *Neuroreport* **2000**, *11*, 1721–1727. [CrossRef] [PubMed]

34. Jakowec, M.W.; Fox, A.J.; Martin, L.J.; Kalb, R.G. Quantitative and qualitative changes in AMPA receptor expression during spinal cord development. *Neuroscience* **1995**, *67*, 893–907. [CrossRef]

35. Baccei, M.L.; Fitzgerald, M. Development of GABAergic and glycinergic transmission in the neonatal rat dorsal horn. *J. Neurosci.* **2004**, *24*, 4749–4757. [CrossRef] [PubMed]

36. Fitzgerald, M. The neurobiology of chronic pain in children. In *Handbook of Pediatric Chronic Pain*; Springer: New York, NY, USA, 2011; pp. 15–25.

37. Rajaofetra, N.; Sandillon, F.; Geffard, M.; Privat, A. Pre-and post-natal ontogeny of serotonergic projections to the rat spinal cord. *J. Neurosci. Res.* **1989**, *22*, 305–321. [CrossRef] [PubMed]

38. Fitzgerald, M.; Koltzenburg, M. The functional development of descending inhibitory pathways in the dorsolateral funiculus of the newborn rat spinal cord. *Dev. Brain Res.* **1986**, *24*, 261–270. [CrossRef]

39. Hathway, G.J.; Koch, S.; Low, L.; Fitzgerald, M. The changing balance of brainstem–spinal cord modulation of pain processing over the first weeks of rat postnatal life. *J. Physiol.* **2009**, *587*, 2927–2935. [CrossRef] [PubMed]

40. Koch, S.C.; Fitzgerald, M. The selectivity of rostroventral medulla descending control of spinal sensory inputs shifts postnatally from A fibre to C fibre evoked activity. *J. Physiol.* **2014**, *592*, 1535–1544. [CrossRef] [PubMed]

41. Burgess, S.E.; Gardell, L.R.; Ossipov, M.H.; Malan, T.P.; Vanderah, T.W.; Lai, J.; Porreca, F. Time-dependent descending facilitation from the rostral ventromedial medulla maintains, but does not initiate, neuropathic pain. *J. Neurosci.* **2002**, *22*, 5129–5136. [PubMed]

42. Hartley, C.; Moultrie, F.; Gursul, D.; Hoskin, A.; Adams, E.; Rogers, R.; Slater, R. Changing balance of spinal cord excitability and nociceptive brain activity in early human development. *Curr. Biol.* **2016**, *26*, 1998–2002. [CrossRef] [PubMed]

43. Beggs, S.; Salter, M.W. Microglia-neuronal signalling in neuropathic pain hypersensitivity 2.0. *Curr. Opin. Neurobiol.* **2010**, *20*, 474–480. [CrossRef] [PubMed]

44. Walker, S.M.; Tochiki, K.K.; Fitzgerald, M. Hindpaw incision in early life increases the hyperalgesic response to repeat surgical injury: Critical period and dependence on initial afferent activity. *Pain* **2009**, *147*, 99–106. [CrossRef] [PubMed]

45. Walker, S.M.; Meredith-Middleton, J.; Lickiss, T.; Moss, A.; Fitzgerald, M. Primary and secondary hyperalgesia can be differentiated by postnatal age and ERK activation in the spinal dorsal horn of the rat pup. *Pain* **2007**, *128*, 157–168. [CrossRef] [PubMed]

46. Jennings, E.; Fitzgerald, M. Postnatal changes in responses of rat dorsal horn cells to afferent stimulation: A fibre-induced sensitization. *J. Physiol.* **1998**, *509*, 859–868. [CrossRef] [PubMed]

47. Ririe, D.G.; Liu, B.; Clayton, B.; Tong, C.; Eisenach, J.C. Electrophysiologic characteristics of large neurons in dorsal root ganglia during development and after hind paw incision in the rat. *Anesthesiology* **2008**, *109*, 111–117. [CrossRef] [PubMed]

48. Andrews, K.; Fitzgerald, M. The cutaneous withdrawal reflex in human neonates: Sensitization, receptive fields, and the effects of contralateral stimulation. *Pain* **1994**, *56*, 95–101. [CrossRef]

49. Andrews, K.A.; Desai, D.; Dhillon, H.K.; Wilcox, D.T.; Fitzgerald, M. Abdominal sensitivity in the first year of life: Comparison of infants with and without prenatally diagnosed unilateral hydronephrosis. *Pain* **2002**, *100*, 35–46. [CrossRef]

50. Andrews, K.; Fitzgerald, M. Cutaneous flexion reflex in human neonates: A quantitative study of threshold and stimulus-response characteristics after single and repeated stimuli. *Dev. Med. Child Neurol.* **1999**, *41*, 696–703. [CrossRef] [PubMed]

51. Fitzgerald, M.; Millard, C.; McIntosh, N. Cutaneous hypersensitivity following peripheral tissue damage in newborn infants and its reversal with topical anaesthesia. *Pain* **1989**, *39*, 31–36. [CrossRef]

52. Woolf, C.J. Central sensitization: Implications for the diagnosis and treatment of pain. *Pain* **2011**, *152* (Suppl. S3), S2–S15. [CrossRef] [PubMed]

53. Costigan, M.; Scholz, J.; Woolf, C.J. Neuropathic pain: A maladaptive response of the nervous system to damage. *Annu. Rev. Neurosci.* **2009**, *32*, 1–32. [CrossRef] [PubMed]

54. Howard, R.F.; Walker, S.M.; Mota, P.M.; Fitzgerald, M. The ontogeny of neuropathic pain: Postnatal onset of mechanical allodynia in rat spared nerve injury (SNI) and chronic constriction injury (CCI) models. *Pain* **2005**, *115*, 382–389. [CrossRef] [PubMed]

55. Moss, A.; Beggs, S.; Vega-Avelaira, D.; Costigan, M.; Hathway, G.J.; Salter, M.W.; Fitzgerald, M. Spinal microglia and neuropathic pain in young rats. *Pain* **2007**, *128*, 215–224. [CrossRef] [PubMed]

56. Costigan, M.; Moss, A.; Latremoliere, A.; Johnston, C.; Verma-Gandhu, M.; Herbert, T.A.; Barrett, L.; Brenner, G.J.; Vardeh, D.; Woolf, C.J.; et al. T-cell infiltration and signaling in the adult dorsal spinal cord is a major contributor to neuropathic pain-like hypersensitivity. *J. Neurosci.* **2009**, *29*, 14415–14422. [CrossRef] [PubMed]

57. Vega-Avelaira, D.; McKelvey, R.; Hathway, G.; Fitzgerald, M. The emergence of adolescent onset pain hypersensitivity following neonatal nerve injury. *Mol. Pain* **2012**, *8*, 1. [CrossRef] [PubMed]

58. McKelvey, R.; Berta, T.; Old, E.; Ji, R.R.; Fitzgerald, M. Neuropathic pain is constitutively suppressed in early life by anti-inflammatory neuroimmune regulation. *J. Neurosci.* **2015**, *35*, 457–466. [CrossRef] [PubMed]

59. Anand, P.; Birch, R. Restoration of sensory function and lack of long-term chronic pain syndromes after brachial plexus injury in human neonates. *Brain* **2002**, *125*, 113–122. [CrossRef] [PubMed]

60. McCann, M.E.; Waters, P.; Goumnerova, L.C.; Berde, C. Self-mutilation in young children following brachial plexus birth injury. *Pain* **2004**, *110*, 123–129. [CrossRef] [PubMed]

61. Brett, E.M. *Pediatric Neurology*, 2nd ed.; Churchill Livingston: Edinburgh, UK, 1998; pp. 209–233.

62. Wilkins, K.L.; McGrath, P.J.; Finley, G.A.; Katz, J. Phantom limb sensations and phantom limb pain in child and adolescent amputees. *Pain* **1998**, *78*, 7–12. [CrossRef]

63. Krane, E.J.; Heller, L.B. The prevalence of phantom sensation and pain in pediatric amputees. *J. Pain Symptom Manag.* **1995**, *10*, 21–29. [CrossRef]

64. Nikolajsen, L.; Jensen, T.S. Phantom limb pain. *Br. J. Anaesth.* **2001**, *87*, 107–116. [CrossRef] [PubMed]

65. Aasvang, E.K.; Kehlet, H. Chronic pain after childhood groin hernia repair. *J. Pediatr. Surg.* **2007**, *42*, 1403–1408. [CrossRef] [PubMed]

66. Tsai, Y.C.; Ho, C.H.; Tai, H.C.; Chung, S.D.; Chueh, S.C. Laparoendoscopic single-site versus conventional laparoscopic total extraperitoneal hernia repair: A prospective randomized clinical trial. *Surg. Endosc.* **2013**, *27*, 4684–4692. [CrossRef] [PubMed]

67. Kristensen, A.D.; Ahlburg, P.; Lauridsen, M.C.; Jensen, T.S.; Nikolajsen, L. Chronic pain after inguinal hernia repair in children. *Br. J. Anaesth.* **2012**, *109*, 603–608. [CrossRef] [PubMed]

68. Lauridsen, M.H.; Kristensen, A.D.; Hjortdal, V.E.; Jensen, T.S.; Nikolajsen, L. Chronic pain in children after cardiac surgery via sternotomy. *Cardiol. Young* **2014**, *24*, 893–899. [CrossRef] [PubMed]

69. Turk, D.C.; Okifuji, A. Pain terms and taxonomies of pain. In *Bonica's Management of Pain*, 3rd ed.; Lippincott Williams & Wilkins: Philadelphia, PA, USA, 2001; pp. 17–25.

70. Stevens, B.J.; Pillai Riddell, R. Looking beyond acute pain in infancy. *Pain* **2006**, *124*, 11–12. [CrossRef] [PubMed]

71. Hall, R.W.; Boyle, E.; Young, T. Do ventilated neonates require pain management? *Semin. Perinatol.* **2007**, *31*, 289–297. [CrossRef] [PubMed]
72. Raeside, L. Physiological measures of assessing infant pain: A literature review. *Br. J. Nurs.* **2011**, *20*, 1370–1376. [CrossRef] [PubMed]
73. Boyle, E.M.; Freer, Y.; Wong, C.M.; McIntosh, N.; Anand, K.J.S. Assessment of persistent pain or distress and adequacy of analgesia in preterm ventilated infants. *Pain* **2006**, *124*, 87–91. [CrossRef] [PubMed]
74. Van Dijk, M.; Roofthooft, D.W.; Anand, K.J.; Guldemond, F.; de Graaf, J.; Simons, S.; de Jager, Y.; van Goudoever, J.B.; Tibboel, D. Taking up the challenge of measuring prolonged pain in (premature) neonates: The COMFORTneo scale seems promising. *Clin. J. Pain* **2009**, *25*, 607–616. [CrossRef] [PubMed]
75. Debillion, T.; Zupan, V.; Ravault, N.; Magny, J.F.; Dehan, M. Development and initial validation of the EDIN scale, a new tool for assessing prolonged pain in preterm infants. *Arch. Dis Child. Fetal* **2001**, *85*, F36–F41. [CrossRef]

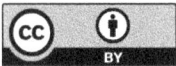

Review

Rewiring of Developing Spinal Nociceptive Circuits by Neonatal Injury and Its Implications for Pediatric Chronic Pain

Mark L. Baccei

Pain Research Center, Department of Anesthesiology, University of Cincinnati Medical Center, 231 Albert Sabin Way, Cincinnati, OH 45267, USA; mark.baccei@uc.edu

Academic Editor: Carl L. von Baeyer
Received: 8 August 2016; Accepted: 16 September 2016; Published: 20 September 2016

Abstract: Significant evidence now suggests that neonatal tissue damage can evoke long-lasting changes in pain sensitivity, but the underlying cellular and molecular mechanisms remain unclear. This review highlights recent advances in our understanding of how injuries during a critical period of early life modulate the functional organization of synaptic networks in the superficial dorsal horn (SDH) of the spinal cord in a manner that favors the excessive amplification of ascending nociceptive signaling to the brain, which likely contributes to the generation and/or maintenance of pediatric chronic pain. These persistent alterations in synaptic function within the SDH may also contribute to the well-documented "priming" of developing pain pathways by neonatal tissue injury.

Keywords: pain; neonate; spinal cord; dorsal horn; synapse; glutamate; GABA; glycine; incision; rodent

1. Introduction

Pain processing in the central nervous system (CNS) begins in the dorsal horn of the spinal cord which receives direct input from peripheral sensory neurons that are activated by noxious stimuli, defined as stimuli that damage or threaten to damage normal tissue. These signals are integrated with other types of incoming sensory information, including touch, before being transmitted to nociceptive circuits in the brain where the perception of pain ultimately emerges. This need for complex integration of sensory stimuli across multiple modalities is reflected in the functional organization of the dorsal horn network, in that >95% of neurons are propriospinal neurons or local circuit interneurons (both excitatory and inhibitory) whose axons do not leave the spinal cord. Meanwhile, nociceptive information is conveyed to the brain by an exclusive group of projection neurons concentrated mainly in laminae I and V [1], whose firing is strongly controlled by the balance of activity in the different excitatory (glutamatergic) and inhibitory (expressing gamma-aminobutyric acid (GABA) and/or glycine) populations of interneurons. For example, it has long been known that blocking synaptic inhibition within the spinal cord causes robust mechanical allodynia [2–4] and unmasks a novel excitatory input to lamina I projection neurons [5–7]. Recent evidence suggests that inhibitory interneurons expressing parvalbumin or dynorphin may tonically suppress the activation of ascending projection neurons by innocuous mechanical stimuli, and pharmacogenetic silencing of these interneurons evokes mechanical pain hypersensitivity including allodynia [8,9]. Therefore, a complete mechanistic understanding of pathological pain cannot be obtained without detailed knowledge of how peripheral nerve or tissue damage modifies synaptic transmission within spinal dorsal horn circuits. It is also essential to elucidate the extent to which age determines the effects of injury on synaptic signaling in the spinal superficial dorsal horn. The major aim of this review is to highlight recent work demonstrating that synaptic function within spinal nociceptive networks is persistently influenced by tissue damage during early life.

2. Spinal Mechanisms Contributing to Central Sensitization

"Central sensitization" has been operationally defined as an increased responsiveness of nociceptive neurons in the CNS to their normal or subthreshold afferent input, and can drive the generation of chronic pain under pathological conditions [10,11]. It is now clear that a reduction in the efficacy of synaptic inhibition within the spinal dorsal horn is an important contributor to central sensitization after injury. The decreased inhibitory tone in the dorsal horn after nerve or tissue damage reflects a multitude of underlying changes in synaptic function. This includes a dampening of glycinergic transmission [12–14] which has been linked to a prostaglandin E2 (PGE2)- and protein kinase A (PKA)-dependent phosphorylation of glycine receptors (GlyRs) containing the α_3 subunit [15,16]. Following nerve damage, a subset of glycinergic neurons expressing parvalbumin also exhibit a weaker innervation of excitatory protein kinase C gamma (PKCγ)-expressing interneurons in the dorsal horn [8], which likely leads to the disinhibition of this neuronal population previously implicated in neuropathic pain [7,17]. The efficacy of GABAergic and glycinergic inhibition also critically depends on the maintenance of low intracellular Cl$^-$ levels within the postsynaptic neuron [18,19], which in turn depends on the activity of the K-Cl co-transporter potassium-chloride transporter member 5 (KCC2) [20–22]. Importantly, the expression of KCC2 in adult dorsal horn neurons is significantly reduced by peripheral nerve injury leading to weaker GABAergic inhibition, and in some cases the influence of GABA can switch to being excitatory in nature [23,24]. This injury-evoked shift mimics the situation during early development, where low levels of KCC2 in the dorsal horn [25] lead to a reduced ability to extrude intracellular Cl$^-$ [26] and the occurrence of depolarizing responses to GABA [27].

Mounting evidence suggests that while central sensitization occurs at all stages of postnatal development as a consequence of injury, the underlying mechanisms may be at least partially dependent on the age at which the injury occurs [28]. For example, peripheral inflammation or surgical incision of the rodent hindpaw during the first days of life leads to a transient elevation in glutamate release within the superficial dorsal horn (SDH) that is not observed following the same injury at later ages [29]. This enhanced glutamate release includes a strengthening of high-threshold (i.e., putative nociceptive) primary afferent synapses onto lamina II interneurons that requires nerve growth factor (NGF) activation of tropomyosin receptor kinase A (trkA) receptors [30]. The short-term potentiation in glutamatergic function is also activity-dependent, as it is prevented by blocking sciatic nerve activity from the time of injury [31]. In contrast, inflammation during early life failed to compromise synaptic inhibition within the immature dorsal horn [29,31], although Cl$^-$ homeostasis was not specifically examined. Peripheral nerve damage also evokes distinct changes in the neonatal versus adult dorsal horn, as no alterations in spontaneous excitatory or inhibitory signaling are seen in the days following sciatic nerve damage at postnatal day (P) 10 [32]. This is interesting in light of behavioral studies showing a delayed onset of neuropathic pain after peripheral nerve injury during early life [33,34].

3. Neonatal Injury "Primes" Developing Nociceptive Circuits in the CNS

Tissue damage during a critical period of early life can evoke prolonged changes in nociceptive processing and pain sensitivity. Quantitative sensory testing (QST) approaches have shown that children with a prior stay in a neonatal intensive care unit (NICU) display greater pain sensitivity in response to prolonged noxious stimulation compared to a control, non-hospitalized group, even a decade later [35,36]. These persistent changes were more pronounced in patients that also required neonatal surgery [37]. Nonetheless, the complex nature of the NICU experience makes it difficult to conclusively attribute such long-term changes in pain processing to tissue damage per se, as these infants also experience a high number of stressors [38] that can also modulate nociceptive processing in the CNS. Therefore, it is important to note that preclinical investigations have produced qualitatively similar results. Numerous studies have demonstrated that hindpaw injury during the neonatal period leads to an exacerbated degree of pain hypersensitivity following repeat injury of the affected paw, an effect which persists throughout life [39–42]. This reflects, at least in part, a localized "priming" of spinal nociceptive circuits following early trauma [43]. Consistent with a role for the spinal cord, neonatal inflammation is sufficient to significantly alter the pattern of gene expression across the adult dorsal horn, including genes that are known to be involved in synaptic transmission [44].

Recent work has explored the long-term effects of neonatal tissue damage on synaptic signaling within the mature SDH. Hindpaw surgical incision at P3 led to a significant dampening of phasic glycinergic transmission onto both GABAergic and presumed glutamatergic interneurons in lamina II of the adult mouse SDH [45]. While this phasic (or "fast") synaptic inhibition involves the activation of GlyRs located at the synapse [46], the activation of extrasynaptic GlyRs by ambient levels of glycine can evoke a strong tonic inhibition of neuronal excitability in the SDH [47]. Notably, P3 incision also produced a long-lasting decrease in the density of tonic GlyR-mediated current within excitatory lamina II interneurons of the adult spinal cord [45], which is predicted to enhance their firing (via a process of disinhibition). Such deficits in inhibition could be exacerbated if the neonatal injury also persistently reduces KCC2 expression in the dorsal horn, as seen acutely after adult peripheral nerve injury [23,24], although this has yet to be directly investigated. Overall, these results suggest that neonatal tissue injury alters the delicate balance between excitation and inhibition within the mature SDH circuit towards excessive excitation, which in turn would predict an increased level of ascending nociceptive transmission to the brain. However, given that lamina II consists entirely of propriospinal or local circuit interneurons [48,49], the consequences of these changes in synaptic function for pain perception will ultimately depend on the degree to which they influence synaptic signaling onto the spinal projection neurons which convey noxious sensory information to the brain.

4. Neonatal Tissue Damage Shapes Synaptic Integration in Adult Spinal Projection Neurons

Primary afferent inputs to the SDH not only directly excite ascending lamina I projection neurons [50,51] but also evoke polysynaptic inhibition of this same population, termed "feedforward" inhibition [52,53], via their synapses onto inhibitory interneurons in the region. Importantly, surgical injury during the neonatal period significantly weakens both GABAergic and glycinergic feedforward inhibition onto adult spinal projection neurons [52]. This cannot be explained by a disruption in the normal innervation of mature projection neurons by local inhibitory interneurons, as early injury failed to alter the number of synaptic boutons expressing known markers of GABAergic and glycinergic presynaptic terminals that were in apposition to adult projection neurons [52]. Instead, the weaker feedforward inhibition could reflect an injury-evoked reduction in the intrinsic membrane excitability of GABAergic interneurons in the mature SDH [54]. Meanwhile, the strength of the direct (i.e., monosynaptic) primary afferent input to adult projection neurons was significantly enhanced by hindpaw incision at P3 [52]. Therefore, early tissue damage significantly alters the balance of synaptic excitation vs. inhibition onto the major output neurons of the spinal nociceptive circuit. This would predict that adult projection neurons would fire more robustly in response to sensory input when preceded by an injury during early life. Consistent with this prediction, adult spino-parabrachial (PB) neurons exhibited a greater number of action potentials in response to primary afferent stimulation in mice with neonatal surgical injury as compared to naïve littermate controls [52]. This demonstrates that neonatal tissue damage persistently increases the signaling "gain" of the mature SDH network, such that peripheral nociceptive input is amplified to a greater degree within the spinal cord before being transmitted to higher pain centers in the brain. Nonetheless, it should be noted that these prior studies have exclusively focused on the lamina I projection neurons innervating the PB nucleus in the brain. It will be important to also elucidate the long-term effects of early injury on synaptic integration within other populations of spinal projection neurons, such as those targeting the periaqueductal gray (PAG) or thalamus [1], as the electrophysiological properties of projection neurons can vary significantly depending on their target in the brain [55–57].

5. Long-Term Potentiation at Sensory Synapses onto Spinal Projection Neurons

Primary afferent synapses onto spinal projection neurons can be strengthened by repetitive activation [51,55]. This synaptic long-term potentiation (LTP) represents a major mechanism by which ascending nociceptive transmission to the brain can be amplified within the spinal dorsal horn network (for review see [58]). Numerous lines of evidence point to the functional relevance of spinal LTP for chronic pain. For example, LTP can be evoked by both electrical stimulation of sensory inputs to the dorsal horn as well as peripheral tissue or nerve damage [59,60], and the same electrical stimulation protocols that evoke LTP can produce hyperalgesia in rodents [61,62]. Furthermore, pharmacological agents that prevent the generation of spinal LTP also reduce behavioral pain hypersensitivity after injury [58]. Critically, the administration of LTP induction protocols involving high-frequency stimulation has been shown to increase pain sensitivity in humans [63–65]. Therefore, one potential mechanism by which neonatal injury could "prime" mature nociceptive circuits is by persistently facilitating LTP at sensory synapses onto lamina I projection neurons. This could occur by enhancing the magnitude of LTP at these synapses and/or increasing the likelihood that LTP occurs in response to a given sensory input by modulating the timing rules governing activity-dependent synaptic plasticity within the mature dorsal horn.

It is now abundantly clear that the relative timing of presynaptic versus postsynaptic activity profoundly influences synaptic strength in the CNS, a phenomenon referred to as "spike timing-dependent plasticity" or "STDP" [66,67]. While the precise temporal rules governing STDP vary across different brain regions, the majority of studies report that presynaptic inputs which precede postsynaptic action potential discharge by a brief interval (10–50 ms) undergo LTP (termed "spike timing-dependent LTP" or "t-LTP"), while those that follow postsynaptic firing undergo long-term depression (LTD) [68]. This raises the possibility that neonatal tissue damage could facilitate LTP at afferent synapses onto adult projection neurons by: (1) increasing the magnitude of synaptic potentiation produced by highly correlated pre- and postsynaptic firing occurring within the optimum timing window for t-LTP; and/or (2) widening the timing window during which the presynaptic and postsynaptic firing must occur in order to evoke t-LTP.

6. Neonatal Injury Relaxes the Timing Rules Governing Spike Timing-Dependent LTP in Adult Spinal Pain Circuits

To address this issue, a recent study [69] evoked action potential firing in lamina I projection neurons at defined intervals either before (i.e., Post → Pre) or after (Pre → Post) the arrival of a presynaptic input mediated by sensory afferents (with the pairing protocol repeated 30 times at 0.2 Hz). The resultant change in synaptic strength was measured and compared between adult mice that had experienced surgical injury as a neonate and naïve littermate controls. In projection neurons from naïve mice, Pre → Post pairings at an interval between 10–20 ms produced significant t-LTP, while the reverse (i.e., Post → Pre) pairings failed to change the amplitude of the synaptic response (i.e., produced neither t-LTP nor t-LTD). Strikingly, hindpaw incision at P3 significantly widened the timing window for evoking t-LTP (Figure 1), as a greater potentiation of excitatory postsynaptic current (EPSC) amplitude was seen in projection neurons from these mice at Pre → Post intervals of 20 and 50 ms compared to the naïve group [69]. In addition, reverse (i.e., Post → Pre) pairings produced marked t-LTP in neonatally-injured mice, suggesting that early tissue damage removes the temporal requirement for the sensory input to precede the firing of adult projection neurons. Such a change is predicted to persistently increase the likelihood that LTP occurs at a given primary afferent synapse, and thus elevate the overall number of synapses that are strengthened following sensory input to the spinal cord. This could favor the excessive amplification of ascending nociceptive transmission to the mature brain in response to subsequent injury and thereby exacerbate chronic pain.

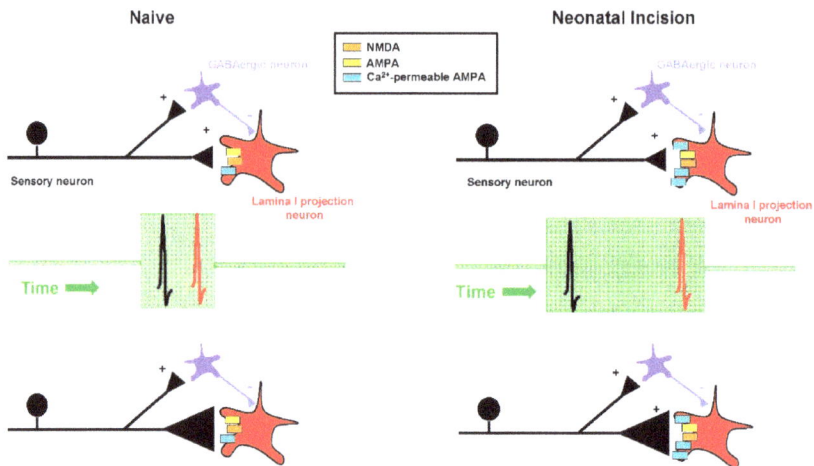

Figure 1. Early tissue damage widens the timing window for evoking spike timing-dependent long-term potentiation (t-LTP) at sensory synapses onto adult spinal projection neurons. **Left column (Naïve)**: In naïve adult mice, highly correlated presynaptic (black) and postsynaptic (red) action potential firing (i.e., occurring within a window of 10–20 ms; green box) led to a strengthening of primary afferent synapses onto ascending lamina I projection neurons. This reflected an increase in the probability of glutamate release from the presynaptic terminals of the sensory neurons, as illustrated here by a larger size of the presynaptic terminals (black triangles in bottom panels). **Right column (Neonatal Incision)**: In adult mice subjected to neonatal surgical injury, the timing window for generating t-LTP (green box) at afferent synapses onto spinal projection neurons significantly widened, such that poorly correlated presynaptic and postsynaptic firing (at pairing intervals $\geq$50 ms; middle panel) was still able to generate t-LTP. This enhanced propensity to generate t-LTP likely results, at least in part, from an elevated expression of Ca^{2+}-permeable α-amino-3-hydroxy-5-methyl-4-isoxazolepropionic acid (AMPA) receptors (AMPARs) (blue rectangles) in mature projection neurons following early tissue damage, since blocking these glutamate receptors prevented t-LTP in neonatally-injured mice but not naïve littermate controls [69]. NMDA: *N*-methyl-D-aspartate.

Under normal conditions, the need for sequential Pre → Post activation to produce t-LTP is thought to reflect the biophysical properties of the *N*-methyl-D-aspartate (NMDA) subtype of glutamate receptor (NMDAR), which requires both glutamate binding and membrane depolarization in order to be activated due to a voltage-dependent block of the channel by Mg^{2+} ions at resting membrane potentials [70]. As a result, Pre → Post pairings produce greater Ca^{2+} influx through the NMDAR [71] which is essential for producing t-LTP in many types of CNS neurons [72–74]. Interestingly, while the block of NMDARs abolishes t-LTP in adult spinal projection neurons from naïve mice, it fails to do so in neonatally incised mice [69], suggesting a reduced dependence on NMDAR activation in the aftermath of early life injury. Nonetheless, preventing an elevation in intracellular Ca^{2+} within projection neurons prevented t-LTP in both the naïve and P3 incision groups, demonstrating that postsynaptic Ca^{2+} remains a critical mediator of LTP regardless of the presence of noxious sensory experience during the neonatal period. Collectively, these observations raised the possibility that a supplemental source of postsynaptic Ca^{2+} influx is recruited following early tissue injury, thus reducing the reliance on NMDAR activation in order to achieve the intracellular Ca^{2+} levels necessary to drive t-LTP at sensory synapses onto mature projection neurons [69].

Significant glutamate-evoked Ca^{2+} influx into neurons can also occur through a subset of α-amino-3-hydroxy-5-methyl-4-isoxazolepropionic acid (AMPA) receptors (AMPAR) that lack the

GluR2 subunit [75,76]. These Ca^{2+}-permeable AMPARs are known to be expressed in the superficial dorsal horn and can contribute to the generation of both spinal LTP [77] and chronic pain after injury [78], thereby making them strong candidates to regulate synaptic plasticity within adult spinal nociceptive circuits after early life injury. Indeed, neonatal surgical incision elevated the relative expression of Ca^{2+} permeable AMPARs at sensory synapses onto mature lamina I projection neurons [69]. Furthermore, while blocking Ca^{2+}-permeable AMPARs had no effect on timing-dependent LTP (t-LTP) in projection neurons from naïve mice, it completely suppressed t-LTP at the same synapses in neonatally-injured mice [69]. Collectively, the results suggest that early tissue damage unmasks a novel role of Ca^{2+}-permeable AMPARs in the regulation of STDP at primary afferent synapses onto ascending projection neurons in the adult spinal cord.

7. Future Directions

Despite recent progress towards elucidating the short- and long-term effects of neonatal tissue injury on synaptic signaling within developing spinal nociceptive circuits, many important questions remain unanswered. For example, how does early tissue damage alter the synaptic "microcircuits" within the mature SDH? While prior work has demonstrated reduced feedforward synaptic inhibition onto adult projection neurons after neonatal surgical injury, how this injury influences neurotransmitter release from specific subpopulations of inhibitory dorsal horn interneurons (i.e., those expressing parvalbumin, neuropeptide Y, galanin or nitric oxide synthase) remains unknown. In addition, since immune cells play an important role in shaping synaptic development in the CNS [79] and early tissue damage alters neuroimmune signaling in the mature spinal cord [43], it will be interesting to examine the potential role of spinal microglia in orchestrating the short- and long-term alterations in synaptic function within the SDH after neonatal injury. Microglia could also contribute to the changes in spike timing-dependent plasticity within adult spinal projection neurons after early tissue damage, as they are known to modulate other forms of LTP in the SDH [80].

The t-LTP characterized at primary afferent synapses onto ascending projection neurons appears to involve the release of a retrograde messenger which enhances glutamate release from the sensory neurons [69]. However, the identity of the retrograde signal, and whether neonatal injury alters this signaling pathway, has yet to be investigated. Another intriguing question is whether early tissue damage evokes a novel timing window at afferent synapses onto adult projection neurons, or whether this more permissive environment for t-LTP normally exists during early life and the injury somehow prevents a developmental sharpening (or "tuning") of the timing window. Notably, the prolonged changes in pain sensitivity [41,42] and synaptic plasticity [69] both require that the initial injury occur during a critical period of early postnatal development, corresponding to the first postnatal week in the rodent. However, the mechanisms which underlie the closure of this critical period are currently a mystery. A better understanding of why tissue damage at later ages fails to evoke the same permanent alterations in spinal nociceptive processing could yield valuable insight into novel strategies to minimize the persistent effects of neonatal injuries on developing nociceptive pathways.

Acknowledgments: This work was supported by the National Institutes of Health (NS080889 to M.L.B.).

Conflicts of Interest: The author declares no conflict of interest.

References

1. Todd, A.J. Neuronal circuitry for pain processing in the dorsal horn. *Nat. Rev. Neurosci.* **2010**, *11*, 823–836. [CrossRef] [PubMed]
2. Sherman, S.E.; Loomis, C.W. Morphine insensitive allodynia is produced by intrathecal strychnine in the lightly anesthetized rat. *Pain* **1994**, *56*, 17–29. [CrossRef]
3. Sivilotti, L.; Woolf, C.J. The contribution of GABAA and glycine receptors to central sensitization: Disinhibition and touch-evoked allodynia in the spinal cord. *J. Neurophysiol.* **1994**, *72*, 169–179. [PubMed]

4.   Yaksh, T.L. Behavioral and autonomic correlates of the tactile evoked allodynia produced by spinal glycine inhibition: Effects of modulatory receptor systems and excitatory amino acid antagonists. *Pain* **1989**, *37*, 111–123. [CrossRef]

5.   Torsney, C.; MacDermott, A.B. Disinhibition opens the gate to pathological pain signaling in superficial neurokinin 1 receptor-expressing neurons in rat spinal cord. *J. Neurosci.* **2006**, *26*, 1833–1843. [CrossRef] [PubMed]

6.   Peirs, C.; Williams, S.P.; Zhao, X.; Walsh, C.E.; Gedeon, J.Y.; Cagle, N.E.; Goldring, A.C.; Hioki, H.; Liu, Z.; Marell, P.S.; et al. Dorsal Horn Circuits for Persistent Mechanical Pain. *Neuron* **2015**, *87*, 797–812. [CrossRef] [PubMed]

7.   Lu, Y.; Dong, H.; Gao, Y.; Gong, Y.; Ren, Y.; Gu, N.; Zhou, S.; Xia, N.; Sun, Y.Y.; Ji, R.R.; et al. A feed-forward spinal cord glycinergic neural circuit gates mechanical allodynia. *J. Clin. Investig.* **2013**, *123*, 4050–4062. [CrossRef] [PubMed]

8.   Petitjean, H.; Pawlowski, S.A.; Fraine, S.L.; Sharif, B.; Hamad, D.; Fatima, T.; Berg, J.; Brown, C.M.; Jan, L.Y.; Ribeiro-da-Silva, A.; et al. Dorsal Horn Parvalbumin Neurons Are Gate-Keepers of Touch-Evoked Pain after Nerve Injury. *Cell Rep.* **2015**, *13*, 1246–1257. [CrossRef] [PubMed]

9.   Duan, B.; Cheng, L.; Bourane, S.; Britz, O.; Padilla, C.; Garcia-Campmany, L.; Krashes, M.; Knowlton, W.; Velasquez, T.; Ren, X.; et al. Identification of spinal circuits transmitting and gating mechanical pain. *Cell* **2014**, *159*, 1417–1432. [CrossRef] [PubMed]

10.   Woolf, C.J. Central sensitization: Implications for the diagnosis and treatment of pain. *Pain* **2011**, *152* (Suppl. 3), S2–S15. [CrossRef] [PubMed]

11.   Latremoliere, A.; Woolf, C.J. Central sensitization: A generator of pain hypersensitivity by central neural plasticity. *J. Pain* **2009**, *10*, 895–926. [CrossRef] [PubMed]

12.   Ahmadi, S.; Lippross, S.; Neuhuber, W.L.; Zeilhofer, H.U. PGE(2) selectively blocks inhibitory glycinergic neurotransmission onto rat superficial dorsal horn neurons. *Nat. Neurosci.* **2002**, *5*, 34–40. [CrossRef] [PubMed]

13.   Foster, E.; Wildner, H.; Tudeau, L.; Haueter, S.; Ralvenius, W.T.; Jegen, M.; Johannssen, H.; Hosli, L.; Haenraets, K.; Ghanem, A.; et al. Targeted ablation, silencing, and activation establish glycinergic dorsal horn neurons as key components of a spinal gate for pain and itch. *Neuron* **2015**, *85*, 1289–1304. [CrossRef] [PubMed]

14.   Muller, F.; Heinke, B.; Sandkühler, J. Reduction of glycine receptor-mediated miniature inhibitory postsynaptic currents in rat spinal lamina I neurons after peripheral inflammation. *Neuroscience* **2003**, *122*, 799–805. [CrossRef] [PubMed]

15.   Harvey, R.J.; Depner, U.B.; Wassle, H.; Ahmadi, S.; Heindl, C.; Reinold, H.; Smart, T.G.; Harvey, K.; Schutz, B.; Bo-Salem, O.M.; et al. GlyR alpha3: An essential target for spinal PGE2-mediated inflammatory pain sensitization. *Science* **2004**, *304*, 884–887. [CrossRef] [PubMed]

16.   Acuna, M.A.; Yevenes, G.E.; Ralvenius, W.T.; Benke, D.; Di, L.A.; Lara, C.O.; Munoz, B.; Burgos, C.F.; Moraga-Cid, G.; Corringer, P.J.; et al. Phosphorylation state-dependent modulation of spinal glycine receptors alleviates inflammatory pain. *J. Clin. Investig.* **2016**, *126*, 2547–2560. [CrossRef] [PubMed]

17.   Malmberg, A.B.; Chen, C.; Tonegawa, S.; Basbaum, A.I. Preserved acute pain and reduced neuropathic pain in mice lacking PKCgamma. *Science* **1997**, *278*, 279–283. [CrossRef] [PubMed]

18.   Doyon, N.; Vinay, L.; Prescott, S.A.; De Koninck, Y. Chloride Regulation: A Dynamic Equilibrium Crucial for Synaptic Inhibition. *Neuron* **2016**, *89*, 1157–1172. [CrossRef] [PubMed]

19.   Ben-Ari, Y. Excitatory actions of gaba during development: The nature of the nurture. *Nat. Rev. Neurosci.* **2002**, *3*, 728–739. [CrossRef] [PubMed]

20.   Rohrbough, J.; Spitzer, N.C. Regulation of intracellular Cl− levels by Na(+)-dependent Cl− cotransport distinguishes depolarizing from hyperpolarizing GABAA receptor-mediated responses in spinal neurons. *J. Neurosci.* **1996**, *16*, 82–91. [PubMed]

21.   Ehrlich, I.; Lohrke, S.; Friauf, E. Shift from depolarizing to hyperpolarizing glycine action in rat auditory neurones is due to age-dependent Cl− regulation. *J. Physiol.* **1999**, *520 Pt 1*, 121–137. [CrossRef] [PubMed]

22.   Rivera, C.; Voipio, J.; Payne, J.A.; Ruusuvuori, E.; Lahtinen, H.; Lamsa, K.; Pirvola, U.; Saarma, M.; Kaila, K. The K+/Cl− co-transporter KCC2 renders GABA hyperpolarizing during neuronal maturation. *Nature* **1999**, *397*, 251–255. [PubMed]

23. Coull, J.A.M.; Beggs, S.; Boudreau, D.; Boivin, D.; Tsuda, M.; Inoue, K.; Gravel, C.; Salter, M.W.; De Koninck, Y. BDNF from microglia causes the shift in neuronal anion gradient underlying neuropathic pain. *Nature* **2005**, *438*, 1017–1021. [CrossRef] [PubMed]

24. Coull, J.A.; Boudreau, D.; Bachand, K.; Prescott, S.A.; Nault, F.; Sik, A.; De Koninck, P.; De Koninck, Y. Trans-synaptic shift in anion gradient in spinal lamina I neurons as a mechanism of neuropathic pain. *Nature* **2003**, *424*, 938–942. [CrossRef] [PubMed]

25. Hubner, C.A.; Stein, V.; Hermans-Borgmeyer, I.; Meyer, T.; Ballanyi, K.; Jentsch, T.J. Disruption of KCC2 reveals an essential role of K-Cl cotransport already in early synaptic inhibition. *Neuron* **2001**, *30*, 515–524. [CrossRef]

26. Cordero-Erausquin, M.; Coull, J.A.; Boudreau, D.; Rolland, M.; De Koninck, Y. Differential maturation of GABA action and anion reversal potential in spinal lamina I neurons: Impact of chloride extrusion capacity. *J. Neurosci.* **2005**, *25*, 9613–9623. [CrossRef] [PubMed]

27. Baccei, M.L.; Fitzgerald, M. Development of GABAergic and glycinergic transmission in the neonatal rat dorsal horn. *J. Neurosci.* **2004**, *24*, 4749–4757. [CrossRef] [PubMed]

28. Schwaller, F.; Fitzgerald, M. The consequences of pain in early life: Injury-induced plasticity in developing pain pathways. *Eur. J. Neurosci.* **2014**, *39*, 344–352. [CrossRef] [PubMed]

29. Li, J.; Baccei, M.L. Excitatory synapses in the rat superficial dorsal horn are strengthened following peripheral inflammation during early postnatal development. *Pain* **2009**, *143*, 56–64. [CrossRef] [PubMed]

30. Li, J.; Baccei, M.L. Neonatal tissue damage facilitates nociceptive synaptic input to the developing superficial dorsal horn via NGF-dependent mechanisms. *Pain* **2011**, *152*, 1846–1855. [CrossRef] [PubMed]

31. Li, J.; Walker, S.M.; Fitzgerald, M.; Baccei, M.L. Activity-dependent modulation of glutamatergic signaling in the developing rat dorsal horn by early tissue injury. *J. Neurophysiol.* **2009**, *102*, 2208–2219. [CrossRef] [PubMed]

32. Li, J.; Xie, W.; Zhang, J.M.; Baccei, M.L. Peripheral nerve injury sensitizes neonatal dorsal horn neurons to tumor necrosis factor-alpha. *Mol. Pain* **2009**, *5*, 10. [CrossRef] [PubMed]

33. McKelvey, R.; Berta, T.; Old, E.; Ji, R.R.; Fitzgerald, M. Neuropathic pain is constitutively suppressed in early life by anti-inflammatory neuroimmune regulation. *J. Neurosci.* **2015**, *35*, 457–466. [CrossRef] [PubMed]

34. Vega-Avelaira, D.; McKelvey, R.; Hathway, G.; Fitzgerald, M. The emergence of adolescent onset pain hypersensitivity following neonatal nerve injury. *Mol. Pain* **2012**, *8*, 30. [CrossRef] [PubMed]

35. Hermann, C.; Hohmeister, J.; Demirakca, S.; Zohsel, K.; Flor, H. Long-term alteration of pain sensitivity in school-aged children with early pain experiences. *Pain* **2006**, *125*, 278–285. [CrossRef] [PubMed]

36. Hohmeister, J.; Kroll, A.; Wollgarten-Hadamek, I.; Zohsel, K.; Demirakca, S.; Flor, H.; Hermann, C. Cerebral processing of pain in school-aged children with neonatal nociceptive input: An exploratory fMRI study. *Pain* **2010**, *150*, 257–267. [CrossRef] [PubMed]

37. Walker, S.M.; Franck, L.S.; Fitzgerald, M.; Myles, J.; Stocks, J.; Marlow, N. Long-term impact of neonatal intensive care and surgery on somatosensory perception in children born extremely preterm. *Pain* **2009**, *141*, 79–87. [CrossRef] [PubMed]

38. Newnham, C.A.; Inder, T.E.; Milgrom, J. Measuring preterm cumulative stressors within the NICU: The Neonatal Infant Stressor Scale. *Early Hum. Dev.* **2009**, *85*, 549–555. [CrossRef] [PubMed]

39. Hohmann, A.G.; Neely, M.H.; Pina, J.; Nackley, A.G. Neonatal chronic hind paw inflammation alters sensitization to intradermal capsaicin in adult rats: A behavioral and immunocytochemical study. *J. Pain* **2005**, *6*, 798–808. [CrossRef] [PubMed]

40. Chu, Y.C.; Chan, K.H.; Tsou, M.Y.; Lin, S.M.; Hsieh, Y.C.; Tao, Y.X. Mechanical pain hypersensitivity after incisional surgery is enhanced in rats subjected to neonatal peripheral inflammation: Effects of N-methyl-D-aspartate receptor antagonists. *Anesthesiology* **2007**, *106*, 1204–1212. [CrossRef] [PubMed]

41. Ren, K.; Anseloni, V.; Zou, S.P.; Wade, E.B.; Novikova, S.I.; Ennis, M.; Traub, R.J.; Gold, M.S.; Dubner, R.; Lidow, M.S. Characterization of basal and re-inflammation-associated long-term alteration in pain responsivity following short-lasting neonatal local inflammatory insult. *Pain* **2004**, *110*, 588–596. [CrossRef] [PubMed]

42. Walker, S.M.; Tochiki, K.K.; Fitzgerald, M. Hindpaw incision in early life increases the hyperalgesic response to repeat surgical injury: Critical period and dependence on initial afferent activity. *Pain* **2009**, *147*, 99–106. [CrossRef] [PubMed]

43. Beggs, S.; Currie, G.; Salter, M.W.; Fitzgerald, M.; Walker, S.M. Priming of adult pain responses by neonatal pain experience: Maintenance by central neuroimmune activity. *Brain* **2012**, *135 Pt 2*, 404–417. [CrossRef] [PubMed]

44. Ren, K.; Novikova, S.I.; He, F.; Dubner, R.; Lidow, M.S. Neonatal local noxious insult affects gene expression in the spinal dorsal horn of adult rats. *Mol. Pain* **2005**, *1*, 27. [CrossRef] [PubMed]

45. Li, J.; Blankenship, M.L.; Baccei, M.L. Deficits in glycinergic inhibition within adult spinal nociceptive circuits after neonatal tissue damage. *Pain* **2013**, *154*, 1129–1139. [CrossRef] [PubMed]

46. Farrant, M.; Nusser, Z. Variations on an inhibitory theme: Phasic and tonic activation of GABA(A) receptors. *Nat. Rev. Neurosci.* **2005**, *6*, 215–229. [CrossRef] [PubMed]

47. Takazawa, T.; MacDermott, A.B. Glycinergic and GABAergic tonic inhibition fine tune inhibitory control in regionally distinct subpopulations of dorsal horn neurons. *J. Physiol.* **2010**, *588 Pt 14*, 2571–2587. [CrossRef] [PubMed]

48. Bice, T.N.; Beal, J.A. Quantitative and neurogenic analysis of neurons with supraspinal projections in the superficial dorsal horn of the rat lumbar spinal cord. *J. Comp. Neurol.* **1997**, *388*, 565–574. [CrossRef]

49. Bice, T.N.; Beal, J.A. Quantitative and neurogenic analysis of the total population and subpopulations of neurons defined by axon projection in the superficial dorsal horn of the rat lumbar spinal cord. *J. Comp. Neurol.* **1997**, *388*, 550–564. [CrossRef]

50. Dahlhaus, A.; Ruscheweyh, R.; Sandkühler, J. Synaptic input of rat spinal lamina I projection and unidentified neurones in vitro. *J. Physiol.* **2005**, *566 Pt 2*, 355–368. [CrossRef] [PubMed]

51. Ikeda, H.; Heinke, B.; Ruscheweyh, R.; Sandkühler, J. Synaptic plasticity in spinal lamina I projection neurons that mediate hyperalgesia. *Science* **2003**, *299*, 1237–1240. [CrossRef] [PubMed]

52. Li, J.; Kritzer, E.; Craig, P.E.; Baccei, M.L. Aberrant synaptic integration in adult lamina I projection neurons following neonatal tissue damage. *J. Neurosci.* **2015**, *35*, 2438–2451. [CrossRef] [PubMed]

53. Nakatsuka, T.; Chen, M.; Takeda, D.; King, C.; Ling, J.; Xing, H.; Ataka, T.; Vierck, C.; Yezierski, R.; Gu, J.G. Substance P-driven feed-forward inhibitory activity in the mammalian spinal cord. *Mol. Pain* **2005**, *1*, 20. [CrossRef] [PubMed]

54. Li, J.; Baccei, M.L. Neonatal tissue injury reduces the intrinsic excitability of adult mouse superficial dorsal horn neurons. *Neuroscience* **2014**, *256*, 392–402. [CrossRef] [PubMed]

55. Ikeda, H.; Stark, J.; Fischer, H.; Wagner, M.; Drdla, R.; Jager, T.; Sandkühler, J. Synaptic amplifier of inflammatory pain in the spinal dorsal horn. *Science* **2006**, *312*, 1659–1662. [CrossRef] [PubMed]

56. Li, J.; Baccei, M.L. Developmental regulation of membrane excitability in rat spinal lamina I projection neurons. *J. Neurophysiol.* **2012**, *107*, 2604–2614. [CrossRef] [PubMed]

57. Ruscheweyh, R.; Ikeda, H.; Heinke, B.; Sandkühler, J. Distinctive membrane and discharge properties of rat spinal lamina I projection neurones in vitro. *J. Physiol.* **2004**, *555 Pt 2*, 527–543. [CrossRef] [PubMed]

58. Ruscheweyh, R.; Wilder-Smith, O.; Drdla, R.; Liu, X.G.; Sandkühler, J. Long-term potentiation in spinal nociceptive pathways as a novel target for pain therapy. *Mol. Pain* **2011**, *7*, 20. [CrossRef] [PubMed]

59. Sandkühler, J.; Liu, X. Induction of long-term potentiation at spinal synapses by noxious stimulation or nerve injury. *Eur. J. Neurosci.* **1998**, *10*, 2476–2480. [CrossRef] [PubMed]

60. Zhou, L.J.; Ren, W.J.; Zhong, Y.; Yang, T.; Wei, X.H.; Xin, W.J.; Liu, C.C.; Zhou, L.H.; Li, Y.Y.; Liu, X.G. Limited BDNF contributes to the failure of injury to skin afferents to produce a neuropathic pain condition. *Pain* **2010**, *148*, 148–157. [CrossRef] [PubMed]

61. Hathway, G.J.; Vega-Avelaira, D.; Moss, A.; Ingram, R.; Fitzgerald, M. Brief, low frequency stimulation of rat peripheral C-fibres evokes prolonged microglial-induced central sensitization in adults but not in neonates. *Pain* **2009**, *144*, 110–118. [CrossRef] [PubMed]

62. Zhang, X.C.; Zhang, Y.Q.; Zhao, Z.Q. Involvement of nitric oxide in long-term potentiation of spinal nociceptive responses in rats. *Neuroreport* **2005**, *16*, 1197–1201. [CrossRef] [PubMed]

63. Klein, T.; Magerl, W.; Hopf, H.C.; Sandkühler, J.; Treede, R.D. Perceptual correlates of nociceptive long-term potentiation and long-term depression in humans. *J Neurosci.* **2004**, *24*, 964–971. [CrossRef] [PubMed]

64. Klein, T.; Magerl, W.; Nickel, U.; Hopf, H.C.; Sandkühler, J.; Treede, R.D. Effects of the NMDA-receptor antagonist ketamine on perceptual correlates of long-term potentiation within the nociceptive system. *Neuropharmacology* **2007**, *52*, 655–661. [CrossRef] [PubMed]

65.	Schilder, A.; Magerl, W.; Hoheisel, U.; Klein, T.; Treede, R.D. Electrical high-frequency stimulation of the human thoracolumbar fascia evokes long-term potentiation-like pain amplification. *Pain* **2016**. [CrossRef] [PubMed]

66.	Dan, Y.; Poo, M.M. Spike timing-dependent plasticity of neural circuits. *Neuron* **2004**, *44*, 23–30. [CrossRef] [PubMed]

67.	Larsen, R.S.; Rao, D.; Manis, P.B.; Philpot, B.D. STDP in the Developing Sensory Neocortex. *Front. Synaptic. Neurosci.* **2010**, *2*, 9. [CrossRef] [PubMed]

68.	Feldman, D.E. The spike-timing dependence of plasticity. *Neuron* **2012**, *75*, 556–571. [CrossRef] [PubMed]

69.	Li, J.; Baccei, M.L. Neonatal Tissue Damage Promotes Spike Timing-Dependent Synaptic Long-Term Potentiation in Adult Spinal Projection Neurons. *J. Neurosci.* **2016**, *36*, 5405–5416. [CrossRef] [PubMed]

70.	Mayer, M.L.; Westbrook, G.L.; Guthrie, P.B. Voltage-dependent block by Mg^{2+} of NMDA responses in spinal cord neurones. *Nature* **1984**, *309*, 261–263. [CrossRef] [PubMed]

71.	Koester, H.J.; Sakmann, B. Calcium dynamics in single spines during coincident pre- and postsynaptic activity depend on relative timing of back-propagating action potentials and subthreshold excitatory postsynaptic potentials. *Proc. Natl. Acad. Sci. USA* **1998**, *95*, 9596–9601. [CrossRef] [PubMed]

72.	Cho, K.; Aggleton, J.P.; Brown, M.W.; Bashir, Z.I. An experimental test of the role of postsynaptic calcium levels in determining synaptic strength using perirhinal cortex of rat. *J. Physiol.* **2001**, *532 Pt 2*, 459–466. [CrossRef] [PubMed]

73.	Cormier, R.J.; Greenwood, A.C.; Connor, J.A. Bidirectional synaptic plasticity correlated with the magnitude of dendritic calcium transients above a threshold. *J. Neurophysiol.* **2001**, *85*, 399–406. [PubMed]

74.	Yang, S.N.; Tang, Y.G.; Zucker, R.S. Selective induction of LTP and LTD by postsynaptic [Ca2+]i elevation. *J. Neurophysiol.* **1999**, *81*, 781–787. [PubMed]

75.	Hollmann, M.; Hartley, M.; Heinemann, S. Ca^{2+} permeability of KA-AMPA-gated glutamate receptor channels depends on subunit composition. *Science* **1991**, *252*, 851–853. [CrossRef] [PubMed]

76.	Washburn, M.S.; Numberger, M.; Zhang, S.; Dingledine, R. Differential dependence on GluR2 expression of three characteristic features of AMPA receptors. *J. Neurosci.* **1997**, *17*, 9393–9406. [PubMed]

77.	Youn, D.H.; Royle, G.; Kolaj, M.; Vissel, B.; Randic, M. Enhanced LTP of primary afferent neurotransmission in AMPA receptor GluR2-deficient mice. *Pain* **2008**, *136*, 158–167. [CrossRef] [PubMed]

78.	Hartmann, B.; Ahmadi, S.; Heppenstall, P.A.; Lewin, G.R.; Schott, C.; Borchardt, T.; Seeburg, P.H.; Zeilhofer, H.U.; Sprengel, R.; Kuner, R. The AMPA receptor subunits GluR-A and GluR-B reciprocally modulate spinal synaptic plasticity and inflammatory pain. *Neuron* **2004**, *44*, 637–650. [CrossRef] [PubMed]

79.	Wu, Y.; Dissing-Olesen, L.; MacVicar, B.A.; Stevens, B. Microglia: Dynamic Mediators of Synapse Development and Plasticity. *Trends Immunol.* **2015**, *36*, 605–613. [CrossRef] [PubMed]

80.	Clark, A.K.; Gruber-Schoffnegger, D.; Drdla-Schutting, R.; Gerhold, K.J.; Malcangio, M.; Sandkühler, J. Selective activation of microglia facilitates synaptic strength. *J. Neurosci.* **2015**, *35*, 4552–4570. [CrossRef] [PubMed]

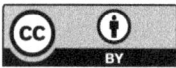

children

MDPI

Article

Perinatal Risk Factors and Genu Valgum Conducive to the Onset of Growing Pains in Early Childhood

Angelos Kaspiris [1,*], **Efstathios Chronopoulos** [2] **and Elias Vasiliadis** [3]

[1] Department of Trauma and Orthopaedics, Thriasio General Hospital—NHS, G. Gennimata av, Magoula 19600, Athens, Greece

[2] Second Department of Orthopaedic Surgery, Konstantopoulio General Hospital and Medical School, University of Athens, Athens 14233, Greece; stathi24@yahoo.gr

[3] Third Department of Orthopaedic Surgery, KAT General Hospital and Medical School, University of Athens, Kifissia 14561, Athens, Greece; eliasvasiliadis@yahoo.gr

* Correspondence: angkaspiris@hotmail.com; Tel.: +30-213-2028-258; Fax: +30-261-0623-049

Academic Editor: Carl L. von Baeyer
Received: 10 August 2016; Accepted: 9 November 2016; Published: 18 November 2016

Abstract: The most prevalent musculoskeletal disorder of childhood with unclear aetiology is growing pains (GPs). Anatomic deformities and factors that change bone turnover are implicated in GP pathophysiology. Perinatal risk factors alter the bone metabolism affecting the bone mineral density and content. The aim of our study was to analyze the relationship between GPs, knock knees and perinatal factors. The examined population consisted of 276 children aged 3–7 years. Among them, ten pairs of dizygotic twins were evaluated. The data were collected by using a combination of semi-structured questionnaires, clinical examinations and medical charts of the children and the obstetric history of the mothers. A total of 78 children presenting GPs met Peterson's criteria. Genu valgum severity was a significant factor for GP manifestation and for their increased frequency and intensity. Subsequently, perinatal factors regarding gestational age, Apgar score, head circumference (lower than 33 cm) and birth length or weight (smaller than 50 cm and 3000 g, respectively) made a remarkable contribution to the development of GPs. Conversely, antenatal corticosteroid treatment, increased maternal age and maternal smoking during pregnancy were not predictive of the disorder. Our data are potentially supportive for the "bone strength" theory and for the contribution of anatomical disturbances in GP appearance.

Keywords: growing pains; genu valgum; perinatal factors; bone metabolism

---

1. Introduction

Growing pains (GPs) are the most common form of episodic musculoskeletal pains during childhood. GPs mainly affect children between the ages of 3–12 years [1–4], but their highest frequency is detected in the age-group of 4–6 years [3]. Although GPs were first described by the French physician Duchamp in 1823 [5], their underlying pathophysiological mechanism still remains an enigma. In order to explain their development, various theories have been supported. The first theory was anatomical and centered on the observation that lower limb deformities (flat-feet or valgus knee) induce the appearance of pains [6]. Despite the fact that this theory has been recently weakened, it is still under investigation [2]. The second theory is the nocturnally accelerated bone theory [7] that analyzes the association between increased growth spurts and the appearance of GPs. However, there are no validated findings confirming that bone growth can be reason for pain [2]. Other theories include the local overuse syndrome theory which remains untested [8], the non-inflammatory pain syndrome theory [9], which is supported by reports for increased activity levels of children in more than 40% of the publications [2], and the hypothesis of early childhood's pain amplification syndrome [10].

Furthermore, a twin family survey [11] provided evidence that GPs appear to bear genetic susceptibility and present genetic association with restless leg syndrome. However, as there is no reliable and valid assessment tool testing hypermobility in children, the last hypothesis remains unproven [2]. Currently, many studies focus on the correlation of growing pains with bone density [8] and with factors affecting paediatric bone metabolism regarding serum levels of vitamin D or calcium [8] and omega-3 fatty acid intake [12–16]. The bone strength theory, which is closely related to the non-inflammatory pain syndrome theory, is based on the observation that the tibial bone density in children with GPs, as it was measured by quantitative ultrasound, was significantly reduced compared to healthy children [8]. Furthermore, the serum levels of vitamin D3 in GPs patients were remarkably low [12,13,15,16]. Similarly, in the affected children, the bone mineral status of the phalanx was low and accompanied by increased serum levels of parathyroid hormone (PTH), whereas the alkaline phosphatase levels were normal [12]. However, the bone strength theory is still subject to further research.

It is recognized from animal-based and clinical studies that perinatal risk factors including gestational age [17,18], birth length [18,19], birth weight [19,20] and maternal smoking or ethanol consumption [21] as well as the antenatal use of corticosteroids [18,22–25], contribute towards alterations in a newborn's bone metabolism having a direct impact on the mineralization of osteoid tissue during infancy. As the skeletal development is strongly related with bone changes during fetal and newborn periods, evaluation of the factors influencing mineral metabolism during early childhood can lead to useful conclusions about skeletal functionality in later life.

The aim of this study is to analyze the possible association between the development and intensity of GPs with perinatal characteristics in children 3–7 years old. Moreover, this research examines the possible interaction between the severity of valgus knee deformity and perinatal risk factors in the development of GPs in children.

2. Materials and Methods

2.1. Study Design

This is a retrospective study that was conducted based on the combination of semi-structured questionnaires (a mixture of open and closed questions), clinical examinations and clinical data collected by the medical charts of the children and the obstetric history of the mothers. Particularly, our methodological approach was as follows: First we selected and evaluated the GP cases based on Peterson's criteria and afterwards we reviewed the medical charts for children's perinatal characteristics. It took place from January 2014 to January 2015 during the children's visits to the paediatric department of the co-operated National Primary Care Trust. These visits took place for routine check-ups and vaccinations. Overall, 276 children aged 3–7 years old, including ten pairs of dizygotic twins, were examined on a daily basis. To determine the correct sample size for our survey, Cochran's formula was used: $n = Z^2 pq/e^2$, where Z is the confidence level (1.96), p is the variability (0.50), q (0.50) and e is the precision (7%). Our sample size was 30% larger than the minimum number of participants ($n = 196$) required to ensure accurate results based on the above parameters. The sample was also representative of sex, social economic status and geographical distribution, including children from local urban, suburban and rural areas, as it was based on the social insurance of the participants.

The children's parents or guardians were fully informed about the nature and the aim of the study and written consent was obtained (reference number of National's Primary Health Care Board approval: 3305/01-6-2013). The study complies with the Helsinki Declaration of 1964.

2.2. Inclusion and Exclusion Criteria

The inclusion criteria of our research were based on Peterson's [26] definition standards for GPs. These are as follows: recurrent pains in both lower extremities, with duration of up to 72 h, usually in the late afternoon or evening, with no arthritic localization or impaired joint mobility, in the absence of rubor, oedema, sensitivity, lesions, infections or other disorders. Exclusion criteria were history of known bone disease or musculoskeletal disorders such as fractures or chronic inflammation, clinical signs of articular disease including swelling, redness, reduced joint range, or trauma. Additionally, children with bone metabolism diseases (i.e., chronic renal syndrome, osteogenesis imperfecta, diastrophic dwarfism) or being under treatment with drugs that increase bone metabolism (i.e., glucocorticoids, anticonvulsants, antiretroviral therapy) were excluded from the study.

2.3. The Questionnaire

The questionnaire used included questions concerning the appearance of GPs during the year before the children visit our department, their frequency, and information about their age, sex, ethnicity, medical or orthopaedic history and medication. The questionnaire of the study was developed by the validated survey of Evans and Scutter [27]. The Wong-Baker FACES Pain Rating Scale (FACES scale) was used in order to assess pain intensity. The FACES scale is displayed on a horizontal line of six hand-drawn faces that ranged from a smiling face on the left to a crying face on the right, being scored from zero to ten respectively. We use this scale because its accuracy during the self-report pain intensity in children [28] that develop GPs [12] is well documented.

The zygosity of the twin pairs was assessed after applying the 12-question formula concerning the general similarity between twins, as it was introduced by Jackson et al. [29,30].

Finally, the height and weight of the children were measured and their body mass index (BMI) was calculated. A BMI within the 5th and 95th sex-specific and age-specific percentiles using the Center for Disease Control and Prevention (CDC) revised growth charts was considered normal.

2.4. Tibiofemoral Angle and Intermalleolar Distance

The tibiofemoral (TF) angle and the intermalleolar (IM) distance were measured with a clinical method introduced by Cheng et al. [31] that was also used by our team as thoroughly described in a previous study [32]. Specifically, the lower limbs were carefully positioned during the assessment. The children were made to stand, ensuring full extension and neutral rotation at the hips and knees, with the knees or ankles touching each other closely. The superior iliac spines, the region and the centre of the knee and the midpoint of the ankle joint were marked with a dermographic pen. Subsequently, the TF angle was measured very carefully in both legs. The valgus angle was measured with a positive sign. The distance between the malleoli was measured in an upright position using a tape measure and was also expressed with a positive sign. In assessing the IM distance, the knees were pressed at the medial condyles of both limbs against each other. This was helpful in the measurement of obese children with fat thighs [32]. The examination was performed by an experienced paediatric orthopaedic surgeon.

2.5. Perinatal Factors

The perinatal characteristics were based on the medical charts of the children and the maternal obstetrical history. Specifically, we retrieved information regarding gestational age, birth weight, length, head circumference, Apgar score, maternal infection, mode of delivery and use of medication, alcohol or smoking during pregnancy. Gestational age had been estimated from the first day of the last menstrual period. Children with birth weight between the 10th and 90th percentiles for gestational age were deemed appropriate for gestational age.

Furthermore, data were retrieved for the antenatal use of corticosteroids from the obstetrical files concerning the gestational age at administration of corticosteroids and the number of corticosteroid courses. A complete course of corticosteroid therapy was defined as at least one course of therapy 24 h before delivery [33].

2.6. Statistical Analysis

The data were initially entered on a Microsoft Excel 2007 (Microsoft, Redmond, WA, USA) spreadsheet and then analyzed statistically using SPSS version 21.0 (IBM Corporation, New York, NY,

USA). Initially, the data were summarized using descriptive statistics (mean, standard deviation (SD) and 95% confidence interval). Subsequently, the normality of the variables was studied using the Kolmogorov-Smirnov and the Shapiro-Wilk tests. Additionally, Levene's test was used to assess the equality of variances. Where the distribution of variables was normal, the Student's *t*-test was used, whereas in cases of divergence in the distribution of a variable, we proceeded with the Mann-Whitney U-test. The contribution of the independent variables to the development of GPs was also studied using logistic regression analysis. Due to the limited number of dizygotic twins, the non-parametric Wilcoxon signed-rank test was used. Pearson chi-square test was also used. The level of statistical significance was set to 5% ($p = 0.05$).

3. Results

3.1. Growing Pains and Demographic Characteristics

A total of 261 Caucasian children (124 boys and 137 girls) were eligible for inclusion in the study, whereas 15 children were excluded. There were 78 children (49 boys and 29 girls) who met the criteria of Peterson [25] for GPs (prevalence = 29.9%). The children's demographics are shown in Table 1.

Table 1. Demographic characteristics of the study population.

	Total Sample (*n* = 261)				With Growing Pains (*n* = 78)				Without Growing Pains (*n* = 183)				Dizygotic Twins (*n* = 20)			
	Mean	Min	Max	SD	Mean	Min	Max	SD	Mean	Min	Max	SD	Mean	Min	Max	SD
Age (years)	5.07	3.00	7.50	1.22	5.15	3.00	7.00	1.21	5.04	3.00	7.50	1.22	4.95	3.00	7.00	1.10
Weight (kg)	21.2	13.0	50.0	5.42	22.1	13.5	50.0	6.59	20.9	13.0	38.5	4.81	19.5	13.5	30.0	4.35
Height (cm)	114	91.0	139	9.58	115	97.5	139	9.58	113	91.0	134	9.50	111	97.5	127	7.62
BMI (kg/m^2)	16.2	11.4	27.9	3.53	16.2	11.4	27.9	2.64	10.2	11.4	22.7	1.97	15.7	12.5	19.6	1.83

SD: standard deviation.

3.2. GPs and Tibiofemoral Angle/Intermalleolar Distance

The mean values, SDs, Min/Max and confidence interval for the anatomic femoral-tibial angles and for the IM distance in both groups are presented in Table 2. Increased degree of genu valgum was positively correlated with the development of GPs in children (Table 2). Specifically, TF angle and IM distance are statistically associated with the appearance of GPs ($p < 0.01$ and $p < 0.01$, respectively).

3.3. GPs and Perinatal Factors

Statistical analysis revealed that perinatal risk factors are positively correlated with the development of GPs during childhood. In particular, a short gestation period ($p < 0.01$), low Apgar score ($p < 0.02$)and small birth length ($p < 0.01$), or birth weight ($p < 0.01$) and head circumference ($p < 0.01$) (Table 2) increase the risk of GPs. Interestingly, the risk of GP development increased when the birth weight of the child was lower than 3000 g. According to the study's data (Table 3) 36 out of 187 (19.3%) children suffering from GPs weighed over 3000 g at birth, while 42 out of 74 (56.8%) weighed less than 3000 g ($p < 0.01$). Similarly (Table 3), the birth head circumference in 53 out of 219 (24.2%) children suffering from GPs was greater than 33 cm while in 25 out of 42 (59.5%) was less than 33 cm ($p < 0.01$). On the contrary, maternal age ($p = 0.91$), maternal smoking during pregnancy ($p = 0.05$) and the antenatal use of corticosteroids ($p = 0.57$) does not seem to be implicated in the development of GPs (Tables 2 and 3).

Conclusively, the logistic regression analysis confirms that male sex, children's increased age, severity of genu valgum and gestational age of the affected children are statistically correlated with the appearance of GPs (Table 4). On the contrary, low Apgar score, increased maternal age and smoke exposure are not statistically related with GP development.

Table 2. Descriptive clinical features and statistical analysis of the study participants.

Clinical Characteristics	With Growing Pains						Without Growing Pains						Statistical Significance		
	Mean	Min	Max	SD	95% CI Lower Bound	Upper Bound	Mean	Min	Max	SD	95% CI Lower Bound	Upper Bound	t	Z	p Value
Genu valgum															
TF angle (degrees)	5.30	0.00	9.00	2.30	4.49	6.12	2.90	0.00	4.00	1.15	2.34	3.45		−7.07	<0.01
IM distance (cm)	3.32	0.00	6.00	1.54	2.77	3.86	1.34	0.00	3.00	0.96	0.88	1.80	−9.61		<0.01
Perinatal factors															
Gestational age (weeks)	36.8	28.0	40.0	2.49	35.9	37.6	37.7	34.0	40.0	1.63	36.9	38.5		−4.44	<0.01
Corticosteroid treatment (doses)	1.91	1.00	4.00	0.77	1.64	2.18	1.84	1.00	4.00	0.83	1.44	2.24		−0.43	0.57
Apgar score	8.42	6.00	10.0	1.12	7.88	8.96	8.76	6.00	10.0	1.15	8.35	9.16		−2.36	0.02
Birth length (cm)	47.9	40.0	54.0	2.78	47.0	48.9	49.9	45.0	54.0	2.09	48.9	50.9		−5.18	<0.01
Birth weight (g)	2727	1395	3880	579	2522	2932	2983	1650	4040	489	2747	3219	3.66		<0.01
Head circumference (cm)	33.2	28.0	37.5	1.90	32.5	33.8	34.4	31.4	38.0	1.57	33.6	35.2	3.51		<0.01
Maternal age (years)	31.7	21.0	40.0	4.60	30.1	33.4	33.2	26.0	41.0	3.72	31.4	35.0	−0.12		0.91

CI: confidence interval; TF angle: tibiopfemoral angle; IM distance: intermalleolar distance.

Table 3. Growing pains and their association with perinatal factors.

Variable	Present Pains (*n* = 78)	Do Not Present Pains (*n* = 183)	Total (*n* = 261)	*p* Value
		Birth weight		
<3000 g	*n* = 42 (56.8%)	*n* = 32 (43.2%)	*n* = 74	<0.01
>3000 g	*n* = 36 (19.3%)	*n* = 151 (80.7%)	*n* = 187	
		Head circumference		
<33 cm	*n* = 25 (59.5%)	*n* = 17 (40.5%)	*n* = 42	<0.01
>33 cm	*n* = 53 (24.2%)	*n* = 166 (75.8%)	*n* = 219	
		Maternal smoking		
Non-smokers	*n* = 63 (27.8%)	*n* = 164 (72.2%)	*n* = 227	0.05
Smokers	*n* = 15 (44.1%)	*n* = 19 (55.9%)	*n* = 34	

Table 4. Results of statistically significant factors for the development of growing pains derived after logistic regression analysis.

Risk Factors	B	SE	Wald	95% CI Lower	95% CI Upper	*p* Value
Sex	−0.86	0.37	5.33	0.21	0.88	0.02
Children's age (years)	0.31	0.15	4.21	1.02	1.84	0.04
IM distance (cm)	0.99	0.15	45.5	2.02	3.61	<0.01
Gestational age (weeks)	1.95	0.50	15.3	0.71	1.26	<0.01
Apgar score	−0.33	0.22	2.14	0.46	1.12	0.14
Maternal age (years)	−0.02	0.04	0.29	0.91	1.06	0.54
Smoking	0.33	0.56	0.34	0.46	4.18	0.56

SE: standard error, Wald: Wald chi-square test.

3.4. Types, Frequency and Intensity of GPs

We also studied the impact of genu valgum severity and perinatal risk factors on the form and frequency of GPs. As shown in Table 4, IM distance and maternal age are not statistically associated with the type of GP (Table 5).

Table 5. Comparison of growing pains intensity with the perinatal factors' characteristics and knock-knee severity of the affected children.

Type of Pain	Mean	SD	SE	*t*	*p* Value
		Nocturnal waking (n = 42)			
IM distance (cm)	3.43	1.36	0.21	−0.43	0.67
Birth length (cm)	48.5	2.81	0.43	3.47	<0.01
Head circumference (cm)	33.4	1.89	0.29	3.35	<0.01
Maternal age (years)	31.6	3.75	0.58	−1.47	0.15
		Crying (n = 36)			
IM distance (cm)	3.47	1.43	0.24	−0.63	0.53
Birth length (cm)	48.6	3.05	0.51	2.37	0.02
Head circumference (cm)	33.4	1.91	0.32	2.93	0.02
Maternal age (years)	31.7	3.74	0.62	−1.52	0.14
		Pains in both legs (n = 51)			
IM distance (cm)	3.32	1.45	0.20	0.38	0.71
Birth length (cm)	48.6	2.57	0.36	4.47	<0.01
Head circumference (cm)	33.4	1.57	0.22	5.30	<0.01
Maternal age (years)	31.7	4.67	0.65	−2.46	0.01

On the contrary, the perinatal characteristics including small birth length, head circumference and weight are strongly correlated with GPs (Tables 4 and 5). In particular, birth length smaller than 50 cm, birth weight lower than 3000 g and head circumference less than 33 cm are statistically correlated with nocturnal waking, crying and pains in both legs (Table 6).

Table 6. Statistical analysis for the relationship between types of growing pains, perinatal factors and use of corticosteroids.

Type of Pain	Birth Length		*p* Value	Birth Weight		*p* Value	Head Circumference		*p* Value	Use of Corticosteroids		*p* Value	Total
	<50 cm	>50 cm		<3000 g	>3000 g		<33 cm	>33 cm		Yes	No		
Nocturnal waking	$n = 32$ (76.2%)	$n = 10$ (23.8%)	0.05	$n = 31$ (73.8%)	$n = 11$ (26.2%)	<0.01	$n = 22$ (52.4%)	$n = 20$ (47.6%)	<0.01	$n = 27$ (64.3%)	$n = 15$ (35.7%)	<0.01	$n = 42$
Crying	$n = 26$ (72.2%)	$n = 10$ (27.8%)	0.47	$n = 28$ (77.8%)	$n = 8$ (22.2%)	<0.01	$n = 19$ (52.8%)	$n = 17$ (47.2%)	<0.01	$n = 21$ (58.3%)	$n = 15$ (41.7%)	<0.01	$n = 36$
Pains in both legs	$n = 40$ (78.4%)	$n = 11$ (21.6%)	<0.01	$n = 34$ (66.7%)	$n = 17$ (33.3%)	<0.01	$n = 23$ (45.1%)	$n = 28$ (54.9%)	<0.01	$n = 28$ (54.9%)	$n = 23$ (45.1%)	<0.01	$n = 51$

Furthermore, the weekly appearance of GPs (Tables 6 and 7) is statistically linked with reduced head circumference ($p < 0.01$) and birth weight ($p < 0.01$), though it is not associated with IM distance ($p = 0.86$), birth length ($p = 0.19$) or maternal age ($p = 0.45$). We must underline that although the antenatal administration of corticosteroids was not a contributing factor to the development of GPs, the frequency and the intensity of GPs were elevated in the children who had been exposed to dexamethasone (Tables 6 and 8).

Table 7. Comparison of the frequency of growing pains appearance with perinatal factors' characteristics and knock-knee severity of the affected children.

Frequency of Pain	Mean	SD	SE	Min	Max	F Value	*p* Value
			Weekly (n = 19)				
IM distance (cm)	3.37	1.55	0.36	0.00	5.50	0.25	0.86
Birth length (cm)	48.7	2.31	0.53	45.0	53.0	1.63	0.19
Head circumference (cm)	33.5	1.75	0.40	31.0	37.0	5.22	<0.01
Maternal age (years)	31.8	3.49	0.80	27.0	37.0	0.90	0.45
			Monthly (n = 33)				
IM distance (cm)	3.33	1.27	0.22	1.00	6.00		
Birth length (cm)	49.1	3.05	0.53	40.0	54.0		
Head circumference (cm)	33.5	1.74	0.30	28.0	37.0		
Maternal age (years)	31.3	4.38	0.76	23.0	39.0		
			Every three months (n = 19)				
IM distance (cm)	3.26	1.48	0.34	0.00	6.00		
Birth length (cm)	50.2	1.56	0.36	48.0	53.0		
Head circumference (cm)	35.0	0.97	0.22	33.5	37.5		
Maternal age (years)	30.1	4.99	1.15	21.0	40.0		
			Every six months (n = 7)				
IM distance (cm)	3.79	1.38	0.52	2.00	6.00		
Birth length (cm)	50.3	1.05	0.40	49.3	52.0		
Head circumference (cm)	34.7	0.76	0.30	33.5	35.8		
Maternal age (years)	29.1	5.43	2.05	24.0	40.0		

Pain intensity was examined using the FACES scale (Table 9). The statistical analysis revealed a correlation between GP severity and gestational age ($p < 0.01$), birth length ($p < 0.01$), birth weight ($p < 0.01$) and head circumference ($p < 0.01$).

Table 8. Association between the frequency of growing pains, birth weight and perinatal corticosteroid administration.

Frequency of Pain	Birth Weight		*p* Value	Administration of Corticosteroids		*p* Value	Total
	<3000 g	>3000 g	<0.01	With Corticosteroids	Without Corticosteroids	<0.01	
Weekly	*n* = 14 (73.7%)	*n* = 5 (26.3%)		*n* = 10 (52.6%)	*n* = 9 (47.4%)		*n* = 19
Monthly	*n* = 21 (63.6%)	*n* = 12 (36.4%)		*n* = 17 (51.5%)	*n* = 16 (48.5%)		*n* = 33
Every three months	*n* = 4 (21.1%)	*n* = 12 (78.9%)		*n* = 6 (31.6%)	*n* = 13 (68.4%)		*n* = 19
Every six months	*n* = 3 (42.9%)	*n* = 4 (57.1%)		*n* = 0 (0%)	*n* = 7 (100%)		*n* = 7

Table 9. Results derived after the Spearman correlation test examined the association between the FACES scale and the risk factors for the development of growing pains.

Risk Factors	FACES Scale		
	n	Correlation Coefficient	*p* Value
TF angle (degrees)	78	0.07	0.52
IM distance (cm)	78	0.11	0.35
Gestational age (weeks)	78	−0.32	0.01
Administration of corticosteroids (doses)	33	0.32	0.07
Apgar score	78	0.03	0.78
Birth length (cm)	78	−0.48	<0.01
Birth weight (g)	78	−0.49	<0.01
Head circumference (cm)	78	−0.43	<0.01
Maternal age (years)	78	0.03	0.78

3.5. GPs in Dizygotic Twins

In our study, ten pairs of dizygotic twins were included and all of the above-mentioned variables were examined. Under the assumption that twin pairs share, to a significant extent, environmental and genetic influences, we aim to test if anatomic differences are related with the appearance of GPs. Interestingly, the appearance of GPs in the twins was not affected by the anthropometric characteristics including current weight, height or BMI nor the perinatal factors (Table 10). Contrariwise, elevated TF angle and IM distance (Table 10) are positively associated with the appearance of GPs (*p* = 0.02 and *p* = 0.02, respectively).

Table 10. Statistical analysis of the dizygotic twins' clinical characteristics.

Clinical Characteristics	Present Growing Pains (*n* = 9)				Do Not Present Growing Pains (*n* = 11)				Statistical Significance	
	Mean	Min	Max	SD	Mean	Min	Max	SD	Z	*p* Value
Current weight (kg)	19.0	13.5	30.0	5.46	19.9	14.0	26.0	3.42	−0.10	0.92
Current height (cm)	109	97.5	127	9.05	112	102	123	6.17	−1.66	0.10
Current BMI (kg/m^2)	15.8	12.5	19.6	2.30	15.6	12.5	17.2	1.45	−0.66	0.51
TF angle (degrees)	6.22	3.00	8.00	1.48	2.91	1.00	4.00	1.04	−2.33	0.02
IM distance (cm)	3.89	2.50	5.50	0.96	1.36	0.00	3.00	0.92	−2.41	0.02
Birth length (cm)	47.5	42.0	52.0	2.89	49.1	45.0	51.0	2.23	−1.07	0.28
Birth weight (g)	2444	1600	2910	417	2786	1650	3260	471	−1.23	0.22
Head circumference (cm)	33.7	31.5	37.5	1.79	33.7	31.4	36.5	1.57	−0.60	0.57
Apgar score	7.89	6.00	10.0	1.62	7.91	6.00	9.00	1.14	−0.14	0.89

4. Discussion

The most common cause of musculoskeletal pain during childhood are GPs, which remain largely inexplicable. Despite the fact that GPs are widely considered a benign syndrome and their resolution occurs during late childhood, they may have deleterious effects leading many researchers to explore their underlying pathophysiological mechanism. To the best of our knowledge, this is the first study that investigates the association of children's perinatal characteristics with the appearance of GPs and examines the correlation of genu valgum severity using clinical methodology, with the frequency and intensity of GPs. However, our research has a number of limitations. First, it is retrospective and the data rely on the information accuracy of the interviewed children or parents. Moreover, inherited design limitations appear in retrospective studies such as inability to collect missing or unreported data, parental difficulties in recalling information and the studies not being blind. However, they allow accumulation of data for a significant number of patients, thus minimizing possible errors. Secondly, the evaluation of valgus deformity was performed by a clinical method which raises concerns about its reliability and reproducibility. However, the clinical method of measuring the knee angle is validated [31], widely accepted, easily reproducible and is inexpensive and radiation-free [34]. Moreover, it was performed by an experienced paediatric orthopaedic surgeon using fixed bony points to calculate the TF angle and the IM distance. Additionally, the palpation of bony landmarks is practical and easy, diminishing the possibility of an erroneous measurement even in obese children [34]. Third, the results are not accompanied by supportive analysis of biological data. Finally, the small number of dizygotic twins did not allow us to draw definite conclusions.

In the present study, GP prevalence is high, corresponding to 29.88% of children aged 3–7 years. The reported prevalence differs between various surveys. Evans et al. estimated that the frequency of GPs was 36.9% in children 4–6 years of age [3]. In a Mediterranean population of children 3–12 years old the frequency of the disorder was 24.5% [4], while Oster found that 15% of school children have occasional limb pain [35]. In a very large British cohort study, but without applying Peterson's criteria for GP assessment, the referred prevalence was 21.4% [14]. Overall, their prevalence varies from 2.6% to 49.4% [36]. Differences not only in sample size or age range and definition criteria but also in ethnicity features may explain this discordance.

Anatomical or mechanical factors were always considered in the research of GPs [2,35]. In our study, the severity of genu valgum (increased IM distance and TF angle) was statistically associated with the development of GPs in children, though it was not correlated with their frequency or intensity. Additionally, increased IM distance and TF angle were strongly related with GPs in dizygotic twins. As we assume that dizygotic twins stem from the same gene pool and are exposed to similar environmental factors [37], the knee deformity may have a critical contribution in the appearance of the pains. This finding is in agreement with Brenning's observation that anatomical deformities which cause mechanical instability of the lower limbs including scoliosis, pes planus or genu valgum are closely related with GPs [38]. This is also supported by the study of Evans [6] where the correction of the lower extremity malalignment with shoe inserts reduces the frequency and the severity of GPs. Furthermore, the application of customized foot orthoses that control overpronation and decrease the secondary genu valgum of the knee joint in children with overpronated feet led to significant improvement in pain degree and frequency after 1 and 3 months [39]. On the contrary, in the study of Evans and Scatter, although the navicular height was weakly correlated with foot functional indexes, the overall foot posture examination measurements did not reveal any statistical significance with GPs [40].

Perinatal risk factors were closely related not only with the appearance of GPs but also with their frequency and magnitude. Specifically, the risk of GP appearance was statistically increased when the birth weight of the child was lower than 3000 g. Additionally, the possibility of GP development was increased in children with birth head circumference smaller than 33 cm. In children that present GPs, the possibilities of nocturnal waking or crying and suffering from pain in both legs was also increased in the aforementioned groups. Several studies have shown that whole-body bone mineral content (BMC) correlates with gestational age, body length and body weight. Moreover, growth of head circumference in infants was found to be synchronized with long bone growth and integrity [41]. Research data suggest that there was a decrease in bone mineral density (BMD) in animals with intrauterine growth restriction [42]. These animals also had reduced serum concentrations of vitamin D during their first 20 weeks of life which is in line with the observations of Monangi et al. [43], whereby the odds of low serum concentrations of vitamin D was increased 2.6-fold in infants born less than 28 weeks postmenstrual age. Newborns with low birth weight also had lower BMC [44]. Similarly, postnatal measurements with quantitative ultrasound confirm that the values of tibial speed of sound are affected by a short gestation period [45]. This is consistent with the results of Kurl et al. [17] which demonstrated that remarkably lower BMC and BMD were detected in preterm infants than the term group. It is noteworthy that adolescents with idiopathic short stature had a reduction in their BMD [46]. Wang et al. reported that very low birth weight infants had reduced bone mass at ages 5 to 10 years, even after adjustment for height, lean mass, or bone area [47], whereas in the same study, short gestation period was correlated with unfavorable skeletal health among prepubertal boys [47]. Predicated on the concept that vitamin D deficiency [12–16] and BMD [8] are key factors for the development of GPs, further research may reveal if the implication of perinatal risk factors in the bone metabolism process results in the onset of the disorder.

Contrariwise, antenatal corticosteroid treatment, increased maternal age and maternal smoking during pregnancy were not predictive of GPs. Despite the fact that antenatal administration of corticosteroids was not a contributing factor to the development of GPs, the frequency and the intensity of GPs were elevated in the children who had been exposed to dexamethasone. In children that present GPs, the use of corticosteroids was closely related with nocturnal waking or crying and suffering from pain in both legs. Furthermore, our data indicates that in these children the frequency of GP episodes was as high as once per week. Although corticosteroids are implicated in bone metabolism, many studies have failed to show distinct differences in BMC values between dexamethasone infants and controls [18,48,49]. Furthermore, Korakaki et al. reported that bone formation serum marker concentration was unaffected or slightly reduced at birth in neonates of mothers treated with corticosteroids compared to control subjects, while the bone resorption markers did not differ among the two groups [24]. Furthermore, the bone collagen markers in the newborns exposed to dexamethasone were restored during the first ten days of life [24]. Based on the above findings, we can hypothesize that the antenatal administration of corticosteroids does not affect the onset of GPs due to the minor impact of dexamethasone on bone turnover in infants.

5. Conclusions

The findings of the present study demonstrate that perinatal risk factors can be predictive of the development of growing pains. The close association of gestational age, head circumference and birth length or weight with bone turnover could support the bone strength theory for this disorder, indicating to clinicians a detailed bone monitoring of this subgroup. Furthermore, our results also support the anatomical theory as the degree of genu valgum has a significant effect on the development of GPs, leading to the notion that an orthotic correction of severe valgus deformity may be an efficient intervention for the prevention or the treatment of this condition.

Acknowledgments: The authors would like to thank Crisi Zafiropoulou, pediatrician of the National Organization for Primary Care Health Services, for her valuable contribution and her assistance in the clinical examination and in the collection of the questionnaires.

Author Contributions: A.K. conceived and authored most of the study, carried out the statistical analysis and reviewed the literature. A.K., E.C. and E.V. performed the clinical examination. E.C. and E.V. were involved in the drafting and conceptualization of the study and the experimental design. All the authors have read and approved the final manuscript.

Conflicts of Interest: There are no conflicts of interest.

References

1. Abu-Arafeh, I.; Russell, G. Recurrent limb pain in schoolchildren. *Arch. Dis. Child.* **1996**, *74*, 336–339. [CrossRef] [PubMed]

2. Evans, A.M. Growing pains: Contemporary knowledge and recommended practice. *J. Foot Ankle Res.* **2008**, *1*, 1–5. [CrossRef] [PubMed]

3. Evans, A.M.; Scutter, S.D. Prevalence of "growing pains" in young children. *J. Pediatr.* **2004**, *145*, 255–258. [CrossRef] [PubMed]

4. Kaspiris, A.; Zafiropoulou, C. Growing pains in children: Epidemiological analysis in a Mediterranean population. *Jt. Bone Spine* **2009**, *76*, 486–490. [CrossRef] [PubMed]

5. Duchamp, M. Maladies de la croissance. In *Mémoires de Médecine Practique*; Levrault, F.G., Ed.; Jean-Frédéric Lobstein: Paris, France, 1823.

6. Evans, A.M. Relationship between "growing pains" and foot posture in children: Single-case experimental designs in clinical practice. *J. Am. Podiatr. Med. Assoc.* **2003**, *93*, 111–117. [CrossRef] [PubMed]

7. Noonan, K.J.; Farnum, C.E.; Leiferman, E.M.; Lampl, M.; Markel, M.D.; Wilsman, N.J. Growing pains: Are they due to increased growth during recumbency as documented in a lamb model? *J. Pediatr. Orthop.* **2004**, *24*, 726–731. [CrossRef] [PubMed]

8. Friedland, O.; Hashkes, P.J.; Jaber, L.; Cohen, H.A.; Eliakim, A.; Wolach, B.; Uziel, Y. Decreased bone speed of sound in children with growing pains measured by quantitative ultrasound. *J. Rheumatol.* **2005**, *32*, 1354–1357. [PubMed]

9. Hashkes, P.J.; Friedland, O.; Jaber, L.; Cohen, H.A.; Wolach, B.; Uziel, Y. Decreased pain threshold in children with growing pains. *J. Rheumatol.* **2004**, *31*, 610–613. [PubMed]

10. Uziel, Y.; Chapnick, G.; Jaber, L.; Nemet, D.; Hashkes, P.J. Five-year outcome of children with "growing pains": Correlations with pain threshold. *J. Pediatr.* **2010**, *156*, 838–840. [CrossRef] [PubMed]

11. Champion, D.; Pathirana, S.; Flynn, C.; Taylor, A.; Hopper, J.L.; Berkovic, S.F.; Jaaniste, T.; Qiu, W. Growing pains: Twin family study evidence for genetic susceptibility and a genetic relationship with restless legs syndrome. *Eur. J. Pain* **2012**, *16*, 1224–1231. [CrossRef] [PubMed]

12. Morandi, G.; Maines, E.; Piona, C.; Monti, E.; Sandri, M.; Gaudino, R.; Boner, A.; Antoniazzi, F. Significant association among growing pains, vitamin D supplementation, and bone mineral status: Results from a pilot cohort study. *J. Bone Min. Metab.* **2015**, *33*, 201–206. [CrossRef] [PubMed]

13. Park, M.J.; Lee, J.; Lee, J.K.; Joo, S.Y. Prevalence of Vitamin D Deficiency in Korean Children Presenting with Nonspecific Lower-Extremity Pain. *Yonsei Med. J.* **2015**, *56*, 1384–1388. [CrossRef] [PubMed]

14. Golding, J.; Northstone, K.; Emmett, P.; Steer, C.; Hibbeln, J.R. Do ω-3 or other fatty acids influence the development of 'growing pains'? A prebirth cohort study. *BMJ Open* **2012**, *2*, 1–7. [CrossRef] [PubMed]

15. Szalay, E.A.; Tryon, E.B.; Pleacher, M.D.; Whisler, S.L. Pediatric vitamin D deficiency in a southwestern luminous climate. *J. Pediatr. Orthop.* **2011**, *31*, 469–473. [CrossRef] [PubMed]

16. Qamar, S.; Akbani, S.; Shamim, S.; Khan, G. Vitamin D levels in children with growing pains. *J. Coll. Phys. Surg. Pak.* **2011**, *21*, 284–287.

17. Tshorny, M.; Mimouni, F.B.; Littner, Y.; Alper, A.; Mandel, D. Decreased neonatal tibial bone ultrasound velocity in term infants born after breech presentation. *J. Perinatol.* **2007**, *27*, 693–696. [CrossRef] [PubMed]

18. Kurl, S.; Heinonen, K.; Länsimies, E. Effects of prematurity, intrauterine growth status, and early dexamethasone treatment on postnatal bone mineralisation. *Arch. Dis. Child. Fetal Neonatal Ed.* **2000**, *83*, F109–F111. [CrossRef] [PubMed]

19. Jones, G.; Dwyer, T. Birth weight, birth length, and bone density in prepubertal children: Evidence for an association that may be mediated by genetic factors. *Calcif. Tissue Int.* **2000**, *67*, 304–308. [CrossRef] [PubMed]

20. Koklu, E.; Akcakus, M.; Narin, F.; Saraymen, R. The relationship between birth weight, oxidative stress and bone mineral status in newborn infants. *J. Paediatr. Child Health* **2007**, *43*, 667–672. [CrossRef] [PubMed]

21. Namgung, R.; Tsang, R.C. Factors affecting newborn bone mineral content: In utero effects on newborn bone mineralization. *Proc. Nutr. Soc.* **2000**, *59*, 55–63. [CrossRef] [PubMed]

22. Tatara, M.R.; Sliwa, E.; Krupski, W. Prenatal programming of skeletal development in the offspring: Effects of maternal treatment with beta-hydroxy-beta-methylbutyrate (HMB) on femur properties in pigs at slaughter age. *Bone* **2007**, *40*, 1615–1622. [CrossRef] [PubMed]

23. Korakaki, E.; Damilakis, J.; Gourgiotis, D.; Katonis, P.; Aligizakis, A.; Yachnakis, E.; Stratakis, J.; Manoura, A.; Hatzidaki, E.; Saitakis, E.; et al. Quantitative ultrasound measurements in premature infants at 1 year of age: The effects of antenatal administered corticosteroids. *Calcif. Tissue Int.* **2011**, *88*, 215–222. [CrossRef] [PubMed]

24. Korakaki, E.; Gourgiotis, D.; Aligizakis, A.; Manoura, A.; Hatzidaki, E.; Giahnakis, E.; Marmarinos, A.; Kalmanti, M.; Giannakopoulou, C. Levels of bone collagen markers in preterm infants: Relation to antenatal glucocorticoid treatment. *J. Bone Min. Metab.* **2007**, *25*, 172–178. [CrossRef] [PubMed]

25. Sliwa, E.; Tatara, M.R.; Nowakowski, H.; Pierzynowski, S.G.; Studziński, T. Effect of maternal dexamethasone and alpha-ketoglutarate administration on skeletal development during the last three weeks of prenatal life in pigs. *J. Matern. Fetal Neonatal Med.* **2006**, *19*, 489–493. [CrossRef] [PubMed]

26. Peterson, H. Growing pains. *Pediatr. Clin. N. Am.* **1986**, *33*, 1365–1372. [CrossRef]

27. Evans, A.M.; Scutter, S.D. Development of a questionnaire for parental rating of leg pain in young children: Internal validity and reliability testing following triangulation. *Foot* **2004**, *14*, 42–48. [CrossRef]

28. Tomlinson, D.; von Baeyer, C.L.; Stinson, J.N.; Sung, L. A systematic review of faces scales for the self-report of pain intensity in children. *Pediatrics* **2010**, *126*, e1168–e1198. [PubMed]

29. Jackson, R.W.; Snieder, H.; Davis, H.; Treiber, F.A. Determination of twin zygosity: A comparison of DNA with various questionnaire indices. *Twin Res.* **2001**, *4*, 12–18. [CrossRef] [PubMed]

30. Champion, D.; Pathirana, S.; Flynn, C.; Taylor, A.; Hopper, J.L.; Berkovic, S.F.; Jaaniste, T.; Qiu, W. Growing pains: Twin family study evidence for genetic susceptibility and a genetic relationship with restless legs syndrome. *Eur. J. Pain* **2012**, *16*, 1224–1231. [PubMed]

31. Cheng, J.C.; Chan, P.S.; Chiang, S.C.; Hui, P.W. Angular and rotational profile of the lower limb in 2630 Chinese children. *J. Pediatr. Orthop.* **1991**, *11*, 154–161. [CrossRef] [PubMed]

32. Kaspiris, A.; Zaphiropoulou, C.; Vasiliadis, E. Range of variation of genu valgum and association with anthropometric characteristics and physical activity: Comparison between children aged 3–9 years. *J. Pediatr. Orthop. B* **2013**, *22*, 296–305. [PubMed]

33. Wijnberger, L.D.; Mostert, J.M.; van Dam, K.I.; Mol, B.W.; Brouwers, H.; Visser, G.H. Comparison of single and repeated antenatal corticosteroid therapy to prevent neonatal death and morbidity in the preterm infant. *Early Hum. Dev.* **2002**, *67*, 29–36. [CrossRef]

34. Saini, U.C.; Bali, K.; Sheth, B.; Gahlot, N.; Gahlot, A. Normal development of the knee angle in healthy Indian children: A clinical study of 215 children. *J. Child. Orthop.* **2010**, *4*, 579–586. [CrossRef] [PubMed]

35. Oster, J.; Nielson, A. Growing pain: A clinical investigation of a school population. *Acta Paediatr. Scand.* **1972**, *61*, 329–334. [CrossRef] [PubMed]

36. Uziel, Y.; Hashkes, P.J. Growing pains in children. *Pediatr. Rheumatol. Online J.* **2007**, *5*, 1–4. [CrossRef] [PubMed]

37. Townsend, G.; Hughes, T.; Luciano, M.; Bockmann, M.; Brook, A. Genetic and environmental influences on human dental variation: A critical evaluation of studies involving twins. *Arch. Oral Biol.* **2009**, *54*, S45–S51. [CrossRef] [PubMed]

38. Brenning, R. Growing pain. *Acta Soc. Med. Ups* **1960**, *65*, 185–201.

39. Lee, H.J.; Lim, K.B.; Yoo, J.; Yoon, S.W.; Jeong, T.H. Effect of foot orthoses on children with lower extremity growing pains. *Ann. Rehabil. Med.* **2015**, *39*, 285–293. [CrossRef] [PubMed]

40. Evans, A.M.; Scutter, S.D. Are foot posture and functional health different in children with growing pains? *Pediatr. Int.* **2007**, *49*, 991–996. [CrossRef] [PubMed]

41. Caino, S.; Kelmansky, D.; Adamo, P.; Lejarraga, H. Short-term growth in head circumference and its relationship with supine length in healthy infants. *Ann. Hum. Biol.* **2010**, *37*, 108–116. [CrossRef] [PubMed]

42. Lanham, S.A.; Roberts, C.; Perry, M.J.; Cooper, C.; Oreffo, R.O. Intrauterine programming of bone. Part 2: Alteration of skeletal structure. *Osteoporos. Int.* **2008**, *19*, 157–167. [CrossRef] [PubMed]

43. Monangi, N.; Slaughter, J.L.; Dawodu, A.; Smith, C.; Akinbi, H.T. Vitamin D status of early preterm infants and the effects of vitamin D intake during hospital stay. *Arch. Dis. Child. Fetal Neonatal Ed.* **2014**, *99*, F166–F168. [CrossRef] [PubMed]

44. Beltrand, J.; Alison, M.; Nicolescu, R.; Verkauskiene, R.; Deghmoun, S.; Sibony, O.; Sebag, G.; Lévy-Marchal, C. Bone mineral content at birth is determined both by birth weight and fetal growth pattern. *Pediatr. Res.* **2008**, *64*, 86–90. [CrossRef] [PubMed]

45. Ipek, M.S.; Zenciroglu, A.; Aydin, M.; Okumus, N.; Erol, S.S.; Karagol, B.S.; Hakan, N. The role of antenatal factors on tibial speed of sound values in newborn infants. *J. Matern. Fetal Neonatal Med.* **2012**, *25*, 2122–2125. [CrossRef] [PubMed]

46. Leunissen, R.W.; Stijnen, T.; Hokken-Koelega, A.C. Influence of birth size on body composition in early adulthood: The programming factors for growth and metabolism (PROGRAM)-study. *Clin. Endocrinol.* **2009**, *70*, 245–251. [CrossRef] [PubMed]

47. Wang, D.; Vandermeulen, J.; Atkinson, S.A. Early life factors predict abnormal growth and bone accretion at prepuberty in former premature infants with/without neonatal dexamethasone exposure. *Pediatr. Res.* **2007**, *61*, 111–116. [CrossRef] [PubMed]

48. Ryan, S.; Congdon, P.J.; Horsman, A.; James, J.R.; Truscott, J.; Arthur, R. Bone mineral content in bronchopulmonary dysplasia. *Arch. Dis. Child.* **1987**, *62*, 889–894. [CrossRef] [PubMed]

49. Greer, F.R.; McCormick, A. Bone mineral content and growth in very-low-birth-weight premature infants. Does bronchopulmonary dysplasia make a difference? *Am. J. Dis. Child.* **1987**, *141*, 179–183. [CrossRef] [PubMed]

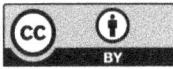

Section 2:
Psychological Factors

Review

A Broad Consideration of Risk Factors in Pediatric Chronic Pain: Where to Go from Here?

Hannah N. McKillop [1,*] and Gerard A. Banez [2]

1   Case Western Reserve University, 11220 Bellflower Rd, Cleveland, OH 44106, USA
2   Cleveland Clinic Children's Hospital for Rehabilitation, Pediatric Pain Rehabilitation Program,
    CR 11/ 2801 MLK Jr. Drive, Cleveland, OH 44104, USA; banezg@ccf.org
*   Correspondence: hannah.mckillop@case.edu, Tel.: +1-216-368-0721

Academic Editor: Lynn S. Walker
Received: 1 September 2016; Accepted: 22 November 2016; Published: 30 November 2016

Abstract: Pediatric chronic pain is a significant problem associated with substantial functional impairment. A variety of risk factors have been found to be associated with chronic pain in youth. The greatest amount of evidence appears to support that temperament, anxiety, depression, subjective experience of stress, passive coping strategies, sleep problems, other somatic-related problems, and parent and/or family factors are important variables. However, a great deal of this research focuses on a single risk factor or on multiple risk factors in isolation. Much of the literature utilizes older diagnostic criteria and would benefit from replication, larger sample sizes, and comparison across pain disorders. Problems also exist with disagreement across definitions, resulting in inconsistency or unclear use of terms. Furthermore, recent consideration has suggested that outcome measures should include functional disability in addition to pain. A second generation of research is needed to shed light on the complex interactions that likely play a role in the transition from acute to chronic pain. Building on recent calls for changes in research in this area, we propose the next steps for this research, which involve consideration of both biopsychosocial and developmental contexts.

Keywords: chronic pain; pediatrics; risk factors; family factors; peer factors; biopsychosocial; development

1. Introduction

Chronic pain is a significant problem among children and adolescents and is associated with significant functional disability and other poor outcomes, including problems with school attendance and performance, difficulties with peer relationships, disruptions in family life, appetite, sleep, and participation in enjoyable activities [1–3]. Children and adolescents with chronic pain also report frequent use of medications, placing the child at risk for future overuse [2]. Although prevalence estimates fluctuate drastically across studies, geographic location, and medical diagnoses, chronic and recurrent pain is thought to be very common in youth [4]. For example, one large-scale international study demonstrated prevalence of headache as 54.1%, stomachache as 49.8%, and backache as 37% [5].

The impact of chronic pain extends beyond the individual as well. Families of children with chronic pain frequently seek professional medical or mental health services [2], which are likely to be very expensive for the family and the healthcare system. With a stronger understanding of the mechanisms that contribute to the development of chronic pain from acute pain, the possibility of developing successful treatment methods could contribute to a reduction in the attendant psychological, social, learning-related, developmental, and monetary costs.

Although there have been many studies of specific risk factors that may contribute to chronic pain, the mechanisms that lead to a progression from acute pain to chronic pain are not well understood. A more nuanced understanding of the complex interactions among a variety of factors has the potential for providing valuable information about the development and maintenance of these conditions, as well as for developing more effective treatments for children in this situation. The focus of this narrative review is on risk factors associated with the most common chronic pain diagnoses seen in pediatric practice.

2. Methods

Articles for consideration in this narrative review were identified through a computerized search of electronic databases primarily including PsycINFO, PubMed, and Google Scholar. The search requested all citations that included either a specific chronic pain diagnosis (e.g., complex regional pain syndrome, chronic migraine) or the term "chronic pain" as one identifier and "pediatric," "children," "adolescent," "youth," "risk factor," or "predictor" as a second identifier. Diagnoses where pain is the secondary issue (e.g., cancer, cerebral palsy) were not included. Given the broader search capacity of Google Scholar, the first five to ten pages of results (the equivalent of 50–100 articles) were manually scanned for relevant material for each specific search. The search was narrowed to include papers only published within the past 15 years where possible, unless recent research was sparse and/or seminal articles had been published prior to the year 2000.

The literature search yielded a preliminary database of approximately 13,184 published articles. Abstracts were manually scanned for relevance to the review. Approximately 234 articles were obtained for consideration. Articles were then reviewed for inclusion in the review, from which 135 were selected for inclusion in this review.

3. Current Status of the Literature on Risk Factors for Pediatric Chronic Pain

The extant literature on pediatric chronic pain has identified a variety of potential risk factors, including demographic factors such as age and sex, factors related to the individual such as coping style, and familial or environmental factors. These studies represent an excellent first generation of research that has helped to identify potential risk factors for further study. Interestingly, many of the risk factors identified were predicted in an early survey study comparing children with recurrent abdominal pain to children without these symptoms from the 1950s, including family history of pain, temperament, and anxiety symptoms, as well as higher incidence in females and onset during adolescence [6]. However, it is important to move forward to a next stage of research to better understand the role of these factors in the mechanisms that lead acute pain to become chronic, as well as contribute to the maintenance of chronic pain.

The literature at present has often focused on one medical chronic pain diagnosis at a time, which is useful in the understanding of that particular disorder but is difficult to generalize to chronic pain diagnoses in general. In addition, issues with diagnostic criteria have been raised with the implementation of the fifth edition of the Diagnostic and Statistical Manual of Mental Disorders (DSM) [7]. Many of the studies also have small sample sizes (e.g., often ranging from 15–35 participants), inconsistent definitions or use of unclear terms (e.g., variation across studies in terms of the definition of headache), and static forms of measurement (e.g., self-report questionnaire). Few studies examine the longitudinal impact. In addition, studies often focus on a single risk factor or explore multiple risk factors in isolation. This type of research design, while necessary for the original identification of these risk factors, cannot provide information about causality or the complex interactions among variables that may explain a larger portion of the variance in chronic pain.

This article first provides an overview of the current state of this "first generation" of research, which can serve as a starting point for consideration of potential variables to be included in more complex models. In line with this idea, we next identify studies that embody the second generation of research, and then propose next steps to continue in this direction (see Figure 1). These next steps consider the development of chronic pain from acute pain, taking into account: (1) developmental stages; (2) family and peer factors; (3) physiological components; and (4) will integrate the interplay of multiple risk factors. It is proposed that functioning represents as much importance in outcome as the presence of pain.

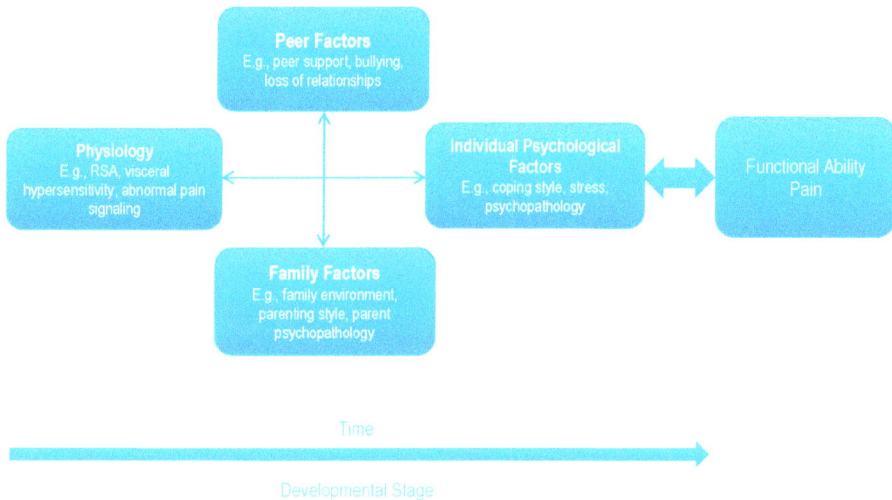

Figure 1. Incorporation of biopsychosocial factors into a developmental framework. RSA: respiratory sinus arrhythmia.

3.1. A Review of Risk Factors

A large number of risk factors of pediatric pain have been studied, and this literature spans a variety of categories. Many studies have focused on within-person factors, that is, factors specific to the child himself or herself, such as temperament and coping style. Between-person factors, such as parent psychopathology and social functioning, are considered. Demographic factors are also included, such as sex, age, and ethnicity.

3.2. Within-Person Factors

3.2.1. Demographic Factors

Briefly, several demographic factors are considered in relation to pediatric chronic pain, including age, sex, and ethnicity.

Increased age (typically early adolescence rather than early childhood) is associated with various pediatric chronic pain disorders, including low back pain [8] and musculoskeletal pain [9]. That is, chronic pain appears to most often occur in adolescence rather than earlier in childhood. However, recurrent abdominal pain appears to peak below 5 years of age and again between ages 8–10 years [10]. This particular finding speaks to the potential relationship between pain and developmental stage, which will be discussed later in this article.

The literature suggests that female youth report more severe headache and back pain [11–14], chronic musculoskeletal pain [9], temporomandibular pain disorders [15], and recurrent or functional abdominal pain than male youth [16]. However, some studies have found only minimal support for this relationship, demonstrating small effect sizes for duration and intensity of pain for girls versus boys [17].

A sex by age relationship has been observed in children and adolescents with chronic migraine. Based on the extant literature, chronic migraines appear to be more common in boys than girls prior to puberty [18]. Thus, onset of migraines in boys is likely earlier than for girls. This estimate changes by the onset of puberty, and the prevalence of chronic migraines in girls is estimated to double that of boys at that stage [18].

Race and ethnicity have rarely been the sole focus of research on pediatric chronic pain disorders, although it is well studied in adults. Briefly, studies have found the following: (1) participants of European descent were more likely to have juvenile idiopathic arthritis than children of other descent [19]; (2) American Indian adolescents had the highest rate of recurrent headaches followed by white adolescents [20], and Asian and Pacific Island adolescents were the least likely to experience recurrent headaches [20]; (3) African American youths were more likely to experience a variety of pains related to temporomandibular joint disorders than their Caucasian counterparts [21]; (4) Hispanic ethnicity was associated with higher widespread pain scores in children with acute pain, presurgical, and chronic pain [22]; and (5) Jewish children experienced significantly more headaches than Arab children in a sample from Northern Israel [23]. Other groups have found no significant differences among ethnic groups in samples of children with a variety of chronic pain diagnoses [24,25]. In addition, ethnicity did not emerge as a risk factor for disability in a study of children with chronic back pain [26].

In sum, demographic factors including age, sex, and ethnicity evidence some support of potential risk factors for pediatric chronic pain. These variables warrant continued research in their potential as risk factors for youth. Studies that assess demographic factors in combination with other identified variables are important for improving our understanding of risk pathways.

3.2.2. Temperament

Broadly defined temperamental factors have been cited in the literature as potential risk factors [27]. For example, infants who were more active and struggled to develop important routines were more likely to develop recurrent abdominal pain later in childhood [28]. Children with recurrent abdominal pain were more "temperamentally difficult" than those without pain, such that girls had more of an irregular temperament style and boys were more likely to withdraw in novel situations [29].

In a study of children with juvenile primary fibromyalgia syndrome, temperament was described as a combination between mood, daily habits, and attentional abilities [30]. The study demonstrated that these children displayed lower mood, irregularity of daily habits, lower task orientation, and higher distractibility than a comparison group (participants had arthritis) as well as a control group [30]. Thus, a difficult temperament may represent a mechanism by which acute pain becomes chronic and/or plays a role in maintenance of impairing pain. Temperament may also influence what eventually becomes a child's coping style [31], which could have important implications for the way a child responds to prolonged experience with pain. While temperament itself is not modifiable by definition, if high-risk temperamental styles are identified early on in children with pain, the first targets of intervention could focus on the development of adaptive coping strategies before pain becomes chronic. However, other factors, outlined below, may represent more promising avenues for prevention and early intervention efforts.

3.2.3. Psychological Disorders

Chronic pain has been found to be associated with a variety of psychological issues, including anxiety, depression, anger, conduct problems, and mental health issues in general.

Anxiety. Anxiety has been frequently studied as a risk factor for numerous chronic pain disorders. While the issue of causality is often cited as a problem with this area of research, a recent study demonstrated a strong temporal association, with anxiety disorders preceding reports of chronic back/neck pain, headaches, and "any chronic pain" [32]. However, another study of predictive factors for recurrent abdominal pain in children specifically did not find such a temporal relationships [33].

Cross-sectional studies do appear to show a somewhat consistent relationship between anxiety and chronic pain. Anxiety has been significantly associated with general musculoskeletal pain for girls [34], migraine with aura [35], and recurrent abdominal pain [36,37]. A recent study supported this finding in a general chronic pain sample and demonstrated that youth with abdominal pain reported higher overall anxiety as well as more panic-somatic symptoms relative to other pain groups [38]. Other studies demonstrate no relationship between anxiety and pain, including studies of juvenile idiopathic arthritis [39] and headache or abdominal pain [40].

Sensitivity to anxiety has also been posited as a factor that contributes to the maintenance of postsurgical pain in children and adolescents [41]. Anxiety sensitivity is defined in terms of the degree to which an individual interprets or predicts anxiety symptoms as being related to significantly harmful somatic, psychological, and/or social outcomes [41], and was the only predictor of maintenance of or recovery from moderate/severe chronic postsurgical pain 12 months after the surgery [41]. Anxiety, when it becomes impairing, could be considered a maladaptive response to pain, if that is indeed the order of occurrence. Longitudinal studies could lend predictive power to the current understanding of the chronicity of pain and the role of anxiety.

Depression. Depression is strongly related to anxiety [42] and is worth examination in relation to chronic pain in its own right. Depression appears to be an important factor in pediatric chronic pain disorders. As with anxiety, the question of whether we can infer causality between depression and pain is often cited. However, a temporal relationship was found between preceding depression diagnoses and headaches or "any chronic pain" [32]. Another study explored childhood predictors of abdominal pain in adolescents over the course of 13 years at six different time points and found that the presence of depressive symptoms in childhood (at age 12) predicted recurrent abdominal pain two years later [16]. This finding suggests that depression may play a role in the transition from acute to chronic pain. Cross-sectional studies have also demonstrated associations between depression and irritable bowel syndrome [43], as well as with chronic daily headache when compared to control samples [35].

Two studies used nationally representative community samples to understand the connection between chronic pain and psychopathology in youth who are not receiving treatment for chronic pain. First, an association was found between musculoskeletal pains and depression in both boys and girls [34]. A second study found that 16% of all adolescents are at risk for developing depression, but this risk increases to 45% when adolescents have daily pain [44]. Studies with larger sample sizes in pediatric clinical populations are needed to further our understanding of the interplay between depression, anxiety, and pain.

Other disorders and mood problems. A small body of literature emphasizes a connection between trauma and chronic pain, primarily focusing on abuse (physical or sexual) or injury (e.g., sports injury, accident) [45]. These studies suggest that early posttraumatic stress disorder (PTSD) or trauma-related symptoms predict later functional impairment and pain [45]. However, more research is needed to understand the connection between trauma and pain in the pediatric population.

Other studies have highlighted issues related to anger [46], oppositional defiant disorder and attention-deficit hyperactivity disorder [34], conduct problems, [47] and a broader "psychopathology" variable [11,48–50]. Furthermore, "negative emotions" have been identified as a risk factor of moderate quality for headache in youth [13]. Broad terms such as "psychopathology" and "negative emotions" are likely too vague and difficult to replicate, and they may not be particularly useful in a clinical setting. Longitudinal studies will be particularly useful in guiding our understanding of the role of psychological factors in the development of chronic pain.

3.2.4. Stress

The subjective experience of stress demonstrates a strong relationship with pain. One study found that perceived stress explained a significant amount of the variance in present and worst pain intensity for younger children [25]. For adolescents, perceived stress was associated with present pain intensity only [25]. These findings are consistent with the adult literature on perceived stress and pain.

Houle and Nash [51] posit that stress is a risk factor in the "chronification" of headache in adults through several mechanisms, including daily stressors and chronic hyperarousal. Stress is also posited to indirectly relate to a series of other potential variables that can impact pain, such as fear of pain, locus of control, dysregulation of sleep and eating routines, overuse of medications, and psychopathology [51]. Thus, stress may play a crucial role in both the etiology and maintenance of pain problems. Finally, the experience of negative or stressful life events appears to be related to chronic pain [16,52–54]. Future research is needed to understand these complex interactions among stress and other variables as they relate to pain, especially in the pediatric population.

3.2.5. Coping Style

Compas et al. [55] define coping as "conscious volitional efforts to regulate emotion, cognition, behavior, physiology, and the environment in response to stressful events or circumstances". This widely accepted definition, especially as it relates to children and adolescents, takes developmental level into account, stating that an individual's development might facilitate or hinder the type of coping strategy that is available to and/or used by the individual [55]. Furthermore, unlike adults, children may not have developed a fully formed "coping style" or approach that they typically rely upon [26]. Children and adolescents may be more likely to employ a larger variety of coping strategies than adults as they attempt to form their own individual coping style. Developmental stage, therefore, is important to take into consideration when designing studies. Some strategies are seen as positive or adaptive and others are seen as maladaptive.

In a study of pediatric pain patients, coping was correlated with depression and disability [56]. The most common strategies were broken down into maladaptive (internalizing and catastrophizing) and adaptive (problem-solving and behavioral distraction) [56]. A strong relationship was found between the maladaptive coping strategies (e.g., dependency, denial, catastrophizing) and chronic pain for adolescents, and is consistent with findings in the adult literature [57–60]. Differences in coping strategies across diagnoses have also been found [56]. A musculoskeletal group reported greater disability and more difficulty coping than the headache group [56]. Further support relates pain catastrophizing to pediatric chronic pain conditions [61]. Together, these findings suggest that coping strategies represent an important area of focus for prevention and intervention strategies for chronic pain. Some promising studies, which are reviewed in depth below, have utilized more sophisticated methodology in order to improve our understanding of the role of different coping strategies.

3.2.6. Fear, Avoidance, and Beliefs

Asmundson et al. [62] argue that fear, anxiety, and avoidance appear to play a circular role in chronic pain. An original injury or experience of pain may lead to fear, which leads to avoidance of activities that may cause more pain. Avoidance of the anxiety felt in situations where an individual might expect to feel pain may strengthen the behavioral avoidance response as well [63]. Anxiety and avoidance may increase the fear. However, with avoidance of activity, eventual involvement in such activities is likely to involve a great deal of pain. Like a self-fulfilling prophecy, the fear of pain is confirmed, leading to continued avoidance of activities. Thus, Asmundson et al. [62] argue that the paradoxical and cyclical nature of the fear and avoidance relationship in chronic pain is problematic.

This problematic cycle includes fear-avoidance behaviors, which have been cited as potential risk factors for adults in the transition from acute to chronic pain with musculoskeletal pain [64], low back pain [65], and back and neck pain [66], as well as with maintenance of chronic pain [67]. In addition, fear of pain on its own has been identified as a risk factor in youth [61]. Studies such as these need to be replicated in pediatric populations to help understand these pathways in children.

A variety of specific beliefs have also been attributed to poor pain outcomes. In a controlled study of adolescents with recurrent abdominal pain (RAP), participants reported significantly greater concerns about undiagnosed physical disease and greater belief in susceptibility to functional impairment by pain and other physical symptoms [36]. Children with recurrent abdominal pain also appear to have significant hypochondriacal beliefs [36]. In the case of headache, locus of control and self-efficacy appear to be important risk factors [46]. A helplessness–hopelessness factor predicted adjustment to low back pain in adults one year later [68]. Thus, some studies support the idea that different types of negative beliefs about the self are related to chronic pain.

3.2.7. Sleep Problems

Related to psychological well-being, the relationship between pain and sleep is well established. Sleep problems are reported by over half of youth with chronic pain [3,69] and are consistently associated with a variety of pain syndromes, including headache [12], musculoskeletal pain [70], fibromyalgia [71], and pain in general [72]. Relatedly, fatigue is often a comorbid complaint of children with chronic pain, which is likely related to poor sleep [70]. Mood and depression appear to complicate this relationship [3,72], and likely require more sophisticated models to understand the full nature of this multivariate relationship.

3.2.8. Summary

The greatest amount of evidence suggests a number of risk factors in relation to pediatric chronic pain, including difficult temperament, anxiety, depression, subjective experience of stress, passive coping strategies, and sleep problems. Some evidence suggests that fear and avoidance behaviors as well as negative beliefs about the self may be risk factors for the development and/or maintenance of pediatric chronic pain. Mixed results for increased age, female sex, and a general psychopathology variable warrant further investigation. However, as discussed, there are a number of problems with the current literature. Small sample sizes, imprecise terminology, lack of comparison studies, and correlational analyses make it difficult to generalize results to the pediatric pain population as a whole. All studies reviewed primarily utilize pain as their outcome measure as well. A second generation of research is needed to build upon this first generation that incorporates more sophisticated methodology and sound research design, examining functional ability as an additional outcome measure.

3.3. Between-Person Factors

Several factors outside of the individual patient have also been found to be influential in pediatric pain, including parent and family variables. Palermo et al. [73] state that there are many gaps in the existing literature on family and parent influences in pediatric chronic pain, and that longitudinal studies are needed to understand the family impact on the development of a child's chronic pain. This section provides a brief overview of the current research on between-person risk factors, providing a context for the proposed next steps in research.

3.3.1. Parental Psychopathology

Depression and anxiety disorders among mothers and fathers are particularly prevalent for parents of children with chronic pain [16,28,74–76]. Thus, this is likely an important consideration in the context of chronic pain. In fact, in a sample of preschool children, maternal depression was the only significant factor of a variety of psychosocial stressors and demographic factors that were examined in association with pediatric chronic pain [76]. Mothers of children with recurrent abdominal pain were significantly more likely than mothers of healthy controls to have a lifetime history of and current anxiety, depressive, and somatoform disorders and poorer overall quality of life [77]. A "parent distress" distress also appears to impact youth chronic pain [78]. Notably, little research on fathers has been conducted in this population [73]. Finally, Palermo et al. [73] point to research suggesting that maternal distress and child chronic pain are bidirectional in nature, but this dynamic needs to be examined further. While some interesting associations have been found, it is clear that more research is needed to understand the role of each of these factors in pediatric chronic pain.

3.3.2. Parenting

Some studies have focused on parenting factors such as parental reactions to their child's pain and parental reinforcement of pain behaviors. Protective parenting and solicitous reactions towards their child's pain behaviors (e.g., reinforcement of pain behaviors, whether intentional or not) are associated with risk of poor adjustment [79,80]. Maternal but not paternal pain catastrophizing is related to pain intensity in children, but neither is related to disability [73]. For children who recently experienced a surgery, reactions by parents who demonstrate more pain catastrophizing within 48–72 h after the surgery predicted greater pain intensity reports in their child 12 months later [41]. One study found that differences in parental bonding style (with the child) were related to rates of chronic pain in children [81]. In addition, the modeling of pain behaviors by parents has also been suggested as a risk factor for youth [82]. Parent protectiveness mediates the relationship between parental cognitions (e.g., pain catastrophizing) and school functioning, including attendance and global ratings of school function [83]. The topic of parent–child interactions represents a promising area of study that may provide fruitful information about the development from acute to chronic pain and/or mechanisms of maintenance.

3.3.3. Family Pain History

Family history of pain has been shown to predict pain in children and adolescents. Children of parents with a specific type of pain are at risk for developing either the same type of pain [8,10,11,50] or other pain-related diagnoses [84,85]. More generally, poor maternal health is related to poor health and function in children with chronic conditions [73]. Family health history is likely to be important in a clinical context, particularly relating to pain, and it appears to be an important avenue for continued research.

3.3.4. Family Environment

A few risk factors related to the family environment have been proposed, including insufficient adult contact [12], single parent household [10], family conflict [86], and low socioeconomic status [18,54]. Disturbances in family functioning have been associated with pain and disability in children [87]. Unexpectedly, family harmony and cohesion has been associated with higher pain in children, although it was hypothesized that the experience of chronic pain in a child may unite families [87]. Anthony and Schanberg [84] posit that family environment plays a crucial role in the experience of juvenile arthritis, although this remains at a theoretical level for this particular disorder. Palermo and Chambers [88] recommend that family communication styles be examined in depth, as little research exists about this particular risk factor. They also highlight the importance of the consideration of family factors in general in a broader model [88].

3.3.5. Social Problems Outside of the Family Context

Poor social functioning has been linked to several chronic pain diagnoses in children and adolescents, including recurrent abdominal pain [36], low back pain [47], fibromyalgia [3], and pain in general [12]. Being bullied is also associated with chronic pain in adolescents [86]. Children with chronic pain often significantly decrease the amount of time spent in activities with peers, including sports and other extracurricular activities [1]. Children who miss significant periods of school due to pain may experience loss of friendships, feel more isolated, are less well-liked, and are less socially accepted than their healthy peers [3,89]. Across a variety of studies, children with chronic pain have reported having fewer friends, were more likely to be victimized by peers, were more isolated, and were evaluated as less likable than healthy peers [90]. In adolescents with chronic pain, pain intensity had a negative impact on independence, emotional adjustment, and identity formation [91].

Perceptions of social functioning also seem to matter. Children who perceived themselves as having poor social competence were more likely to have continued recurrent abdominal pain 5 years later [92]. Adolescents with chronic pain may judge themselves as being less socially developed than their healthy peers [91]. The current research on peer relationships seems to suggest that chronic pain often has a negative impact on the lives of these children and adolescents. However, strong peer relationships may also be protective [91]. Thus, more research on social functioning is needed to provide information about the complex interplay between developmental stage, peer relationships, and pain.

3.3.6. Summary

Research on between-person factors has demonstrated the most support for certain aspects of parenting (e.g., parental response to pain, parental attention), parental psychopathology and family pain history. More research using consistent definitions is needed to fully understand the relationships between family functioning, peer/social functioning, and pediatric chronic pain. The research reviewed here bears similar methodological issues raised in the section on within-person factors. More sophisticated methodology that considers a combination of within- and between-person factors would provide more information about the mechanisms of risk for development of chronic pain to acute pain in children and adolescents.

3.4. The Start of a Second Generation of Research

Cummings et al. [93] argue for a second generation of research in child development, particularly relating to childhood psychopathology. The goals of this research are to: (1) identify and understand the causal agents underlying child disorders as dynamic organizations of social, emotional, physiological, genetic, cognitive, and/or other processes; (2) explicate the broader causal net (e.g., multiple processes, risk and protective factors) that accounts for child disorders and the nature of the interrelations between these factors as causal agents; and (3) identify the familial, community, ethnic, cultural, interpersonal, and other contexts that influence causal processes and interrelations between the various dimensions and levels of social contexts [93].

If these goals are applied to pediatric chronic pain research, it appears evident that next steps in research should involve not only larger sample sizes and the replication of outdated studies, but consideration of relationships among risk factors and the utilization of more complex statistical modeling such as group comparison, exploration of mediation and moderation, and hierarchical linear modeling.

Of equal importance, as highlighted by Cummings et al. [93], is the integration of developmental considerations into this second generation of research. Certain stages of development may represent periods of increased susceptibility to either the development or maintenance of chronic pain issues. For example, research demonstrates that children are most vulnerable to the effects of parental depression during specific periods of infancy and adolescence [93]. Such ideas could be extended to chronic pain research in order to determine heightened areas of risk for youth when exposed to significant pain, which could guide preventive and early intervention efforts.

Cummings et al. [93] suggest that, as an individual experiences cumulative successes or failures in stage-salient tasks or developmental transitions, these processes may represent a mechanism by which the individual becomes "stuck" in increasingly stable, diverging trajectories. This is particularly relevant in youth with chronic pain, as some evidence suggests that certain children are at risk for following trajectories with negative prognoses. For example, Mulvaney et al. [53] identified three unique trajectories of recurrent abdominal pain in pediatric patients in a 5-year longitudinal study, including a "long-term risk group". The long term-risk group did not report the most severe of pain, but had significantly more anxiety, depression, lower perceived self-worth, and more negative life events [53]. Recognition that children face "stage-salient challenges" and incorporation of this information into study designs are crucial for understanding developmental processes and are likely important for understanding the mechanisms that contribute to chronic pain [93].

3.4.1. Examples of Extending the First Generation of Research

One factor that has emerged in the first generation of research on pediatric chronic pain is that of the experience of negative life events [16,52–54]. With the presence of negative life events identified as a possible risk factor, we can use this information to explore this risk more deeply. For example, closely related to the experience of stressful life events is one's ability to cope with that stress. Studies that examine the interaction between the experience of stress and one's coping style, as measured by physiological response, for example, can provide a deeper understanding of differential responses to pain. Thus, future research that examines the relationships between stressful life events, coping strategies, and pain may provide insight into the mechanisms by which acute pain becomes chronic, and can help to identify targets for treatment. In addition, differences among youth across varying developmental stages could be incorporated into research programs. Understanding the role of development in the transition from acute to chronic pain could potentially shed light on factors that place youth at higher risk for developing chronic pain, as well as those that maintain it.

3.4.2. Prospective, Longitudinal Studies

Another way in which the research on risk factors can carry forward is to design longitudinal studies that examine identified variables over time. Some research groups have already begun to do this by exploring community samples of school children longitudinally in order to understand prevalence of chronic pain. Longitudinal models also allow for the examination of predictor variables that may influence pain later in a child's life.

One longitudinal study followed children with pain at three time-points across 15 years [94]. At the second phase of data collection, results suggested that youth with pain were more likely than their healthy peers to demonstrate ineffective coping strategies for dealing with stress and to have poor self-esteem [94]. High frequency of nervousness as children predicted pain in adulthood [94]. In addition, 7% of the overall sample reported at the third time point that they were taking antidepressants, and another 3% used sedatives on a regular basis [94]. The incidence of stress reported by the participants also increased over time. Participants attributed their stress to time pressure (38%), occupation (23%), and social relationships (16%). In addition, participants reported significant restlessness (43%), signs of pathological anxiety (34%), and depressive symptoms (13%) [94].

In another study, Walker et al. [95] identified three distinct subtypes of children with recurrent abdominal pain that yielded significant differences in functional disability over time. The three subtypes were labeled high pain dysfunctional, high pain adaptive, and low pain adaptive [95]. The subtypes differed across several characteristics at baseline assessment, including reported levels of abdominal pain, gastrointestinal (GI) and non-GI symptoms, perceptions of threat related to pain, belief of coping ability, levels of pain catastrophizing, negative affect, and health-related impairment. The high pain dysfunctional group appeared to have the greatest of level of difficulty, with the low pain adaptive experiencing the least [95].

At follow-up, the high pain dysfunctional group was characterized by significantly more impairment in a variety of ways. This group was also significantly more likely to meet criteria for a functional GI disorder (FGID) with pain, an FGID with chronic non-abdominal pain, or an FGID with a comorbid anxiety or depressive disorder [95]. In addition, the high pain dysfunctional group showed significantly greater "thermal wind-up" than low pain adaptive patients in laboratory pain testing at follow-up, suggesting greater central nervous system sensitization [95]. Future studies with similar methods, including a physiological component, could provide valuable insight into subtypes of pediatric pain patients with other pain disorders such as complex regional pain syndrome or chronic migraine. Longitudinal study designs such as these are needed to understand causal effects in the transition from acute to chronic pain, as well as maintenance, in children and adolescents.

3.4.3. Mediating Factors

Another important way in which the field can move to a second generation of research is to examine the relationships among various risk factors. Understanding the interactions among variables, using models such as mediation and moderation, will provide more information than single risk factor models. Grunau et al. [96] hypothesize that mother–child interactions may be a mediating factor in children learning to cope with pain. They suggest that sensitive parenting may enhance appropriate interpretation of pain later in childhood for children who are exposed to a great deal of pain earlier in life. Using this theory, transactional processes between parent responses to pain and children's coping strategies may represent an important process in the transition from acute to chronic pain.

Some studies have moved beyond theory and examined relationships among identified variables. For example, in a community sample of adolescents, anxiety was found to partially mediate the relationship between psychosocial stress and abdominal pain, such that the influence of stress on children's pain was partially diminished after controlling for anxiety [40]. Involving the family context, Claar et al. [97] found that child anxiety was a moderating factor such that for those with greater anxiety, higher levels of parental protective behavior were associated with higher levels of disability in the child. Child anxiety and depression also separately moderated the relationship between parental pain minimization and children's somatic symptoms [97].

Packham et al. [58] found that, in combination, five predictors, including, age and pain coping strategies, accounted for 53% of the variance in pain related to pediatric arthritis [58]. By using more sophisticated methodology, such as the interactions among several variables identified in the first generation of research, we can begin to understand the important factors in the mechanisms of the transition from acute to chronic pain. Studies such as this one need to be conducted in pediatric samples. Such advanced modeling provides a context for results of single risk factors from the first generation of research and may provide clues as to the mechanisms of the transition from acute to chronic pain.

3.4.4. Profiles of Response

Sophisticated methodology to determine differential responses to pain or to treatment is another example of research that exemplifies a second generation in research. Walker et al. [95] used hierarchical cluster analyses to determine distinct patterns of coping profiles in pediatric patients with abdominal pain. Six distinct coping profiles were identified: infrequent copers, self-reliant copers, engaged copers, inconsistent copers, avoidant copers, and dependent copers [98]. The method of determining coping strategy profiles involved a 60-item inventory measure that is easily completed by children. An efficient method for categorizing adaptive and maladaptive coping responses in patients was identified, which can be used in clinical settings to help determine treatment goals. For example, if a child relies primarily on poor coping strategies, a greater focus of early treatment could target more effective coping strategies for that child. This research has important implications both for understanding possible mechanisms of the transition from acute to chronic pain as well as maladaptive behaviors that may contribute to maintenance of poor functioning.

4. Discussion

This review identified a variety of intra- and interpersonal risk factors that represent the first generation of research on risk for pediatric chronic pain. These studies provide a foundation for a next generation of more sophisticated research on risk mechanisms associated with the transition from acute to chronic pain as well as the maintenance of pain-related functional disability. Several limitations of the current research were identified, including the need for larger sample sizes, multiple formats of measurement (e.g., self- and parent-report, physiological measures), consistent definitions, and replication. Furthermore, longitudinal studies and more complex methodologies are needed to understand temporal and other relationships among these variables.

Importantly, as laid out by the Pediatric Initiative on Methods, Measurement, and Pain Assessment in Clinical Trials (PedIMMPACT) [99], a closer look at functional ability is needed to fully understand mechanisms of chronic pain. The majority of the studies reviewed here consider some characteristic of pain (e.g., presence, severity) as the outcome variable. However, it could be argued that the reason most children and adolescents present for treatment is due to the disability that the pain has caused in their lives, whether it be a decline in school attendance, lessened participation in preferred sports activities, loss of important relationships, and/or other disruptions to day-to-day functioning. Indeed, some researchers have begun following these guidelines in treatment studies, arguing that the primary goal of cognitive-behavioral treatment, a common form of treatment used for chronic pain, is to reduce disability [100].

Future Directions

Despite the problems listed, a first generation of research is needed to provide the basis for the next generation. In other words, the studies reviewed here are a necessary step to identify variables that can then be explored in a more complex manner. A second generation of research must then be generated to elucidate knowledge gained from the first generation [101]. A second generation would include efforts in two main areas: (1) improvement from the existing research, including replication with larger sample sizes, the addition of physiology and developmental stage into conceptual models, and further research in family and peer factors related to the development of chronic pain, and (2) more sophisticated methodological approaches, including the use of comparison studies, examination of interactions among previously identified variables, use of longitudinal design, and analyses such as hierarchical linear modeling and cluster analyses to determine bidirectional influences and trajectories, respectively. Hierarchical linear modeling can be used to account for dynamic interactions between two individuals (e.g., parent–child) and changes over time (e.g., different developmental stages, actor–partner influence in real time) [102]. Finally, once the second generation is complete, a third generation of research may be needed to identify causal relationships [103].

A biopsychosocial perspective in a developmental context is proposed (see Figure 1), which would extend beyond the limitations of the first generation of research. In addition to the risk factors identified thus far, we first propose that interactions among these factors be explored in relation to the development of chronic pain.

The "biological" piece of biopsychosocial considerations has not received as much attention in the literature. In the context of mediating and moderating relationships, the youth's own physiological functioning may be an important area of consideration. For example, respiratory sinus arrhythmia, or heart rate variability, as well as skin conductance are promising areas of research. These underlying physiological processes may further complete the picture of the transition from acute to chronic pain. Respiratory sinus arrhythmia is thought to be an index of emotion regulation on a physiological level [104,105], which may play a role in children's and parents' responses to chronic pain. Indeed, a study of adults with fibromyalgia and temporomandibular disorder found that patients demonstrated greater changes in respiratory sinus arrhythmia than controls, which was thought to reflect hyperarousal in an inappropriate context [106]. Other examples of biological contributors or processes that have been associated with pediatric chronic pain include visceral sensitivity [107,108] seen in children who have recurrent abdominal pain and abnormal pain signaling in complex regional pain [109].

Furthermore, in the treatment literature, a number of studies assess the efficacy of biofeedback for children and adolescents with chronic pain. Biofeedback typically involves therapist-assisted measurement and observation of physiology as well as suggestions for improvement from the therapist [110]. Several studies have demonstrated promising results in treatment of youth with biofeedback procedures [111,112], suggesting the physiology plays an important role in chronic pain and may be modified to improve the quality of life of individuals dealing with chronic pain. Underlying physiological mechanisms, particularly in the context of chronic pain disorders, which are very closely tied to medical issues, would be a valuable addition to Palermo and Chambers' [88] model.

Regarding the "social" piece of biopsychosocial considerations, in addition to inclusion of family and/or parent factors, peer relationships require further examination. Peer relationships or social functioning may play a role in the transition from acute to chronic pain, as many pediatric patients are likely to be in a stage of adolescence where peer relationships are incredibly salient. This area of focus also touches upon the developmental framework proposed, as the "tasks" of development differ depending upon age and stage of development. For example, adolescence marks an important time for development of significant peer relationships and identity formation. Certain aspects of peer relationships, such as the quality of these relationships, social support, victimization, and other salient elements could be included in mediation and moderation models. Coping strategies, thought to change across childhood, are another area of potentially fruitful, developmentally oriented research. Thus, development is an important context that must be included in consideration of risk in pediatric pain.

The "psychological" piece of the biopsychosocial model has perhaps received the most attention in the literature. The proposed next steps integrate all aspects of the biopsychological model, as well as developmental considerations. This proposal extends beyond Palermo and Chamber's [88] important model by adding psychophysiological, peer, and developmental variables (see Figure 1). Furthermore, complex methodology can provide a more thorough understanding of the interactions among variables related to the development, and maintenance, of pediatric chronic pain. These next steps represent the second generation of research in pediatric chronic pain, which can inform prevention and early intervention efforts.

Acknowledgments: The authors have no funding to disclose related to this study.

Author Contributions: Both authors conceived and wrote the paper.

Conflicts of Interest: The authors declare no conflict of interest.

References

1. Palermo, T.M. Impact of recurrent and chronic pain on child and family daily functioning: A critical review of the literature. *Dev. Behav. Pediatr.* **2000**, *21*, 58–69. [CrossRef]
2. Roth-Isigkeit, A.; Thyen, U.; Stöven, H.; Schwarzenberger, J.; Schmucker, P. Pain among children and adolescents: Restrictions in daily living and triggering factors. *Pediatrics* **2005**, *115*, e152–e162. [CrossRef] [PubMed]
3. Schechter, N.L.; Palermo, T.M.; Walco, G.A.; Berde, C.B. Persistent pain in children. In *Bonica's Management of Pain*, 4th ed.; Fishman, S.M., Ballantyne, J.C., Rathmell, J.P., Eds.; Lippincott Williams & Wilkins: Philadelphia, PA, USA, 2009; pp. 767–782.
4. King, S.; Chambers, C.T.; Huguet, A.; MacNevin, R.C.; McGrath, P.J.; Parker, L.; MacDonald, A.J. The epidemiology of chronic pain children and adolescents revisited: A systematic review. *Pain* **2011**, *152*, 2729–2738. [CrossRef] [PubMed]
5. Swain, M.S.; Henschke, N.; Kamper, S.J.; Gobina, I.; Ottová-Jordan, V.; Maher, C.G. An international survey of pain in adolescents. *BMC Public Health* **2014**, *14*, 447–453. [CrossRef] [PubMed]
6. Apley, J.; Naish, N. Recurrent abdominal pains: A field survey of 1000 school children. *Arch. Dis. Child.* **1958**, *33*, 165–170. [CrossRef] [PubMed]
7. Schieveld, J.N.M.; Wolters, A.M.H.; Blankespoor, R.J.; van de Riet, E.H.C.W.; Vos, G.D.; Leroy, P.L.J.M.; van Os, J. The forthcoming DSM-5 critical care medicine, and pediatric neuropsychiatry: Which new concepts do we need? *J. Neuropsychiatr. Clin. Neurosci.* **2013**, *25*, 111–114. [CrossRef] [PubMed]
8. Balagué, F.; Troussier, B.; Salminen, J.J. Non-specific low back pain in children and adolescents: Risk factors. *Eur. Spine J.* **1999**, *8*, 429–438. [CrossRef] [PubMed]
9. Speretto, F.; Brachi, S.; Vittadello, F.; Zulian, F. Musculoskeletal pain in schoolchildren across puberty: A 3-year follow-up study. *Pediatr. Rheumatol.* **2015**, *13*, 16. [CrossRef] [PubMed]
10. Chitkara, D.K.; Rawat, D.J.; Talley, N.J. The epidemiology of childhood recurrent abdominal pain in Western countries: A systematic review. *Am. J. Gastroenterol.* **2005**, *100*, 1868–1875. [CrossRef] [PubMed]

11. Balagué, F.; Skovron, M.; Nordin, M.; Dutoit, G.; Pol, L.R.; Waldburger, M. Low back pain in schoolchildren: A study of familial and psychological factors. *Spine* **1995**, *20*, 1265–1270. [CrossRef] [PubMed]
12. Brattberg, G. The incidence of back pain and headache among Swedish school children. *Qual. Life Res.* **1994**, *3*, S27–S31. [CrossRef] [PubMed]
13. Huguet, A.; Tougas, M.E.; Hayden, J.; McGrath, P.J.; Chambers, C.T.; Stinson, J.N.; Wozney, L. Systematic review of childhood and adolescent risk and prognostic factors for recurrent headaches. *J. Pain* **2016**, *17*, 855–873. [CrossRef] [PubMed]
14. Wang, S.; Fuh, J.; Lu, S.; Juang, K. Chronic daily headache in adolescents: Prevalence, impact, and medication overuse. *Neurology* **2006**, *66*, 193–197. [CrossRef] [PubMed]
15. LeResche, L.; Manci, L.A.; Drangsholt, M.T.; Huang, G.; Von Korff, M. Predictors of onset of facial pain and temporomandibular disorders in early adolescence. *Pain* **2007**, *129*, 269–278. [CrossRef] [PubMed]
16. Helgeland, H.; Sandvik, L.; Mathiesen, K.S.; Kristensen, H. Childhood predictors of recurrent abdominal pain in adolescence: A 13-year population-based prospective study. *J. Psychosom. Res.* **2010**, *68*, 359–367. [CrossRef] [PubMed]
17. Østerås, B.; Sigmundsson, H.; Haga, M. Pain is prevalent among adolescents and equally related to stress across genders. *Scand. J. Pain* **2016**, *12*, 100–107. [CrossRef]
18. Lipton, R.B.; Bigal, M.E. Migraine: Epidemiology, impact, and risk factors for progression. *Headache* **2005**, *45*, S3–S13. [CrossRef] [PubMed]
19. Saurenmann, R.K.; Rose, J.B.; Tyrrell, P.; Feldman, B.M.; Laxer, R.M.; Schneider, R.; Silverman, E.D. Epidemiology of juvenile idiopathic arthritis in a multiethnic cohort. *Arthritis Rheum.* **2007**, *56*, 1974–1984. [CrossRef] [PubMed]
20. Rhee, H. Prevalence and predictors of headaches in US adolescents. *Headache* **2000**, *40*, 528–538. [CrossRef] [PubMed]
21. Widmalm, S.E.; Christiansen, R.L.; Gunn, S.M. Race and gender as TMD risk factors in children. *CRANIO: J. Craniomandib. Sleep Pract.* **1995**, *13*, 163–166. [CrossRef]
22. Rabbitts, J.A.; Holley, A.L.; Groenewald, C.B.; Palermo, T.M. Association between widespread pain scores and functional impairment and health-related quality of life in clinical samples of children. *J. Pain* **2016**, *17*, 678–684. [CrossRef] [PubMed]
23. Genizi, J.; Srugo, I.; Kerem, N.C. The cross-ethnic variations in the prevalence of headache and other somatic complaints among adolescents in Northern Israel. *J. Headache Pain* **2013**, *14*, 21–26. [CrossRef] [PubMed]
24. Gold, J.I.; Mahrer, N.E.; Yee, J.; Palermo, T.M. Pain, fatigue, and health-related quality of life in children and adolescents with chronic pain. *Clin. J. Pain* **2009**, *25*, 407–412. [CrossRef] [PubMed]
25. Varni, J.W.; Rapoff, M.A.; Waldron, S.A.; Gragg, R.A.; Bernstein, B.H.; Lindsley, C.B. Effects of perceived stress on pediatric chronic pain. *J. Behav. Med.* **1996**, *19*, 515–528. [CrossRef] [PubMed]
26. Lynch, A.M.; Kashikar-Zuck, S.; Goldschneider, K.R.; Jones, B.A. Sex and age differences in coping styles among children with chronic pain. *J. Pain Symp. Manag.* **2007**, *33*, 208–216. [CrossRef] [PubMed]
27. Malleson, P.N.; Connell, H.; Bennett, S.M.; Eccleston, C. Chronic musculoskeletal and other idiopathic pain syndromes. *Arch. Dis. Child.* **2001**, *84*, 189–192. [CrossRef] [PubMed]
28. Ramchandani, P.G.; Stein, A.; Hotopf, M.; Wiles, N.J.; the ALSPAC Study Team. Early parental and child predictors of recurrent abdominal pain at school age: Results of a large population-based study. *J. Am. Acad. Child. Adolesc. Psychiatr.* **2006**, *45*, 729–736. [CrossRef] [PubMed]
29. Davison, I.S.; Faull, C.; Nicol, A.R. Research note: Temperament and behaviour in six-year-olds with recurrent abdominal pain: A follow up. *J. Child. Psychol. Psychiatr.* **1986**, *27*, 539–544. [CrossRef]
30. Conte, P.M.; Walco, G.A.; Kimura, Y. Temperament and stress response in children with juvenile primary fibromyalgia syndrome. *Arthritis Rheum.* **2003**, *48*, 2923–2930. [CrossRef] [PubMed]
31. Compas, B.E. Coping with stress during childhood and adolescence. *Psychol. Bull.* **1987**, *101*, 393–403. [CrossRef] [PubMed]
32. Tegethoff, M.; Belardi, A.; Stalujanis, E.; Meinlschmidt, G. Comorbidity of mental disorders and chronic pain: Chronology of onset in adolescents of a national representative cohort. *J. Pain* **2015**, *16*, 1054–1064. [CrossRef] [PubMed]

33. Di Lorenzo, C.; Colletti, R.B.; Lehmann, P.; Boyle, J.T.; Gerson, W.T.; Hyams, J.S.; Squires, R.H., Jr.; Walker, L.S.; Kanda, P.T. Chronic abdominal pain in children: A technical report of the American Academy of Pediatrics and the North American Society for Pediatric Gastroenterology, Hepatology and Nutrition. *J. Pediatr. Gastroenterol. Nutr.* **2005**, *40*, 249–261. [CrossRef] [PubMed]

34. Egger, H.L.; Costello, E.J.; Erkanli, A.; Angold, A. Somatic complaints and psychopathology in children and adolescents: Stomach aches, musculoskeletal pains, and headaches. *J. Am. Acad. Child. Adolesc. Psychiatr.* **1999**, *38*, 852–860. [CrossRef] [PubMed]

35. Rousseau-Salvador, C.; Amouroux, R.; Annequin, D.; Salvodor, A.; Tourniaire, B.; Rusinek, S. Anxiety, depression and school abseentism in youth with chronic or episodic headache. *Pain Res. Manag.* **2014**, *19*, 235–240. [CrossRef] [PubMed]

36. Campo, J.V.; Lorenzo, C.D.; Chiappetta, L.; Bridge, J.; Colborn, D.K.; Gartner, J.C.; Gaffney, P.; Kocoshis, S.; Brent, D. Adult outcomes of pediatric recurrent abdominal pain: They just grow out of it? *Pediatrics* **2001**, *108*, 502. [CrossRef]

37. Campo, J.V.; Bridge, J.; Ehmann, M.; Altman, S.; Lucas, A.; Birmaher, B.; Di Lorenzo, C.; Iyengar, S.; Brent, D.A. Recurrent abdominal pain, anxiety, and depression in primary care. *Pediatrics* **2004**, *113*, 817–824. [CrossRef] [PubMed]

38. Tran, S.T.; Jastrowski Mano, K.E.; Anderson Khan, K.; Davies, W.H.; Hainsworth, K.R. Patterns of anxiety symptoms in pediatric chronic pain as reported by youth, mothers, and fathers. *Clin. Pract. Pediatr. Psychol.* **2016**, *4*, 51–62. [CrossRef]

39. Margetić, B.; Aukst-Margetić, B.; Bilić, E.; Jelušić, M.; Bukovac, L.T. Depression, anxiety and pain in children with juvenile idiopathic arthritis (JIA). *Eur. Psychiatr.* **2005**, *20*, 274–276. [CrossRef] [PubMed]

40. White, K.S.; Farrell, A.D. Anxiety and psychosocial stress as predictors of headache and abdominal pain in urban early adolescents. *J. Pediatr. Psychol.* **2006**, *31*, 582–596. [CrossRef] [PubMed]

41. Pagé, M.G.; Stinson, J.; Campbell, F.; Isaac, L.; Katz, J. Identification of pain-related psychological risk factors for the development and maintenance of pediatric chronic postsurgical pain. *J. Pain Res.* **2013**, *6*, 167–180. [CrossRef] [PubMed]

42. Clark, L.E.; Watson, D. Tripartite model of anxiety and depression: Psychometric evidence and taxonomic implications. *J. Abnorm. Psychol.* **1991**, *100*, 316–336. [CrossRef] [PubMed]

43. Hyams, J.F.; Burke, G.; Davis, P.M.; Rzepski, B.; Andrulonis, P.A. Abdominal pain and irritable bowel syndrome in adolescents: A community-based study. *J. Pediatr.* **1996**, *129*, 220–226. [CrossRef]

44. Youssef, N.N.; Atienza, K.; Langseder, A.L.; Strauss, R.S. Chronic abdominal pain and depressive symptoms: Analysis of the National Longitudinal Study of Adolescent Health. *Clin. Gastroenterol. Hepatol. Off. Clin. Pract. J. Am. Gastroenterol. Assoc.* **2008**, *6*, 329–332. [CrossRef] [PubMed]

45. Holley, A.L.; Wilson, A.C.; Noel, M.; Palermo, T.M. Post-traumatic stress symptoms in children and adolescents with chronic pain: A topical review of the literature and a proposed framework for future research. *Eur. J. Pain* **2016**, *20*, 1371–1383. [CrossRef] [PubMed]

46. Nicholson, R.A.; Houle, T.T.; Rhudy, J.L.; Norton, P.J. Psychological risk factors in headache. *Headache* **2007**, *47*, 413–426. [CrossRef] [PubMed]

47. Jones, G.T.; Watson, K.D.; Silman, A.J.; Symmons, D.P.M.; Macfarlane, G.J. Predictors of low back pain in British schoolchildren: A population-based prospective cohort study. *Pediatrics* **2003**, *111*, 822–828. [CrossRef] [PubMed]

48. Feldman, D.E.; Shrier, I.; Rossignol, M.; Abenheim, L. Risk factors for the development of neck and upper limb pain in adolescents. *Spine* **2002**, *27*, 523–528. [CrossRef]

49. Hotopf, M.; Carr, S.; Mayou, R.; Wadsworth, M.; Wessely, S. Why do children have chronic abdominal pain, and what happens to them when they grow up? Population based cohort study. *Br. Med. J.* **1998**, *316*, 1196–1200. [CrossRef]

50. Wiendels, N.J.; Neven, A.K.; Rosendaal, F.R.; Spinhoven, P.; Zitman, F.G.; Assendelft, W.J.J.; Ferrari, M.D. Chronic frequent headache in the general population: Prevalence and associated factors. *Cephalalgia* **2006**, *26*, 1434–1442. [CrossRef] [PubMed]

51. Houle, T.; Nash, J.M. Stress and headache chronification. *Headache* **2008**, *48*, 40–44. [CrossRef] [PubMed]

52. Geertzen, J.H.B.; de Bruijn-Kofman, A.T.; de Bruijn, H.P.; van de Wiel, H.B.M.; Dijkstra, P.U. Stressful life events and psychological dysfunction in complex regional pain syndrome type I. *Clin. J. Pain* **1998**, *14*, 143–147. [CrossRef] [PubMed]

53. Mulvaney, S.; Lambert, E.W.; Garber, J.; Walker, L.S. Trajectories of symptoms and impairment for pediatric patients with functional abdominal pain: A 5-year longitudinal study. *J. Am. Acad. Child. Adolesc. Psychiatr.* **2006**, *45*, 737–744. [CrossRef] [PubMed]
54. Scher, A.I.; Midgette, L.A.; Lipton, R.B. Risk factors for headache chronification. *Headache* **2008**, *48*, 16–25. [CrossRef] [PubMed]
55. Compas, B.E.; Connor-Smith, J.K.; Saltzman, H.; Thomsen, A.H.; Wadsworth, M.E. Coping with stress during childhood and adolescence: Problems, progress, and potential in theory and research. *Psychol. Bull.* **2001**, *127*, 87–127. [CrossRef] [PubMed]
56. Kashikar-Zuck, S.; Goldschneider, K.R.; Powers, S.W.; Vaught, M.H.; Hershey, A.D. Depression and functional disability in chronic pediatric pain. *Clin. J. Pain* **2001**, *17*, 341–349. [CrossRef] [PubMed]
57. Litt, M.D.; Shafer, D.M.; Ibanez, C.R.; Kreutzer, D.L.; Tawfik-Yonkers, Z. Momentary pain and coping in temporomandibular disorder pain: Exploring mechanisms of cognitive behavioral treatment for chronic pain. *Pain* **2009**, *145*, 160–168. [CrossRef] [PubMed]
58. Packham, J.C.; Hall, M.A.; Pimm, T.J. Long-term follow-up of 246 adults with juvenile idiopathic arthritis: Predictive factors for mood and pain. *Paediatr. Rheumatol.* **2002**, *41*, 1444–1449. [CrossRef]
59. Sacheti, A.; Szemere, J.; Bernstein, B.; Tafas, T.; Schechter, N.; Tsipouras, P. Chronic pain is a manifestation of the Ehlers–Danlos syndrome. *J. Pain Symp. Manag.* **1997**, *14*, 88–93. [CrossRef]
60. Turner, J.A.; Clancy, S. Strategies for coping with chronic low back pain: Relationship to pain and disability. *Pain* **1986**, *24*, 355–364. [CrossRef]
61. Cousins, L.A.; Cohen, L.L.; Venable, C. Risk and resilience in pediatric chronic pain: Exploring the protective role of optimism. *J. Pediatr. Psychol.* **2015**, *40*, 934–942. [PubMed]
62. Asmundson, G.J.G.; Norton, P.H.; Norton, G.R. Beyond pain: The role of fear and avoidance in chronicity. *Clin. Psychol. Rev.* **1999**, *19*, 97–119. [CrossRef]
63. Walker, L.S. An evolution of research on recurrent abdominal pain: History, assumptions, and a conceptual model. In *Chronic and Recurrent Pain in Children and Adolescents*; McGrath, P.J., Finley, G.A., Eds.; IASP Press: Seattle, WA, USA, 1999; pp. 141–172.
64. Vlaeyen, J.W.S.; Linton, S.J. Fear-avoidance and its consequences in chronic musculoskeletal pain: A state of the art. *Pain* **2000**, *85*, 317–332. [CrossRef]
65. Vlaeyen, J.W.S.; Kole-Snijders, A.M.J.; Boeren, R.G.B.; van Eek, H. Fear of movement/(re)injury in chronic low back pain and its relation to behavioral performance. *Pain* **1995**, *62*, 363–372. [CrossRef]
66. Linton, S.J. A review of psychological risk factors in back and neck pain. *Spine* **2000**, *25*, 1148–1156. [CrossRef] [PubMed]
67. Philips, H.C. Avoidance behaviour and its role in sustaining chronic pain. *Behav. Res. Ther.* **1987**, *25*, 273–279. [CrossRef]
68. Koleck, M.; Mazaux, J.; Rascle, N.; Bruchon-Schweitzer, M. Psycho-social factors and coping strategies as predictors of chronic evolution and quality of life in patients with low back pain: A prospective study. *Eur. J. Pain* **2006**, *10*, 1–11. [CrossRef] [PubMed]
69. Long, A.C.; Krishnamurthy, V.; Palermo, T.C. Sleep disturbances in school-age children with chronic pain. *J. Pediatr. Psychol.* **2008**, *33*, 258–268. [CrossRef] [PubMed]
70. Mikkelsson, M.; Salminen, J.J.; Sourander, A.; Kautianen, H. Contributing factors to the persistence of musculoskeletal pain in preadolescents: A prospective 1-year follow-up study. *Pain* **1998**, *77*, 67–72. [CrossRef]
71. Kashikar-Zuck, S.; Lynch, A.M.; Slater, S.; Graham, T.B.; Swain, N.F.; Noll, R.B. Family factors, emotional functioning, and functional impairment in juvenile fibromyalgia syndrome. *Arthritis Rheum.* **2008**, *59*, 1392–1398. [CrossRef] [PubMed]
72. Palermo, T.M.; Kiska, R. Subjective sleep disturbances in adolescents with chronic pain: Relationship to daily functioning and quality of life. *J. Pain* **2005**, *6*, 201–207. [CrossRef] [PubMed]
73. Palermo, T.M.; Valrie, C.R.; Karlson, C.W. Family and parent influences on pediatric chronic pain: A developmental perspective. *Am. Psychol.* **2014**, *69*, 142–152. [CrossRef] [PubMed]
74. Garber, J.; Zeman, J.; Walker, L.S. Recurrent abdominal pain in children: Psychiatric diagnoses and parental psychopathology. *J. Am. Acad. Child. Adolesc. Psychiatr.* **1990**, *29*, 648–656. [CrossRef] [PubMed]
75. Hodges, K.; Kline, J.J.; Barbero, G.; Woodruff, C. Anxiety in children with recurrent abdominal pain and their parents. *Psychosomatics* **1985**, *26*, 859–866. [CrossRef]

76. Zuckerman, B.; Stevenson, J.; Bailey, V. Stomachaches and headaches in a community sample of preschool children. *Pediatrics* **1987**, *79*, 677–682. [PubMed]

77. Campo, J.V.; Bridge, J.; Lucas, A.; Savorelli, S.; Walker, L.; Di Lorenzo, C.; Satish, I.; Brent, D.A. Physical and emotional health of mothers of youth with functional abdominal pain. *Arch. Pediatr. Adolesc. Med.* **2007**, *161*, 131–137. [CrossRef] [PubMed]

78. Chow, E.T.; Otis, J.D.; Simons, L.E. The longitudinal impact of parent distress and behavior on functional outcomes among youth with chronic pain. *J. Pain* **2016**, *17*, 729–738. [CrossRef] [PubMed]

79. Palermo, T.M.; Eccleston, C. Parents of children and adolescents with chronic pain. *Pain* **2009**, *146*, 15–17. [CrossRef] [PubMed]

80. Peterson, C.C.; Palermo, T.M. Parental reinforcement of recurrent pain: The moderating impact of child depression and anxiety on functional disability. *J. Pediatr. Psychol.* **2004**, *29*, 331–341. [CrossRef] [PubMed]

81. Anno, K.; Shibata, M.; Ninomiya, T.; Iwaki, R.; Kawata, H.; Sawamoto, R.; Kubo, C.; Kiyohara, Y.; Sudo, N.; Hosoi, M. Paternal and maternal bonding styles in childhood are associated with the prevalence of chronic pain in a general adult population: The Hisayama Study. *BMC Psychiatr.* **2015**, *15*, 1–8. [CrossRef] [PubMed]

82. Stone, A.L.; Walker, L.S. Adolescents' observations of parent pain behaviors: Preliminary measure validation and test of social learning theory in pediatric chronic pain. *J. Pediatr. Psychol.* **2016**, *41*. [CrossRef] [PubMed]

83. Logan, D.E.; Simons, L.E.; Carpino, E.A. Too sick for school? Parent influences on school functioning among children with chronic pain. *Pain* **2012**, *153*, 437–443. [CrossRef] [PubMed]

84. Anthony, K.K.; Schanberg, L.E. Pediatric pain syndromes and management of pain in children and adolescents with rheumatic disease. *Pediatr. Clin. N. Am.* **2005**, *52*, 611–639. [CrossRef] [PubMed]

85. Schanberg, L.E.; Anthony, K.A.; Gil, K.M.; Lefebvre, J.C.; Kredich, D.W.; Macharoni, L.M. Family pain history predicts child health status in children with chronic rheumatic disease. *Pediatrics* **2001**, *108*, 1–7. [CrossRef]

86. Voerman, J.S.; Vogel, I.; Waart, F.; Westendorp, T.; Timman, R.; Busschbach, J.J.V.; van de Looij-Jansen, P.; Klerk, C. Bullying, abuse and family conflict as risk factors for chronic pain among Dutch adolescents. *Eur. J. Pain* **2015**, *19*, 1544–1551. [CrossRef] [PubMed]

87. Lewandowski, A.S.; Palermo, T.M.; Stinson, J.; Handley, S.; Chambers, C.T. Systematic review of family functioning in families of children and adolescents with chronic pain. *J. Pain* **2010**, *11*, 1027–1038. [CrossRef] [PubMed]

88. Palermo, T.M.; Chambers, C.T. Parent and family factors in pediatric chronic pain and disability: An integrative approach. *Pain* **2005**, *119*, 1–4. [CrossRef] [PubMed]

89. Assa, A.; Ish-Tov, A.; Rinawi, F.; Shamir, R. School attendance in children with functional abdominal pain and inflammatory bowel diseases. *J. Pediatr. Gastroenterol. Nutr.* **2015**, *61*, 553–557. [CrossRef] [PubMed]

90. Forgeron, P.A.; King, S.; Stinson, J.N.; McGrath, P.J.; MacDonald, A.J.; Chambers, C.T. Social functioning and peer relationships in children and adolescents with chronic pain: A systematic review. *Pain Res. Manag.* **2010**, *15*, 27–41. [CrossRef] [PubMed]

91. Eccleston, C.; Wastell, S.; Crombez, G.; Jordan, A. Adolescent social development and chronic pain. *Eur. J. Pain* **2008**, *12*, 765–774. [CrossRef] [PubMed]

92. Walker, L.S.; Guite, J.W.; Duke, M.; Barnard, J.A.; Greene, J.W. Recurrent abdominal pain: A potential precursor of irritable bowel syndrome in adolescents and young adults. *J. Pediatr.* **1998**, *132*, 1010–1015. [CrossRef]

93. Cummings, E.M.; Davies, P.T.; Campbell, S.B. *Developmental Psychopathology and Family Process: Theory, Research, and Clinical Implications*; Guilford Press: New York, NY, USA, 2000.

94. Brattberg, G. Do pain problems in young school children persist into early adulthood? A 13-year follow-up. *Eur. J. Pain* **2004**, *8*, 187–199. [CrossRef] [PubMed]

95. Walker, L.S.; Sherman, A.L.; Bruehl, S.; Garber, J.; Smith, C.A. Functional abdominal pain patient subtypes in childhood predict functional gastrointestinal disorders with chronic pain and psychiatric comorbidities in adolescence and adulthood. *Pain* **2012**, *153*, 1798–1806. [CrossRef] [PubMed]

96. Grunau, R.V.E.; Whitfield, M.F.; Petrie, J.H.; Fryer, E.L. Early pain experience, child and family factors, as precursors of somatization: A prospective study of extremely premature and full-term children. *Pain* **1994**, *56*, 353–359. [CrossRef]

97. Claar, R.L.; Simons, L.E.; Logan, D.E. Parental response to children's pain: The moderating impact of children's emotional distress on symptoms and disability. *Pain* **2008**, *138*, 172–179. [CrossRef] [PubMed]

98. Walker, L.S.; Baber, K.F.; Garber, J.; Smith, C.A. A typology of pain coping strategies in pediatric patients with chronic abdominal pain. *Pain* **2008**, *137*, 266–275. [CrossRef] [PubMed]

99. McGrath, P.J.; Walco, G.A.; Turk, D.C.; Dworkin, R.H.; Brown, M.T.; Davidson, K.; Eccleston, C.; Finley, G.A.; Goldschneider, K.; Haverkos, L.; et al. Core outcome domains and measures for pediatric acute and chronic/recurrent pain clinical trials: PedIMMPACT recommendations. *J. Pain* **2008**, *9*, 771–783. [CrossRef] [PubMed]

100. Kashikar-Zuck, S.; Ting, T.V.; Arnold, L.M.; Bean, J.; Powers, S.T.; Graham, T.B.; Passo, M.H.; Schikler, K.N.; Hashkes, P.J.; Spalding, S.; et al. Cognitive behavioral therapy for the treatment of juvenile fibromyalgia: A multisite, single-blind, randomized, controlled clinical trial. *Pediatr. Rheumatol.* **2012**, *64*, 297–305. [CrossRef] [PubMed]

101. Hoyle, R.H. Introduction to the special section: Structural equation modeling in clinical research. *J. Consult. Clin. Psychol.* **1994**, *62*, 427–428. [CrossRef] [PubMed]

102. Kenny, D.A.; Kashy, D.A.; Cook, W.L. *Dyadic Data Analysis*; The Guilford Press: New York, NY, USA, 2006.

103. Friedman, M.A.; Brownell, K.D. Psychological correlates of obesity: Moving to the next research generation. *Psychol. Bull.* **1995**, *117*, 3–20. [CrossRef] [PubMed]

104. Beauchaine, T. Vagal tone, development, and Gray's motivational theory: Toward an integrated model of autonomic nervous system functioning in psychopathology. *Dev. Psychopathol.* **2001**, *13*, 183–214. [CrossRef] [PubMed]

105. Butler, E.A.; Wilhelm, F.H.; Gross, J.J. Respiratory sinus arrhythmia, emotion, and emotion regulation during social interaction. *Psychophysiology* **2006**, *43*, 612–622. [CrossRef] [PubMed]

106. Eisenlohr-Moul, T.A.; Crofford, L.J.; Howard, T.W.; Yepes, J.F.; Carlson, C.R.; de Leeuw, R. Parasympathetic reactivity in fibromyalgia and temporomandibular disorder: Associations with sleep problems, symptom severity, and functional impairment. *J. Pain* **2015**, *16*, 247–257. [CrossRef] [PubMed]

107. Van Ginkel, R.; Voskuijl, W.P.; Benninga, M.A.; Boeckxstaens, G.E. Alterations in rectal sensitivity and motility in childhood irritable bowel syndrome. *Gastroenterology* **1999**, *120*, 31–38. [CrossRef]

108. Di Lorenzo, C.; Youssef, N.N.; Sigurdsson, L.; Scharff, L.; Griffiths, J.; Wald, A. Visceral hyperalgesia in children with functional abdominal pain. *J. Pediatr.* **2001**, *139*, 838–843. [CrossRef] [PubMed]

109. Harden, R.N.; Oaklander, A.L.; Burton, A.W.; Perez, R.S.G.M.; Richardson, K.; Swan, M.; Barthel, J.; Costa, B.; Graciosa, J.R.; Bruehl, S. Complex regional pain syndrome: Practical diagnostic and treatment guidelines, 4th edition. *Pain Med.* **2013**, *14*, 180–229. [CrossRef] [PubMed]

110. Haynes, S.N.; Griffin, P.; Mooney, D.; Parise, M. Electromyographic biofeedback and relaxation instructions in the treatment of muscle contraction headaches. *Behav. Ther.* **1975**, *6*, 672–678. [CrossRef]

111. Allen, K.D.; Shriver, M.D. Role of parent-mediated pain behavior management strategies in biofeedback treatment of childhood migraines. *Behav. Ther.* **1998**, *29*, 477–490. [CrossRef]

112. Yetwin, A.; Marks, K.; Bell, T.; Gold, J. Heart rate variability biofeedback therapy for children and adolescents with chronic pain. *J. Pain* **2012**, *13*, S93. [CrossRef]

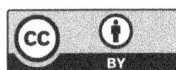

![children logo] **MDPI**

Review
Goal Pursuit in Youth with Chronic Pain

Emma Fisher [1,*] and **Tonya M. Palermo [1,2]**

[1] Center for Child Health, Behavior, and Development, Seattle Children's Research Institute, Seattle, WA 98122, USA; Tonya.Palermo@seattlechildrens.org

[2] Department of Anesthesiology and Pain Medicine, University of Washington, Seattle, WA 98195, USA

*   Correspondence: Emma.Fisher@seattlechildrens.org; Tel.: +1-206-884-0147

Academic Editor: Sari A. Acra

Received: 18 August 2016; Accepted: 11 November 2016; Published: 22 November 2016

Abstract: Children and adolescents frequently experience chronic pain that can disrupt their usual activities and lead to poor physical and emotional functioning. The fear avoidance model of pain with an emphasis on the maladaptive behaviors that lead to activity avoidance has guided research and clinical practice. However, this model does not take into consideration variability in responses to pain, in particular the active pursuit of goals despite pain. This review aims to introduce a novel conceptualization of children's activity engagement versus avoidance using the framework of goal pursuit. We propose a new model of Goal Pursuit in Pediatric Chronic Pain, which proposes that the child's experience of pain is modified by child factors (e.g., goal salience, motivation/energy, pain-related anxiety/fear, and self-efficacy) and parent factors (e.g., parent expectations for pain, protectiveness behaviors, and parent anxiety), which lead to specific goal pursuit behaviors. Goal pursuit is framed as engagement or avoidance of valued goals when in pain. Next, we recommend that research in youth with chronic pain should be reframed to account for the pursuit of valued goals within the context of pain and suggest directions for future research.

Keywords: adolescents; children; chronic pain; goal pursuit

1. Introduction and Purpose of Review

Children and adolescents frequently experience pain, most commonly headache, abdominal pain, and musculoskeletal pain [1]. Pain can range in intensity, frequency, and duration. For some children and adolescents, pain can persist, interrupting daily routines and activities. Pain that persists for longer than three months is defined as chronic [2]. Between 5%–8% of children experience chronic pain that is severe and disabling [3]. Chronic pain during childhood is a risk factor for chronic pain in adulthood, with studies showing that 35% of adolescents with chronic pain go on to report chronic pain in adulthood [4] and experience emotional distress [5]. Thus, understanding and treating pain in childhood is critical for interrupting a potential lifelong trajectory of pain and disability.

Children and adolescents with chronic pain report that pain is disruptive to many aspects of their daily functioning, such as decreasing physical functioning, impacting school attendance, and interactions with peers, leading to emotional distress [6–8]. In particular, children and adolescents with chronic pain report high levels of anxiety, depression, and maladaptive coping strategies [9–12]. Greater anxiety symptoms have been linked to avoidance of activities [13]. Unlike acute pain where children are encouraged to rest, or avoid activities that may aggravate the injury, treatment of chronic pain requires encouraging children to engage with physical activities and normal functioning despite their pain. Avoidance of everyday activities leads to increased disability, increased depression, higher fear, and increased pain sensitivity [7,13–15].

The fear avoidance model demonstrates this pathway linking anxiety and avoidance, and was proposed to aid research and clinical understanding of the maintenance of pain and disability [14].

In a second pathway, confrontation is predicted to lead to recovery; however, this has received less research attention. This model has been more recently adapted to describe development and mechanisms of pain in children and adolescents [13]. However, there are some limitations to this model, particularly in the underlying assumption that avoidance is a single pathway that leads to disability. Children and adolescents may or may not avoid activities because of pain, and there is evidence to suggest that many children and adolescents persist with activities despite their pain. As documented in epidemiological papers, around 25%–40% of children report experiencing chronic pain [3,16]. However, only 5%–8% of children have moderate to severe chronic pain, which impacts their daily functioning [3]. Therefore, many children and adolescents have frequent pain that is not disabling, and there may be unique protective factors that lead to recovery or adaptation to pain. The fear avoidance model does not conceptualize the experiences of children and adolescents with chronic pain who demonstrate more adaptive functioning or who are not fearful. This gap in understanding of adaptation to pain may be critical to expanding and informing psychological treatment models for children and adolescents with chronic pain.

Recognizing this variability in children's responses to chronic pain, we propose a new conceptual model that characterizes an individual's reaction to pain in the context of their engagement and pursuit of personal goals. We propose to reframe our thinking about young people with chronic pain to specifically understand those factors that lead to engagement and avoidance, which better reflects the active and dynamic process of responding to challenges in the pursuit of personal goals. Specifically, we focus on the interplay of child individual processes (such as the child's motivation and fear of pain) and parent factors (such as parent expectations and anxiety) in the pursuit of goal achievement that results in approach or avoidance of activities. In this review, we describe the work to date that has investigated goal pursuit, importance, and frustration within the context of pediatric chronic pain/illness. Next, we propose a new conceptual model that integrates this research. Finally, we suggest next steps for future research on this topic.

2. An Overview of Goals, Goal Achievement, and Goal Frustration

Goals, defined by Austin and Vancouver [17], are "internal representations of desired states, where states are broadly construed as outcomes, events, or processes" (p. 338). Goals can be short or long-term and can pertain to any area such as academics, social, and sporting. Some goals may transcend health and illness; however, chronic pain may lead to a re-prioritization of goals, the creation of new goals, or the termination of existing goals.

When pain is experienced, some goals may become unattainable. For example, a painful limb due to a fracture may prevent a child from taking part in a sports tournament. When pain persists, the consequences may include a lack of attainment of the child's short-term and long-term goals. For example, pain may prevent regular attendance at school, impacting later educational attainment. Research in adults has suggested that giving up unattainable goals can be positive for mental health outcomes [18]; however, it is unknown when it is appropriate or desirable for children to "give up" their goals, even if deemed unattainable or difficult to attain. Nevertheless, the conflict between having pain and wanting to engage in desired activities is not well understood in this field and is central to developing effective treatment strategies to motivate young people to pursue goal-directed activities despite their pain.

Experiencing pain for a long period of time can lead to goal frustration, regardless of goal importance. Two studies have investigated goal frustration in youth with chronic pain, one including youth with and without headaches [19] and one including youth with and without musculoskeletal pain [20]. In both studies, youth rated goal importance and frustration on six categories including personal values, social acceptance, self-acceptance, school, health, and self-development. In a study by Massey, Garnefski and Gebhardt [19], youth with weekly headaches allocated a higher importance to personal goals (e.g., treating others fairly and having a good relationship with parents) compared with those without headaches. Goal importance did not differ for other categories (e.g., social acceptance, self-acceptance, school, and health). Adolescents with weekly headaches reported higher frustration on social- and self-acceptance, school, and health goals compared with adolescents without headaches. However, adolescents with weekly headaches did not report higher frustration for personal goals compared to those without headaches.

Stommen, Verbunt, and Goossens [20] similarly found no significant differences in how adolescents allocated the importance of goals between those with and without musculoskeletal pain. However, adolescents with musculoskeletal pain reported higher frustration with goals pertaining to personal values, social acceptance, self-acceptance, and health compared with adolescents without musculoskeletal pain. In both studies, increased goal frustration was associated with higher depression and lower quality of life [19,20]. These findings suggest that, while there are few differences in adolescent perceptions of goal importance, there seems to be a relationship between higher goal frustration and poorer well-being. However, it is unknown whether frustration is associated with a lower pursuit of goals, or whether it encourages adolescents to strive more persistently towards their goals. More likely, other individual differences will predict the pursuit or avoidance of these goals.

Goals have a specific context that is important to understand. There are often multiple, competing, and conflicting goals that must be weighed by the individual in determining their action toward those goals. In a study with 170 adolescents from a community sample, Fisher et al. [21] investigated conflicting goals. Adolescents were asked to report their likelihood of approaching or avoiding situations where pain conflicted with a goal (e.g., having a headache but wanting to meet up with friends). Vignettes described either high (the headache is very painful) or low (the headache is quite mild) pain intensity situations. Afterwards, adolescents were asked to report the personal importance they ascribed to each goal described in the vignettes. Results showed that activities with a higher goal importance were more likely to be approached. However, individuals who had higher levels of pain anxiety were more likely to avoid high pain intensity situations even if the goal was very important to them. General anxiety was also assessed, but this was not a significant predictor of avoidance, suggesting that pain-specific anxiety may more directly influence goal engagement.

Although adolescence is a time of increasing emotional and behavioral autonomy and separateness from parents [22], parents are still important role models and their communication and modeling are critical in the context of chronic pain. Chronic pain has a bi-directional impact on parents, as proposed in the integrated parent and family model. Specifically, this model outlines that the individual child characteristics lie within broader dyadic and family level factors that influence a child's experience of pain and associated disability [23]. Parents of youth with chronic pain report a higher burden of parenting, higher emotional distress, and lower social functioning when their child has chronic pain [22,24]. However, specific parenting behaviors and modeling also influence a child's interpretation of pain and pain-related behaviors [25]. Some parent behaviors have been associated with poorer child adaptation to chronic pain, such as communicating too much about pain to their child, catastrophizing about their child's pain, modeling illness behaviors, or any combination of these. For example, parents who reported higher levels of catastrophizing were more likely to stop their child from doing a task earlier than parents with lower catastrophizing [26]. Moreover, a relationship has been demonstrated between parents' higher degree of attending behaviors toward their child's pain and higher levels of child symptom complaints, disability, and depression [25,27].

Parents can be a source of support and motivation when their child is striving for their desired goals. Research in children with diabetes has found that parents who supported their children in their treatment were more likely to reach their blood glucose targets compared with those children whose parents did not [28]. Similarly, Fisher et al. [29] found in a self-management cognitive-behavioral therapy intervention for youth with chronic pain and their parents that dyads who chose matching goals (i.e., identical goal content) at the start of treatment were more likely to report lower pain intensity post-treatment and at follow-up. In particular, dyads with identical physical activity goals were more likely to have lower pain intensity at post-treatment and follow-up were comparable to those dyads who selected less physically active goals or did not agree on goal content.

Within the context of pain, most prior research investigating goals has been conducted within adult populations. These studies found that pain severity and catastrophizing about pain consistently predicted task interference [30] and that fear of pain mediated associations between goal self-efficacy/conflict and depression/disability in adults with chronic low back pain [31]. Other research has proposed theoretical models of problem-solving during goal pursuit [32]. This model proposes that worry is a key psychological factor in problem-solving around chronic pain.

Further, there have been several adaptations of the fear avoidance model using a motivational perspective to understand adults with chronic pain [32–35]. An updated fear-avoidance model incorporating the role of goals has been published [36]. This model predicts that pain can be either high or low threat to an individual, who will then choose to engage valued life goals or pain control goals. When priority is given to valued goals, this leads to approach behaviors and then recovery. When priority is given to pain control goals, it is predicted that this leads to the fear, avoidance, and disability pathway of the fear avoidance model [36]. Investigations into valued goals vs. pain control goals have been explored in adults [37,38], but not in children. The model proposed by Vlaeyen, Crombez, and Linton [36] is the first to explicitly incorporate goals within the fear avoidance model; however, it does not account for the developmental context (i.e., parent factors and developmentally relevant child factors) that is important to understanding chronic pain and goal pursuit in children and adolescents. There is also research within the context of chronic illnesses theorizing goal pursuit and health behavior change [39,40]. However, our model presented here differs from other models in the field as we focus specifically on factors that might promote or inhibit goal pursuit when children experience pain, rather than using goal pursuit to understand disability or to describe behavior change, goal setting, or other related process.

3. Description of a New Goal Pursuit Model for Pediatric Chronic Pain

We propose a new goal pursuit model for pediatric chronic pain (Figure 1), which incorporates the child's pain experience, child and parent factors, and goal pursuit behaviors. The child's pain experience is moderated by both child and parent responses to pain, which accumulatively influences goal pursuit behavior. In our proposed model, the child is placed within the broader context of the parent, consistent with a social-environmental framework. Here, we focus on the factors that could inhibit or encourage goal pursuit behavior in youth with chronic pain.

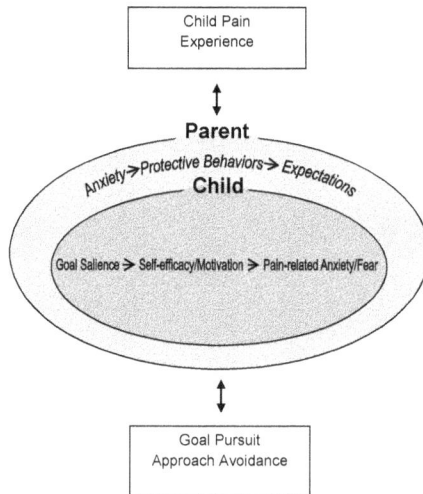

Figure 1. Goal Pursuit Model of Pediatric Chronic Pain.

3.1. Child's Pain Experience

The child's experience of pain is presented as the first step in our model. Definitions of chronic pain in children and adolescents are focused only on the length of time that the child has experienced the pain (i.e., longer than three months [2]). However, many other factors are important to consider about the pain experience such as the child's perceived intensity/severity of pain, amount of interference, pain frequency, as well as pain duration. The child's experience of their pain may directly influence whether they engage or avoid a specific goal. Perceptions of more intense or worse pain experiences are more likely to lead to avoidance of goals, compared with less severe pain experiences, as demonstrated in the vignette study conducted by Fisher et al. [41]. However, as shown in Figure 1, the pain experience of the child is also likely to interact with child and parent factors and thus influence goal pursuit behaviors.

3.2. Child Factors

Three individual child factors are highlighted in the model including goal salience, self-efficacy/motivation, and pain-related anxiety/fear. Goal saliency, which describes the importance that a child or adolescent allocates to a goal may directly influence motivation toward goal engagement. Goals will differ in salience for each child and may also be context-dependent. Goals with higher salience are more likely to be motivationally pursued and therefore approached compared with those goals that are less salient. However, even if a goal is deemed salient, high pain anxiety or low self-efficacy may influence the child's pursuit of the goal. Higher levels of pain intensity have also been associated with lower motivation in this population, which may translate into the child avoiding a goal despite having a high level of personal importance (e.g., seeing friends). Of course, goal salience and pain experience may conflict, meaning that, even though a child wants to pursue a goal, pain severity may inhibit goal engagement.

Self-efficacy, or one's belief in their ability to manage pain, may also be an important individual factor that influences goal pursuit behaviors. Self-efficacy has been studied more frequently in adults with chronic pain, finding consistently that higher self-efficacy is associated with lower levels of disability, distress, and pain severity in a review of 86 studies [42]. Although only a few studies assessing self-efficacy have been conducted in youth with chronic pain, patterns are similar; higher self-efficacy was associated with lower pain intensity [43] and better school functioning, lower disability, and lower depression in youth with chronic headaches [44]. Although there is limited pediatric research on self-efficacy, we predict that higher levels of self-efficacy are more likely to be associated with engagement of goals.

Even if goals are salient and the child has a high level of motivation and self-efficacy, the child's pain anxiety or fear of pain may inhibit goal pursuit and lead to avoidance behaviors. Since the publication of the fear avoidance model [14], a plethora of research has been conducted to show the association between pain intensity, pain anxiety, fear of pain, and disability. Research has demonstrated that higher levels of pain anxiety and fear of pain increase avoidance behaviors when in pain [13,45–47]. In addition, adolescents with higher pain anxiety were likely to avoid activities despite rating goals as important [41]. Pain anxiety/fear of pain may moderate the relationship between goal salience and goal pursuit behaviors.

There are likely many other individual child factors such as neurobiological factors that may also moderate a child's pain experience and therefore their goal pursuit engagement or avoidance behaviors. However, we chose to focus on several child psychosocial factors that have received research attention and could be specifically targeted in psychological interventions for pediatric chronic pain and disability.

3.3. Parent Factors

The influence of parents on the child's goal pursuit behaviors is critical in a developmentally informed model of childhood chronic pain. Parent factors will influence child factors directly, and any goal pursuit behavior will be a conflict or balance between child and parent factors, and the pain experience.

Parent anxiety, including worry and catastrophizing about their child's pain has been found to be associated with maladaptive behaviors, such as protectiveness and modeling of illness behaviors [48,49]. Children with chronic pain, whose parents report higher anxiety and are more protective, are also more likely to report higher levels of anxiety and disability [49–51]. Similarly, parents who report higher catastrophizing, which is comprised of magnification, rumination, and helplessness about their child's pain condition, are more likely to stop their child from engaging in activity when they have pain [26]. These parent factors have been associated with higher disability in children reporting chronic pain, and are likely to influence children's goal pursuit.

Parents with higher anxiety and protective behaviors are likely to reduce their expectations of their child. Parent expectations which are realistic of their child's abilities are predicted to increase goal approach. Unrealistic expectations such that expectations are set too high or too low are predicted to increase goal avoidance. For example, going to school may be of low salience to the child, but parent expectation may be appropriate and realistic. Such expectations may drive parent behaviors (i.e., reduced protectiveness behaviors) that support the likelihood of the child pursuing the goal. Chronic pain presents in variable ways and often children and those around them have to temporarily shift their expectations of what the child can achieve until pain intensity is manageable. Research to date has predominantly focused on maladaptive parent behaviors (rather than how positive behaviors can support children). For example, research has shown that when parents reduce their expectations considerably, such as excuse children from chores, fail to enforce school, and allow additional rest time, children experience increased pain-related disability [52]. We hypothesize that expectations from others are likely to influence goal salience, with realistic and positive expectations encouraging engagement of goals, while too low or too high expectations likely lead to the avoidance of goals.

3.4. Goal Pursuit

When faced with a goal conflict, the individuals' avoidance or engagement of goals is an observable and measurable behavior. Avoidance can be expressed as the delay of a goal or the termination of the goal such that the goal is not accomplished. Engagement, on the other hand, can be expressed in terms of the extent of involvement in or accomplishment of the goal (i.e., partial or full engagement). After pursuing a goal, the child may experience direct or indirect consequences. For example, when a child or adolescent engages with an activity to achieve a goal, they may experience increased pain intensity as a consequence, which may influence their goal pursuit behavior in the future. Equally, if the child or adolescent engages in goal behavior and experiences rewarding consequences, then they may be more likely to engage in this behavior in the future. Each child will weigh the risk–benefit ratio of rewards to consequences differently. As documented by the fear avoidance model, avoidance is strongly associated with higher pain-related disability in this population. However, there is little research on the positive impact of engagement behaviors and how to promote these behaviors in youth with chronic pain. It is likely that engagement behaviors reduce pain intensity, anxiety, and depression and promote social interaction and normal functioning. However, engagement behaviors are not synonymous with positive outcomes and equally, avoidance behaviors may not be a proxy for disability. Indeed, in studies of adults with chronic pain, the engagement and persistence of activities has been linked to higher pain intensity [53]. Research investigating the consequences of goal pursuit is likely to be complex and involve dynamic processes that may change over the course of a child's pain condition.

4. Future Directions

We present a new social-environmental model of goal pursuit behavior in order to advance research on understanding children's and parent's responses to chronic pain and potential strategies to promote engagement behaviors and return to normal functioning. In particular, we identified three areas in the model that are important to understand. First, research is needed to understand what inhibits and motivates important goals for youth with chronic pain, apart from the pain context itself. Child and parent factors outlined in the model are suggested as a starting point. For example, relevant research questions are whether parent protectiveness or expectations influence the pursuit of salient goals; how much motivation is needed for a child to approach a goal instead of avoid it; and whether there are associations between self-efficacy, the child's pain experience, and their goal pursuit behaviors. Further exploration of the interaction between child and parent factors will provide a more comprehensive understanding of children's goal-driven behavior in the context of chronic pain. Further, more research is needed to determine whether approach and avoidance behaviors lead to negative or positive outcomes for this population. As discussed previously, engagement can lead to higher pain and disability in adults [53], but this has not been studied in youth. Similarly, identifying whether goals are realistic or have been "given up" by youth may also be important within the context of approaching and avoiding. Goals can be both short- and long-term, and we do not differentiate between these in our model. Frequent everyday activity may be both a short-term goal to stay active, but also a long-term goal to have good physical conditioning. However, youth may not always recognize long-term goals, or that immediate actions may lead to the attainment of long-term goals.

Second, research investigating goal conflict is important in order to understand the tipping balance between engagement and avoidance of goals when experiencing pain. There is emerging research in adults using experimental methods of pain and altering goals using monetary rewards to investigate this question [38,54]. Within pediatrics, vignettes have been used to understand goal conflict and approach–avoidance behaviors in healthy youth [41]. However, little research has been conducted with youth with chronic pain on goal conflict to understand whether youth with chronic pain have frequent goal conflict and how they attempt to resolve it. Studies might employ experimental methodologies or ecological momentary assessment to investigate situations where high pain intensity conflicts with highly salient goals and to determine which individual factors predict engagement or avoidance.

Third, psychological therapies for youth with chronic pain could be developed or refined to reduce goal frustration and conflict and to aid problem solving when a goal cannot be engaged. Factors outlined in the Goal Pursuit model could be targeted. For example, treatments could target increasing children's self-efficacy and motivation, which we predict will increase the likelihood of goal engagement. Strategies could also employ already established strategies to decrease pain-related anxiety and general anxiety [55], which may in turn reduce goal pursuit barriers. Parent factors are also crucial to address, and treatments are increasingly including parent interventions to improve communication, coping skills, and parenting behaviors [56]. Parent treatments have recently been piloted for this population and have shown benefit for reducing parent distress as well as positive but preliminary "downward" effects for improving children's emotional functioning [57]. So far, the active ingredients that lead to change within these psychological treatments are unknown; a more frequent use of conceptual models such as the one proposed here to design and evaluate treatments could enhance understanding and inform modifications to enhance the effectiveness of these therapies.

Another avenue of investigation is goal setting within the context of psychological or other pain management treatments. Within cognitive behavioral treatments, therapists may set goals directly with children and parents and may encourage parents to appropriately support the chosen goal and even provide a reward system for reaching targeted goals. As discussed, parents may be particularly important in supporting youth in reaching their goals by providing encouragement and setting behavioral expectations consistent with engagement. There is some evidence to suggest that treatment goals are more effective if mutually agreed between parent and teen [29]. However, further research is needed to explore the content of goals as well as their salience in children and their parents entering treatment to understand their potential influence on treatment engagement and outcomes.

Finally, our model is not exhaustive of all factors that could be investigated when considering goal pursuit. We have specifically targeted psychosocial factors in our conceptualization of goal pursuit, but there are other neurobiological factors (e.g., sex, genetics, and cognition) that may also be important to consider.

5. Conclusions

In summary, we propose a new model of goal pursuit in pediatric chronic pain to guide research and clinical assessment of children's responses to chronic pain. This model offers a broader perspective on youth engagement versus avoidance of activities among youth who are actively seeking goals despite their pain. A more complete understanding of child and parent factors that influence goal pursuit and goal salience is needed to further advance and motivate treatment development to enhance the effectiveness of psychological treatments for youth with chronic pain.

Acknowledgments: This work was supported by the National Institutes of Health (Grant: K24HD060068).

Author Contributions: E.F. conceived the ideas included in the manuscript in collaboration with T.P., E.F. wrote the first draft of, and edited, the manuscript. T.P. edited drafts of the manuscript and approved it for submission.

Conflicts of Interest: The authors declare no conflict of interest.

References

1. King, S.; Chambers, C.T.; Huguet, A.; MacNevin, R.C.; McGrath, P.J.; Parker, L.; MacDonald, A.J. The epidemiology of chronic pain in children and adolescents revisited: A systematic review. *Pain* **2011**, *152*, 2729–2738. [CrossRef] [PubMed]
2. Merskey, H.; Bogduk, N. *Classification of Chronic Pain: Descriptions of Chronic Pain Syndromes and Definitions of Pain Terms*; IASP Press: Seattle, WA, USA, 1994.
3. Huguet, A.; Miró, J. The severity of chronic pediatric pain: An epidemiological study. *J. Pain* **2008**, *9*, 226–236. [CrossRef] [PubMed]
4. Walker, L.S.; Dengler-Crish, C.M.; Rippel, S.; Bruehl, S. Functional abdominal pain in childhood and adolescence increases risk for chronic pain in adulthood. *Pain* **2010**, *150*, 568–572. [CrossRef] [PubMed]
5. Kashikar-Zuck, S.; Cunningham, N.; Sil, S.; Bromberg, M.H.; Lynch-Jordan, A.M.; Strotman, D.; Peugh, J.; Noll, J.; Ting, T.V.; Powers, S.W.; et al. Long-term outcomes of adolescents with juvenile-onset fibromyalgia in early adulthood. *Pediatrics* **2014**, *133*, e592–e600. [CrossRef] [PubMed]
6. Forgeron, P.A.; Evans, J.; McGrath, P.J.; Stevens, B.; Finley, G.A. Living with difference: Exploring the social self of adolescents with chronic pain. *Pain Res. Manag.* **2013**, *18*, e115–e123. [CrossRef] [PubMed]
7. Gauntlett-Gilbert, J.; Eccleston, C. Disability in adolescents with chronic pain: Patterns and predictors across different domains of functioning. *Pain* **2007**, *131*, 132–141. [CrossRef] [PubMed]
8. Logan, D.E.; Simons, L.E.; Stein, M.J.; Chastain, L. School impairment in adolescents with chronic pain. *J. Pain* **2008**, *9*, 407–416. [CrossRef] [PubMed]
9. Kaczynski, K.J.; Simons, L.E.; Claar, R.L. Anxiety, coping, and disability: A test of mediation in a pediatric chronic pain sample. *J. Pediatr. Psychol.* **2011**, *36*, 932–941. [CrossRef] [PubMed]
10. Cohen, L.L.; Vowles, K.E.; Eccleston, C. The impact of adolescent chronic pain on functioning: Disentangling the complex role of anxiety. *J. Pain* **2010**, *11*, 1039–1046. [CrossRef] [PubMed]
11. Kashikar-Zuck, S.; Parkins, I.S.; Graham, T.B.; Lynch, A.M.; Passo, M.; Johnston, M.; Schikler, K.N.; Hashkes, P.J.; Banez, G.; Richards, M.M. Anxiety, mood, and behavioral disorders among pediatric patients with juvenile fibromyalgia syndrome. *Clin. J. Pain* **2008**, *24*, 620–626. [CrossRef] [PubMed]
12. Walker, L.S.; Smith, C.A.; Garber, J.; Claar, R.L. Appraisal and coping with daily stressors by pediatric patients with chronic abdominal pain. *J. Pediatr. Psychol.* **2007**, *32*, 206–216. [CrossRef] [PubMed]
13. Simons, L.E.; Kaczynski, K.J. The fear avoidance model of chronic pain: Examination for pediatric application. *J. Pain* **2012**, *13*, 827–835. [CrossRef] [PubMed]

14. Vlaeyen, J.W.S.; Linton, S.J. Fear-avoidance and its consequences in chronic musculoskeletal pain: A state of the art. *Pain* **2000**, *85*, 317–332. [CrossRef]
15. Caes, L.; Fisher, E.; Clinch, J.; Tobias, J.H.; Eccleston, C. The role of pain-related anxiety in adolescents' disability and social impairment: Alspac data. *Eur. J. Pain* **2015**, *19*, 842–851. [CrossRef] [PubMed]
16. Perquin, C.W.; Hazebroek-Kampschreur, A.A.J.M.; Hunfeld, J.A.; Bohnen, A.M.; van Suijlekom-Smit, L.W.A.; Passchier, J.; van der Wouden, J.C. Pain in children and adolescents: A common experience. *Pain* **2000**, *87*, 51–58. [CrossRef]
17. Austin, J.T.; Vancouver, J.B. Goal constructs in psychology: Structure, process, and content. *Psychol. Bull.* **1996**, *120*, 338–375. [CrossRef]
18. Wrosch, C.; Miller, G.E.; Scheier, M.F.; De Pontet, S.B. Giving up on unattainable goals: Benefits for health? *Personal. Soc. Psychol. Bull.* **2007**, *33*, 251–265. [CrossRef] [PubMed]
19. Massey, E.K.; Garnefski, N.; Gebhardt, W.A. Goal frustration, coping and well-being in the context of adolescent headache: A self-regulation approach. *Eur. J. Pain* **2009**, *13*, 977–984. [CrossRef] [PubMed]
20. Stommen, N.C.; Verbunt, J.A.; Goossens, M.E. Future goals of adolescents and young adults with chronic musculoskeletal pain. *Eur. J. Pain* **2016**, *20*, 564–572. [CrossRef] [PubMed]
21. Fisher, E.; Keogh, E.; Eccleston, C. Adolescents' approach-avoidance behaviour in the context of pain. *Pain* **2016**, *157*, 370–376. [CrossRef] [PubMed]
22. Palermo, T.M.; Valrie, C.R.; Karlson, C.W. Family and parent influences on pediatric chronic pain: A developmental perspective. *Am. Psychol.* **2014**, *69*, 142–152. [CrossRef] [PubMed]
23. Palermo, T.M.; Chambers, C.T. Parent and family factors in pediatric chronic pain and disability: An integrative approach. *Pain* **2005**, *119*, 1–4. [CrossRef] [PubMed]
24. Jordan, A.L.; Eccleston, C.; Osborn, M. Being a parent of the adolescent with complex chronic pain: An interpretative phenomenological analysis. *Eur. J. Pain* **2007**, *11*, 49. [CrossRef] [PubMed]
25. Walker, L.S.; Williams, S.E.; Smith, C.A.; Garber, J.; Van Slyke, D.A.; Lipani, T.A. Parent attention versus distraction: Impact on symptom complaints by children with and without chronic functional abdominal pain. *Pain* **2006**, *122*, 43–52. [CrossRef] [PubMed]
26. Caes, L.; Vervoort, T.; Eccleston, C.; Vandenhende, M.; Goubert, L. Parental catastrophizing about child's pain and its relationship with activity restriction: The mediating role of parental distress. *Pain* **2011**, *152*, 212–222. [CrossRef] [PubMed]
27. Claar, R.L.; Simons, L.E.; Logan, D.E. Parental response to children's pain: The moderating impact of children's emotional distress on symptoms and disability. *Pain* **2008**, *138*, 172–179. [CrossRef] [PubMed]
28. Grey, M.; Davidson, M.; Boland, E.A.; Tamborlane, W.V. Clinical and psychosocial factors associated with achievement of treatment goals in adolescents with diabetes mellitus. *J. Adolesc. Health* **2001**, *28*, 377–385. [CrossRef]
29. Fisher, E.; Bromberg, M.; Tai, G.; Palermo, T.M. Adolescent and parent treatment goals in an internet delivered chronic pain self-management program: Does agreement of treatment goals matter? *J. Pediatr. Psychol.* **2016**, in press.
30. Karoly, P.; Ruehlman, L.S. Psychosocial aspects of pain-related life task interference: An exploratory analysis in a general population sample. *Pain Med.* **2007**, *8*, 563–572. [CrossRef] [PubMed]
31. Karoly, P.; Okun, M.A.; Ruehlman, L.S.; Pugliese, J.A. The impact of goal cognition and pain severity on disability and depression in adults with chronic pain: An examination of direct effects and mediated effects via pain-induced fear. *Cogn. Ther. Res.* **2008**, *32*, 418–433. [CrossRef]
32. Eccleston, C.; Crombez, G. Worry and chronic pain: A misdirected problem solving model. *Pain* **2007**, *132*, 233–236. [CrossRef] [PubMed]
33. Crombez, G.; Eccleston, C.; Van Damme, S.; Vlaeyen, J.W.S.; Karoly, P. Fear-avoidance model of chronic pain: The next generation. *Clin. J. Pain* **2012**, *28*, 475–483. [CrossRef] [PubMed]
34. Van Damme, S.; Crombez, G.; Eccleston, C. Coping with pain: A motivational perspective. *Pain* **2008**, *139*, 1–4. [CrossRef] [PubMed]
35. Van Damme, S.; Kindermans, H. A self-regulation perspective on avoidance and persistence behavior in chronic pain: New theories, new challenges? *Clin. J. Pain* **2015**, *31*, 115–122. [CrossRef] [PubMed]

36. Vlaeyen, J.W.S.; Crombez, G.; Linton, S.J. The fear-avoidance model of pain. *Pain* **2016**, *157*, 1588–1589. [CrossRef] [PubMed]
37. Schrooten, M.G.S.; Wiech, K.; Vlaeyen, J.W.S. When pain meets . . . Pain-related choice behavior and pain perception in different goal conflict situations. *J. Pain* **2014**, *15*, 1166–1178. [CrossRef] [PubMed]
38. Van Damme, S.; Van Ryckeghem, D.M.; Wyffels, F.; Van Hulle, L.; Crombez, G. No pain no gain? Pursuing a competing goal inhibits avoidance behavior. *Pain* **2012**, *153*, 800–804. [CrossRef] [PubMed]
39. Maes, S.; Karoly, P. Self-regulation assessment and intervention in physical health and illness: A review. *Appl. Psychol.* **2005**, *54*, 267–299. [CrossRef]
40. Schwarzer, R.; Lippke, S.; Luszczynska, A. Mechanisms of health behavior change in persons with chronic illness or disability: The health action process approach (HAPA). *Rehabil. Psychol.* **2011**, *56*, 161–170. [CrossRef] [PubMed]
41. Fisher, E.; Caes, L.; Clinch, J.; Tobias, J.H.; Eccleston, C. Anxiety at 13 and its effect on pain, pain-related anxiety, and pain-related disability at 17: An ALSPAC cohort longitudinal analysis. *Psychol. Health Med.* **2016**, *21*, 1–9. [CrossRef] [PubMed]
42. Jackson, T.; Wang, Y.; Wang, Y.; Fan, H. Self-efficacy and chronic pain outcomes: A meta-analytic review. *J. Pain* **2014**, *15*, 800–814. [CrossRef] [PubMed]
43. Carpino, E.; Segal, S.; Logan, D.; Lebel, A.; Simons, L.E. The interplay of pain-related self-efficacy and fear on functional outcomes among youth with headache. *J. Pain* **2014**, *15*, 527–534. [CrossRef] [PubMed]
44. Kalapurakkel, S.; Carpino, E.A.; Lebel, A.; Simons, L.E. "Pain can't stop me": Examining pain self-efficacy and acceptance as resilience processes among youth with chronic headache. *J. Pediatr. Psychol.* **2015**, *40*, 926–933. [CrossRef] [PubMed]
45. Tran, S.T.; Jastrowski Mano, K.E.; Hainsworth, K.R.; Medrano, G.R.; Anderson Khan, K.; Weisman, S.J.; Davies, W.H. Distinct influences of anxiety and pain catastrophizing on functional outcomes in children and adolescents with chronic pain. *J. Pediatr. Psychol.* **2015**, *40*, 744–755. [CrossRef] [PubMed]
46. Vervoort, T.; Eccleston, C.; Goubert, L.; Buysse, A.; Crombez, G. Children's catastrophic thinking about their pain predicts pain and disability 6 months later. *Eur. J. Pain* **2010**, *14*, 90–96. [CrossRef] [PubMed]
47. Vervoort, T.; Goubert, L.; Eccleston, C.; Bijttebier, P.; Crombez, G. Catastrophic thinking about pain is independently associated with pain severity, disability, and somatic complaints in school children and children with chronic pain. *J. Pediatr. Psychol.* **2006**, *31*, 674–683. [CrossRef] [PubMed]
48. Caes, L.; Vervoort, T.; Devos, P.; Verlooy, J.; Benoit, Y.; Goubert, L. Parental distress and catastrophic thoughts about child pain: Implications for parental protective behavior in the context of child leukemia-related medical procedures. *Clin. J. Pain* **2014**, *30*, 787–799. [CrossRef] [PubMed]
49. Sieberg, C.B.; Williams, S.; Simons, L.E. Do parent protective responses mediate the relation between parent distress and child functional disability among children with chronic pain? *J. Pediatr. Psychol.* **2011**, *36*, 1043–1051. [CrossRef] [PubMed]
50. Guite, J.W.; McCue, R.L.; Sherker, J.L.; Sherry, D.D.; Rose, J.B. Relationships among pain, protective parental responses, and disability for adolescents with chronic musculoskeletal pain: The mediating role of pain catastrophizing. *Clin. J. Pain* **2011**, *27*, 775–781. [CrossRef] [PubMed]
51. Cunningham, N.R.; Lynch-Jordan, A.; Barnett, K.; Peugh, J.; Sil, S.; Goldschneider, K.; Kashikar-Zuck, S. Child pain catastrophizing mediates the relation between parent responses to pain and disability in youth with functional abdominal pain. *J. Pediatr. Gastroenterol. Nutr.* **2014**, *59*, 732–738. [CrossRef] [PubMed]
52. Lipani, T.A.; Walker, L.S. Children's appraisal and coping with pain: Relation to maternal ratings of worry and restriction in family activities. *J. Pediatr. Psychol.* **2006**, *31*, 667–673. [CrossRef] [PubMed]
53. Hasenbring, M.I.; Hallner, D.; Klasen, B.; Streitlein-Bohme, I.; Willburger, R.; Rusche, H. Pain-related avoidance versus endurance in primary care patients with subacute back pain: Psychological characteristics and outcome at a 6-month follow-up. *Pain* **2012**, *153*, 211–217. [CrossRef] [PubMed]
54. Claes, N.; Crombez, G.; Vlaeyen, J.W.S. Pain-avoidance versus reward-seeking: An experimental investigation. *Pain* **2015**, *156*, 1449–1457. [CrossRef] [PubMed]
55. James, A.C.; James, G.; Cowdrey, F.A.; Soler, A.; Choke, A. Cognitive behavioural therapy for anxiety disorders in children and adolescents. In *Cochrane Database of Systematic Reviews*; John Wiley & Sons, Ltd.: Hoboken, NJ, USA, 2015.

56. Palermo, T.M.; Law, E.F.; Fales, J.; Bromberg, M.H.; Jessen-Fiddick, T.; Tai, G. Internet-delivered cognitive-behavioral treatment for adolescents with chronic pain and their parents: A randomized controlled multicenter trial. *Pain* **2016**, *157*, 174–185. [CrossRef] [PubMed]
57. Palermo, T.M.; Law, E.F.; Essner, B.; Jessen-Fiddick, T.; Eccleston, C. Adaptation of problem-solving skills training (PSST) for parent caregivers of youth with chronic pain. *Clin. Pract. Pediatr. Psychol.* **2014**, *2*, 212–223. [CrossRef] [PubMed]

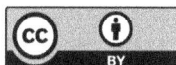

children MDPI

Review

Mental Health Comorbidities in Pediatric Chronic Pain: A Narrative Review of Epidemiology, Models, Neurobiological Mechanisms and Treatment

Jillian Vinall [1], Maria Pavlova [2], Gordon J. G. Asmundson [3], Nivez Rasic [1] and Melanie Noel [2,4,*]

[1] Department of Anesthesia, University of Calgary, Calgary, AB T3B 6A8, Canada; jillian.vinall@ahs.ca (J.V.); nivez.rasic@ahs.ca (N.R.)
[2] Department of Psychology, University of Calgary, Calgary, AB T2N 1N4, Canada; mpavlova@ucalgary.ca
[3] Department of Psychology, University of Regina, Regina, SK S4S 0A2, Canada; Gordon.Asmundson@uregina.ca
[4] Division of Behaviour and the Developing Brain, Alberta Children's Hospital Research Institute, Calgary, AB T3B 6A8, Canada
* Correspondence: melanie.noel@ucalgary.ca; Tel.: +1-403-955-7969

Academic Editor: Sari A. Acra
Received: 15 September 2016; Accepted: 21 November 2016; Published: 2 December 2016

Abstract: Chronic pain during childhood and adolescence can lead to persistent pain problems and mental health disorders into adulthood. Posttraumatic stress disorders and depressive and anxiety disorders are mental health conditions that co-occur at high rates in both adolescent and adult samples, and are linked to heightened impairment and disability. Comorbid chronic pain and psychopathology has been explained by the presence of shared neurobiology and mutually maintaining cognitive-affective and behavioral factors that lead to the development and/or maintenance of both conditions. Particularly within the pediatric chronic pain population, these factors are embedded within the broader context of the parent–child relationship. In this review, we will explore the epidemiology of, and current working models explaining, these comorbidities. Particular emphasis will be made on shared neurobiological mechanisms, given that the majority of previous research to date has centered on cognitive, affective, and behavioral mechanisms. Parental contributions to co-occurring chronic pain and psychopathology in childhood and adolescence will be discussed. Moreover, we will review current treatment recommendations and future directions for both research and practice. We argue that the integration of biological and behavioral approaches will be critical to sufficiently address why these comorbidities exist and how they can best be targeted in treatment.

Keywords: chronic pain; posttraumatic stress disorder; anxiety; depression; neurobiology; stress; brain; comorbidity; parent; intervention

1. Introduction

Chronic pain, defined as pain occurring constantly or frequently for 3 months or more, is very prevalent in adolescence [1] and poses high costs to society ($11.8 billion/year) [2]. Poorly managed pain in childhood can lead to persistent pain problems and mental health disorders into adulthood [3,4]. In a longitudinal study, youth with chronic abdominal pain were found to be at greater risk of developing anxiety and depressive disorders as compared to youth without chronic pain [3,5]. Importantly, the risk of anxiety and depressive disorders were higher than controls regardless of whether or not chronic pain persisted into adulthood, suggesting that chronic pain in adolescence heightens the risk of developing mental health disorders, even when pain resolves [5]. Epidemiological research also suggests that youth with chronic pain have higher rates of anxiety disorders in adulthood [4]. This provides compelling evidence that youth with chronic pain are at risk for having and developing mental health conditions. Nevertheless, there remains limited understanding of the mechanisms associated with these comorbid mental health disorders that might impact children's response to pain and pain treatment.

The co-occurrence of chronic pain and mental health conditions (i.e., posttraumatic stress disorder (PTSD)), anxiety and depressive disorders) is high, and has been explained by the presence of shared neurobiology (e.g., genes, hormones, brain networks) and mutually maintaining cognitive (e.g., attention and memory biases) and behavioral (e.g., sleep disturbance) factors that lead to the development and/or maintenance of both conditions [6–8]. However, existing interventions generally fail to effectively target co-morbid mental health disorders and underlying mechanisms that maintain both conditions [9]. It is becoming increasingly clear that there is a need for treatments of pediatric chronic pain to move away from the "one-size-fits-all" approach, which may not sufficiently help a substantial portion of youth with mental health co-morbidities. Indeed, treatment effects for psychological therapies for pediatric chronic pain have generally been small [10], which could be due to heterogeneity within pediatric samples in terms of these underlying mental health conditions. It has been suggested that by increasing our understanding of the genetic and neurobiological mechanisms underlying these comorbidities, we may be able to better predict trajectories of pain and tailor interventional strategies [11]. Moreover, particularly in youth, one cannot underestimate the interaction and influence of the environment (e.g., the parents' influence) on children's pain and mental health conditions.

This review will explore the epidemiology of mental health disorders in pediatric chronic pain populations, and present current working models that have been put forth to explain this comorbidity. Given that the vast majority of work on this topic has emphasized cognitive, affective, and behavioral mechanisms, we will highlight recent research investigating the shared neurobiological mechanisms that may underlie these comorbidities. Parental contributions to comorbid chronic pain and psychopathology in childhood will also be discussed. Finally, we will discuss current treatment recommendations and future directions for both research and practice. Given the high prevalence [1], large economic burden [12], and sometimes debilitating nature of pediatric chronic pain on physical and mental health [13] that can persist into adulthood [4], identifying and modifying mechanisms underlying these conditions has powerful implications for preventing adult-onset chronic pain and mental health disorders.

2. Epidemiology of Internalizing Mental Health Disorders in Pediatric Chronic Pain Population

2.1. Longitudinal Studies of Pediatric Chronic Pain and Internalizing Mental Health Issues in Adulthood

Evidence demonstrating the comorbidity of chronic pain and mental health disorders is accumulating (Table 1). One of the seminal epidemiological studies examining the co-occurrence of pediatric chronic pain and psychiatric disorders was undertaken by Hotopf et al. [5]. The 1946 birth cohort, followed for over two decades examined the relationship between chronic abdominal pain in childhood and medically unexplained symptoms, and mental health disorders in adulthood. They found that while the presence of pediatric abdominal pain was not associated with physical symptoms in adulthood, the risk of developing a psychiatric disorder by the age of 36 years was higher in children who had recurrent abdominal pain versus those who did not [5]. A similar study reported recurrent headaches in childhood to be related to an increased risk of psychiatric morbidity and multiple physical symptoms at the age of 33 years [3]. Despite the reliance on maternal and self-report, and failure to use a conventional definition of chronic pain (e.g., that included pain frequency in addition to pain duration), these studies laid an important foundation for the field of pediatric pain. They provided evidence that while pediatric chronic pain may or may not persist into adulthood, it confers risk of developing mental health disorders in adulthood.

Table 1. Summary of epidemiological studies of internalizing mental health issues in youth with chronic pain.

Study	n	Design	Age (Year)	Assessment Time Points	Pain assessment	Internalizing Disorders/Symptoms Assessment	Findings
Longitudinal studies of pediatric chronic pain and internalizing mental health issues into adulthood							
Egger et al., 1998 [14]	1013	Longitudinal cohort study	5–15	Assessed annually over 3 years	CAPA somatization section	CAPA	40.8% of girls with depression reported headaches as compared to girls without depression (10.5%). 34.1% of girls with an anxiety disorder reported having headaches as compared with girls without an anxiety disorder (10%). 19.2% of boys with CD and 10% of boys with ODD reported having headaches as compared to boys without externalizing disorders (9.6%).
Egger et al., 1999 [15]	3733	Longitudinal cohort study	9–16	Assessed annually over 3 years	CAPA somatization section	CAPA	Girls with stomach aches (OR 7.2, CI 2.8–18.5) and musculoskeletal pain (OR 3.4, CI 1.5–8.0) were more likely to have anxiety as compared to pain-free girls. Boys with stomach aches were likely to have ODD (OR 3.6, CI 1.6–8.1) and ADHD (OR 3.5, CI 1.8–7.1) as compared to boys without stomach aches. Both girls (OR 12.9, CI 4.5–37.0) and boys (OR 10.5, CI 2.3–48.0) with musculoskeletal pain were more likely to report depression compared to children without musculoskeletal pain.
Hotopf et al., 1998 [5]	3637	Longitudinal cohort study	7–36	7, 11, 15 years old / 36 years old	Parent report of abdominal pain at ages 7, 11 and 15 years / Self-report of physical symptoms (back pain, headache, abdominal pain, chest pain, dizziness, and rheumatism)	N/A / Semi-structured psychiatric interview (Present State Examination)	Youth who had abdominal pain were more likely to develop a psychiatric disorder by Time 2 (OR 2.72, CI 1.65–4.49). Pain in childhood was not associated with heightened risk of physical symptoms in adulthood (OR 1.39, CI 0.83–2.36).
Fearon et al., 2001 [3]	11,407	Longitudinal cohort study	7–33	7, 11, 16, 23 years old / 33 years old	Parent report of headache at ages 7 and 11 (binary variable) / Self-report of physical symptoms (back pain, headache, twitches, rheumatism, indigestion, heart racing, worries about health)	Bristol Social Adjustment Guide / Presence of four or more symptoms on a psychiatric morbidity self-report scale	Youth suffering from frequent headaches were more likely to have recurrent headaches in adulthood (OR 2.22, CI 1.62–3.06), physical symptoms (OR 1.75, CI 1.46–2.10), and psychiatric disorders (OR 1.41, CI 1.20–1.66).
Walker et al., 2012 [16]	843	Longitudinal cohort study	12–21	12 years old / 21 years old	API, CSI / Rome III, PPQ	N/A / ADIS	At 21 years, participants with High Pain Dysfunctional profile were at a higher risk of having a pain-related FGID (OR 3.45, CI 1.95–6.11), FGID and non-abdominal chronic pain (OR 2.6, CI 1.45–4.66), FGID and anxiety or depressive disorder (OR 2.84, CI 1.35–6.00) as compared with Low Pain Adaptive profile participants.

Table 1. *Cont.*

Study	*n*	Design	Age (Year)	Assessment Time Points	Pain assessment	Internalizing Disorders/Symptoms Assessment	Findings
Longitudinal studies of pediatric chronic pain and internalizing mental health issues into adulthood							
Shelby et al., 2013 [4]	491	Longitudinal cohort study	8–21	8–17 years old	Vanderbilt Pediatric Gastroenterology Service evaluation of FAP	N/A	At follow-up, participants with FAP were more likely to meet criteria for lifetime (OR 4.9, CI 2.83–7.43) and current (OR 3.57, CI 2.00–6.36) anxiety disorder and lifetime depressive disorder (OR 2.62, CI 1.56–4.40) as compared to controls. Participants with FAP, who developed FGID by follow-up, were more likely to meet criteria for any lifetime (OR 7.31, CI 4.17–12.81) or current (OR 5.09, CI 2.70–9.59) anxiety disorder and any lifetime depressive disorder (OR 4.14, CI 2.31–7.40) as compared to controls. Participants with FAP, who have not met criteria for FGID by follow-up, were still more likely to have any lifetime (OR 3.36, CI 2.01–5.63) or current (OR 2.68, CI 1.44–4.99) anxiety disorder as compared to controls.
				4 years after initial assessment	Rome III	ADIS	
Shanahan et al., 2015 [17]	1420	Longitudinal cohort study	9–26	9–16 years old, assessed 4–7 times	Self- and parent-report of recurrent (at least one one-hour episode at least once a week in the past three months) pain (headache, abdominal or muscle pain)	CAPA	34.4% of children reported somatic complaints. Participants with somatic complaints were more likely to have depressive (OR 6.90, CI 3.57–13.34) or anxiety (OR2.75, CI 1.55–4.89) disorders in childhood versus pain-free peers. Children with somatic complaints in childhood were more likely to develop depressive (OR 3.21, CI 1.54–6.70) or any anxiety disorders (CI 2.32, CI 1.30–4.14) by young adulthood as compared to pain-free participants. Sex differences in the likelihood of developing psychiatric disorders in adulthood following somatic complaints in childhood were not revealed.
				19, 21, 24–26	Recurrent headache binomial variable within the YAPA	YAPA	
Noel et al., 2016 [18]	14,790	Longitudinal cohort study	12–32	Wave I and II: 12–18	Self-report general health survey—frequency of headache, stomach ache, muscle/joints pain. Chronic pain was defined as pain at wave I and/or wave II	N/A	21.9% of participants reported having chronic pain during adolescence. Youth with chronic pain reported higher rates of lifetime depressive (24.5%) and anxiety (21.1%) disorders versus youth without chronic pain. Chronic pain in youth was associated with a greater likelihood of having lifetime anxiety (OR 1.33, CI 1.09–1.63) and depressive (OR 1.38, CI 1.16–1.64) disorders.
				Wave IV: ages 24–32	N/A	Diagnosis of PTSD, anxiety, and/or depression by a health care provider	

Table 1. *Cont.*

Studies of co-occurring pediatric chronic pain and internalizing mental health issues

Study	n	Design	Age (Year)	Assessment Time Points	Pain assessment	Internalizing Disorders/Symptoms Assessment	Findings
Balottin et al., 2013 [19]	1124	Meta-analysis	Mean ages: 11.6 (migraine), 12.3 (tension-type headache), 11.75 controls	N/A	ICHD I or II	CBCL	Having tension-type headaches was associated with higher internalizing symptoms (Hedge's *g* = 2.344).
Blaauw et al., 2014 [20]	4872	Cross-sectional study	12–17	N/A	Headache interview assessing frequency of migraine, tension-type headache or unclassifiable headache over the last year	SCL-5	Recurrent headache of any type (migraine, tension-type) was associated with anxiety and depression symptoms (at the age of 12–14 years, OR 2.50, CI 1.61–2.61; at the age of 15–17 years, OR 1.64, CI 1.39–1.93).
Coffelt et al., 2013 [21]	3752	Retrospective cohort study	Mean age 13.54	N/A	Hospital record of chronic pain diagnoses (e.g., psychogenic pain not otherwise specified, chronic pain syndrome, complex regional pain syndrome)	Hospital record of a psychiatric diagnosis.	44% of youth with chronic pain have been diagnosed with a psychiatric condition, specifically, an affective (28%), anxiety (18%), somatization (6%) disorder or PTSD (2.4%).
Noel et al., 2016 [22]	195	Cross-sectional study	10–17	N/A	Self-report of pain characteristics (i.e., pain intensity, frequency, location, unpleasantness, and duration over the previous seven days); pain interference sub-scale of the PROMIS-25 Pediatric Profile	CPSS-5	32% of youth with chronic pain reported clinically significant PTSD symptoms as compared to 8% of pain-free peers. Parents of youth with chronic pain had higher levels of clinically significant PTSD symptoms (8%) as compared with parents' of youth without chronic pain (1%). Among the chronic pain group, PTSD symptoms were significantly associated with pain intensity, unpleasantness, interference, and quality of life.
Simons et al., 2012 [23]	655	Retrospective chart review	8–17	N/A	11-point NRS	RCMAS	11% of youth with chronic pain reported clinically significant levels of anxiety, 31% underreported their anxiety levels.
Tegethoff et al., 2015 [24]	6483	Cross-sectional study	13–18 years	N/A	Self-report chronic pain conditions checklist	CIDI; parent-report SAQ	25.93% of youth reported having chronic pain and mental health disorder in their lifetime. Any type or chronic pain increased the risk of developing eating (OR 2.63, CI 1.63–4.24), anxiety (OR 2.42, CI 2.03–2.88), affective (OR 2.32, CI 1.85–2.91), or any mental (OR 2.51, CI 2.12–2.98) disorder. The onset of any mental health disorder preceded any chronic pain (OR 1.64, CI 1.44–1.86).

ADHD: attention-deficit/hyperactivity disorder; ADIS: Anxiety Disorders Interview Schedule-IV, Adult Lifetime and Child and Parent Versions; API: Abdominal pain index; CAPA: Child and Adolescent Psychiatric Assessment; CBCL: Child Behavior Checklist; CD: conduct disorder; CI: confidence interval; CIDI: Composite International Diagnostic interview; CPSS-5: Child PTSD Symptom Scale; CSI: Children's Somatization Inventory; FAP: functional abdominal pain; FGID: functional gastrointestinal disorders; ICHD: International Classification of Headache Disorders; NRS: Numerical Rating Scale; ODD: oppositional defiant disorder; OR: odds ratio; PPQ: Persistent Pain Questionnaire; PROMIS-25: Patient-Reported Outcomes Measurement Information System; PTSD: posttraumatic stress disorder; Rome III: diagnostic questionnaire for functional gastrointestinal disorders; RCMAS: Revised Children's Manifest Anxiety Scale; SAQ: self-administered questionnaire; SCL-5: Symptom Checklist; YAPA: Young Adult Psychiatric Assessment.

Building upon these previous epidemiological studies, Walker et al. [16] conducted a longitudinal study of youth diagnosed with chronic abdominal pain followed into adulthood, at which time their pain and mental health status was assessed. The authors used cluster analysis to categorize youth with persistent abdominal pain into three groups based on pain ratings, gastrointestinal and non-gastrointestinal symptoms, beliefs about pain threat, pain coping efficacy, pain catastrophizing, negative affect and functional disability assessed in adolescence (i.e., Low Pain Adaptive, High Pain Adaptive, and High Pain Dysfunctional) [16]. Follow-up clinical interviews at the mean age of 21 years revealed that high pain ratings in conjunction with poorer coping skills and psychological functioning (i.e., characteristic of the High Pain Dysfunctional group) were associated with higher risk of developing functional gastrointestinal disorder (FGID) and non-abdominal chronic pain in adulthood [16]. The odds of having an anxiety or depressive disorder comorbid with FGID in adulthood were significantly higher only in the High Pain Dysfunctional group [16]. These findings provided further evidence of reciprocal relationships between pediatric chronic pain and mental health disorders. This study demonstrated for the first time that it is not pain per se but, rather, the combination of pain and psychological functioning that predicts the co-occurrence of pain and mental health disorders into adulthood. In a second investigation, Shelby et al. [4] examined the same cohort of youth with functional abdominal pain (FAP), as well as a pain-free controls whose mental health was assessed in adulthood. Fifty-one percent of youth with a childhood history of FAP developed an anxiety disorder over their lifetime, and 30% of youth had a current anxiety disorder at follow-up [4]. Depressive symptoms followed a different pattern; lifetime, but not current, risk of developing a depressive disorder was higher for individuals with chronic abdominal pain in childhood [4]. Risk of developing anxiety or depressive disorders was heightened for youth with chronic pain (versus controls) even when their pain resolved by adulthood. Temporal associations (based on retrospective recall) between mental health status and chronic pain suggested that anxiety disorders preceded the onset of chronic pain, whereas a depressive disorder followed it [4].

Recent data from a cohort study found that in a sample of 1420 youth, somatic complaints during childhood predicted generalized anxiety and depressive disorders at the age of 19–26 years [17]. Findings of the most recent epidemiological study by Noel et al. [18] revealed a consistent pattern. The study conducted a secondary data analysis of a sample of 14,790 individuals from the National Longitudinal Study of Adolescent to Adult Health to examine the co-occurrence of adolescent chronic pain and lifetime rates of mental health disorders [18]. In contrast to previous research, a broader range of chronic pain conditions (i.e., headache, abdominal and musculoskeletal pain) were assessed in adolescence, and lifetime history of mental health disorders (i.e., depressive and anxiety disorders) were subsequently assessed in adulthood. Individuals with, versus without, chronic pain in adolescence subsequently reported significantly higher lifetime rates of anxiety (21.1%) and depressive (24.5%) disorders [18]. After controlling for established confounding factors (e.g., age, sex, insufficient sleep, general health), chronic pain in adolescence was associated with a greater likelihood of having anxiety (odds ratio (OR) 1.33) and depressive (OR 1.38) disorders over the lifetime [18].

2.2. Co-Occurrence of Pediatric Chronic Pain and Internalizing Mental Health Issues

Other studies have focused on establishing concurrent rates of mental health disorders and chronic pain status in youth. Coffelt et al. [21] analyzed retrospective data from 3752 youth admitted with a primary diagnosis of chronic pain. Forty-four percent of adolescents had a comorbid mental health condition [21]. The diagnoses included mood disorders (28%), anxiety disorders (18%), conversion and somatization disorders (6%), and PTSD (2.4%) [21]. Simons et al. [23] also investigated the prevalence of anxiety symptoms in a large sample of youth with chronic pain. While only 11% of the participants reported clinically significant levels of total anxiety, 31% may have underreported their anxiety symptoms given their heightened scores on a social desirability scale [23]. Children with diffuse pain reported significantly higher levels of anxiety as compared to youth with musculoskeletal, abdominal or neuropathic pain [23]. Recently, Noel et al. [25] compared prevalence of PTSD symptoms in a sample of youth with chronic pain and their parents to pain-free peers. Findings revealed significantly higher levels of PTSD symptoms (including clinically significant symptoms) in youth with chronic pain and their parents [25].

Similar patterns of co-occurring pain and mental health disorders were found among youth with chronic headaches. In a large sample of youth, recurrent headaches were positively related to higher levels of anxiety and depressive symptoms across two broad age groups (12–14 years, OR 2.05; 15–17 years, OR 1.64) [20]. These results are consistent with those of a meta-analysis of mental health conditions in pediatric headache populations, which revealed higher levels of psychopathology symptoms in children and adolescents with headache as compared to healthy controls [19]. Tension-type headaches were associated with higher internalizing symptoms, which included anxiety and depressive symptoms, withdrawal and somatic complaints [19]. A meta-analysis of FAP revealed that levels of concurrent anxiety, depression and psychological distress were significantly higher in youth with FAP as compared to pain-free youth [26].

The co-occurrence of pediatric chronic pain and mental health disorders has been shown to differ by child sex [14,27]. In a representative sample of 3733 youth, abdominal pain and headaches were associated with co-occurring anxiety disorders in girls, but not boys [27]. Musculoskeletal pain exhibited a similar pattern, showing a strong association with anxiety disorders in girls, but not boys [27]. Conversely, boys were more likely than girls to develop externalizing mental health disorders comorbid with recurrent abdominal pain [14,27]. Both girls and boys were at risk for developing depression in the presence of musculoskeletal pains [27].

In addition to establishing prevalence rates of pediatric chronic pain and mental disorders, Tegethoff et al. [24] sought to determine the temporal primacy of each condition using structured clinical interviews assessing mental health disorders, parental reports of youth mental health disorders and adolescent self-reports of chronic pain in a sample of 6000 youth. More than a quarter of youth reported having both a mental health disorder and chronic pain in their lifetime [24]. Most youth who experienced any type of chronic pain (i.e., back/neck pain, headache, or other chronic pain) reported having an anxiety disorder (17.4%) and an affective disorder (10.06%) [24]. Having experienced any type of chronic pain increased the risk of developing anxiety (OR 2.42), eating (OR 2.63) and depressive (OR 2.32) disorders [24]. Temporal associations (albeit assessed via retrospective report) were reported between the onset of mental health disorders in childhood and the subsequent onset of chronic pain. There were no significant temporal associations between the preceding onset of chronic pain and the subsequent onset of psychological disorders later in life.

Taken together, the available literature demonstrates high levels of co-occurrence of pediatric chronic pain and mental health disorders and symptoms. A major limitation of much of the epidemiological work to date has been the suboptimal assessment of pain. Indeed, chronic or recurrent pain status has often been limited to a single binary question that fails to capture crucial aspects of chronic pain assessment, such as pain frequency, distress due to pain, and pain interference or disability. Moreover, over-reliance on retrospective self-report of symptoms has precluded reliable conclusions about risk and temporal relationships between the onset of chronic pain and mental health issues. The few studies examining temporality suggest that anxiety issues may indeed precede the development of chronic pain; however, rigorous prospective research is needed. Arguably the most striking finding from this body of research is that, irrespective of whether or not pediatric chronic pain resolves by adulthood, the long-term risk for developing mental health disorders remains. This has important clinical implications and suggests that treatments for chronic pain that only target pain, may not be sufficient for interrupting a trajectory of illness into adulthood.

3. Models of Chronic Pain and Comorbid Anxiety, Depression and PTSD

Several models have been proposed to understand the mechanisms underlying comorbidities between various mental health disorders and chronic pain in adults. Sharp and Harvey's mutual maintenance model accounted for seven mechanisms through which PTSD and chronic pain might mutually maintain each other [8]. They proposed that cognitive (e.g., attentional biases), affective (e.g., depression) and behavioral (e.g., reduced activity levels) factors, characteristic of chronic pain, serve to exacerbate PTSD symptoms. Similarly, physiological (e.g., heightened alarm response to trauma reminder), affective (e.g., negative alterations on mood and cognitions) and behavioral (e.g., avoidance) aspects of PTSD contribute to the exacerbation of chronic pain [8]. The model, however, does not account for potential causal connections between those factors.

Liedl et al. [28] subsequently proposed the Perpetual Avoidance Model (PAM). The authors posited that trauma catalyzes dysfunctional cognitions and sensations of intrusion which lead to heightened arousal [28]. The role of hyperarousal is thought to be two-fold: it promotes avoidance behaviors that feed into PTSD-related dysfunctional cognitions and it amplifies pain sensations [28]. Intensified pain sensations further drive pain-related cognitions (e.g., catastrophizing, fear-avoidance beliefs), in turn, promoting avoidance of pain-inducing activities [28]. Avoidance (an element shared with PTSD) further intensifies pain sensations [28]. Hence, individuals get trapped in a cycle of perpetual avoidance that serves to maintain both PTSD and chronic pain. The PAM assumes no direct relationship between an inciting traumatic event and chronic pain. The pain model by Norman et al. [29] postulates that pain drives PTSD onset, whereas PTSD does not contribute to pain maintenance. Brown et al. [30] used structural equation modelling to test three theoretical models with a pediatric population (i.e., the PAM, mutual maintenance model, and the pain model). The authors used diagnostic interviews to assess PTSD and self-report to assess physical pain in a clinical sample of youth with traumatic brain injuries (TBIs) 3, 6 and 18 months after their injuries [30]. Sharp and Harvey's model fit the acquired data significantly better as compared to the Norman et al. pain model. The PAM did not differ significantly in terms of fit as compared to Sharp and Harvey's model, suggesting equally good fit [30]. The authors concluded that PTSD drives the presence of physical pain in this particular pediatric population.

Sharp and Harvey's mutual maintenance model was later expanded to distinguish between mutual maintaining versus shared vulnerability factors, the latter of which serve to precipitate both conditions [7]. The shared vulnerability model postulates that certain psychological symptom clusters (e.g., anxiety sensitivity) and physiological factors (e.g., lower alarm threshold) can precipitate the emergence of both chronic pain and PTSD and be causally related to cognitive and behavioral mechanisms [6,7]. Moreover, the model posits that the conditions only develop when an individual with such a diathesis is exposed to a traumatic life event [7]. Trauma initiates a diathesis-amplified psychological response that includes maladaptive levels of fear and anxiety, and results in an array of detrimental behavioral (e.g., avoidance), cognitive (e.g., hypervigilance) and physiological (e.g., autonomic nervous system responsivity) consequences [7]. These consequences, which are thought to be bi-directionally related, account for the development of PTSD, chronic pain and/or both comorbidities [7]. The shared vulnerability model is the first model to include anxiety disorders, in addition to PTSD. Just as symptoms of mental health disorders (e.g., physiological arousal in anxiety, lack of positive emotions in anxiety or anhedonia in depression) may intensify pain symptoms [7], pain-related cognitive biases, physiological responses and maladaptive behaviors may serve to aggravate symptoms of mental health disorders [7]. It is, therefore, likely that mental health conditions and chronic pain share certain predisposing factors that form a common diathesis.

Until only recently, existing models of co-occurring mental health disorders and chronic pain were specific to adults. In a recent topical review, Holley et al. [31] proposed a new pediatric model of PTSD and chronic pain comorbidity in youth. Central to this model are shared vulnerability and mutually maintaining factors that are thought to influence PTSD, chronic pain and the disorders' comorbidity in bi-directional ways. While many of the proposed factors are similar to those covered in the previous models (e.g., anxiety sensitivity, avoidance, hyperarousal), the authors drew evidence from pediatric research, confirming the important roles that these factors play in pain and mental health trajectories in childhood and adolescence [31]. Unique to this model is the integration of individual (e.g., trauma and pain-related variables), interpersonal (e.g., parent traumatic stress, peer victimization) and neurobiological (e.g., PTSD and pain influences on the developing brain) factors, all couched within a developmental context [31]. At all levels, PTSD and pain symptomatology are thought to reciprocally influence one another. For instance, catastrophic thoughts about pain in youth may lead to behavioral avoidance, and similar cognitions in parents may serve to exacerbate these cognitions and behaviors in their child [31]. Likewise, depressive symptoms characteristic of chronic pain and PTSD might be aggravated or even induced by peer difficulties and social isolation that are also commonly found in both conditions [31]. Overall, the proposed model fills a gap in the literature by being the first to integrate evidence from the pediatric PTSD and pain literatures, and positing developmentally relevant mechanisms that might underlie and serve to maintain both conditions in youth.

4. Potential Neurobiological Mechanisms Underlying Comorbid Chronic Pain and Anxiety, Depression or PTSD

As outlined in some of the models previously described (e.g., [6,7,31]), shared neurobiology of chronic pain and mental health conditions may in part explain the high co-occurrence of these disorders. Nevertheless, biological underpinnings of comorbidity have largely been overlooked relative to cognitive, affective and behavioral factors. There is accumulating evidence to suggest that genes, hormones and neural networks contribute to both the predisposition and maintenance of, chronic pain, PTSD, anxiety and depressive disorders. The following will provide a brief overview of some of the neurobiological factors that may underlie chronic pain and these associated mental health conditions. Presently, there are a limited number of studies that have examined mechanisms contributing to the development and maintenance of pediatric chronic pain and comorbid internalizing mental health issues. Therefore, in this particular section of the review, where there is an absence of child research, we draw from adult and animal literatures. We acknowledge that work in this area is preliminary. It is important that future research further investigate these factors and their developmental specificity to children and adolescents, so that interventions can be developed to effectively target the underlying mechanisms that maintain these conditions during the pediatric period.

4.1. The Hypothalamic–Pituitary–Adrenal Axis

Both stress and pain incite a cascade of neurobiological events, leading to the activation of the hypothalamic–pituitary–adrenal (HPA) axis and production of stress hormones (glucocorticoids (cortisol in humans)), which regulate the transcription of genes [32]. The process through which cortisol is secreted begins with the activation of the hypothalamus. This leads to the co-release of hormones [33–36] that stimulate the synthesis and release of adrenocorticotropin (ACTH) from the anterior pituitary gland. ACTH secretion influences the release of glucocorticoids from the adrenal cortex into general circulation [33–36]. Cortisol binds with glucocorticoid receptors in the hypothalamus, hippocampus and other brain regions to inhibit further production of cortisol (negative feedback) [33,34]. However, early and/or prolonged exposure to stress and/or pain can disrupt this cortisol feedback loop. Individuals with chronic pain often demonstrate HPA dysfunction [37,38], including altered glucocorticoid negative feedback [39,40] and abnormal cortisol levels [41–44]. Similarly, co-occurring stress-related mental health conditions (PTSD, anxiety and depressive disorders) are also associated with disruptions to the HPA axis [45–47].

Priming of the HPA axis begins in utero. Prenatal exposure to stress hormones leads to greater stress responses in adults, by reducing glucocorticoid receptors in the hippocampus [48,49]. Fewer glucocorticoid receptors in the hippocampus, leads to poorer negative feedback, and greater anxiety-related behavior during adulthood [48,49]. The postnatal environment also has considerable influence on the programming of the HPA axis. Natural variations in maternal behavior, such as the amount a rat licks and grooms their pups in the first week of life [50], incites a cascade of serotonin-mediated changes affecting hippocampal glucocorticoid receptor expression [51–57]. Adult offspring of low licking and grooming rat mothers showed reduced hippocampal glucocorticoid receptor expression, poorer glucocorticoid feedback sensitivity, and greater glucocorticoid production in comparison to pups reared by high licking and grooming mothers [52,53]. These changes in physiology are related to alterations in behavior as adults. Offspring of low licking and grooming mothers show greater anxiety-like behavior and alterations in cognitive functioning during adulthood [51,55,58–60], factors commonly associated with chronic pain [7]. Comparable disruption of cortisol reactivity in response to maternal behavior has been observed in humans. Early disruptions in the parent–child relationship have been associated with increased levels of cortisol in preschoolers [61]. Moreover, these heighted glucocorticoid responses were associated with increased behavioral and emotional problems both at school-age and adulthood [61,62]. Therefore, normal variations in early life experience and parent–child interactions can subsequently alter stress reactivity and behavior; this may contribute to the vulnerability and or mutual maintenance of psychopathology and chronic pain [7].

Cumulative life trauma also influences the development of chronic pain and psychopathology [63–65], which may, in part, be explained by dysregulation of the HPA axis. Youth with chronic pain report having a greater number of stressful life events compared to those without chronic pain, and cumulative trauma was associated with higher PTSD symptoms [25]. The timing and duration of traumatic events appears to largely influence glucocorticoid and behavioral responses to trauma. Both in humans and animals, prolonged pain and distress appears to be associated with a dampening of cortisol responses, in contrast to acute stressors that are associated with hyper-secretion of cortisol [52,53,66–70]. For example, among rhesus monkeys during the first month of life, when abuse is most prevalent, abused infants had elevated plasma cortisol levels as compared to non-abused infants [71]. However, by 6 months of age, the monkeys exhibited lower basal cortisol levels and attenuated ACTH to corticotropin-releasing factor (CRF) compared to control monkeys [71]. In humans, children who experienced abuse in their home environments, showed enhanced ACTH responses and normal cortisol levels [72]. However, adult survivors of childhood abuse or those with PTSD demonstrate lower ACTH responses following CRF injections [73]. Moreover, in a sample of youth exposed to interpersonal violence, if the trauma occurred in the last year of assessment, higher levels of salivary cortisol were positively associated with PTSD [74]. Conversely, in individuals with traumas exceeding a year prior to assessment, PTSD symptoms were associated lower levels of cortisol [74]. Ultimately, previous and/or prolonged physiological arousal associated with stress initiated by exposure to the threat of or actual death, serious injury, or violence can have detrimental effects on activation of neural and hormonal processes, and may contribute to the development of chronic pain and mental health disorders. This research also suggests that timing of exposure to traumatic/stressful events as well as assessment can influence the patterns of activation found.

Therefore, prolonged activation of the HPA axis may lead to stress-related conditions as chronic pain, PTSD, anxiety and depressive disorders. At this time, the mechanisms underlying the relationships between chronic pain and mental health conditions have not been well characterized. However, given the widespread actions of cortisol on multiple neurobiological systems, prolonged exposure to glucocorticoids may lead to changes in gene expression, the immune system and to the developing brain, thereby increasing the vulnerability and maintenance of these conditions.

4.2. Serotonin

Serotonin (5-hydroxytryptamine (5-HT)) is a widely distributed neurotransmitter that is a key modulator of stress responses (i.e., HPA axis) [75,76]. It is also an important molecule for pain processing, and is centrally involved in chronic pain states [77,78]. Previous studies have shown that individuals with chronic pain have decreased levels of 5-HT in their serum and cerebrospinal fluid [79,80]. This led to an investigation as to whether variants of 5-HT genes were associated with increased risk of developing chronic pain. One of the major 5HT receptor subtypes is the serotonin 2A receptor (5-HT2AR). It was found that following nerve injury, 5-HT2AR promotes spinal hyper-excitation and impairs spinal μ-opioid mechanisms, thereby contributing to the development of mechanical allodynia [81]. Using 2 population-based cohorts, Nicholl et al. [82] were able to demonstrate for the first time that single-nucleotide polymorphisms (SNP) of the 5-HT2AR gene were associated with musculoskeletal pain in adult males, even after adjustment for symptoms of depressive disorders. Therefore, 5-HT availability appears to have a role in the development of chronic pain conditions. Central to the reuptake of 5-HT is the transporter protein (5-HTT). Genetic variants of the transporter promoter region (5-HTTLPR) play a critical role in determining intra-synaptic 5-HT signaling [83]. In humans it has been found that the short (S) allele of 5-HTTLPR results in ~50% reduction in 5-HT reuptake compared to the long (L) allele [84]. The S allele has been found to increase the risk of chronic pain [85,86]. Chronic pain patients with the S allele also demonstrated higher levels of anxiety and depressive disorders [85]. It has been theorized that the inability for rapid 5-HT clearance from the synaptic cleft may result in serotonin 1A receptor (5-HT1A) subtype negative feedback, causing an overall decreased in 5-HT neurotransmission for individuals with the S allele [85]. Converging evidence from both human and nonhuman primates suggests that S allele carriers may also have greater vulnerability for anxiety and depressive disorders [87]. Indeed, a recent meta-analysis found a significant association between 5-HTTLPR genotype and HPA-axis reactivity to acute psychosocial stress, with homozygous carriers of the S allele displaying increased stress hormone reactivity compared with individuals with the S/L and L/L genotype [88]. The 5-HTTLPR genotype also modulates brain activation during emotional processing tasks [89,90]. Human adult functional magnetic resonance imaging (fMRI) studies have found consistent associations between the short allele and greater amygdala reactivity to aversive versus neutral stimuli [91,92]. This is important given that the amygdala plays a key role in activating the HPA axis. Altogether, it would appear that 5-HT availability modifies brain responses and predisposes individuals to developing chronic pain and/or mental health conditions.

4.3. Brain-Derived Neurotrophic Factor

Serotonin interacts closely with brain-derived neurotrophic factor (BDNF), a neurotrophin that is widely expressed in stress-related brain regions (e.g., prefrontal cortex and hippocampus) and is intrinsic to neurogenesis and synaptogenesis [93]. Both human and animal studies have demonstrated that stress hormones modify BDNF expression, such that there is decreased BDNF expression in the hippocampus and increased expression in the amygdala [94–96]. This finding is consistent with recent neuroimaging studies, which have reported significant loss in hippocampal neuroconnectivity with the medial prefrontal cortex [97], and exaggerated amygdalar connectivity with the central executive network (dorsolateral prefrontal cortex and posterior parietal cortex) in individuals with chronic pain compared to healthy controls [98]. Therefore, genetically determined BDNF availability may modify brain connections contributing to the development and maintenance of chronic pain conditions. To that effect, it has been shown that induced chronic inflammatory pain dampens hippocampal *BDNF* gene expression in rats [99]. Deletion of *BDNF* also produces chronic pain and depressive-like behavior in mice [100], and stimulators of BDNF synthesis have been shown to have an analgesic effect and reduce depression-like behavior in rats with chronic pain [101]. Similar to 5-HT, there are variants of *BDNF*, which are important determinants of intracellular processing and secretion [102]. Unlike Val66Met (rs6265), the 66Met allele results in lower BDNF availability, and is associated with alterations of human hippocampal function [103]. Both human and mouse 66Met allele carriers have been shown to have smaller bilateral hippocampi, in addition to lower gray mater volumes (e.g., prefrontal cortex), and reduced white matter tract integrity when compared to 66Val homozygote controls [104–110]. Furthermore, adult human and rat studies have shown that 66Met carriers may be at higher risk for developing chronic pain, PTSD, anxiety and depressive disorders [111–119]. Therefore, stress-regulated *BDNF* may be another mechanism through which genes may increase susceptibility to chronic pain and comorbid mental health conditions.

4.4. Inflammation

Another important factor to consider in the co-occurrence of chronic pain and mental health disorders is the effect that chronic pain and stress can have on immune function. Injury leads to the activation of microglia in the dorsal horn of the spinal cord, which results in the release of cytokines and growth factors that excite nociceptive dorsal horn neurons, contributing to the development of central sensitization and hyperalgesia [120] as well as the pathogenesis of chronic pain [121,122]. It is important to note that chronic inflammatory processes are not specific to pain (e.g., autoimmune diseases, aging) [123,124] and may arise from acute immune challenges [125]. Therefore, other conditions that incite neuro-inflammatory responses may also lead to chronic pain and comorbid conditions. Post-mortem immunohistochemical studies of the spinal cord in patients with complex regional pain syndrome [126] and human immunodeficiency virus-related neuropathic pain [127], and cerebral spinal fluid sampling of patients with fibromyalgia and chronic low back pain [128,129], have provided support for the involvement of glia in the pathogenesis of chronic pain. A recent study using positron emission tomography–magnetic resonance imaging showed for the first time, in vivo, that the occurrence of glial activation, as measured by an increase in [^{11}C]PBR28 binding, was greater in the thalamus of patients with chronic pain as compared to controls [130]. Preclinical research involving nerve injury models have shown that chronic pain evokes anatomically specific neuroinflammation in brain regions that is causally linked to anxiety and depressive-like symptoms [131]. Specifically, nerve injury elicits the production of pro-inflammatory cytokines both in the periphery and centrally, which can cause a reduction in BDNF (neurogenesis) and glucocorticoid receptor expression and function, and an increase in excitoxicity in brain regions that are critical for behavior regulation (i.e., hippocampus, hypothalamus, amygdala, prefrontal cortex) [131–135]. Altering the connectivity of these regions can lead to alterations in function and behavioral disturbances. In humans, the production capacity of several cytokines has been positively associated with severity of depressive and anxiety symptoms, even while taking lifestyle and health factors into account [136]. Furthermore, it has been shown that among chronic pain patients, higher levels of tumor necrosis factor-α (TNF-α) and interleukin-6 (IL-6) were associated with less improvement in pain intensity, greater psychological inflexibility and lower mental health-related quality of life following a pain intervention, compared to patients with lower levels of these cytokines [137]. Therefore, inflammation may not only act as a precipitating factor for pain and mental health conditions, but also may be a perpetuating factor that deters patient recovery.

To date, very little research has been completed examining inflammatory factors and its contribution to the chronicity of pediatric pain and comorbid mental health disorders. Therefore, this represents an important, cutting-edge area for future research. We know that early life pain and/or stress also appears to dysregulate the developing immune system. Rat pups surgically incised on postnatal day 3 show priming of the central neuroimmune response, such that upon re-injury during adulthood, they demonstrate an enhanced degree and duration of microglial reactivity [138]. This is one of the first studies to demonstrate how early tissue injury can modify the neuroimmune profile to shape nociceptive processing throughout life, and may yield valuable insights into the potential link between pediatric and adult chronic pain conditions [138]. To the best of our knowledge, this has not yet been demonstrated in humans. However, Mitchell and Goldstein [139] reviewed 67 studies including nearly 4000 youth with mental health conditions and found preliminary evidence for elevated markers of inflammation in this population. In particular, associations with depressive disorders and PTSD converge with the extant adult literature demonstrating associations with inflammatory markers [139]. Early-life stress leads to a suppression of inflammatory markers during development, but causes a shift towards a pro-inflammatory state in later life [140]. For children born extremely preterm, this change in inflammatory responses may coincide with the dampening of HPA activity over time [69,70]. Prolonged stress appears to have a similar effect on inflammatory responses, such that in adult patients with comorbid PTSD and major depressive disorder demonstrated higher IL-6 activity concurrent with reduced sensitivity to glucocorticoids as compared to PTSD patients alone [141]. Furthermore, another study found that combat veterans with PTSD demonstrated abnormally elevated neuroinflammatory responses to deep pain stimuli relative to combat veterans without PTSD [142]. Taken together, inflammatory responses appear to play an important role in the development and maintenance of comorbid chronic pain and mental health disorders. Currently, many new pharmacological agents that target cytokines are being synthesized for different clinical indicators [143], which may result in better control of chronic inflammation, as well as improved treatment outcomes for patients with chronic pain and PTSD, anxiety and depressive disorder comorbidities.

4.5. Neuroimaging Chronic Pain and Psychopathology

In recent years, several neuroimaging studies have attempted to characterize nociceptive systems, their central nervous system targets (e.g., primary and secondary somatosensory cortices, insula, anterior cingulate cortex, and thalamus) [144–148], and correlate these regions with the modality and intensity of noxious input [144,149–151]. For example, in a recent fMRI study involving 114 healthy adult participants, Wager et al. [151] found a highly sensitive and specific neurologic signature of physical pain. It included both medial (e.g., affective; anterior cingulate cortex) and lateral (e.g., sensory; somatosensory cortices) pain systems that were consistent across individuals [151]. However, in the transition from an acute and adaptive pain state to a chronic, maladaptive neuropathic disease state, there is extensive functional and metabolic reorganization in pain-related brain circuitry. A recent study by Hubbard et al. [152] examined functional brain changes over time in response to acetone application to the left hindpaw in rats that either received a spared nerve injury (SNI) or sham surgery. The SNI rats demonstrated early hyperactivity of sensory areas (ventroposterior lateral nucleus of the thalamus, primary somatosensory cortex) and later hyperactivity of affective areas (anterior cingulate cortex, prelimbic cortex), and early and sustained hypoactivity of the medial thalamus and periaqueductal gray matter [152]. Moreover, for the SNI rats, these functional brain changes were associated with early and sustained increases in behavioral measures of mechanical and cold sensitivity [152]. Therefore, it would appear that as an individual transitions from an acute to chronic pain state, activations within the brain move from primarily somatosensory regions to limbic regions, indicating a shift from primarily physical to emotional neural processing. These findings were recently corroborated by Jensen et al. [153]. Using an activation likelihood estimate to analyze 138 independent data sets, they demonstrated that chronic pain patients were less likely to activate key nociceptive regions compared to healthy controls [153]. In low back pain patients followed longitudinally, Mutso et al. [97] showed that over the course of 1 year, patients acquired significant losses in hippocampal connectivity with the medial prefrontal cortex. This cellular loss between the hippocampus and cortex seemed to contribute to the transition from subacute to chronic pain and was thought to be a factor in the known aversive learning and heightened anxiety associated with chronic pain. Baliki et al. [154] also noted over the same time course that gray matter brain density decreased in patients with low back pain relative to healthy controls. However, adult chronic low back pain patients also tended to have exaggerated amygdalar connectivity with the central executive network (dorsolateral prefrontal cortex and posterior parietal cortex) as compared to healthy controls [98]. Moreover, this greater connectivity has been associated with increased tendencies to engage in catastrophic thinking about pain [98]. In support of this finding, in adolescents with irritable bowel syndrome, disease duration is associated with cortical thickness in bilateral dorsolateral prefrontal cortex and left supramarginal gyri [155]. Additionally, higher levels of pain intensity were associated with significant cortical thickening in the bilateral orbitofrontal cortex [155]. Thus, similar to the animal research described above, in humans, the transition from acute to chronic pain is characterized by reorganization within the limbic structures, thereby altering cognitive and emotional processes. This also supports the potential role of cognitive (e.g., memory and attentional biases) and affective (e.g., depressive symptoms) factors as potential mechanisms that may maintain the comorbidity between chronic pain and mental health conditions.

To date, very few neuroimaging studies have been conducted in pediatric chronic pain populations. However, among the few pediatric studies, similar findings to studies in adults have been reported. Youth with complex regional pain syndrome have been shown to have greater connectivity of the left and right amygdala to several cortical and subcortical areas as compared to healthy controls [156]. However, despite this greater connectivity, Simons et al. [157] found decreased evoked responses to fearful stimuli in patients with complex regional pain syndrome compared to healthy sex- and age-matched controls in prefrontal and limbic regions, particularly within the striatum, amygdala, insula and dorsolateral prefrontal cortex. Furthermore, blunted responses to fearful expressions in the caudate, putamen, centromedial amygdala, and anterior insula were associated with pain-related fear levels. Simons et al. [157] postulated that these results corroborate accumulating research demonstrating alterations in cognitive-affective brain regions in the chronic pain state [158] and may reflect either allostatic over-load [159,160] or pain avoidance, a maladaptive behavior often used in an effort to manage chronic pain [157].

Although the majority of neuroimaging studies of pediatric chronic pain have focused on the amygdala and its functional connections, pain is a multidimensional experience, with sensory, cognitive, and evaluative aspects. Therefore, other networks may be simultaneously activated during the transmission of pain signals in the brain. Differences in intrinsic brain networks were observed in pediatric complex regional pain syndrome patients as compared to controls, with the most prominent differences in the central executive, default mode, sensorimotor, and salience (anterior insula, mid-cingulate cortex, temperoparietal junction, and dorsolateral prefrontal cortex) networks [161]. Given the extent of neural networks that are affected by chronic pain, it is not surprising that comorbidities (i.e., PTSD, anxiety and depressive disorders) exist among individuals with chronic pain. Indeed, these same networks have also been shown to be altered in individuals with PTSD, anxiety and depressive disorders [162–165]. The majority of neuroimaging studies to date have only examined one to two of these disorders in conjunction with pain and their effects on the brain. Therefore, the specificity of the overlap within the brain between each of these disorders requires further investigation. However, it is becoming increasingly clear that chronic pain, anxiety, depression and/or PTSD, are not completely independent and the predisposing factors and neurobiological mechanisms, which lead to the presence and/or comorbidity of these disorders, are intrinsically related.

5. Parental Mental Health Disorders in Pediatric Chronic Pain Population

As previously mentioned, the neurobiology of pediatric chronic pain is deeply embedded in the broader social context of the family and parent–child relationship. It is, therefore, essential to examine parental factors that co-occur with pediatric pain or that might contribute to the development of chronic pain and comorbid mental health conditions. Several studies and reviews have confirmed a strong relationship between familial history of chronic pain with pediatric chronic pain [166,167]. Hoftun et al. [168] used a large community sample of Norwegian youth and at least one of their parents to examine the relationship between parental chronic pain history and pediatric chronic pain. The youth were more likely to have chronic pain if their mother or father reported recurrent pain issues; the risk was much higher if both parents were suffering from chronic pain [168].

There is evidence to suggest that genes, in combination with early environments, contribute to the risk of developing chronic pain and comorbid mental health conditions. Parents with the *5-HTTLPR* S allele exhibit significantly less observed positive parenting than those with the L genotype [169]. The S allele results in ~50% reduction in 5-HT reuptake compared to the long (L) allele [84], which is thought to cause an overall decrease of 5-HT neurotransmission in individuals with the short *5-HTTLPR* allele [85]. Lower 5-HT availability, leads to reduced glucocorticoid receptor expression, and greater circulating cortisol [51–57]. As previously described, children of mothers that have increased stress hormones during pregnancy are more likely to have greater stress responses as adults [48,49]. However, the postnatal environment is also important for HPA axis programming, such that parent behaviors can either reduce or increase cortisol activity, thereby modifying gene expression [52,53,170,171]. Glucocorticoid dysfunction is associated with chronic pain and mental health conditions (PTSD, anxiety and depressive disorders) [45–47]. Therefore, parent factors contribute to their child's risk of subsequently developing chronic pain and comorbid mental health conditions.

Other studies have also reported associations between parental mental health and chronic pain in children. Garber et al. [167] examined children with recurrent abdominal pain (RAP) with and without known "organic cause", children with psychiatric issues and a healthy control group. Parental self-reports of psychiatric symptoms were significantly different between the groups. Mothers (but not fathers) of children with RAP were more anxious than mothers of children who had pain with a known "organic" origin and mothers in the control group [167]. Mothers of children who had RAP without a known "organic cause" reported more depressive and somatization symptoms than mothers of healthy controls. Walker et al. [172] reported similar findings: mothers of children with RAP reported higher levels of depressive, anxiety, and somatization symptoms as compared to mothers of healthy children. Parental reports did not differ significantly between the groups. Campo et al. [173] examined a clinical sample of children with FAP and their mothers, finding the latter were significantly more likely to report a lifetime incidence of anxiety or depressive disorders as compared to mothers of children without recurrent pain. The UK child development cohort study mirrored those findings: high levels of maternal neuroticism was a risk factor for pediatric abdominal pain [5], and family history of mental health issues were linked to recurrent headaches in childhood [3,21]. Williamson et al. [174] examined a small clinical sample of youth with chronic pain and their mothers. In addition to child ratings of pain, another significant predictor of child-reported depression was maternal depression. Similarly, Wolff et al. [175] assessed anxiety and depressive symptoms in pregnant women as a part of a population-based cohort study (the Generation R). Among other factors (e.g., maternal stress and child temperament), higher anxiety symptoms in mothers increased the risk of somatic complaints in their 18 month old children [175]. While the number of studies in this area is rather limited, a pattern of high co-occurrence between pediatric chronic pain and parental mental health disorders and symptoms is evident.

Moreover, as reported in a recent meta-analysis, children of parents who have versus who do not have chronic pain are more likely to develop a host of physical and mental health problems from early in life [176]. Starting as early as perinatal period, children of mothers with chronic pain were at higher risk for preterm delivery, C-section, and adverse birth outcomes (e.g., low birth weight, congenital abnormalities) [176]. In addition to increased pain problems, offspring of parents with chronic pain were at higher risk for poorer mental health outcomes [176]. Limited evidence was found for higher rates of externalizing problems [176]; however, consistent patterns were found for internalizing problems. Levels of both parent- and youth-reported internalizing problems (including symptoms of depression, anxiety and obsessive–compulsive disorder) in youth whose parents had chronic pain were higher as compared to controls (i.e., children of pain-free parents) [176]. Other research has examined parent–child transmission of gastrointestinal illness (GI) behaviors and psychosocial mechanisms underlying this transmission [177,178]. In a study of parents with and without irritable bowel syndrome and their children, a stronger relationship between maternal and child psychological distress was found among the clinical group [178].

Stone and Wilson [179] recently developed an integrative conceptual model addressing the apparent clustering of chronic pain within families. The model outlines possible mechanisms (e.g., pain-specific social learning, general parenting style) and child vulnerabilities (e.g., altered pain processing, pain-related cognitions, pain coping behaviors, physical health, emotion regulation) that contribute to intergenerational transmission of chronic pain risk and may lead to adverse pain-related child outcomes (chronic pain, poor psychological functioning, disability) [179]. The authors also identified potential moderators that exacerbate the risk of transmitting chronic pain to offspring. Thus, chronic pain status of the second parent increases the risk of child developing chronic pain, whereas a pain-free second parent may buffer this risk [179]. Earlier and longer exposure to parental chronic pain, that is, in the same location as child pain is more detrimental as it increases the chances of child learning and adopting pain-related behaviors and beliefs [179]. Girls, African American youth and youth exposed to parental chronic pain at earlier ages may be at higher risk for developing chronic pain as compared to boys, non-Hispanic White youth, and youth who were exposed to parental chronic pain during late adolescence [179]. Importantly, it was proposed that positive affectivity in the child might buffer against the negative influence of parental chronic pain on children, whereas negative affectivity and attention control (i.e., effortful control) in the child may have the opposite effect [179].

Many of the same mechanisms that have been proposed to underlie parental and child chronic pain may also underlie the familial transmission of chronic pain and internalizing mental health symptoms between parents and youth. These proposed mechanisms include: (1) genetic contributions; (2) modeling of behavior (i.e., mothers with higher levels of anxiety model associated patterns of behavior to their children) and pain-specific learning; (3) changes in parenting style, behavior, and interactions with the child (e.g., withdrawal associated with depression, excessive attention to child's pain in cases of heightened anxiety); (4) early neurobiological changes; (5) general familial health; and (6) exposure to stressful environment [167,179]. However, it remains unclear whether parental mental health is a risk factor for development of pediatric pain or a result of having a child with a pain problem. Certainly, parenting a child with chronic pain is associated with high emotional burden to the parent and the broader family system, and recent efforts have been made to directly target parental distress in pediatric chronic pain for this very reason [180]. Twenty percent of parents of youth with chronic pain (versus 1% of parents of pain free peers) have been found to experience clinically significant levels of PTSD [25], however, their PTSD symptoms were not related to those of their child [25].

Any temporal and/or causal connections between pediatric chronic pain and parental psychological health are premature and require further longitudinal and epidemiological investigations. It will also be important to consider that parental mental health might be comorbid and have a bi-directional influence on youth's psychological functioning in chronic pain populations. Palermo et al. [181] developed a conceptual three-level model that elucidates factors at play in pediatric chronic pain. Parental level variables (mental health and emotions, behaviors, physical health status) connect to the other two levels including family variables and developmental factors, by the means of bi-directional relationships. Clearly there is a necessity to further investigate parental factors to gain a more comprehensive understanding of their role in the onset and trajectories of pediatric chronic pain and mental health.

6. Treatments for Comorbid Chronic Pain in Youth

Despite growing recognition of the high co-occurrence of mental health disorders in children and adolescents with chronic pain, treatment approaches to address this growing problem have lagged behind. Currently, psychological treatments for chronic pain have taken a "one-size-fits-all" approach and predominantly focus on changing pain-related cognitions and behaviors without adequately addressing elevations in anxiety and depressive symptoms that often accompany the pain. This could, in part, explain the small and non-significant treatment effects that have been found for face-to-face psychological interventions in reducing pain and disability among headache and non-headache pain populations, respectively. While it may also account for a lack of lasting reductions found in anxiety and depressive symptoms following treatment, this could also reflect the small number of trials that have analyzed mental health conditions as outcomes [10]. Similarly, in a recent meta-analysis of remotely delivered psychological interventions (e.g., via the internet, computers, smartphone applications or telephone), there were no beneficial effects found in reducing depressive symptoms and only small effects in reducing headache pain in the short-term [182]. However, it should be noted that there were only a small number of (small) trials conducted, and, like the face-to-face trials, many did not assess both anxiety and depressive symptoms as primary outcomes. Taken together, the evidence to date suggests that our existing interventions for chronic pain emphasize changing pain cognitions and behaviors without adequate emphasis on co-occurring mental health conditions. Although more trials assessing pain and mental health disorders as primary outcomes are needed, it is possible that existing treatments may not be sufficient for interrupting a trajectory of pain and comorbid mental health conditions from persisting long-term.

Recent research suggests that mental health comorbidities and symptoms can impede recovery among youth with chronic pain. Cunningham et al. [183] examined 175 children seen in a pediatric pain management center, 40 of who completed cognitive–behavioral therapy for chronic pain. Findings revealed that children who had clinically significant symptoms of anxiety at the time of initial evaluation (albeit similar levels of pain and functioning) showed greater initiation in and completion of the pain intervention but poorer treatment response (i.e., less reductions in pain intensity and functional disability) as compared to youth with subclinical anxiety symptoms. Research also suggests that modifying anxiety is important for reducing pain and improving functioning during intensive interdisciplinary rehabilitation pain programs. Specifically, Benore et al. [184] found that over and above the effect of age, sex and pain at admission and 1-month post-discharge, reductions in general anxiety, pain-specific anxiety and pain catastrophizing predicted improved physical quality of life, as well as pain intensity, but, not the number of missed school days. Taken together, this evidence demonstrates that mental health (anxiety) symptom elevations impede recovery in psychological pain treatments and should be reduced in order to see improvements in pain and functional outcomes. This suggests that youth with chronic pain are not a homogenous group and treatment approaches that are tailored to addressing co-morbid anxiety symptoms are likely necessary for subgroups of youth who exhibit clinically significant anxiety symptoms. Moreover, youth who appear to be most engaged in treatment (i.e., those with clinically significant anxiety symptoms) might be the very ones who are least likely to recover. Research on treatment response among youth with other mental health conditions (e.g., depression, PTSD) is needed.

Like Cunningham et al. [183], recent authors have argued for the use of mental health screening tools to identify mental health disorder co-morbidities [31,185,186] in order to predict outcomes and inform clinician-use of treatment approaches. Some authors have also provided treatment recommendations [31,185], albeit largely based on adult research. Adult guidelines recommend treating overlapping pain and PTSD symptoms (e.g., fears and avoidance behaviors) concurrently [9,187]. Dually targeted interventions have been developed for adults that combine PTSD behavioral activation, pain education and emphasis on exercise [9,188]. Similarly, other programs developed for adult veterans have combined cognitive processing therapy for PTSD with CBT for chronic pain [9,189]. Pediatric researchers have stressed the importance of understanding comorbid PTSD and chronic pain within a developmental context [31] and cautioned against simply downwardly extending adult recommendations to pediatric populations. Attempts have been made to apply a unified, transdiagnostic treatment for adolescents with chronic pain and comorbid anxiety and depressive disorders (Unified Protocol for the Treatment of Emotions in Youth With Pain (UP-YP)) [190]. The UP-YP is a modular-based individual treatment protocol [190]. Treatment is offered between 8 to 21 50-min sessions over a front-loaded 6-month period [190]. The UP-YP modules include: (a) psychoeducation about emotions and pain; (b) awareness of emotions and pain; (c) flexibility in thinking; (d) modifying emotion-driven behaviors through exposures; and (e) treatment review and relapse prevention [190]. Several optional modules are available as well (e.g., parenting the emotional adolescent with pain) [190]. Although similar in its application to traditional CBT therapy, the UP-YP aims to modify both pain and emotions [190]. Using two case studies, Allen et al. [190] provided initial evidence that the UP-YP can be used to broaden the scope of treatment to include both emotion regulation skills and cognitive–behavioral treatment strategies to assist individuals with complex medical and psychological conditions. After completing the training modules, case 1 was back at school nearly full-time, engaging in social activities, and showed significant improvement in his anxiety and disability, although his pain levels remained more or less the same. Case 2, was somewhat less successful as her pain symptoms were initially being addressed by the program, but her physical illness towards the end of treatment precluded her from the continued benefits of UP-YP. As an alternative to this method of intervention, clinicians may choose to stagger treatment delivery by treating the condition that causes the most distress first and then addressing remaining symptoms of the other condition; however, treatment algorithms based on evidence are needed. Clearly, knowing when and how to integrate versus stagger treatment is a critical area for future research in this area.

Another reason why existing interventions may not help a substantial portion of youth may be due to the fact that they do not effectively target the underlying mechanisms that maintain these conditions. Genetic screening for alleles associated with these conditions may help to identify patients at risk for developing chronic pain and a comorbid mental health condition, allowing clinicians to intervene prior to significant neural remodeling. A better understanding of the neural "signature(s)" associated with chronic pain, PTSD, anxiety and depressive disorders will also help to evaluate the effectiveness of clinical interventions for altering this neural circuitry. New therapies, which directly target the underlying mechanisms of these conditions, may also be a promising new direction for clinical intervention. For example, transcranial magnetic stimulation (rTMS) involves using a magnetic field generator to stimulate small regions of the affected brain region. Thus far, rTMS has been shown to be an effective treatment for burning mouth syndrome [191], complex regional pain syndrome [192], fibromyalgia [193,194], neuropathic pain [195–197], depressive disorders [198] and to a lesser degree PTSD and other anxiety disorders [199,200]. It has been proposed to prevent or revert the ongoing maladaptive plasticity within the pain matrix [201], and modify opioidergic, glutamatergic, gamma-aminobutyric acidergic, and serotoninergic neurotransmissions [202]. The application of screening, implementation of early interventions at the individual and familial level (e.g., teaching coping mechanisms, parent sensitivity training), refining current intervention strategies, and the innovation of new, targeted therapies, holds promise for addressing and reducing these comorbidities.

7. Discussion

High levels of comorbid chronic pain and mental health conditions have been reported in pediatric populations, and persistent pain reportedly increases the risk of PTSD, anxiety and depressive disorders later in adulthood [3–5,16,17]. Chronic pain and mental health disorders (as well as their subclinical symptoms) reciprocally influence each other, significantly decrease youth quality of life and impose a large health care and economic burden in childhood and adulthood [2,7,18,31]. While studies have attempted to identify mechanisms underlying these relationships, they often focus on one to two factors, which cannot account for the complex interplay between genetic, epigenetic, chemical, neuronal and environmental factors that may interact synergistically to influence the development and maintenance of chronic pain and mental health conditions. This review highlights some of the ways in which pre-determined and concurrent neurobiology and genetics interact with parental influences to influence chronic pain and mental health conditions in youth (Figure 1). It extends previous pediatric and adult work on mental health conditions/symptoms and chronic pain, which have focused primarily on cognitive, affective, and behavioral mechanisms. We suggest that an integrative approach combining biological and behavioral factors is needed to push forward this important line of inquiry, and ultimately inform how to interrupt this trajectory, to prevent issues from persisting into adulthood. However, systematic review methodology is warranted as more evidence accumulates on this topic.

Theoretical work is critical for synthesizing existing (and often disparate) bodies of evidence and guiding future scientific inquiry. Existing models that address comorbidity of mental health disorders and chronic pain are scarce. Moreover, they focus primarily on the relationship between PTSD and chronic pain, and are primarily based on adult populations [7,8,28]. While mutual maintenance [8] and shared vulnerability [6] models account for the relationship between PTSD and persistent pain in adults, they do not account for an array of dynamic changes that occur during childhood and adolescence and the unique influence of parents. The new developmentally informed model of Holley et al. [31] begins to fill this gap by placing shared PTSD and chronic pain factors within interpersonal (e.g., parent context) and neurobiological (e.g., impact of pain and PTSD on the developing brain) developmental contexts. A more generalized model addressing the comorbidity between several mental health disorders/symptoms (depression, anxiety and PTSD) and chronic pain in youth would help guide future research and inform clinical practice in this area.

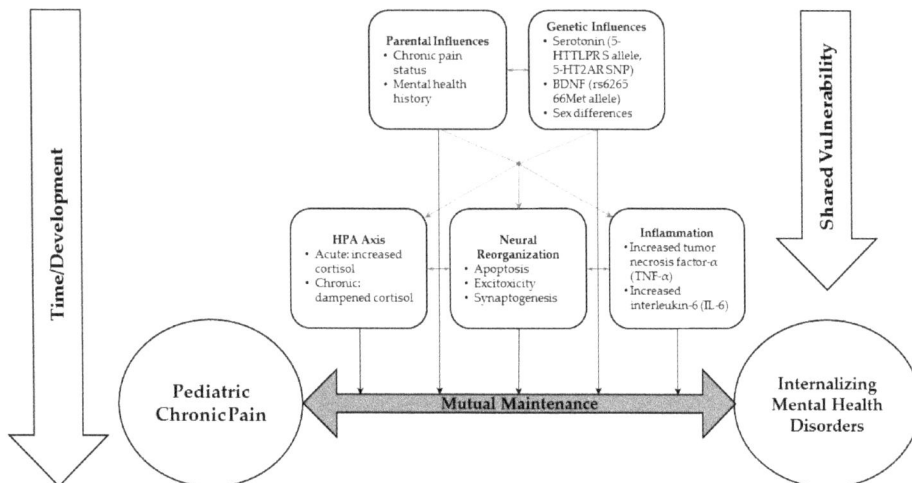

Figure 1. Possible mechanisms underlying the shared vulnerability and mutual maintenance of pediatric chronic pain and internalizing mental health disorders. 5-HTTLPR: Serotonin-transporter-linked polymorphic region; BDNF: Brain-derived neurotrophic factor; HPA: hypothalamic–pituitary–adrenal; S allele: Short allele.

There has been extensive literature examining the contribution of specific genes and neurobiological pathways underlying chronic pain, anxiety, depression and PTSD in adults and animals. However, these studies are often conducted in isolation of one another and focus specifically on the neurobiological influence on one or two outcomes in particular. We have demonstrated in this review that many of the same genes (e.g., 5-HT, *BDNF*), hormones (e.g., cortisol), neurotransmitters (e.g., 5-HT), cytokines (e.g., TNF-α, IL-6) have been implicated in each of these conditions and are inextricably related to one another, either directly or indirectly through the HPA axis. For example, individuals with the short (S) allele of 5-HTTLPR have ~50% reduction in 5-HT reuptake compared to the long (L) allele [84], which may result in decreased 5-HT neurotransmission [85]. Reduced 5-HT availability leads to lower glucocorticoid receptor expression, which results in poorer negative feedback and greater cortisol secretion [51–57]. Stress hormones modify BDNF expression, such that there is decreased BDNF expression in the hippocampus and increased expression in the amygdala [94–96]. BDNF is intrinsic to neurogenesis and synaptogenesis [93], therefore, BDNF availability may contribute to the patterns of neuroconnectivity that develop as pain becomes comorbid and chronic [97,98]. Prolonged exposure to pain leads to a dampening of cortisol responses [52,53,66–70]. Inhibition of the HPA axis leads to heightened inflammatory/immune responses [203,204]. Therefore, following exposure to pain, large inflammatory responses in both the periphery and central systems may cause a reduction in neurogenesis and an increase in excitoxicity leading to both the chronification of pain and its comorbidities. Furthermore, glucocorticoids are involved in normal brain maturation and cell survival [205–207], and both an excess of or too low levels of cortisol can have deleterious effects on the brain, leading to long-term changes in behavior. HPA activity is programmed at birth [48,49], modified by the environment (e.g., parent behavior) [51–57,72], has significant effects in the developing brain [52,53], and influences responses to pain and behavior [63–65]. Pain, anxiety, depression and PTSD are all stress-related conditions influenced by either hyper- or hypo-glucocorticoid activity [63–65]. Evidence suggests that the combination of predisposing factors, along with the timing and duration of environmental influences, modifies HPA activity, which has widespread effects on the neurobiological (e.g., brain organization/function), physiological (e.g., arousal), and psychological systems (e.g., stress, anxiety sensitivity), and may lead to the maintenance of these conditions.

Precedence of mental health disorders onset prior to chronic pain have been reported [24,30]; however, the studies examining temporal relationships between the conditions are scarce, conflicting [208], and come with methodological limitations (e.g., reliance on retrospective report). Clinician-administered interviews (as opposed to self- and parental report) to prospectively assess mental and physical health in childhood, adolescence and early to middle adulthood would be a methodological advance that would help determine temporal relationships between chronic pain and psychiatric disorders.

When examining mental health and chronic pain in youth, it is crucial to take into account the parent–child relational context and the influential role of parental factors. Indeed, parents of youth with chronic pain report more anxiety, depression, and somatization symptoms than pain-free peers [167,173]. Moreover, maternal anxiety and depressive disorders were associated with depressive and somatic symptoms of children with chronic pain [167,172]. Therefore, it is possible that parents with mental health disorders through interactions with their genes and environment influence the comorbidity of chronic pain and mental health conditions in the child. It is necessary to further investigate the role of parental factors in the development and maintenance of pediatric chronic pain and comorbid mental health disorders and symptoms. Additionally, there is a paucity of research examining mental health in fathers of youth with chronic pain. Given the profound influence that pediatric chronic pain has on the entire family, it will be important to address paternal factors in addition to, and in combination with, maternal contributions to pediatric chronic pain and mental health conditions.

While psychological treatments for chronic pain have led to some changes in pain and disability, there is currently no evidence to suggest that it leads to lasting reductions in mental health symptoms. Moreover, many randomized controlled trials of psychological interventions for pediatric chronic pain have not included (or reported on) measures of PTSD, anxiety and depressive disorders over the course of treatment. These mental health conditions are often comorbid with one another, and many of the proposed mechanisms (e.g., avoidance, cognitive biases, sleep disturbances) underlying them are similar. Research in this area has tended to focus on these conditions and symptoms in isolation. Future research examining all of these mental health symptoms in the context of pediatric chronic pain is needed. Moreover, despite increasing evidence demonstrating that these comorbidities are common and debilitating, there is currently minimal empirically based guidance for how to treat children and adolescents who present with comorbid chronic pain and mental health conditions, and clinicians often rely on adult recommendations and/or clinical intuition. Clearly, treatment development and research on comorbid mental health conditions and chronic pain in youth is critically needed at this time. New therapies, which directly target the underlying neural mechanisms (e.g., rTMS; targeted anti-inflammatories) may also be a promising new direction for clinical intervention. However, whether or not these new treatments will be effective for treating chronic pain together with comorbid mental health disorders will need to be determined. Given potential intergenerational transmission of chronic pain and high levels of mental health symptoms among parents, research is needed to determine how to best address parents' emotional burden. Novel parenting interventions to reduce parent distress in the context of pediatric chronic pain have been developed and tested and show promising evidence for improving parent and child emotional outcomes [180]. Addressing parent mental health conditions is likely a necessary first step before they can engage in behavior change that is often required in psychological treatments for their child's chronic pain.

Sex differences in 5-HT signaling systems, stress responses, and neuroimmune interactions are being increasingly recognized [209,210]. Estrogens are often regarded as a central nervous system stimulant, and androgen receptor-mediated actions are often related to inhibition, which may underlie the lower incidence of many forms of chronic pain in males [211]. However, given the scope of this narrative review, in which we examined developmental trajectories of potentially shared neurobiological mechanisms underlying pain, PTSD, anxiety and depressive disorders, we were not able to describe the influence of sex hormones on each of these conditions, and how this changes across development. This is an important area for future research.

Given the debilitating impact of comorbid chronic pain and mental health disorders on youth there is an increasing need for prospective, interdisciplinary studies to identify the primary mechanisms underlying this co-occurrence in youth. This will inform the development and refinement of evidence-based interventions that can interrupt or possibly prevent the maintenance of these chronic conditions. Developmentally sensitive research integrating biological, behavioral, and social perspectives will be critical in driving forward this field of inquiry and addressing this growing epidemic.

Acknowledgments: Jillian Vinall is supported by a Fellowship in Pediatric Pain Research from the Louise and Allan Edward Foundation, and received a Postdoctoral Scholarship from the Alberta Children's Hospital Research Institute/Cumming School of Medicine at the University of Calgary. Jillian Vinall is also a member of the Pain in Child Health research training initiative. Gordon J.G. Asmundson is supported by the University of Regina President's Chair for Academic Excellence in Adult Mental Health Research. Melanie Noel's research is supported by the Alberta Children's Hospital Research Institute, Canadian Institutes of Health Research, and American Pain Society.

Author Contributions: M.N. and G.J.G.A. conceptualized the manuscript. J.V. M.P. and M.N. drafted the manuscript for review. All authors provided critical review of the manuscript for publication.

Conflicts of Interest: The authors declare no conflict of interest. The founding sponsors had no role in the design of the study; in the collection, analyses, or interpretation of data; in the writing of the manuscript, and in the decision to publish the results.

References

1. King, S.; Chambers, C.T.; Huguet, A.; MacNevin, R.C.; McGrath, P.J.; Parker, L.; MacDonald, A.J. The epidemiology of chronic pain in children and adolescents revisited: A systematic review. *Pain* **2011**, *152*, 2729–2738. [CrossRef] [PubMed]

2. Groenewald, C.B.; Essner, B.S.; Wright, D.; Fesinmeyer, M.D.; Palermo, T.M. The economic costs of chronic pain among a cohort of treatment-seeking adolescents in the united states. *J. Pain* **2014**, *15*, 925–933. [CrossRef] [PubMed]

3. Fearon, P.; Hotopf, M. Relation between headache in childhood and physical and psychiatric symptoms in adulthood: National birth cohort study. *BMJ* **2001**, *322*, 1145. [CrossRef] [PubMed]

4. Shelby, G.D.; Shirkey, K.C.; Sherman, A.L.; Beck, J.E.; Haman, K.; Shears, A.R.; Horst, S.N.; Smith, C.A.; Garber, J.; Walker, L.S. Functional abdominal pain in childhood and long-term vulnerability to anxiety disorders. *Pediatrics* **2013**, *132*, 475–482. [CrossRef] [PubMed]

5. Hotopf, M.; Carr, S.; Mayou, R.; Wadsworth, M.; Wessely, S. Why do children have chronic abdominal pain, and what happens to them when they grow up? Population based cohort study. *BMJ* **1998**, *316*, 1196–1200. [CrossRef] [PubMed]

6. Asmundson, G.J.; Coons, M.J.; Taylor, S.; Katz, J. Ptsd and the experience of pain: Research and clinical implications of shared vulnerability and mutual maintenance models. *Can. J. Psychiatry* **2002**, *47*, 930–937. [PubMed]

7. Asmundson, G.J.; Katz, J. Understanding the co-occurrence of anxiety disorders and chronic pain: State-of-the-art. *Depress. Anxiety* **2009**, *26*, 888–901. [CrossRef] [PubMed]

8. Sharp, T.J.; Harvey, A.G. Chronic pain and posttraumatic stress disorder: Mutual maintenance? *Clin. Psychol. Rev.* **2001**, *21*, 857–877. [CrossRef]

9. Asmundson, G.J. The emotional and physical pains of trauma: Contemporary and innovative approaches for treating co-occurring ptsd and chronic pain. *Depress. Anxiety* **2014**, *31*, 717–720. [CrossRef] [PubMed]

10. Eccleston, C. Systematic review and meta-analysis of psychological therapies for children with chronic pain. *Clin. Pract. Pediatr. Psychol.* **2014**, *39*, 763–782.

11. Shipton, E.A. The transition from acute to chronic post surgical pain. *Anaesth. Intensive Care* **2011**, *39*, 824–836. [PubMed]

12. Groenewald, C.B.; Wright, D.R.; Palermo, T.M. Health care expenditures associated with pediatric pain-related conditions in the united states. *Pain* **2015**, *156*, 951–957. [CrossRef] [PubMed]
13. Palermo, T.M. Impact of recurrent and chronic pain on child and family daily functioning: A critical review of the literature. *J. Dev. Behav. Pediatr.* **2000**, *21*, 58–69. [CrossRef] [PubMed]
14. Egger, H.L.; Angold, A.; Costello, E.J. Headaches and psychopathology in children and adolescents. *J. Am. Acad. Child Adolesc. Psychiatry* **1998**, *37*, 951–958. [CrossRef] [PubMed]
15. Egger, H.L.; Costello, E.J.; Erkanli, A.; Angold, A. Somatic complaints and psychopathology in children and adolescents: Stomach aches, musculoskeletal pains, and headaches. *J. Am. Acad. Child Adolesc. Psychiatry* **1999**, *38*, 852–860.
16. Walker, L.S.; Sherman, A.L.; Bruehl, S.; Garber, J.; Smith, C.A. Functional abdominal pain patient subtypes in childhood predict functional gastrointestinal disorders with chronic pain and psychiatric comorbidities in adolescence and adulthood. *Pain* **2012**, *153*, 1798–1806. [CrossRef] [PubMed]
17. Shanahan, L.; Zucker, N.; Copeland, W.E.; Bondy, C.L.; Egger, H.L.; Costello, E.J. Childhood somatic complaints predict generalized anxiety and depressive disorders during young adulthood in a community sample. *Psychol. Med.* **2015**, *45*, 1721–1730. [CrossRef] [PubMed]
18. Noel, M.; Groenewald, C.B.; Beals-Erickson, S.E.; Gebert, J.T.; Palermo, T.M. Chronic pain in adolescence and internalizing mental health disorders: A nationally representative study. *Pain* **2016**, *157*, 1333–1338. [CrossRef] [PubMed]
19. Balottin, U.; Fusar Poli, P.; Termine, C.; Molteni, S.; Galli, F. Psychopathological symptoms in child and adolescent migraine and tension-type headache: A meta-analysis. *Cephalalgia* **2013**, *33*, 112–122. [CrossRef] [PubMed]
20. Blaauw, B.A.; Dyb, G.; Hagen, K.; Holmen, T.L.; Linde, M.; Wentzel-Larsen, T.; Zwart, J.A. Anxiety, depression and behavioral problems among adolescents with recurrent headache: The young-hunt study. *J. Headache Pain* **2014**, *15*, 38. [CrossRef] [PubMed]
21. Coffelt, T.A.; Bauer, B.D.; Carroll, A.E. Inpatient characteristics of the child admitted with chronic pain. *Pediatrics* **2013**, *132*, e422–e429. [CrossRef] [PubMed]
22. Noel, M.; Beals-Erickson, S.E.; Law, E.F.; Alberts, N.; Palermo, T.M. Characterizing the pain narratives of parents of youth with chronic pain. *Clin. J. Pain* **2016**, *32*, 849–858. [CrossRef] [PubMed]
23. Simons, L.E.; Sieberg, C.B.; Claar, R.L. Anxiety and functional disability in a large sample of children and adolescents with chronic pain. *Pain Res. Manag.* **2012**, *17*, 93–97. [CrossRef] [PubMed]
24. Tegethoff, M.; Belardi, A.; Stalujanis, E.; Meinlschmidt, G. Comorbidity of mental disorders and chronic pain: Chronology of onset in adolescents of a national representative cohort. *J. Pain* **2015**, *16*, 1054–1064. [CrossRef] [PubMed]
25. Noel, M.; Wilson, A.C.; Holley, A.L.; Durkin, L.; Patton, M.; Palermo, T.M. Posttraumatic stress disorder symptoms in youth with versus without chronic pain. *Pain* **2016**, *157*, 2277–2284. [CrossRef] [PubMed]
26. Korterink, J.J.; Diederen, K.; Benninga, M.A.; Tabbers, M.M. Epidemiology of pediatric functional abdominal pain disorders: A meta-analysis. *PLoS ONE* **2015**, *10*, e0126982. [CrossRef] [PubMed]
27. Egger, H.L.; Costello, E.J.; Erkanli, A.; Angold, A. Somatic complaints and psychopathology in children and adolescents: Stomach aches, musculoskeletal pains, and headaches. *J. Am. Acad. Child Adolesc. Psychiatry* **1999**, *38*, 852–860. [CrossRef] [PubMed]
28. Liedl, A.; Knaevelsrud, C. Chronic pain and PTSD: The perpetual avoidance model and its treatment implications. *Torture* **2008**, *18*, 69–76. [PubMed]
29. Norman, S.B.; Stein, M.B.; Dimsdale, J.E.; Hoyt, D.B. Pain in the aftermath of trauma is a risk factor for post-traumatic stress disorder. *Psychol. Med.* **2008**, *38*, 533–542. [CrossRef] [PubMed]
30. Brown, E.A.; Kenardy, J.A.; Dow, B.L. Ptsd perpetuates pain in children with traumatic brain injury. *J. Pediatr. Psychol.* **2014**, *39*, 512–520. [CrossRef] [PubMed]
31. Holley, A.L.; Wilson, A.C.; Noel, M.; Palermo, T.M. Post-traumatic stress symptoms in children and adolescents with chronic pain: A topical review of the literature and a proposed framework for future research. *Eur. J. Pain* **2016**, *20*, 1371–1383. [CrossRef] [PubMed]
32. Chrousos, G.P. Stress and disorders of the stress system. *Nat. Rev. Endocrinol.* **2009**, *5*, 374–381. [CrossRef] [PubMed]
33. Francis, D.D.; Champagne, F.A.; Liu, D.; Meaney, M.J. Maternal care, gene expression, and the development of individual differences in stress reactivity. *Ann. N. Y. Acad. Sci.* **1999**, *896*, 66–84. [CrossRef] [PubMed]

34. Gunnar, M.; Quevedo, K. The neurobiology of stress and development. *Annu. Rev. Psychol.* **2007**, *58*, 145–173. [CrossRef] [PubMed]
35. Heim, C.; Nemeroff, C.B. The role of childhood trauma in the neurobiology of mood and anxiety disorders: Preclinical and clinical studies. *Biol. Psychiatry* **2001**, *49*, 1023–1039. [CrossRef]
36. Peters, K.L. Neonatal stress reactivity and cortisol. *J. Perinat. Neonatal Nurs.* **1998**, *11*, 45–59. [CrossRef] [PubMed]
37. Shanks, N.; Harbuz, M.S.; Jessop, D.S.; Perks, P.; Moore, P.M.; Lightman, S.L. Inflammatory disease as chronic stress. *Ann. N. Y. Acad. Sci.* **1998**, *840*, 599–607. [CrossRef] [PubMed]
38. Lentjes, E.G.; Griep, E.N.; Boersma, J.W.; Romijn, F.P.; de Kloet, E.R. Glucocorticoid receptors, fibromyalgia and low back pain. *Psychoneuroendocrinology* **1997**, *22*, 603–614. [CrossRef]
39. Heim, C.; Ehlert, U.; Hanker, J.P.; Hellhammer, D.H. Abuse-related posttraumatic stress disorder and alterations of the hypothalamic-pituitary-adrenal axis in women with chronic pelvic pain. *Psychosom. Med.* **1998**, *60*, 309–318. [CrossRef] [PubMed]
40. Blumer, D.; Zorick, F.; Heilbronn, M.; Roth, T. Biological markers for depression in chronic pain. *J. Nerv. Ment. Dis.* **1982**, *170*, 425–428. [CrossRef] [PubMed]
41. Tennant, F.; Hermann, L. Normalization of serum cortisol concentration with opioid treatment of severe chronic pain. *Pain Med.* **2002**, *3*, 132–134. [CrossRef] [PubMed]
42. Geiss, A.; Varadi, E.; Steinbach, K.; Bauer, H.W.; Anton, F. Psychoneuroimmunological correlates of persisting sciatic pain in patients who underwent discectomy. *Neurosci. Lett.* **1997**, *237*, 65–68. [CrossRef]
43. Griep, E.N.; Boersma, J.W.; Lentjes, E.G.; Prins, A.P.; van der Korst, J.K.; de Kloet, E.R. Function of the hypothalamic-pituitary-adrenal axis in patients with fibromyalgia and low back pain. *J. Rheumatol.* **1998**, *25*, 1374–1381. [PubMed]
44. Korszun, A.; Young, E.A.; Singer, K.; Carlson, N.E.; Brown, M.B.; Crofford, L. Basal circadian cortisol secretion in women with temporomandibular disorders. *J. Dent. Res.* **2002**, *81*, 279–283. [CrossRef] [PubMed]
45. Blackburn-Munro, G.; Blackburn-Munro, R.E. Chronic pain, chronic stress and depression: Coincidence or consequence? *J. Neuroendocrinol.* **2001**, *13*, 1009–1023. [CrossRef] [PubMed]
46. Yehuda, R. Biology of posttraumatic stress disorder. *J. Clin. Psychiatry* **2001**, *62* (Suppl. 17), 41–46. [PubMed]
47. Boyer, P. Do anxiety and depression have a common pathophysiological mechanism? *Acta Psychiatr. Scand. Suppl.* **2000**, 24–29. [CrossRef]
48. Levitt, N.S.; Lindsay, R.S.; Holmes, M.C.; Seckl, J.R. Dexamethasone in the last week of pregnancy attenuates hippocampal glucocorticoid receptor gene expression and elevates blood pressure in the adult offspring in the rat. *Neuroendocrinology* **1996**, *64*, 412–418. [CrossRef] [PubMed]
49. Harris, A.; Seckl, J. Glucocorticoids, prenatal stress and the programming of disease. *Horm. Behav.* **2011**, *59*, 279–289. [CrossRef] [PubMed]
50. Champagne, F.A.; Francis, D.D.; Mar, A.; Meaney, M.J. Variations in maternal care in the rat as a mediating influence for the effects of environment on development. *Physiol. Behav.* **2003**, *79*, 359–371. [CrossRef]
51. Caldji, C.; Tannenbaum, B.; Sharma, S.; Francis, D.; Plotsky, P.M.; Meaney, M.J. Maternal care during infancy regulates the development of neural systems mediating the expression of fearfulness in the rat. *Proc. Natl. Acad. Sci. USA* **1998**, *95*, 5335–5340. [CrossRef] [PubMed]
52. Francis, D.; Diorio, J.; Liu, D.; Meaney, M.J. Nongenomic transmission across generations of maternal behavior and stress responses in the rat. *Science* **1999**, *286*, 1155–1158. [CrossRef] [PubMed]
53. Liu, D.; Diorio, J.; Tannenbaum, B.; Caldji, C.; Francis, D.; Freedman, A.; Sharma, S.; Pearson, D.; Plotsky, P.M.; Meaney, M.J. Maternal care, hippocampal glucocorticoid receptors, and hypothalamic-pituitary-adrenal responses to stress. *Science* **1997**, *277*, 1659–1662. [CrossRef] [PubMed]
54. Menard, J.L.; Champagne, D.L.; Meaney, M.J. Variations of maternal care differentially influence 'fear' reactivity and regional patterns of cfos immunoreactivity in response to the shock-probe burying test. *Neuroscience* **2004**, *129*, 297–308. [CrossRef] [PubMed]
55. van Hasselt, F.N.; Cornelisse, S.; Zhang, T.Y.; Meaney, M.J.; Velzing, E.H.; Krugers, H.J.; Joels, M. Adult hippocampal glucocorticoid receptor expression and dentate synaptic plasticity correlate with maternal care received by individuals early in life. *Hippocampus* **2012**, *22*, 255–266. [CrossRef] [PubMed]
56. Weaver, I.C.; Cervoni, N.; Champagne, F.A.; D'Alessio, A.C.; Sharma, S.; Seckl, J.R.; Dymov, S.; Szyf, M.; Meaney, M.J. Epigenetic programming by maternal behavior. *Nat. Neurosci.* **2004**, *7*, 847–854. [CrossRef] [PubMed]

57. Zhang, T.Y.; Bagot, R.; Parent, C.; Nesbitt, C.; Bredy, T.W.; Caldji, C.; Fish, E.; Anisman, H.; Szyf, M.; Meaney, M.J. Maternal programming of defensive responses through sustained effects on gene expression. *Biol. Psychol.* **2006**, *73*, 72–89. [CrossRef] [PubMed]

58. Liu, D.; Diorio, J.; Day, J.C.; Francis, D.D.; Meaney, M.J. Maternal care, hippocampal synaptogenesis and cognitive development in rats. *Nat. Neurosci.* **2000**, *3*, 799–806. [PubMed]

59. Pena, C.J.; Neugut, Y.D.; Calarco, C.A.; Champagne, F.A. Effects of maternal care on the development of midbrain dopamine pathways and reward-directed behavior in female offspring. *Eur. J. Neurosci.* **2014**, *39*, 946–956. [CrossRef] [PubMed]

60. Starr-Phillips, E.J.; Beery, A.K. Natural variation in maternal care shapes adult social behavior in rats. *Dev. Psychobiol.* **2014**, *56*, 1017–1026. [CrossRef] [PubMed]

61. Essex, M.J.; Klein, M.H.; Cho, E.; Kalin, N.H. Maternal stress beginning in infancy may sensitize children to later stress exposure: Effects on cortisol and behavior. *Biol. Psychiatry* **2002**, *52*, 776–784. [CrossRef]

62. Barry, T.J.; Murray, L.; Fearon, R.M.; Moutsiana, C.; Cooper, P.; Goodyer, I.M.; Herbert, J.; Halligan, S.L. Maternal postnatal depression predicts altered offspring biological stress reactivity in adulthood. *Psychoneuroendocrinology* **2015**, *52*, 251–260. [CrossRef] [PubMed]

63. McCauley, J.; Kern, D.E.; Kolodner, K.; Dill, L.; Schroeder, A.F.; DeChant, H.K.; Ryden, J.; Derogatis, L.R.; Bass, E.B. Clinical characteristics of women with a history of childhood abuse: Unhealed wounds. *JAMA* **1997**, *277*, 1362–1368. [CrossRef] [PubMed]

64. Yaari, A.; Eisenberg, E.; Adler, R.; Birkhan, J. Chronic pain in holocaust survivors. *J. Pain Symptom Manag.* **1999**, *17*, 181–187. [CrossRef]

65. Young Casey, C.; Greenberg, M.A.; Nicassio, P.M.; Harpin, R.E.; Hubbard, D. Transition from acute to chronic pain and disability: A model including cognitive, affective, and trauma factors. *Pain* **2008**, *134*, 69–79. [CrossRef] [PubMed]

66. Young, E.A.; Haskett, R.F.; Murphy-Weinberg, V.; Watson, S.J.; Akil, H. Loss of glucocorticoid fast feedback in depression. *Arch. Gen. Psychiatry* **1991**, *48*, 693–699. [CrossRef] [PubMed]

67. Yehuda, R. Biology of posttraumatic stress disorder. *J Clin Psychiatry* **2000**, *61* (Suppl. 7), 14–21. [PubMed]

68. Muhtz, C.; Rodriguez-Raecke, R.; Hinkelmann, K.; Moeller-Bertram, T.; Kiefer, F.; Wiedemann, K.; May, A.; Otte, C. Cortisol response to experimental pain in patients with chronic low back pain and patients with major depression. *Pain Med.* **2013**, *14*, 498–503. [CrossRef] [PubMed]

69. Grunau, R.E.; Cepeda, I.L.; Chau, C.M.; Brummelte, S.; Weinberg, J.; Lavoie, P.M.; Ladd, M.; Hirschfeld, A.F.; Russell, E.; Koren, G.; et al. Neonatal pain-related stress and nfkbia genotype are associated with altered cortisol levels in preterm boys at school age. *PLoS ONE* **2013**, *8*, e73926. [CrossRef] [PubMed]

70. Brummelte, S.; Chau, C.M.; Cepeda, I.L.; Degenhardt, A.; Weinberg, J.; Synnes, A.R.; Grunau, R.E. Cortisol levels in former preterm children at school age are predicted by neonatal procedural pain-related stress. *Psychoneuroendocrinology* **2015**, *51*, 151–163. [CrossRef] [PubMed]

71. McCormack, K.; Sanchez, M.M.; Bardi, M.; Maestripieri, D. Maternal care patterns and behavioral development of rhesus macaque abused infants in the first 6 months of life. *Dev. Psychobiol.* **2006**, *48*, 537–550. [CrossRef] [PubMed]

72. Kaufman, J.; Birmaher, B.; Perel, J.; Dahl, R.E.; Moreci, P.; Nelson, B.; Wells, W.; Ryan, N.D. The corticotropin-releasing hormone challenge in depressed abused, depressed nonabused, and normal control children. *Biol. Psychiatry* **1997**, *42*, 669–679. [CrossRef]

73. De Bellis, M.D.; Chrousos, G.P.; Dorn, L.D.; Burke, L.; Helmers, K.; Kling, M.A.; Trickett, P.K.; Putnam, F.W. Hypothalamic-pituitary-adrenal axis dysregulation in sexually abused girls. *J. Clin. Endocrinol. Metab.* **1994**, *78*, 249–255. [PubMed]

74. Weems, C.F.; Carrion, V.G. The association between ptsd symptoms and salivary cortisol in youth: The role of time since the trauma. *J. Trauma. Stress* **2007**, *20*, 903–907. [CrossRef] [PubMed]

75. Laplante, P.; Diorio, J.; Meaney, M.J. Serotonin regulates hippocampal glucocorticoid receptor expression via a 5-ht7 receptor. *Brain Res. Dev. Brain Res.* **2002**, *139*, 199–203. [CrossRef]

76. Charnay, Y.; Leger, L. Brain serotonergic circuitries. *Dialogues Clin. Neurosci.* **2010**, *12*, 471–487. [PubMed]

77. Suzuki, R.; Rygh, L.J.; Dickenson, A.H. Bad news from the brain: Descending 5-ht pathways that control spinal pain processing. *Trends Pharmacol. Sci.* **2004**, *25*, 613–617. [CrossRef] [PubMed]

78. Sommer, C. Is serotonin hyperalgesic or analgesic? *Curr. Pain Headache Rep.* **2006**, *10*, 101–106. [CrossRef] [PubMed]

79. Wolfe, F.; Russell, I.J.; Vipraio, G.; Ross, K.; Anderson, J. Serotonin levels, pain threshold, and fibromyalgia symptoms in the general population. *J. Rheumatol.* **1997**, *24*, 555–559. [PubMed]
80. Russell, I.J.; Vaeroy, H.; Javors, M.; Nyberg, F. Cerebrospinal fluid biogenic amine metabolites in fibromyalgia/fibrositis syndrome and rheumatoid arthritis. *Arthritis Rheumatol.* **1992**, *35*, 550–556. [CrossRef] [PubMed]
81. Aira, Z.; Buesa, I.; Salgueiro, M.; Bilbao, J.; Aguilera, L.; Zimmermann, M.; Azkue, J.J. Subtype-specific changes in 5-ht receptor-mediated modulation of c fibre-evoked spinal field potentials are triggered by peripheral nerve injury. *Neuroscience* **2010**, *168*, 831–841. [CrossRef] [PubMed]
82. Nicholl, B.I.; Holliday, K.L.; Macfarlane, G.J.; Thomson, W.; Davies, K.A.; O'Neill, T.W.; Bartfai, G.; Boonen, S.; Casanueva, F.F.; Finn, J.D.; et al. Association of htr2a polymorphisms with chronic widespread pain and the extent of musculoskeletal pain: Results from two population-based cohorts. *Arthritis Rheumatol.* **2011**, *63*, 810–818. [CrossRef] [PubMed]
83. Hanley, G.E.; Oberlander, T.F. Neurodevelopmental outcomes following prenatal exposure to serotonin reuptake inhibitor antidepressants: A "social teratogen" or moderator of developmental risk? *Birth Defects Res. A Clin. Mol. Teratol.* **2012**, *94*, 651–659. [CrossRef] [PubMed]
84. Heils, A.; Teufel, A.; Petri, S.; Stober, G.; Riederer, P.; Bengel, D.; Lesch, K.P. Allelic variation of human serotonin transporter gene expression. *J. Neurochem.* **1996**, *66*, 2621–2624. [CrossRef] [PubMed]
85. Offenbaecher, M.; Bondy, B.; de Jonge, S.; Glatzeder, K.; Kruger, M.; Schoeps, P.; Ackenheil, M. Possible association of fibromyalgia with a polymorphism in the serotonin transporter gene regulatory region. *Arthritis Rheumatol.* **1999**, *42*, 2482–2488. [CrossRef]
86. Cohen, H.; Buskila, D.; Neumann, L.; Ebstein, R.P. Confirmation of an association between fibromyalgia and serotonin transporter promoter region (5- httlpr) polymorphism, and relationship to anxiety-related personality traits. *Arthritis Rheumatol.* **2002**, *46*, 845–847. [CrossRef] [PubMed]
87. Homberg, J.R.; Lesch, K.P. Looking on the bright side of serotonin transporter gene variation. *Biol. Psychiatry* **2011**, *69*, 513–519. [CrossRef] [PubMed]
88. Miller, R.; Wankerl, M.; Stalder, T.; Kirschbaum, C.; Alexander, N. The serotonin transporter gene-linked polymorphic region (5-httlpr) and cortisol stress reactivity: A meta-analysis. *Mol. Psychiatry* **2013**, *18*, 1018–1024. [CrossRef] [PubMed]
89. Hariri, A.R.; Mattay, V.S.; Tessitore, A.; Kolachana, B.; Fera, F.; Goldman, D.; Egan, M.F.; Weinberger, D.R. Serotonin transporter genetic variation and the response of the human amygdala. *Science* **2002**, *297*, 400–403. [CrossRef] [PubMed]
90. Heinz, A.; Braus, D.F.; Smolka, M.N.; Wrase, J.; Puls, I.; Hermann, D.; Klein, S.; Grusser, S.M.; Flor, H.; Schumann, G.; et al. Amygdala-prefrontal coupling depends on a genetic variation of the serotonin transporter. *Nat. Neurosci.* **2005**, *8*, 20–21. [CrossRef] [PubMed]
91. Hariri, A.R.; Holmes, A. Genetics of emotional regulation: The role of the serotonin transporter in neural function. *Trends Cogn. Sci.* **2006**, *10*, 182–191. [CrossRef] [PubMed]
92. Canli, T.; Lesch, K.P. Long story short: The serotonin transporter in emotion regulation and social cognition. *Nat. Neurosci.* **2007**, *10*, 1103–1109. [CrossRef] [PubMed]
93. Huang, E.J.; Reichardt, L.F. Neurotrophins: Roles in neuronal development and function. *Annu. Rev. Neurosci.* **2001**, *24*, 677–736. [CrossRef] [PubMed]
94. Rasmusson, A.M.; Shi, L.; Duman, R. Downregulation of bdnf mrna in the hippocampal dentate gyrus after re-exposure to cues previously associated with footshock. *Neuropsychopharmacology* **2002**, *27*, 133–142. [CrossRef]
95. Govindarajan, A.; Rao, B.S.; Nair, D.; Trinh, M.; Mawjee, N.; Tonegawa, S.; Chattarji, S. Transgenic brain-derived neurotrophic factor expression causes both anxiogenic and antidepressant effects. *Proc. Natl. Acad. Sci. USA* **2006**, *103*, 13208–13213. [CrossRef] [PubMed]
96. Lakshminarasimhan, H.; Chattarji, S. Stress leads to contrasting effects on the levels of brain derived neurotrophic factor in the hippocampus and amygdala. *PLoS ONE* **2012**, *7*, e30481. [CrossRef] [PubMed]
97. Mutso, A.A.; Petre, B.; Huang, L.; Baliki, M.N.; Torbey, S.; Herrmann, K.M.; Schnitzer, T.J.; Apkarian, A.V. Reorganization of hippocampal functional connectivity with transition to chronic back pain. *J. Neurophysiol.* **2014**, *111*, 1065–1076. [CrossRef] [PubMed]

98. Jiang, Y.; Oathes, D.; Hush, J.; Darnall, B.; Charvat, M.; Mackey, S.; Etkin, A. Perturbed connectivity of the amygdala and its subregions with the central executive and default mode networks in chronic pain. *Pain* **2016**, *157*, 1970–1978. [CrossRef] [PubMed]

99. Duric, V.; McCarson, K.E. Effects of analgesic or antidepressant drugs on pain- or stress-evoked hippocampal and spinal neurokinin-1 receptor and brain-derived neurotrophic factor gene expression in the rat. *J. Pharmacol. Exp. Ther.* **2006**, *319*, 1235–1243. [CrossRef] [PubMed]

100. Heldt, S.A.; Stanek, L.; Chhatwal, J.P.; Ressler, K.J. Hippocampus-specific deletion of bdnf in adult mice impairs spatial memory and extinction of aversive memories. *Mol. Psychiatry* **2007**, *12*, 656–670. [CrossRef] [PubMed]

101. Fukuhara, K.; Ishikawa, K.; Yasuda, S.; Kishishita, Y.; Kim, H.K.; Kakeda, T.; Yamamoto, M.; Norii, T.; Ishikawa, T. Intracerebroventricular 4-methylcatechol (4-mc) ameliorates chronic pain associated with depression-like behavior via induction of brain-derived neurotrophic factor (bdnf). *Cell. Mol. Neurobiol.* **2012**, *32*, 971–977. [CrossRef] [PubMed]

102. Egan, M.F.; Goldberg, T.E.; Kolachana, B.S.; Callicott, J.H.; Mazzanti, C.M.; Straub, R.E.; Goldman, D.; Weinberger, D.R. Effect of comt val108/158 met genotype on frontal lobe function and risk for schizophrenia. *Proc. Natl. Acad. Sci. USA* **2001**, *98*, 6917–6922. [CrossRef] [PubMed]

103. Egan, M.F.; Kojima, M.; Callicott, J.H.; Goldberg, T.E.; Kolachana, B.S.; Bertolino, A.; Zaitsev, E.; Gold, B.; Goldman, D.; Dean, M.; et al. The bdnf val66met polymorphism affects activity-dependent secretion of bdnf and human memory and hippocampal function. *Cell* **2003**, *112*, 257–269. [CrossRef]

104. Pezawas, L.; Verchinski, B.A.; Mattay, V.S.; Callicott, J.H.; Kolachana, B.S.; Straub, R.E.; Egan, M.F.; Meyer-Lindenberg, A.; Weinberger, D.R. The brain-derived neurotrophic factor val66met polymorphism and variation in human cortical morphology. *J. Neurosci.* **2004**, *24*, 10099–10102. [CrossRef] [PubMed]

105. Kennedy, K.M.; Rodrigue, K.M.; Land, S.J.; Raz, N. Bdnf val66met polymorphism influences age differences in microstructure of the corpus callosum. *Front. Hum. Neurosci.* **2009**, *3*, 19. [CrossRef] [PubMed]

106. Montag, C.; Weber, B.; Fliessbach, K.; Elger, C.; Reuter, M. The bdnf val66met polymorphism impacts parahippocampal and amygdala volume in healthy humans: Incremental support for a genetic risk factor for depression. *Psychol. Med.* **2009**, *39*, 1831–1839. [CrossRef] [PubMed]

107. Soliman, F.; Glatt, C.E.; Bath, K.G.; Levita, L.; Jones, R.M.; Pattwell, S.S.; Jing, D.; Tottenham, N.; Amso, D.; Somerville, L.H.; et al. A genetic variant bdnf polymorphism alters extinction learning in both mouse and human. *Science* **2010**, *327*, 863–866. [CrossRef] [PubMed]

108. Hajek, T.; Kopecek, M.; Hoschl, C. Reduced hippocampal volumes in healthy carriers of brain-derived neurotrophic factor val66met polymorphism: Meta-analysis. *World J. Biol. Psychiatry* **2012**, *13*, 178–187. [CrossRef] [PubMed]

109. Molendijk, M.L.; Bus, B.A.; Spinhoven, P.; Kaimatzoglou, A.; Oude Voshaar, R.C.; Penninx, B.W.; van, I.M.H.; Elzinga, B.M. A systematic review and meta-analysis on the association between bdnf val(66)met and hippocampal volume–a genuine effect or a winners curse? *Am. J. Med. Genet. B Neuropsychiatr. Genet.* **2012**, *159B*, 731–740. [CrossRef] [PubMed]

110. Kim, S.N.; Kang, D.H.; Yun, J.Y.; Lee, T.Y.; Jung, W.H.; Jang, J.H.; Kwon, J.S. Impact of the bdnf val66met polymorphism on regional brain gray matter volumes: Relevance to the stress response. *Psychiatry Investig.* **2013**, *10*, 173–179. [CrossRef] [PubMed]

111. Xu, H.; Qing, H.; Lu, W.; Keegan, D.; Richardson, J.S.; Chlan-Fourney, J.; Li, X.M. Quetiapine attenuates the immobilization stress-induced decrease of brain-derived neurotrophic factor expression in rat hippocampus. *Neurosci. Lett.* **2002**, *321*, 65–68. [CrossRef]

112. Chen, Z.Y.; Jing, D.; Bath, K.G.; Ieraci, A.; Khan, T.; Siao, C.J.; Herrera, D.G.; Toth, M.; Yang, C.; McEwen, B.S.; et al. Genetic variant bdnf (val66met) polymorphism alters anxiety-related behavior. *Science* **2006**, *314*, 140–143. [CrossRef] [PubMed]

113. Garcia, L.S.; Comim, C.M.; Valvassori, S.S.; Reus, G.Z.; Barbosa, L.M.; Andreazza, A.C.; Stertz, L.; Fries, G.R.; Gavioli, E.C.; Kapczinski, F.; et al. Acute administration of ketamine induces antidepressant-like effects in the forced swimming test and increases bdnf levels in the rat hippocampus. *Prog. Neuropsychopharmacol. Biol. Psychiatry* **2008**, *32*, 140–144. [CrossRef] [PubMed]

114. Pivac, N.; Kozaric-Kovacic, D.; Grubisic-Ilic, M.; Nedic, G.; Rakos, I.; Nikolac, M.; Blazev, M.; Muck-Seler, D. The association between brain-derived neurotrophic factor val66met variants and psychotic symptoms in posttraumatic stress disorder. *World J. Biol. Psychiatry* **2012**, *13*, 306–311. [CrossRef] [PubMed]

115. Gao, S.; Cui, Y.L.; Yu, C.Q.; Wang, Q.S.; Zhang, Y. Tetrandrine exerts antidepressant-like effects in animal models: Role of brain-derived neurotrophic factor. *Behav. Brain Res.* **2013**, *238*, 79–85. [CrossRef] [PubMed]

116. Lee, L.C.; Tu, C.H.; Chen, L.F.; Shen, H.D.; Chao, H.T.; Lin, M.W.; Hsieh, J.C. Association of brain-derived neurotrophic factor gene val66met polymorphism with primary dysmenorrhea. *PLoS ONE* **2014**, *9*, e112766. [CrossRef] [PubMed]

117. Reddy, S.Y.; Rasmussen, N.A.; Fourie, N.H.; Berger, R.S.; Martino, A.C.; Gill, J.; Longchamps, R.; Wang, X.M.; Heitkemper, M.M.; Henderson, W.A. Sleep quality, bdnf genotype and gene expression in individuals with chronic abdominal pain. *BMC Med. Genom.* **2014**, *7*, 61. [CrossRef] [PubMed]

118. Zhang, L.; Benedek, D.M.; Fullerton, C.S.; Forsten, R.D.; Naifeh, J.A.; Li, X.X.; Hu, X.Z.; Li, H.; Jia, M.; Xing, G.Q.; et al. Ptsd risk is associated with bdnf val66met and bdnf overexpression. *Mol. Psychiatry* **2014**, *19*, 8–10. [CrossRef] [PubMed]

119. Generaal, E.; Milaneschi, Y.; Jansen, R.; Elzinga, B.M.; Dekker, J.; Penninx, B.W. The brain-derived neurotrophic factor pathway, life stress, and chronic multi-site musculoskeletal pain. *Mol. Pain* **2016**, *12*. [CrossRef] [PubMed]

120. Trang, T.; Beggs, S.; Salter, M.W. Brain-derived neurotrophic factor from microglia: A molecular substrate for neuropathic pain. *Neuron. Glia Biol.* **2011**, *7*, 99–108. [CrossRef] [PubMed]

121. Watkins, L.R.; Hutchinson, M.R.; Ledeboer, A.; Wieseler-Frank, J.; Milligan, E.D.; Maier, S.F. Norman cousins lecture. Glia as the "bad guys": Implications for improving clinical pain control and the clinical utility of opioids. *Brain Behav. Immun.* **2007**, *21*, 131–146. [CrossRef] [PubMed]

122. Uceyler, N.; Sommer, C. Cytokine-related and histological biomarkers for neuropathic pain assessment. *Pain Manag.* **2012**, *2*, 391–398. [CrossRef] [PubMed]

123. Ransohoff, R.M. How neuroinflammation contributes to neurodegeneration. *Science* **2016**, *353*, 777–783. [CrossRef] [PubMed]

124. Pankratz, S.; Bittner, S.; Kehrel, B.E.; Langer, H.F.; Kleinschnitz, C.; Meuth, S.G.; Gobel, K. The inflammatory role of platelets: Translational insights from experimental studies of autoimmune disorders. *Int. J. Mol. Sci.* **2016**, *17*. [CrossRef] [PubMed]

125. Benson, S.; Engler, H.; Schedlowski, M.; Elsenbruch, S. Experimental endotoxemia as a model to study neuroimmune mechanisms in human visceral pain. *Ann. N. Y. Acad. Sci.* **2012**, *1262*, 108–117. [CrossRef] [PubMed]

126. Del Valle, L.; Schwartzman, R.J.; Alexander, G. Spinal cord histopathological alterations in a patient with longstanding complex regional pain syndrome. *Brain Behav. Immun.* **2009**, *23*, 85–91. [CrossRef] [PubMed]

127. Shi, Y.; Gelman, B.B.; Lisinicchia, J.G.; Tang, S.J. Chronic-pain-associated astrocytic reaction in the spinal cord dorsal horn of human immunodeficiency virus-infected patients. *J. Neurosci.* **2012**, *32*, 10833–10840. [CrossRef] [PubMed]

128. Brisby, H.; Olmarker, K.; Rosengren, L.; Cederlund, C.G.; Rydevik, B. Markers of nerve tissue injury in the cerebrospinal fluid in patients with lumbar disc herniation and sciatica. *Spine* **1999**, *24*, 742–746. [CrossRef]

129. Kadetoff, D.; Lampa, J.; Westman, M.; Andersson, M.; Kosek, E. Evidence of central inflammation in fibromyalgia-increased cerebrospinal fluid interleukin-8 levels. *J. Neuroimmunol.* **2012**, *242*, 33–38. [CrossRef] [PubMed]

130. Loggia, M.L.; Chonde, D.B.; Akeju, O.; Arabasz, G.; Catana, C.; Edwards, R.R.; Hill, E.; Hsu, S.; Izquierdo-Garcia, D.; Ji, R.R.; et al. Evidence for brain glial activation in chronic pain patients. *Brain* **2015**, *138*, 604–615. [CrossRef] [PubMed]

131. Fiore, N.T.; Austin, P.J. Are the emergence of affective disturbances in neuropathic pain states contingent on supraspinal neuroinflammation? *Brain Behav. Immun.* **2016**, *56*, 397–411. [CrossRef] [PubMed]

132. Goshen, I.; Kreisel, T.; Ben-Menachem-Zidon, O.; Licht, T.; Weidenfeld, J.; Ben-Hur, T.; Yirmiya, R. Brain interleukin-1 mediates chronic stress-induced depression in mice via adrenocortical activation and hippocampal neurogenesis suppression. *Mol. Psychiatry* **2008**, *13*, 717–728. [CrossRef] [PubMed]

133. Goshen, I.; Kreisel, T.; Ounallah-Saad, H.; Renbaum, P.; Zalzstein, Y.; Ben-Hur, T.; Levy-Lahad, E.; Yirmiya, R. A dual role for interleukin-1 in hippocampal-dependent memory processes. *Psychoneuroendocrinology* **2007**, *32*, 1106–1115. [CrossRef] [PubMed]

134. Besedovsky, H.O.; del Rey, A. Immune-neuro-endocrine interactions: Facts and hypotheses. *Endocr. Rev.* **1996**, *17*, 64–102. [CrossRef] [PubMed]

135. Pace, T.W.; Hu, F.; Miller, A.H. Cytokine-effects on glucocorticoid receptor function: Relevance to glucocorticoid resistance and the pathophysiology and treatment of major depression. *Brain Behav. Immun.* **2007**, *21*, 9–19. [CrossRef] [PubMed]

136. Vogelzangs, N.; de Jonge, P.; Smit, J.H.; Bahn, S.; Penninx, B.W. Cytokine production capacity in depression and anxiety. *Transl. Psychiatry* **2016**, *6*, e825. [CrossRef] [PubMed]

137. Lasselin, J.; Kemani, M.K.; Kanstrup, M.; Olsson, G.L.; Axelsson, J.; Andreasson, A.; Lekander, M.; Wicksell, R.K. Low-grade inflammation may moderate the effect of behavioral treatment for chronic pain in adults. *J. Behav. Med.* **2016**. [CrossRef] [PubMed]

138. Beggs, S.; Currie, G.; Salter, M.W.; Fitzgerald, M.; Walker, S.M. Priming of adult pain responses by neonatal pain experience: Maintenance by central neuroimmune activity. *Brain* **2012**, *135*, 404–417. [CrossRef] [PubMed]

139. Mitchell, R.H.; Goldstein, B.I. Inflammation in children and adolescents with neuropsychiatric disorders: A systematic review. *J. Am. Acad. Child Adolesc. Psychiatry* **2014**, *53*, 274–296. [CrossRef] [PubMed]

140. Ganguly, P.; Brenhouse, H.C. Broken or maladaptive? Altered trajectories in neuroinflammation and behavior after early life adversity. *Dev. Cogn. Neurosci.* **2015**, *11*, 18–30. [CrossRef] [PubMed]

141. Gill, J.; Luckenbaugh, D.; Charney, D.; Vythilingam, M. Sustained elevation of serum interleukin-6 and relative insensitivity to hydrocortisone differentiates posttraumatic stress disorder with and without depression. *Biol. Psychiatry* **2010**, *68*, 999–1006. [CrossRef] [PubMed]

142. Lerman, I.; Davis, B.A.; Bertram, T.M.; Proudfoot, J.; Hauger, R.L.; Coe, C.L.; Patel, P.M.; Baker, D.G. Posttraumatic stress disorder influences the nociceptive and intrathecal cytokine response to a painful stimulus in combat veterans. *Psychoneuroendocrinology* **2016**, *73*, 99–108. [CrossRef] [PubMed]

143. Kopf, M.; Bachmann, M.F.; Marsland, B.J. Averting inflammation by targeting the cytokine environment. *Nat. Rev. Drug Discov.* **2010**, *9*, 703–718. [CrossRef] [PubMed]

144. Apkarian, A.V.; Bushnell, M.C.; Treede, R.D.; Zubieta, J.K. Human brain mechanisms of pain perception and regulation in health and disease. *Eur. J. Pain* **2005**, *9*, 463–484. [CrossRef] [PubMed]

145. Bushnell, M.C.; Ceko, M.; Low, L.A. Cognitive and emotional control of pain and its disruption in chronic pain. *Nat. Rev. Neurosci.* **2013**, *14*, 502–511. [CrossRef] [PubMed]

146. Duerden, E.G.; Albanese, M.C. Localization of pain-related brain activation: A meta-analysis of neuroimaging data. *Hum. Brain Mapp.* **2013**, *34*, 109–149. [CrossRef] [PubMed]

147. Iadarola, M.J.; Coghill, R.C. Imaging of pain: Recent developments. *Curr. Opin. Anaesthesiol.* **1999**, *12*, 583–589. [CrossRef] [PubMed]

148. Willis, W.D.; Westlund, K.N. Neuroanatomy of the pain system and of the pathways that modulate pain. *J. Clin. Neurophysiol.* **1997**, *14*, 2–31. [CrossRef] [PubMed]

149. Atlas, L.Y.; Lindquist, M.A.; Bolger, N.; Wager, T.D. Brain mediators of the effects of noxious heat on pain. *Pain* **2014**, *155*, 1632–1648. [CrossRef] [PubMed]

150. Coghill, R.C.; Sang, C.N.; Maisog, J.M.; Iadarola, M.J. Pain intensity processing within the human brain: A bilateral, distributed mechanism. *J. Neurophysiol.* **1999**, *82*, 1934–1943. [PubMed]

151. Wager, T.D.; Atlas, L.Y.; Lindquist, M.A.; Roy, M.; Woo, C.W.; Kross, E. An fmri-based neurologic signature of physical pain. *N. Engl. J. Med.* **2013**, *368*, 1388–1397. [CrossRef] [PubMed]

152. Hubbard, C.S.; Khan, S.A.; Xu, S.; Cha, M.; Masri, R.; Seminowicz, D.A. Behavioral, metabolic and functional brain changes in a rat model of chronic neuropathic pain: A longitudinal mri study. *Neuroimage* **2015**, *107*, 333–344. [CrossRef] [PubMed]

153. Jensen, K.B.; Regenbogen, C.; Ohse, M.C.; Frasnelli, J.; Freiherr, J.; Lundstrom, J.N. Brain activations during pain: A neuroimaging meta-analysis of patients with pain and healthy controls. *Pain* **2016**, *157*, 1279–1286. [CrossRef] [PubMed]

154. Baliki, M.N.; Petre, B.; Torbey, S.; Herrmann, K.M.; Huang, L.; Schnitzer, T.J.; Fields, H.L.; Apkarian, A.V. Corticostriatal functional connectivity predicts transition to chronic back pain. *Nat. Neurosci.* **2012**, *15*, 1117–1119. [CrossRef] [PubMed]

155. Hubbard, C.S.; Becerra, L.; Heinz, N.; Ludwick, A.; Rasooly, T.; Wu, R.; Johnson, A.; Schechter, N.L.; Borsook, D.; Nurko, S. Abdominal pain, the adolescent and altered brain structure and function. *PLoS ONE* **2016**, *11*, e0156545. [CrossRef] [PubMed]

156. Simons, L.E.; Pielech, M.; Erpelding, N.; Linnman, C.; Moulton, E.; Sava, S.; Lebel, A.; Serrano, P.; Sethna, N.; Berde, C.; et al. The responsive amygdala: Treatment-induced alterations in functional connectivity in pediatric complex regional pain syndrome. *Pain* **2014**, *155*, 1727–1742. [CrossRef] [PubMed]

157. Simons, L.E.; Erpelding, N.; Hernandez, J.; Serrano, P.; Zhang, K.; Lebel, A.; Sethna, N.; Berde, C.; Prabhu, S.; Becerra, L.; et al. Fear and reward circuit alterations in pediatric crps. *Front. Hum. Neurosci.* **2016**, *9*, 1–13. [CrossRef] [PubMed]

158. Lebel, A.; Becerra, L.; Wallin, D.; Moulton, E.A.; Morris, S.; Pendse, G.; Jasciewicz, J.; Stein, M.; Aiello-Lammens, M.; Grant, E.; et al. Fmri reveals distinct cns processing during symptomatic and recovered complex regional pain syndrome in children. *Brain* **2008**, *131*, 1854–1879. [CrossRef] [PubMed]

159. McEwen, B.S.; Kalia, M. The role of corticosteroids and stress in chronic pain conditions. *Metabolism* **2010**, *59* (Suppl. 1), S9–S15. [CrossRef] [PubMed]

160. Karatsoreos, I.N.; McEwen, B.S. Psychobiological allostasis: Resistance, resilience and vulnerability. *Trends Cogn. Sci.* **2011**, *15*, 576–584. [CrossRef] [PubMed]

161. Becerra, L.; Sava, S.; Simons, L.E.; Drosos, A.M.; Sethna, N.; Berde, C.; Lebel, A.A.; Borsook, D. Intrinsic brain networks normalize with treatment in pediatric complex regional pain syndrome. *Neuroimage Clin.* **2014**, *6*, 347–369. [CrossRef] [PubMed]

162. Coutinho, J.F.; Fernandesl, S.V.; Soares, J.M.; Maia, L.; Goncalves, O.F.; Sampaio, A. Default mode network dissociation in depressive and anxiety states. *Brain Imaging Behav.* **2016**, *10*, 147–157. [CrossRef] [PubMed]

163. Geng, H.; Li, X.; Chen, J.; Li, X.; Gu, R. Decreased intra- and inter-salience network functional connectivity is related to trait anxiety in adolescents. *Front. Behav. Neurosci.* **2015**, *9*, 350. [CrossRef] [PubMed]

164. Lei, D.; Li, L.; Li, L.; Suo, X.; Huang, X.; Lui, S.; Li, J.; Bi, F.; Kemp, G.J.; Gong, Q. Microstructural abnormalities in children with post-traumatic stress disorder: A diffusion tensor imaging study at 3.0t. *Sci. Rep.* **2015**, *5*, 8933. [CrossRef] [PubMed]

165. Pannekoek, J.N.; van der Werff, S.J.; Meens, P.H.; van den Bulk, B.G.; Jolles, D.D.; Veer, I.M.; van Lang, N.D.; Rombouts, S.A.; van der Wee, N.J.; Vermeiren, R.R. Aberrant resting-state functional connectivity in limbic and salience networks in treatment–naive clinically depressed adolescents. *J. Child Psychol. Psychiatry* **2014**, *55*, 1317–1327. [CrossRef] [PubMed]

166. Schanberg, L.E.; Anthony, K.K.; Gil, K.M.; Lefebvre, J.C.; Kredich, D.W.; Macharoni, L.M. Family pain history predicts child health status in children with chronic rheumatic disease. *Pediatrics* **2001**, *108*, E47. [CrossRef] [PubMed]

167. Garber, J.; Zeman, J.; Walker, L.S. Recurrent abdominal pain in children: Psychiatric diagnoses and parental psychopathology. *J. Am. Acad. Child Adolesc. Psychiatry* **1990**, *29*, 648–656. [CrossRef] [PubMed]

168. Hoftun, G.B.; Romundstad, P.R.; Rygg, M. Factors associated with adolescent chronic non-specific pain, chronic multisite pain, and chronic pain with high disability: The young-hunt study 2008. *J. Pain* **2012**. [CrossRef] [PubMed]

169. Morgan, J.E.; Hammen, C.; Lee, S.S. Parental serotonin transporter polymorphism (5-httlpr) moderates associations of stress and child behavior with parenting behavior. *J. Clin. Child Adolesc. Psychol.* **2016**, 1–12. [CrossRef] [PubMed]

170. Roth, T.L.; Lubin, F.D.; Funk, A.J.; Sweatt, J.D. Lasting epigenetic influence of early-life adversity on the bdnf gene. *Biol. Psychiatry* **2009**, *65*, 760–769. [CrossRef] [PubMed]

171. van der Doelen, R.H.; Arnoldussen, I.A.; Ghareh, H.; van Och, L.; Homberg, J.R.; Kozicz, T. Early life adversity and serotonin transporter gene variation interact to affect DNA methylation of the corticotropin-releasing factor gene promoter region in the adult rat brain. *Dev. Psychopathol.* **2015**, *27*, 123–135. [CrossRef] [PubMed]

172. Walker, L.S.; Greene, J.W. Children with recurrent abdominal pain and their parents: More somatic complaints, anxiety, and depression than other patient families? *J. Pediatr. Psychol.* **1989**, *14*, 231–243. [CrossRef] [PubMed]

173. Campo, J.V.; Bridge, J.; Lucas, A.; Savorelli, S.; Walker, L.; Di Lorenzo, C.; Iyengar, S.; Brent, D.A. Physical and emotional health of mothers of youth with functional abdominal pain. *Arch. Pediatr. Adolesc. Med.* **2007**, *161*, 131–137. [CrossRef] [PubMed]

174. Williamson, G.M.; Walters, A.S.; Shaffer, D.R. Caregiver models of self and others, coping, and depression: Predictors of depression in children with chronic pain. *Health Psychol.* **2002**, *21*, 405–410. [CrossRef] [PubMed]

175. Wolff, N.; Darlington, A.S.; Hunfeld, J.; Verhulst, F.; Jaddoe, V.; Hofman, A.; Passchier, J.; Tiemeier, H. Determinants of somatic complaints in 18-month-old children: The generation r study. *J. Pediatr. Psychol.* **2010**, *35*, 306–316. [CrossRef] [PubMed]

176. Higgins, K.S.; Birnie, K.A.; Chambers, C.T.; Wilson, A.C.; Caes, L.; Clark, A.J.; Lynch, M.; Stinson, J.; Campbell-Yeo, M. Offspring of parents with chronic pain: A systematic review and meta-analysis of pain, health, psychological, and family outcomes. *Pain* **2015**, *156*, 2256–2266. [CrossRef] [PubMed]

177. Levy, R.L.; Whitehead, W.E.; Von Korff, M.R.; Feld, A.D. Intergenerational transmission of gastrointestinal illness behavior. *Am. J. Gastroenterol.* **2000**, *95*, 451–456. [CrossRef] [PubMed]

178. van Tilburg, M.A.; Levy, R.L.; Walker, L.S.; Von Korff, M.; Feld, L.D.; Garner, M.; Feld, A.D.; Whitehead, W.E. Psychosocial mechanisms for the transmission of somatic symptoms from parents to children. *World J. Gastroenterol.* **2015**, *21*, 5532–5541. [CrossRef] [PubMed]

179. Stone, A.L.; Wilson, A.C. Transmission of risk from parents with chronic pain to offspring: An integrative conceptual model. *Pain* **2016**. [CrossRef] [PubMed]

180. Palermo, T.M.; Law, E.F.; Fales, J.; Bromberg, M.H.; Jessen-Fiddick, T.; Tai, G. Internet-delivered cognitive-behavioral treatment for adolescents with chronic pain and their parents: A randomized controlled multicenter trial. *Pain* **2016**, *157*, 174–185. [CrossRef] [PubMed]

181. Palermo, T.M.; Valrie, C.R.; Karlson, C.W. Family and parent influences on pediatric chronic pain: A developmental perspective. *Am. Psychol.* **2014**, *69*, 142–152. [CrossRef] [PubMed]

182. Fisher, E.; Law, E.; Palermo, T.M.; Eccleston, C. Psychological therapies (remotely delivered) for the management of chronic and recurrent pain in children and adolescents. *Cochrane Database Syst. Rev.* **2014**, *2014*.

183. Cunningham, N.R.; Jagpal, A.; Tran, S.T.; Kashikar-Zuck, S.; Goldschneider, K.R.; Coghill, R.C.; Lynch-Jordan, A.M. Anxiety adversely impacts response to cognitive behavioral therapy in children with chronic pain. *J. Pediatr.* **2016**, *171*, 227–233. [CrossRef] [PubMed]

184. Benore, E.; D'Auria, A.; Banez, G.A.; Worley, S.; Tang, A. The influence of anxiety reduction on clinical response to pediatric chronic pain rehabilitation. *Clin. J. Pain* **2015**, *31*, 375–383. [CrossRef] [PubMed]

185. Sullivan, A.; Goodison-Farnsworth, E.; Jaaniste, T. Posttraumatic stress disorder in children with chronic pain. *Pediatr. Pain Lett.* **2015**, *17*, 35–39.

186. Nelson, S.M.; Cunningham, N.R.; Kashikar-Zuck, S. A conceptual framework for understanding the role of adverse childhood experiences in pediatric chronic pain. *Clin. J. Pain* **2016**. [CrossRef] [PubMed]

187. Bosco, M.A.; Gallinati, J.L.; Clark, M.E. Conceptualizing and treating comorbid chronic pain and ptsd. *Pain Res. Treat.* **2013**, *2013*, 174728. [CrossRef] [PubMed]

188. Plagge, J.M.; Lu, M.W.; Lovejoy, T.I.; Karl, A.I.; Dobscha, S.K. Treatment of comorbid pain and ptsd in returning veterans: A collaborative approach utilizing behavioral activation. *Pain Med.* **2013**, *14*, 1164–1172. [CrossRef] [PubMed]

189. Otis, J.D.; Keane, T.M.; Kerns, R.D.; Monson, C.; Scioli, E. The development of an integrated treatment for veterans with comorbid chronic pain and posttraumatic stress disorder. *Pain Med.* **2009**, *10*, 1300–1311. [CrossRef] [PubMed]

190. Allen, L.B.; Tsao, J.C.I.; Seidman, L.C.; Ehrenreich-May, J.; Zeltzer, L.K. A unified, transdiagnositc treatment for adolescents with chronic pain and comorbid anxiety and depression. *Cogn. Behav. Pract.* **2012**, *19*, 56–67. [CrossRef]

191. Umezaki, Y.; Badran, B.W.; DeVries, W.H.; Moss, J.; Gonzales, T.; George, M.S. The efficacy of daily prefrontal repetitive transcranial magnetic stimulation (rtms) for burning mouth syndrome (bms): A randomized controlled single-blind study. *Brain Stimul.* **2016**, *9*, 234–242. [CrossRef] [PubMed]

192. Picarelli, H.; Teixeira, M.J.; de Andrade, D.C.; Myczkowski, M.L.; Luvisotto, T.B.; Yeng, L.T.; Fonoff, E.T.; Pridmore, S.; Marcolin, M.A. Repetitive transcranial magnetic stimulation is efficacious as an add-on to pharmacological therapy in complex regional pain syndrome (crps) type i. *J. Pain* **2010**, *11*, 1203–1210. [CrossRef] [PubMed]

193. Mendonca, M.E.; Simis, M.; Grecco, L.C.; Battistella, L.R.; Baptista, A.F.; Fregni, F. Transcranial direct current stimulation combined with aerobic exercise to optimize analgesic responses in fibromyalgia: A randomized placebo-controlled clinical trial. *Front. Hum. Neurosci.* **2016**, *10*, 68. [CrossRef] [PubMed]

194. Short, E.B.; Borckardt, J.J.; Anderson, B.S.; Frohman, H.; Beam, W.; Reeves, S.T.; George, M.S. Ten sessions of adjunctive left prefrontal rtms significantly reduces fibromyalgia pain: A randomized, controlled pilot study. *Pain* **2011**, *152*, 2477–2484. [CrossRef] [PubMed]

195. Lefaucheur, J.P.; Ayache, S.S.; Sorel, M.; Farhat, W.H.; Zouari, H.G.; Ciampi de Andrade, D.; Ahdab, R.; Menard-Lefaucheur, I.; Brugieres, P.; Goujon, C. Analgesic effects of repetitive transcranial magnetic stimulation of the motor cortex in neuropathic pain: Influence of theta burst stimulation priming. *Eur. J. Pain* **2012**, *16*, 1403–1413. [CrossRef] [PubMed]

196. Fregni, F.; Boggio, P.S.; Lima, M.C.; Ferreira, M.J.; Wagner, T.; Rigonatti, S.P.; Castro, A.W.; Souza, D.R.; Riberto, M.; Freedman, S.D.; et al. A sham-controlled, phase ii trial of transcranial direct current stimulation for the treatment of central pain in traumatic spinal cord injury. *Pain* **2006**, *122*, 197–209. [CrossRef] [PubMed]

197. Defrin, R.; Grunhaus, L.; Zamir, D.; Zeilig, G. The effect of a series of repetitive transcranial magnetic stimulations of the motor cortex on central pain after spinal cord injury. *Arch. Phys. Med. Rehabil.* **2007**, *88*, 1574–1580. [CrossRef] [PubMed]

198. Perera, T.; George, M.S.; Grammer, G.; Janicak, P.G.; Pascual-Leone, A.; Wirecki, T.S. The clinical tms society consensus review and treatment recommendations for tms therapy for major depressive disorder. *Brain Stimul.* **2016**, *9*, 336–346. [CrossRef] [PubMed]

199. Canadian Agency for Drugs and Technologies in Health. Cadth rapid response reports. In *Transcranial Magnetic Stimulation for the Treatment of Adults with Ptsd, Gad, or Depression: A Review of Clinical Effectiveness and Guidelines*; Canadian Agency for Drugs and Technologies in Health: Ottawa, ON, Canada, 2014.

200. Paes, F.; Machado, S.; Arias-Carrion, O.; Velasques, B.; Teixeira, S.; Budde, H.; Cagy, M.; Piedade, R.; Ribeiro, P.; Huston, J.P.; et al. The value of repetitive transcranial magnetic stimulation (rtms) for the treatment of anxiety disorders: An integrative review. *CNS Neurol. Disord. Drug Targets* **2011**, *10*, 610–620. [CrossRef] [PubMed]

201. Naro, A.; Milardi, D.; Russo, M.; Terranova, C.; Rizzo, V.; Cacciola, A.; Marino, S.; Calabro, R.S.; Quartarone, A. Non-invasive brain stimulation, a tool to revert maladaptive plasticity in neuropathic pain. *Front. Hum. Neurosci.* **2016**, *10*, 376. [CrossRef] [PubMed]

202. DosSantos, M.F.; Ferreira, N.; Toback, R.L.; Carvalho, A.C.; DaSilva, A.F. Potential mechanisms supporting the value of motor cortex stimulation to treat chronic pain syndromes. *Front. Neurosci.* **2016**, *10*. [CrossRef] [PubMed]

203. Chrousos, G.P. The hypothalamic-pituitary-adrenal axis and immune-mediated inflammation. *N. Engl. J. Med.* **1995**, *332*, 1351–1362. [PubMed]

204. Elenkov, I.J.; Webster, E.L.; Torpy, D.J.; Chrousos, G.P. Stress, corticotropin-releasing hormone, glucocorticoids, and the immune/inflammatory response: Acute and chronic effects. *Ann. N. Y. Acad. Sci.* **1999**, *876*, 1–11; discussion 11-13. [CrossRef] [PubMed]

205. Meyer, J.S. Early adrenalectomy stimulates subsequent growth and development of the rat brain. *Exp. Neurol.* **1983**, *82*, 432–446. [CrossRef]

206. Meaney, M.J.; Diorio, J.; Francis, D.; Widdowson, J.; LaPlante, P.; Caldji, C.; Sharma, S.; Seckl, J.R.; Plotsky, P.M. Early environmental regulation of forebrain glucocorticoid receptor gene expression: Implications for adrenocortical responses to stress. *Dev. Neurosci.* **1996**, *18*, 49–72. [CrossRef] [PubMed]

207. Korte, S.M. Corticosteroids in relation to fear, anxiety and psychopathology. *Neurosci. Biobehav. Rev.* **2001**, *25*, 117–142. [CrossRef]

208. Knook, L.M.; Lijmer, J.G.; Konijnenberg, A.Y.; Taminiau, B.; van Engeland, H. The course of chronic pain with and without psychiatric disorders: A 6-year follow-up study from childhood to adolescence and young adulthood. *J. Clin. Psychiatry* **2012**, *73*, e134–e139. [CrossRef] [PubMed]

209. Mulak, A.; Tache, Y.; Larauche, M. Sex hormones in the modulation of irritable bowel syndrome. *World J. Gastroenterol.* **2014**, *20*, 2433–2448. [CrossRef] [PubMed]

210. Karshikoff, B.; Lekander, M.; Soop, A.; Lindstedt, F.; Ingvar, M.; Kosek, E.; Olgart Hoglund, C.; Axelsson, J. Modality and sex differences in pain sensitivity during human endotoxemia. *Brain Behav. Immun.* **2015**, *46*, 35–43. [CrossRef] [PubMed]

211. Aloisi, A.M.; Bachiocco, V.; Costantino, A.; Stefani, R.; Ceccarelli, I.; Bertaccini, A.; Meriggiola, M.C. Cross-sex hormone administration changes pain in transsexual women and men. *Pain* **2007**, *132* (Suppl. 1), S60–S67. [CrossRef] [PubMed]

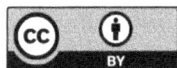

Section 3:
Social Factors: Family, School, Neighborhood

Review

Attachment and Chronic Pain in Children and Adolescents

Theresa J. Donnelly [1] and Tiina Jaaniste [1,2,*]

[1]   Department of Pain & Palliative Care, Sydney Children's Hospital, Randwick, NSW 2031, Australia;
      Theresa.Donnelly@health.nsw.gov.au
[2]   School of Women's and Children's Health, University of New South Wales,
      Kensington, NSW 2052, Australia
*   Correspondence: Tiina.Jaaniste@health.nsw.gov.au; Tel.: +61-2-9382-1818

Academic Editor: Lynn Walker
Received: 9 September 2016; Accepted: 17 October 2016; Published: 25 October 2016

Abstract: Although attachment theory is not new, its theoretical implications for the pediatric chronic pain context have not been thoroughly considered, and the empirical implications and potential clinical applications are worth exploring. The attachment framework broadly focuses on interactions between a child's developing self-regulatory systems and their caregiver's responses. These interactions are believed to create a template for how individuals will relate to others in the future, and may help account for normative and pathological patterns of emotions and behavior throughout life. This review outlines relevant aspects of the attachment framework to the pediatric chronic pain context. The theoretical and empirical literature is reviewed regarding the potential role of attachment-based constructs such as vulnerability and maintaining factors of pediatric chronic pain. The nature and targets of attachment-based pediatric interventions are considered, with particular focus on relevance for the pediatric chronic pain context. The potential role of attachment style in the transition from acute to chronic pain is considered, with further research directions outlined.

Keywords: attachment; chronic pain; child; adolescent

1. Introduction

The term attachment theory has come to loosely refer to a cluster of theories, stemming from the seminal work of Bowlby [1] and Ainsworth [2,3]. Attachment theories broadly focus on interactions between a child's developing self-regulatory systems and their caregiver's responses, and are believed to shed light on an individual's cognitions, emotions and behavior throughout life, helping account for both normative and pathological patterns. The attachment system is considered to be instinctive and biologically based [1], with infants striving to maintain proximity to a caregiver in order to ensure survival needs are attended to [1,4]. The attachment system is understood to be predicated on the goal of increasing the individual's chance of survival and is particularly activated in circumstances where there is a threat such as pain.

The goals of attachment behavior are thought to evolve as a child develops, transitioning from proximity and closeness in infancy and early childhood, through to availability and a secure base from which to explore in middle childhood and adolescence. Infants learn that cries resulting from physical discomfort and needs such as hunger are responded to by a loving caregiver. This is thought to become a template for future relationships. Hence, Bowlby [1,5,6] considered attachment as a relatively stable aspect of personality that is shaped early in life in response to the caregiver's responsivity, consistency, and sensitivity to the child. This is subsequently influenced or reinforced via interactions with caregivers throughout childhood and adolescence [7] and significant others throughout life [8].

Research has generally supported the key premise of attachment theory, namely that early security is beneficial for the developmental adaptation and competence of children, whereas insecurity carries risks for psychopathology (for reviews see [9,10]; for meta-analysis see [11]). Moreover, there is increasing evidence that insecure attachment styles may also carry risks of greater physical symptoms, such as pain [12,13] and greater disability [14,15]. However, the vast majority of this research has been cross-sectional rather than longitudinal, thus making causal inferences difficult.

It has been proposed that an individual's characteristic attachment behaviors are likely to be activated as a result of an illness or threat [16]. Illness, and arguably pain, may trigger an increased need for security and the wish for a close, caring other. This may be an adaptive response within the context of an injury or acute pain. However, in the context of chronic pain this can result in a range of complex and difficult behavioral interactions. Integral to attachment theory are the complex interactions between a child's developing self-regulatory systems and the caregiver's responses, generating a template for the child's emotional and behavioral response patterns throughout life. These systems and interactions are also highly relevant to the chronic pain context and the resulting emotional and behavioral dynamics that become such a central part of the chronic pain experience.

The central aim of this paper is to review the available literature on attachment, specifically with regard to the potential relevance of the attachment framework on enhancing our understanding of children's chronic pain experience and management. The paper will overview some key attachment taxonomies and factor-based attachment structures before exploring the relationship between attachment style and chronic pain. Utilizing a theoretical and empirical perspective, attachment constructs will be considered as possible vulnerability factors or maintaining factors for children's chronic pain. This paper will also provide an overview of the literature on interventions for children and adolescents derived from attachment theory, with particular focus on the potential relevance for the pediatric chronic pain context. Possible directions for future research and clinical application will be considered.

2. Attachment Taxonomies

Since Bowlby [5] highlighted the importance of attachment, attachment systems have been described in terms of resultant behavioral styles reflecting the structure of two internal working models: the model of the self and the model of others. Ainsworth [3], in coding infant behavior in the context of a stressful separation from their caregiver, determined three classifications based on patterns of predictable reactions: 1) secure (exhibited protest on the departure of their caregiver, sought out the caregiver on their return); 2) anxious–ambivalent (exhibited significant distress at the departure of the caregiver and difficulty settling upon their return); and 3) avoidant (did not demonstrate distress on the departure of the caregiver and ignored the caregiver upon their return). Within this conception, a secure style reflects a positive model of both the self and of others. Both the anxious–ambivalent and avoidant styles reflect the manifestation of at least one negative working model, either of others (avoidant), or of the self in conjunction with a positive model of others (anxious-ambivalent). Main [17] instigated the addition of a fourth 'disorganized/disoriented' classification to reflect the use of a combination of both approach and avoidant strategies, typically associated with maltreatment.

Bartholomew and Horowitz [18] were the first to consider all possible combinations of the internal models of self and others to create four discrete factors in an adult sample utilizing self-report measures: (1) secure (self: positive, other: positive; comfortable with intimacy and autonomy); (2) pre-occupied (self: negative, other: positive; preoccupied with relationships); (3) dismissing (self: positive, other: negative; dismissing of intimacy, counter-dependent); (4) fearful (self: negative, other: negative; fearful of intimacy, socially avoidant). The significant addition of this taxonomy is the division of the earlier avoidant (negative model of the other) classification, in terms of the differentiating model of the self. Application of the four-factor structure has also been supported in adolescent populations [19,20].

While a significant portion of the literature has focused on the theoretical models espoused above, recent attention, particularly from within health care settings, has been directed toward the Dynamic

Maturational Model of Attachment [21–23]. According to this model, the focus of attachment processes is largely on the developing child's 'organization' of the self (i.e., self-regulation) via their use and processing of cognitive and affective information available within the caregiving environment [24]. It is important, however, to note that Crittenden [22] uses the term 'cognitive' to refer to the processing of very basic information regarding the temporal ordering of events, which does not necessarily require higher-order thought processes. A three-factor structure has been proposed, reflecting differing degrees of reliance and utilization of cognitive and affective information: 1) Type A (non-attending to affective information, reliance on cognitive information and expected consequences); 2) Type B (balanced processing and use of cognitive and affective information); and 3) Type C (reliance on affective information, non-attending to cognitive information and expected consequences) [21,24]. Crittenden [22] highlighted that both Type A (compulsive) and Type C (obsessive) strategies are associated with psychopathology owing to their tendency to overestimate the probability of danger and act in an unnecessarily self-protective manner. Similarities in these patterns of strategic information processing and behavior can be seen between Type A with avoidant attachment styles and Type C with anxious-ambivalent attachment styles.

A meta-analysis by Fraley [25] found attachment security to be moderately stable in the first 19 years of life. A subsequent large-scale study found that attachment security (measured categorically and dimensionally) was not stable from infancy to late adolescence; however, disorganized attachment at 15 months was predictive of preoccupied attachment at 18 years and security at both 24 and 36 months displayed an association with attachment security in late adolescence [26]. Given that a significant proportion of children and adolescents experiencing chronic and recurrent pains subsequently experience persistence of such into adulthood [27–29], the influence of enduring attachment patterns may be particularly important.

3. Attachment Framework and Vulnerability and Maintenance of Pediatric Chronic Pain

It seems likely that the complex early interactions between a child's developing self-regulatory systems and their caregiver's responses may impact on the vulnerability, onset and offset, or maintenance of chronic pain. The literature on each of these potential roles of attachment systems will be considered.

3.1. Attachment-Based Vulnerability Factors

A case could be made for arguing that attachment-based factors are more likely to render an individual vulnerable to the onset of a functional pain syndrome, with no readily identifiable pathology (e.g., migraines, headaches and abdominal pain), relative to other chronic pain conditions, such as those stemming from injury. Indeed, a large portion of the literature investigating attachment styles and pain has drawn conclusions based on patients with headaches or migraines (e.g., [15,30–32]) and functional abdominal pain (e.g., [33,34]). However, if acute physical threats are likely to activate attachment-based behaviors [16], it seems conceivable that attachment behavior patterns may contribute to an acute pain problem which has resulted from an injury or surgery transitioning into a chronic pain problem. To our knowledge there has not been any research investigating the role of attachment-based factors and the transition from acute to chronic pain. In the absence of any such guiding literature, the current paper will refer to chronic pain regardless of whether or not there is a known cause.

A number of attachment-based factors have been identified in the literature as potential vulnerability factors that may predispose an individual to developing chronic pain. These may include: (1) patterns of emotional expression (inhibitory or excitatory); (2) patterns of behavioral responding to threat; and (3) cognitive appraisal of threat. The literature pertaining to these factors will be reviewed. However, it is important to acknowledge that the studies have typically been cross-sectional, rendering it difficult to draw conclusions regarding cause and effect.

3.1.1. Patterns of Emotional Expression (Inhibitory or Excitatory)

It has been proposed that attachment styles characterized by avoidance of emotional expression (e.g., insecure-avoidant, dismissing and fearful styles, or Type A attachment strategy) may predispose individuals to chronic pain conditions [35]. Children with this attachment style may have parents who respond to expressions of negative affect, including pain, by either withdrawing from their child or responding with displeasure or anger [35]. Children learn to inhibit verbal or nonverbal signs of distress, because they have found these to serve no useful protective function [23]. Attachment styles that are defined by excitatory self-protective mechanisms (i.e., insecure-ambivalent, preoccupied or Type C attachment strategies) are also likely to have implications for pain experiences. Children with this style may have parents who respond unpredictably. Consequently, the child may alternate between signaling various exaggerated expressions of negative affect (e.g., fear, anger, desire for comfort), with the aim of trying to get their unpredictable parent to respond [35]. In a sample of adolescents with somatization disorders, including functional pain syndromes, Kozlowska and Williams [35] observed that patients who utilized inhibitory or excitatory self-protective mechanisms comprised a disproportionately large percentage of the sample population compared to prevalence rates observed in healthy populations.

One possible mechanism to account for the relationships between inhibitory and excitatory emotional expression and pain responses relates to alterations in the body's stress regulatory systems [35,36]. The cumulative adverse effects of chronic activation of the stress system are well documented (e.g., [37,38]), and are largely mediated by dysregulation of the hypothalamus pituitary adrenal (HPA) axis [39–41]. In adults, there is evidence that both anxious and avoidant attachment is associated with heightened reactivity of the HPA axis and autonomic nervous system reactivity to stress [41,42]. In light of the complex interactions between stress and multiple body systems (e.g., immune system, endocrine system), researchers have outlined a potential homeostatic role of increased pain sensitivity, and development of pain disorders characterized by central sensitization, in motivating restorative behavior for the body [43]. In this sense, pain is postulated to be one of a number of symptoms commonly associated with certain chronic pain disorders, e.g., fatigue, dyscognition [44], etc., that may function to promote survival of the organism through the promotion of quiescence. While it is difficult to delineate the direction of these relationships, research suggests the plausibility of both attachment deactivating and hyperactivating strategies contributing to dysregulation of the stress system within the body, and subsequently contributing to pain sensitivity.

The likely involvement of neurobiological processes in the manifestations of chronic or recurrent pains has been illustrated by studies of children with migraine. Insecure attachment has been found to be significantly more common in children with migraine compared to controls [31]. More specifically, the avoidant attachment style was found to have positive associations with migraine characteristics, including frequency, intensity and duration of attacks [31]. The authors highlighted the involvement of neurotransmitter patterns involved in the manifestation of attachment-related behavioral tendencies that also share links with the presence of migraine. Indeed, the literature supports the differential development of neural substrates associated with the caregiving environment and attachment styles [45].

3.1.2. Patterns of Behavioral Responses to Threat

Patterns of behavioral responses to threat may have implications for how individuals respond to painful experiences and consequently the likelihood that acute pain experiences transition to a chronic pain condition. Certain attachment styles and methods of pain signaling may serve as effective and acceptable signals of potential danger or distress, increasing the likelihood of eliciting a protective caregiving response [46]. According to attachment theory, certain attachment styles and patterns of verbal and non-verbal pain communication may serve as effective signals of distress, increasing the likelihood of eliciting a protective caregiving response [46].

The caregiving environment that generates avoidant (fearful/dismissing or Type A) strategies typically results in limited signaling of negative affect in order to avoid characteristically aversive responses. However, it has been suggested that in certain circumstances, the attachment figure in this caregiving environment may tolerate pain (owing to it being understood as a physical symptom) as an acceptable signal of distress compared to fear, anger or sadness [46]. In these circumstances, signaling of pain may elicit a caregiving response serving to reinforce the behavior for any experienced distress [46]. Pain behaviors are also considered useful in ambivalent, preoccupied or Type C strategies, as pain signals that are sufficiently strong may successfully elicit desired caregiving responses from inconsistent caregivers [46]. This is partially supported by results from a study with an adult sample, where preoccupied, dismissing and fearful attachment styles were found to be associated with chronic widespread pain [47]. In this study, the authors suggested that the observed relationship may reflect an increased likelihood of insecurely attached individuals to communicate distress in terms of physical symptoms in lieu of emotional feelings [47–49].

3.1.3. Cognitive Appraisal of Threat

The influence of attachment-related factors on cognitive appraisals of pain as a threat or a challenge affords another potential arena for contributing to vulnerability to chronic pain [50–52]. Pain appraisal is likely to have significant implications in the transition from acute to chronic pain states via its influence on the selection of coping strategies and subsequent adjustment to the pain experience, with known implications for a number of pain-related variables [33,53–55]. In Meredith et al.'s [53] Attachment-Diathesis Model of Chronic Pain, attachment-related primary appraisals of pain interact with secondary appraisals of the self (as equipped or not to cope; worthy or not of social support [56]) and of others (as available and adequate to provide effective support [57]) [52]. The attachment-diathesis model also emphasizes how such appraisals are influential in contributing to both the selection of coping strategies and subsequent emotional states, with threat appraisals likely to result in negative affect states [52,53]. The consequences of the utilization of particular coping strategies are likely to be mediated by contextual variables [52,58]; however, certain strategies have been found to be more commonly associated with poorer pain outcomes and negative emotional states, e.g., emotion-focused strategies that focus primarily on alleviating the experience of negative affect [52], such as pain catastrophizing or wishing [53]. Secure attachment has been shown to increase the likelihood of appraisal of pain as a challenge and subsequent utilization of problem-focused coping strategies such as seeking social support [50]. Conversely, insecure styles characterized by hyperactivating strategies have been shown to influence the appraisal of pain as more threatening [59,60], and in adolescents this was also related to anxiety, pain severity and depression [61]. In another sample of adolescents, Laird et al. [33] demonstrated that insecure attachment was influential in contributing to poorer health-related quality of life via its effect on cognitive appraisals and the subsequent employment of coping strategies.

In summary, there is sound theoretical basis, and some empirical evidence, for a range of attachment-based factors rendering individuals vulnerable to the development of chronic pain conditions, or vulnerable to the transition of acute pain conditions into chronic pain conditions. Patterns of emotional expression and behavioral responses to threat are of particular relevance and form within a developmental context of caregiver interactions. Moreover, the development of attachment style contributes to the manifestation of individual difference factors, such as cognitive appraisals of potential threats, with implications for responding to acute pain experiences. The significant limitation in this area of research is the reliance on cross-sectional rather than longitudinal designs, making issues of causality difficult to determine.

3.2. Attachment-Based Maintaining Factors

Not only do attachment-based factors have the potential to render an individual more vulnerable to the development of chronic pain, factors relevant to an individual's attachment style may serve to maintain the chronic pain condition, regardless of the initial trigger or cause of the pain. Some of the factors identified as possible vulnerability factors for the development of chronic pain may equally serve to maintain a chronic pain condition. This symptom maintenance may occur in a number of ways. Insecurely attached individuals may be: (1) less able to manage the distress associated with pain; (2) more likely to use emotion-focused rather than problem-focused coping strategies; (3) less able to procure and maintain external supports; (4) less able to form therapeutic alliances; (5) less likely to adhere to treatment recommendations; or (6) more likely to evoke and perceive more negative responses from health professionals [53]. These factors may either serve to intensify the pain experience (e.g., through poorer ability to manage distress), or impede effective rehabilitation (e.g., through poorer therapeutic relationships) [62].

Some of these maintaining factors may be more pertinent to adult rather than pediatric pain patients, for example pediatric patients have less personal responsibility for procuring support from health professionals. Nevertheless, adolescents have an increasingly active role in accepting or rejecting potential sources of support. The process of actively seeking support inherently relies on an individual's comfort with closeness to others, the belief that the self is worthy of support and that others are available to provide it [63], all of which are associated with secure attachment [53]. Individuals with dismissing and fearful attachment styles hold a view of others as unavailable or inadequately responsive, and are consequently less likely to acknowledge and seek help for distress related to pain [53,62]. Insecure individuals are therefore more likely to experience poorer pain outcomes.

An individual's use of coping strategies, both in terms of cognitions as well as behaviors, has been found to be related to their attachment style and likely to impact on symptom maintenance. Individuals with secure attachment styles have been found to utilize more diverse, problem-focused and effective coping strategies [12]. In contrast, insecure attachment has been linked with more rigidity in selection of coping strategies and a tendency to employ emotion-focused or avoidant coping techniques [12,64]. Emotion-focused coping strategies have generally been found to be associated with poorer health outcomes in adults with chronic pain [65,66], potentially facilitated by low self-esteem and self-efficacy and the subsequent lessened desire to engage with rehabilitation and pain management programs [67].

In considering the notion of coping in children and adolescence, Schmidt et al. [68] have drawn a distinction between the appropriate selection and use of particular coping strategies, which has been referred to as 'technical competence', and the more interactive process of 'adaptive coping'. Adaptive coping is conceptualized as more than a specific strategy, but as an interactive, developmental process, based on an awareness of context-dependent demands and effective employment of available resources. Attachment processes and interactions are likely to be particularly relevant to the ability to demonstrate competence in adaptive coping, which is considered the best predictor of long-term outcomes [68].

Adolescents with higher pain catastrophizing have been found to have more fearful and preoccupied attachment styles, which is consistent with the adult literature [50,55,69], and subsequently to have greater anxiety, pain severity and depression [61]. In addition to being associated with greater pain and poorer adjustment to chronic pain, pain catastrophizing may contribute to pain maintenance via affective inputs generating neurobiological pain-affect interactions [70]. This explanation is in accordance with the Attachment-Diathesis Model of Chronic Pain [53] which emphasizes factors in the maintenance of the role of attachment-related factors on producing negative emotion states that impact on poorer adjustment to and maintenance of chronic pain.

In summary, a range of attachment-based behaviors may contribute to the maintenance of chronic pain symptoms, most notably a range of interpersonal interaction styles, which when manifested in relationships with health care providers may contribute to the formation of barriers for the provision of effective treatment or adherence to treatment plans [62,71]. As outlined above, other attachment-based factors may also contribute to how a child or adolescent interacts with their primary caregiver and whether or not these interactions facilitate the adoption of clear communication and an active role in their own rehabilitation.

4. Attachment-Based Interventions and Chronic Pain

In light of the broad array of attachment-based factors potentially rendering individuals vulnerable to the transition from acute to chronic pain, as well as attachment factors potentially maintaining chronic pain, it is important to consider the best way that interventions can target these factors. Although a number of researchers have made theoretically-derived treatment recommendations for attachment-based interventions for chronic pain [53,72], such interventions have not been comprehensively outlined, let alone evaluated, within the pediatric chronic pain context. Hence, it is beneficial to consider attachment-based interventions that have been used and evaluated with children and adolescents targeting problems other than pain.

In 2015, a special issue of the journal *Attachment and Human Development* was devoted to articles describing attachment-based treatments for adolescents. These interventions have been used to increase security in the caregiver-adolescent attachment bond, while targeting a range of specific groups, such as depressed and suicidal adolescents [73], hard-to-reach youth [74], and pregnant adolescents [75]. An earlier review was carried out overviewing the attachment-based treatments for use with young children [76]. An underlying assumption for attachment-based treatments is that attachment and caregiving disturbances in some way contribute to the vulnerability, onset or maintenance of psychopathology or the problem in focus. The focus of attachment-based treatments with young children may involve modifying caregiver internal working models of self or others and increasing contingent and sensitive responding to their child's signals and attachment needs. Attachment-based treatments with adolescents need to recognize that by adolescence individuals have become more active partners in maintaining the attachment bond [77–79]. Consequently, there are three possible treatment targets in attachment-based treatments with adolescents: (1) modifying the adolescent's internal working model of self or others (especially their caregiver); (2) modifying the caregiver's internal working model of self or others (especially their adolescent); and (3) promoting emotionally attuned communication between the caregiver and adolescent [80]. The caregiver's ability to maintain a cooperative partnership with an adolescent is likely to be dependent on the caregiver's ability to monitor their own emotions, clearly asserting their own positions, while validating and supporting the adolescent's attachment and autonomy needs [79]. The caregiving environment is thus a necessary consideration in determining both the utility and appropriateness of an attachment-based intervention for pediatric chronic pain patients. As noted in the literature [72], if caregivers are unwilling or unable to engage in the therapeutic process, attempts at altering the working models of children or adolescents in isolation are unlikely to be effective and importantly may undermine the protective function of the established attachment strategy.

Although the attachment-based therapeutic targets outlined above are likely to be pertinent to the context of chronic pain, relatively little research has been done in this area. Numerous pain behaviors have been construed within an attachment framework, potentially rendering them as direct and indirect outcomes of attachment-based treatments. For example, individuals with insecure attachment styles have been found to describe their pain as more threatening and themselves as less able to deal with it [50,81]. Moreover, empirical studies with adults have found insecure attachment styles to be associated with lower trust and satisfaction with their physician [82], greater use of emotion-focused coping and less problem-focused coping [81], lower perceived social support [83], greater pain intensity and disability [14], greater pain-related distress [84], more physical symptoms [12], especially medically unexplained symptoms [13], and higher levels of pain-related stress, anxiety, depression and catastrophizing [50,55,85,86].

In the pediatric literature it has been demonstrated that among a preschool sample of four- and five-year-olds, representations of separation and pain experience were systematically related [87]. Moreover, children with relatively more ambivalent or disorganized attachments have been found to have a greater response to immunization injections and everyday pains [88]. Children with a more controlling attachment have also been found to take more time to calm down after an immunization injection, displaying greater anger [88].

It has been implied by attachment-based theorists that shifting the internal working models of the child/adolescent and the caregiver may help individuals develop more secure attachment styles. Notably, though, studies depicting associations between attachment styles and pain behaviors have generally been cross-sectional. Thus it is not known whether shifting the attachment style of a child/adolescent (and/or their caregiver) will result in changes in pain behaviors or pain outcomes. Longitudinal studies are needed to address such questions. Cognitive-behavioral interventions have, to date, been found to be the most successful treatments for pediatric chronic pain [89,90]. Some support has also been reported for acceptance and commitment interventions [91]. Theoretical and empirical work is needed to consider whether there is scope or value in utilizing attachment-based interventions for a certain group of pediatric chronic pain patients, or whether it is feasible to integrate attachment-based treatment components together with cognitive-behavioral therapy (CBT) or other evidence-based interventions. Despite there being numerous points of contact between attachment theory and the cognitive theory that underlies CBT (see [92] for a review), attachment theory and attachment-based interventions are largely unfamiliar to most cognitive-behavioral therapists. A potentially fruitful future research direction may be to screen pediatric chronic pain patients for insecure attachment styles and to determine whether these individuals benefit from interventions designed to shift the internal working models of the child/adolescent and/or the caregiver. Such interventions may be an adjunct to more established cognitive-behavioral therapies. McBride and Atkinson [92] have argued that attachment theory need not be used to generate new interventions, but may be used to better inform the practice and delivery of existing clinical modalities for the treatment of chronic pain. There is a precedent in incorporating aspects of attachment-based interventions with CBT for anxious adolescents [93]. Kozlowska and Khan [72] outlined a multidisciplinary, multimodal intervention for children and adolescents with medically unexplained pain, incorporating what is postulated regarding information-processing tendencies within the dynamic maturational model of attachment. The intervention highlighted the utility of considering observed deficits in the processing of affective information and addressing these in order to maximize the efficacy of any cognitive-based interventions [72]. The subject intervention reportedly facilitated reductions in pain intensity and improvements in school attendance [94]. Further research is needed in this area within the pediatric chronic pain context.

The inclusion of parent-based treatment components in pediatric chronic pain programs has widely been accepted as being of considerable importance [95]. The efficacy and value of such parent-based interventions may in part be understood from an attachment framework. It is well established that children whose parents engage in more protective behaviors (e.g., excusing their child from the usual roles and responsibilities) have greater functional disability [96,97], more school absences and impairment [98], and greater healthcare utilization [99]. Parental protective behaviors have been found to occur when parents lack confidence in their child's ability to cope with their pain [100]. The context of a medical condition is likely to activate a unique set of caregiver attachment behaviors, motivated by a desire to maintain 'safety [16]. However, when a condition is chronic, it is not helpful for caregivers to remain in a protector role. Adolescence is a time when the need for security must be balanced with an increasing need for autonomy, and a highly protective caregiver is likely to minimize an adolescent's opportunity for autonomy and practice with problem-solving. The goal of emotionally-attuned communication between caregiver and adolescent is likely to be key to providing adolescents with a secure base from which to take ownership of their pain problem and to actively engage in its management, while knowing that they have caring support when needed.

5. Challenges and Future Directions for Research

Although a small number of papers have outlined the potential theoretical relevance of the attachment theory to the chronic pain context [46,53,62], more empirical work is needed to investigate theoretically-derived hypotheses. Questions related to causal direction remain elusive, largely due to the difficulty in carrying out longitudinal research with children who will at some point in the future develop chronic pain. However, even if such longitudinal research were carried out, the causal direction between attachment style and chronic pain might not be unidirectional. Although insecure attachment styles may render individuals vulnerable to developing chronic pain, the pain experience is thought to be likely to bring out an individual's characteristic attachment behaviors, suggesting that a cyclical relationship may exist.

Clinical research investigating attachment styles and treatment outcomes among pediatric chronic pain patients may prove fruitful. There is reason to predict that individuals with insecure attachment styles have poorer treatment outcomes with established evidence-based interventions, perhaps due to lower trust and engagement with health professionals [82] or less use of problem-solving strategies [81]. The next step would be to investigate whether particular patient groups, perhaps differing in attachment variables, would benefit from evidence-based interventions utilizing a more specific attachment focus, or from incorporating an additional attachment-based adjunct treatment component. This would require screening pain patients for attachment-based variables; preliminary investigations are needed to determine which domains of attachment are most closely related to chronic pain outcomes. Self-report questionnaires, such as the Inventory of Parent and Peer Attachment [101], tap into more conscious, strategic aspects of attachment, but may overlook more automatic aspects. Behavioral and observational measures may tap into automatic as well as strategic aspects of attachment, but are more resource-intensive to administer and to code.

Another clinical question which warrants investigation is whether individuals with particular attachment styles are more likely to transition from an acute pain condition to a chronic pain condition. If one is to accept the claim that an individual's attachment style is likely to be activated by a physical threat such as injury or surgery, there would be grounds for hypothesizing that an insecure attachment style may confer a risk for acute or post-operative pains developing into a chronic pain condition. There have been relatively few investigations into potential risk factors associated with a transition from acute to chronic pain in children [102,103], and attachment style has not been considered in these studies.

Finally, it is worth acknowledging that the complex relationship between attachment and pain has also been considered from theoretical perspectives other than attachment theory. Evolutionary perspectives have been used to account for underlying neural similarities between social isolation/exclusion and pain [104,105]. According to this perspective, social isolation, just like physical pain, is designed to trigger an internal alarm, warning of a situation that may be harmful to survival. Just as the unpleasantness of pain prompts an individual to engage in behaviors intended to minimize physical harm, evolutionary pressures may have resulted in social pain or intense negative feelings serving as an indicator of an impending, and potentially dangerous separation or exclusion [106]. Neuroimaging techniques have afforded these theories some support (for a review see [104]).

6. Conclusions

Although there has been relatively little literature relating the attachment framework to the pediatric chronic pain context, there is merit in considering this relationship from a theoretical, empirical and clinical perspective. A range of chronic pain behaviors have been theoretically accounted for by an attachment framework (e.g., [46,62,107,108]); however, the empirical literature to date has been sparse. A number of attachment-based factors have been identified as possible vulnerability factors, predisposing individuals to the onset of chronic pain. These include preoccupied, dismissing and fearful attachment styles, as well as Type A and Type C attachment strategies as defined by the Dynamic Maturational Model. Attachment factors may also serve to maintain chronic pain conditions through a variety of mechanisms, such as poor distress management, maladaptive coping strategies, poor utilization and compliance with healthcare services, and limited access and utilization of social supports. More empirical work is needed before attachment-based treatment targets can be applied to the pediatric chronic pain context. For example, consideration should be given to whether screening chronic pediatric pain patients for particular attachment styles may help identify patient subgroups that might benefit from interventions with a particular attachment focus or as an adjunct attachment-based component to the primary therapeutic approach.

Acknowledgments: Theresa J. Donnelly and Tiina Jaaniste are supported by the Sydney Children's Hospital Foundation.

Author Contributions: Theresa J.Donnelly and Tiina Jaaniste reviewed the literature and wrote the review paper.

Conflicts of Interest: The authors declare no conflict of interest.

References

1. Bowlby, J. *Attachment and Loss: Vol 1. Attachment*; Basic Books: New York, NY, USA, 1969.
2. Ainsworth, M.D. Patterns of attachment behavior shown by the infant in interaction with his mother. *Merrill Palmer Q. Behav. Dev.* **1964**, *10*, 51–58.
3. Ainsworth, M.; Blehar, M.; Waters, E.; Wall, S. *Patterns of Attachment*; Eribaum: Hills-dale, NJ, USA, 1978.
4. Bowlby, J. *A Secure Base: Parent-Child Attachment and Healthy Human Development*; Basic Books: New York, NY, USA, 1988.
5. Bowlby, J. *Attachment and Loss: Vol 2. Separation: Anxiety and Anger*; Basic Books: New York, NY, USA, 1973.
6. Bowlby, J. *Attachment and Loss: Vol 3. Loss*; Basic Books: New York, NY, USA, 1980.
7. Kobak, R.R.; Sceery, A. Attachment in late adolescence: Working models, affect regulation, and representations of self and others. *Child Dev.* **1988**, *59*, 135–146. [CrossRef] [PubMed]
8. Hazan, C.; Shaver, P. Romantic love conceptualised as an attachment process. *J. Personal. Soc. Psychol.* **1987**, *52*, 511–524. [CrossRef]
9. Brumariu, L.E.; Kerns, K.A. Parent-child attachment and internalizing symptoms in childhood and adolescence: A review of empirical findings and future directions. *Dev. Psychopathol.* **2010**, *22*, 177–203. [CrossRef] [PubMed]
10. DeKlyen, M.; Greenberg, M.T. Attachment and psychopathology in childhood. In *Handbook of Attachment: Theory, Research, and Clinical Applications*, 2nd ed.; Guilford Press: New York, NY, USA, 2008.
11. Fearon, R.; Bakermans-Kranenburg, M.J.; Van IJzendoorn, M.H.; Lapsley, A.M.; Roisman, G.I. The significance of insecure attachment and disorganization in the development of children's externalizing behavior: A meta-analytic study. *Child Dev.* **2010**, *81*, 435–456. [CrossRef] [PubMed]
12. Schmidt, S.; Nachtigall, C.; Wuethrich-Martone, O.; Strauss, B. Attachment and coping with chronic disease. *J. Psychosom. Res.* **2002**, *53*, 763–773. [CrossRef]
13. Taylor, R.E.; Marshall, T.; Mann, A.; Goildberg, D.P. Insecure attachment and frequent attendance in primary care: A longitudinal cohort study of medically unexplained symptom presentations in ten UK general practices. *Psychol. Med.* **2012**, *42*, 855–864. [CrossRef] [PubMed]
14. McWilliams, L.A.; Cox, B.J.; Enns, M.W. Impact of adult attachment styles on pain and disability associated with arthritis in a nationally representative sample. *Clin. J. Pain* **2000**, *16*, 360–364. [CrossRef] [PubMed]
15. Rossi, P.; Di Lorenzo, G.; Malpezzi, M.G.; Di Lorenzo, C.; Cesarino, F.; Faroni, J.; Siracusano, A.; Troisi, A. Depressive symptoms and insecure attachment as predictors of disability in a clinical population of patients with episodic and chronic migraine. *Headache J. Head Face Pain* **2005**, *45*, 561–570. [CrossRef] [PubMed]
16. Hunter, J.J.; Maunder, R.G. Using attachment theory to understand illness behavior. *Gen. Hosp. Psychiatr.* **2001**, *23*, 177–182. [CrossRef]
17. Main, M.; Kaplan, N.; Cassidy, J. Security in infancy, childhood, and adulthood: A move to the level of representation. *Monogr. Soc. Res. Child Dev.* **1985**, *50*, 66–104. [CrossRef]
18. Bartholomew, K.; Horowitz, L.M. Attachment styles among young adults: A test of a four-category model. *J. Personal. Soc. Psychol.* **1991**, *61*, 226–244. [CrossRef]
19. Venta, A.; Sharp, C.; Shmueli-Goetz, Y. Assessing attachment in adolescence: A psychometric study of the child attachment interview. *Psychol. Assess.* **2014**, *26*, 238–255. [CrossRef] [PubMed]
20. Allen, J.P.; Land, D. Attachment in adolescence. In *Handbook of Attachment: Theory, Research, and Clinical Applications*; Cassidy, J., Shaver, P.R., Eds.; Guilford Press: New York, NY, USA, 1999; pp. 319–335.
21. Crittenden, P.M. A Dynamic-Maturational Model of Attachment. *Aust. N. Z. J. Fam. Ther.* **2006**, *27*, 105–115. [CrossRef]

22. Crittenden, P.M. Attachment, information processing, and psychiatric disorder. *World Psychiatr.* **2002**, *2*, 72–75.

23. Crittenden, P.M. Danger and Development: The organisation of self-protective strategies. *Monogr. Soc. Res. Child Dev.* **1999**, *64*, 145–171. [CrossRef] [PubMed]

24. Landa, S.; Duschinsky, R. Crittenden's dynamic–maturational model of attachment and adaptation. *Rev. Gen. Psychol.* **2013**, *17*, 326. [CrossRef]

25. Fraley, R.C. Attachment stability from infancy to adulthood: Meta-analysis and dynamic modeling of developmental mechanisms. *Personal. Soc. Psychol. Rev.* **2002**, *6*, 123–151. [CrossRef]

26. Groh, A.M.; Roisman, G.I.; Booth-LaForce, C.; Fraley, R.C.; Owen, M.T.; Cox, M.J.; Burchinal, M.R. IV. Stability of attachment security from infancy to late adolescence. *Monogr. Soc. Res. Child Dev.* **2014**, *79*, 51–66. [CrossRef] [PubMed]

27. Walker, L.S.; Dengler-Crish, C.M.; Rippel, S.; Bruehl, S. Functional abdominal pain in childhood and adolescence increases risk for chronic pain in adulthood. *Pain* **2010**, *150*, 568–572. [CrossRef] [PubMed]

28. Brattberg, G. Do pain problems in young school children persist into early adulthood? A 13-year follow-up. *Eur. J. Pain* **2004**, *8*, 187–199. [CrossRef] [PubMed]

29. Jones, G.T.; Silman, A.J.; Power, C.; Macfarlane, G.J. Are common symptoms in childhood associated with chronic widespread body pain in adulthood. *Arthritis Rheum.* **2007**, *56*, 1669–1675. [CrossRef] [PubMed]

30. Berry, J.K.M.; Drummond, P.D. Does attachment anxiety increase vulnerability to headache? *J. Psychosom. Res.* **2014**, *76*, 113–120. [CrossRef] [PubMed]

31. Esposito, M.; Parisi, L.; Callai, B.; Marotta, R.; Dona, A.D.; Lavano, S.M.; Roccella, M.; Carotenuto, M. Attachment styles in children affected by migraine without aura. *Neuropsychiatr. Dis. Treat.* **2013**, *9*, 1513–1519. [PubMed]

32. Savi, L.; Buccheri, R.; Tambornini, A.; De Martino, P.; Albasi, C.; Pinessi, L. Attachment stules and headache. *J. Headache Pain* **2005**, *6*, 254–257. [CrossRef] [PubMed]

33. Laird, K.T.; Preacher, K.J.; Walker, L.S. Attachment and adjustment in adolescents and young adults with a history of pediatric functional abdominal pain. *Clin. J. Pain* **2015**, *31*, 152–158. [CrossRef] [PubMed]

34. Schulte, I.E.; Petermann, F. Familial risk factors for the development of somatoform symptoms and disorders in children and adolescents: A systematic review. *Child Psychiatr. Hum. Dev.* **2011**, *42*, 569–583. [CrossRef] [PubMed]

35. Kozlowska, K.; Williams, L.M. Self-protective organization in children with conversion and somatoform disorders. *J. Psychosom. Res.* **2009**, *67*, 223–233. [CrossRef] [PubMed]

36. Gunnar, M.; Quevedo, K. The neurobiology of stress and development. *Annu. Rev. Psychol.* **2007**, *58*, 145–173. [CrossRef] [PubMed]

37. Chrousos, G.P.; Gold, P.W. The concepts of stress and stress system disorders. *JAMA* **1992**, *267*, 1244–1252. [CrossRef] [PubMed]

38. McEwen, B.S.; Seeman, T. Protectice and damaging effects of mediators of stress: Elaborating and testing the concepts of allostasis and allostatic load. *Ann. N. Y. Acad. Sci.* **1999**, *896*, 30–47. [CrossRef] [PubMed]

39. Heim, C.; Nater, U.M.; Maloney, E.; Boneva, R.; Jones, J.F.; Reeves, W.C. Childhood trauma and risk for chronic fatigue syndrome: Association with neuroendocrine dysfunction. *Arch. Gen. Psychiatr.* **2009**, *66*, 72–80. [CrossRef] [PubMed]

40. Tak, L.M.; Rosmalen, J.G.M. Dysfunction of the stress responsive systems as a risk factor for functional somatic syndromes. *J. Psychosom. Res.* **2010**, *68*, 461–468. [CrossRef] [PubMed]

41. Luyten, P.; Van Houdenhove, B.; Lemma, A.; Target, M.; Fonagy, P. Vulnerability for functional somatic disorders: A contemporary psychodynamic approach. *J. Psychother. Integr.* **2013**, *23*, 250–262. [CrossRef]

42. Diamond, L.M.; Fagundes, C.P. Psychobiological research on attachment. *J. Soc. Pers. Relatsh.* **2010**, *27*, 218–225. [CrossRef]

43. Gracely, R.H.; Schweinhardt, P. Programmed symptoms: Disparate effects united by purpose. *Curr. Rheumatol. Rev.* **2015**, *11*, 116–130. [CrossRef] [PubMed]

44. Ambrose, K.R.; Gracely, R.H.; Glass, J.M. Fibromyalgia dysognition: Concepts and issues. *Reumatismo* **2012**, *64*, 206–215. [CrossRef] [PubMed]

45. Schore, A.N. Attachment, the regulation of the right brain. *Attach. Hum. Dev.* **2000**, *2*, 23–47. [CrossRef] [PubMed]

46. Kozlowska, K. Attachment relationships shape pain-signalling behaviour. *J. Pain* **2009**, *10*, 1020–1028. [CrossRef] [PubMed]

47. Davies, K.A.; Macfarlane, G.J.; McBeth, J.; Morriss, R.; Dickens, C. Insecure attachment style is associated with chronic widespread pain. *Pain* **2009**, *143*, 200–205. [CrossRef] [PubMed]

48. Salmon, P.; Skaife, K.; Rhodes, J. Abuse, dissociation, and somatization in irritable bowel syndrome: Towards an explanatory model. *J. Behav. Med.* **2003**, *26*, 1–18. [CrossRef] [PubMed]

49. Taylor, R.E.; Mann, A.H.; White, N.J.; Goldberg, D.P. Attachment style in patients with unexplained physical complaints. *Psychol. Med.* **2000**, *30*, 931–941. [CrossRef] [PubMed]

50. Meredith, P.J.; Strong, J.; Feeney, J.A. Evidence of a relationship between adult attachment variables and appraisals of chronic pain. *Pain Res. Manag.* **2005**, *10*, 191–200. [CrossRef] [PubMed]

51. Unruh, A.M.; Ritchie, J.A. Development of the pain appraisal inventory: Psychometric properties. *Pain Res. Manag.* **1998**, *3*, 105–110. [CrossRef]

52. Lazarus, R.S.; Folkman, S. *Stress, Appraisal and Coping*; Springer: New York, NY, USA, 1984.

53. Meredith, P.; Ownsworth, T.; Strong, J. A review of the evidence linking adult attachment theory and chronic pain: Presenting a conceptual model. *Clin. Psychol. Rev.* **2008**, *28*, 407–429. [CrossRef] [PubMed]

54. Turk, D.C.; Okifuji, A. Psychological factors in chronic pain: Evolution and revolution. *J. Consult. Clin. Psychol.* **2002**, *70*, 678–690. [CrossRef] [PubMed]

55. Ciechanowski, P.; Sullivan, M.; Jensen, M.; Romano, J.; Summers, H. The relationship of attachment style to depression, catastrophizing and health care utilization in patients with chronic pain. *Pain* **2003**, *104*, 627–637. [CrossRef]

56. Cohen, S.; Wills, T.A. Stress, social support, and the buffering hypothesis. *Psychol. Bull.* **1985**, *98*, 310–357. [CrossRef] [PubMed]

57. Ognibene, T.C.; Collins, N.L. Adult attachment styles, perceived social support and coping stratgies. *J. Soc. Pers. Relatsh.* **1998**, *15*, 323–345. [CrossRef]

58. Walker, L.S.; Freeman Baber, K.; Garber, J.; Smith, C.A. A typology of pain coping in pediatric patients with chronic abdominal pain. *Pain* **2008**, *137*, 266–275. [CrossRef] [PubMed]

59. Porter, L.S.; Davis, D.; Keefe, F.J. Attachment and Pain: Recent findings and future directions. *Pain* **2007**, *128*, 195–198. [CrossRef] [PubMed]

60. Mikulincer, M.; Shaver, P.R. *Attachment in Adulthood: Structure, Dynamics, and Change*; The Guilford Press: New York, NY, USA, 2007.

61. Tremblay, I.; Sullivan, M.J.L. Attachment and pain outcomes in adolescents: The mediating role of pain catastrophising and anxiety. *J. Pain* **2010**, *11*, 160–171. [CrossRef] [PubMed]

62. Mikail, S.F.; Henderson, P.R.; Tasca, G.A. An interpersonally based model of chronic pain: An application of attachment theory. *Clin. Psychol. Rev.* **1994**, *14*, 1–16. [CrossRef]

63. Simpson, J.A.; Rholes, W.S.; Orina, M.M.; Grich, J. Working models of attachment, support giving, and support seeking in a stressful situation. *Personal. Soc. Psychol. Bull.* **2002**, *28*, 598–608. [CrossRef]

64. Kotler, T.; Buzwell, S.; Romeo, Y.; Bowland, J. Avoidant attachment as a risk factor for health. *Br. J. Med. Psychol.* **1994**, *67*, 237–245. [CrossRef] [PubMed]

65. Jensen, M.P.; Turner, J.A.; Romano, J.M.; Karoly, P. Coping with chronic pain: A critical review of the literature. *Pain* **1991**, *47*, 249–283. [CrossRef]

66. Higgins, N.C.; Bailey, S.J.; LaChapelle, D.L.; Harman, K.; Hadjistavropoulos, T. Coping styles, pain expressiveness, and implicit theories of chronic pain. *J. Psychol.* **2015**, *149*, 737–750. [CrossRef] [PubMed]

67. Dysvik, E.; Natvig, G.K.; Eikeland, O.J.; Lindstrom, T.C. Coping with chronic pain. *Int. J. Nurs. Stud.* **2005**, *42*, 297–305. [CrossRef] [PubMed]

68. Schmidt, S.; Peterson, C.; Bullinger, M. Coping with chronic disease from the perspective of children and adolescents—A conceptual framework and its implications for participation. *Child Care Health Dev.* **2003**, *29*, 63–75. [CrossRef] [PubMed]

69. McWilliams, L.A.; Asmundson, G.J.G. The relationship of adult attachment dimensions to pain-related fear, hypervigilence, and catastrophizing. *Pain* **2007**, *127*, 27–34. [CrossRef] [PubMed]

70. Lumley, M.A.; Cohen, J.L.; Borszcz, G.S.; Cano, A.; Radcliffe, A.M.; Porter, L.S.; Schubiner, H.; Keefe, F.J. Pain and emotion: A biopsychosocial review of recent research. *J. Clin. Psychol.* **2011**, *67*, 942–968. [CrossRef] [PubMed]

71. Ciechanowski, P.S.; Katon, W.J.; Russo, J.E.; Walker, E.A. The patient-provder relationship: Attachment theory and adherence to treatment in diabetes. *Am. J. Psychiatr.* **2001**, *158*, 29–35. [CrossRef] [PubMed]

72. Kozlowska, K.; Khan, R. A developmental, body-oriented intervention for children and adolescents with medically unexplained chronic pain. *Clin. Child Psychol. Psychiatr.* **2011**, *16*, 575–598. [CrossRef] [PubMed]

73. Ewing, E.S.K.; Diamond, G.; Levy, S. Attachment-based family therapy for depressed and suicidal adolescents: Theory, clinical model and empirical support. *Attach. Hum. Dev.* **2015**, *17*, 136–156. [CrossRef] [PubMed]

74. Bevington, D.; Fuggle, P.; Fonagy, P. Applying attachment theory to effective practice with hard-to-reach youth: the AMBIT approach. *Attach. Hum. Dev.* **2015**, *17*, 157–174. [CrossRef] [PubMed]

75. Madigan, S.; Vaillancourt, K.; McKibbon, A.; Benoit, D. Trauma and traumatic loss in pregnant adolescents: The impact of Trauma-Focused Cognitive Behavior Therapy on maternal unresolved states of mind and Posttraumatic Stress Disorder. *Attach. Hum. Dev.* **2015**, *17*, 175–198. [CrossRef] [PubMed]

76. Berlin, L.J.; Zeanah, C.H.; Lieberman, A.F. Prevention and intervention programs for supporting early attachment security. In *Handbook of Attachment: Theory, Research, and Clinical Applications*; Cassidy, J., Shaver, P.R., Eds.; Guilford Press: New York, NY, USA, 2008; pp. 745–761.

77. Allen, J.P. The attachment system in adolescence. In *Handbook of Attachment: Theory, Research, and Clinical Applications*, 2nd ed.; Guilford Press: New York, NY, USA, 2008; pp. 419–435.

78. Kobak, R.; Duemmler, S. Attachment and conversation: Toward a discourse analysis of adolescent and adult security. In *Attachment Processes in Adulthood*; Jessica Kingsley Publishers: London, UK, 1994; pp. 121–149.

79. Kobak, R.R.; Kerig, P.K. Introduction to the special issue: Attachment-based treatments for adolescents. *Attach. Hum. Dev.* **2015**, *17*, 111–118. [CrossRef] [PubMed]

80. Kobak, R.; Zajac, K.; Herres, J.; Krauthamer Ewing, E.S. Attachment based treatments for adolescents: The secure cycle as a framework for assessment, treatment and evaluation. *Attach. Hum. Dev.* **2015**, *17*, 220–239. [CrossRef] [PubMed]

81. Mikulincer, M.; Florian, V. The relationship between adult attachment styles and emotional and cognitive reactions to stressful events. In *Attachment Theory and Close Relationships*; Guilford Press: New York, NY, USA, 1998; pp. 143–165.

82. Holwerda, N.; Sanderman, R.; Pool, G.; Hinnen, C.; Langendijk, J.A.; Bemelman, W.A.; Hagedoorn, M.; Sprangers, M.A. Do patients trust their physician? The role of attachment style in the patient-physician relationship within one year after a cancer diagnosis. *Acta Oncol.* **2013**, *52*, 110–117. [CrossRef] [PubMed]

83. Moreira, J.M.; de Fátima Silva, M.; Moleiro, C.; Aguiar, P.C.; Andrez, M.; Bernardes, S.; Afonso, H. Perceived social support as an offshoot of attachment style. *Personal. Individ. Differ.* **2003**, *34*, 485–501. [CrossRef]

84. Pearce, S.; Creed, P.; Cramond, T. Attachment style and chronic pain syndrome. *Aust. Pain Soc. Newsl.* **2001**, *May*, 2–4.

85. Meredith, P.J.; Strong, J.; Feeney, J.A. The relationship of adult attachment to emotion, catastrophizing, control, threshold and tolerance, in experimentally-induced pain. *Pain* **2006**, *120*, 44–52. [CrossRef] [PubMed]

86. Meredith, P.J.; Strong, J.; Feeney, J.A. Adult attachment variables predict depression before and after treatment for chronic pain. *Eur. J. Pain* **2007**, *11*, 164–170. [CrossRef] [PubMed]

87. Walsh, T.M.; Symons, D.K.; McGrath, P.J. Relations between yound children's responses to the depiction of separation and pain experiences. *Attach. Hum. Dev.* **2004**, *6*, 53–71. [CrossRef] [PubMed]

88. Walsh, T.M.; McGrath, P.J.; Symons, D.K. Attachment dimensions and young children's response to pain. *Pain Res. Manag.* **2008**, *13*, 33–40. [CrossRef] [PubMed]

89. Eccleston, C.; Morley, S.J.; Williams, A.D. Psychological approaches to chronic pain management: Evidence and challenges. *Br. J. Anaesth.* **2013**, *111*, 59–63. [CrossRef] [PubMed]

90. Eccleston, C.; Palermo, T.M.; Williams, A.C.; Lewandowski, A.; Morley, S.; Fisher, E.; Law, E. Psychological therapies for the management of chronic and recurrent pain in children and adolescents. *Cochrane Libr.* **2012**. [CrossRef]

91. Wicksell, R.K.; Melin, L.; Lekander, M.; Olsson, G.L. Evaluating the effectiveness of exposure and acceptance strategies to improve functioning and quality of life in longstanding pediatric pain—A randomized controlled trial. *Pain* **2009**, *141*, 248–257. [CrossRef] [PubMed]

92. McBride, C.; Atkinson, L. Attachment theory and cognitive-behavioral therapy. In *Attachment Theory and Research in Clinical Work with Adults*; Guilford Press: New York, NY, USA, 2009; pp. 434–458.

93. Siqueland, L.; Rynn, M.; Diamond, G.S. Cognitive behavioral and attachment based family therapy for anxious adolescents: Phase I and II studies. *J. Anxiety Disord.* **2005**, *19*, 361–381. [CrossRef] [PubMed]

94. Kozlowska, K.; Rose, D.; Khan, R.; Kram, S.; Lane, L.; Collins, J. A Conceptual Model and Practice Framework for Managing Chronic Pain in Children and Adolescents. *Harv. Rev. Psychiatr.* **2008**, *16*, 136–150. [CrossRef] [PubMed]

95. Palermo, T.M.; Eccleston, C. Parents of children and adolescents with chronic pain. *Pain* **2009**, *146*, 15–17. [CrossRef] [PubMed]

96. Claar, R.L.; Baber, K.F.; Simons, L.E.; Logan, D.E.; Walker, L.S. Pain coping profiles in adolescents with chronic pain. *Pain* **2008**, *140*, 368–375. [CrossRef] [PubMed]

97. Sieberg, C.B.; Williams, S.; Simons, L.E. Do parent protective responses mediate the relation between parent distress and child functional disability among children with chronic pain? *J. Pediatr. Psychol.* **2011**. [CrossRef] [PubMed]

98. Logan, D.E.; Simons, L.E.; Carpino, E.A. Too sick for school? Parent influences on school functioning among children with chronic pain. *Pain* **2012**, *153*, 437–443. [CrossRef] [PubMed]

99. Walker, L.S.; Levy, R.L.; Whitehead, W.E. Validation of a measure of protective parent responses to children's pain. *Clin. J. Pain* **2006**, *22*, 712–716. [CrossRef] [PubMed]

100. Jaaniste, T.; Jia, N.; Lang, T.; Goodison-Farnsworth, E.; McCormick, M.; Anderson, D. The relationship between parental attitudes and behaviours in the context of paediatric chronic pain. *Child Care Health Dev.* **2016**, *42*, 433–438. [CrossRef] [PubMed]

101. Armsden, G.C.; Greenberg, M.T. The inventory of parent and peer attachment: Individual differences and their relationship to psychological well-being in adolescence. *J. Youth Adolesc.* **1987**, *16*, 427–454. [CrossRef] [PubMed]

102. Fortier, M.A.; Chou, J.; Maurer, E.L.; Kain, Z.N. Acute to chronic postoperative pain in children: Preliminary findings. *J. Pediatr. Surg.* **2011**, *46*, 1700–1705. [CrossRef] [PubMed]

103. Pagé, M.G.; Campbell, F.; Isaac, L.; Stinson, J.; Katz, J. Parental risk factors for the development of pediatric acute and chronic postsurgical pain: A longitudinal study. *J. Pain Res.* **2013**, *6*, 727–741. [CrossRef] [PubMed]

104. Eisenberger, N.I.; Lieberman, M.D. Why rejection hurts: A common neural alarm for physical and social pain. *Trends Cogn. Sci.* **2004**, *8*, 294–300. [CrossRef] [PubMed]

105. MacDonald, G.; Leary, M.R. Why does social exclusion hurt? The relationship between social and physical pain. *Psychol. Bull.* **2005**, *131*, 202–223. [CrossRef] [PubMed]

106. Baumeister, R.F.; Leary, M.R. The need to belong: Desire for interpersonal attachments as a fundamental human motivation. *Psychol. Bull.* **1995**, *117*, 497–529. [CrossRef] [PubMed]

107. Anderson, D.; Hines, R. Attachment and pain. In *Psychosocial Vulnerability to Chronic Pain*; Springer: New York, NY, USA, 1994; pp. 137–152.

108. Kolb, L.C. Attachment behavior and pain complaints. *Psychosomatics* **1982**, *23*, 413–425. [CrossRef]

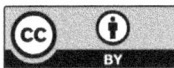

![children logo] *children*

MDPI

Article

Maternal Anxiety and Children's Laboratory Pain: The Mediating Role of Solicitousness

Subhadra Evans [1,*], Laura A. Payne [2], Laura Seidman [2], Kirsten Lung [2], Lonnie Zeltzer [2] and Jennie C. I. Tsao [2]

[1] School of Psychology, Faculty of Health, Deakin University, 221 Burwood Highway, Burwood Victoria 3125, Australia
[2] Pediatric Pain Program, David Geffen School of Medicine, University of California, Los Angeles, CA 90095, USA; lpayne@mednet.ucla.edu (L.A.P.); lseidman@mednet.ucla.edu (L.S.); kirsten.lung@gmail.com (K.L.); lzeltzer@mednet.ucla.edu (L.Z.); jtsao@mednet.ucla.edu (J.C.I.T.)
* Correspondence: subhadra.evans@deakin.edu.au; Tel.: +61-3-924-46270

Academic Editors: Lynn S. Walker and Carl L. von Baeyer
Received: 22 April 2016; Accepted: 13 June 2016; Published: 20 June 2016

Abstract: There has been limited empirical examination of how parent variables such as anxiety and solicitousness collectively impact child pain response. We sought to examine the relationships among maternal anxiety, solicitous parenting, and children's laboratory anxiety and pain intensity in children with chronic pain. Participants included 80 children and adolescents (ages 8–18) with chronic pain and their mothers. Children completed questionnaires and lab pain tasks measuring their parents' solicitous parenting, pressure, cold and heat pain anticipatory anxiety and pain intensity. Using bootstrapping analysis, maternal anxiety predicted child anticipatory anxiety and pain intensity in girls with chronic pain, which was mediated by the child's report of parental solicitousness. For boys with chronic pain, maternal anxiety predicted boys' anticipatory anxiety and pain intensity, with no support for mediation. This study adds to the growing literature demonstrating the impact of maternal anxiety on children's pain. The study highlights the importance of considering parents in treatment designed to reduce children's pain.

Keywords: anxiety; children; chronic pain; parenting

1. Introduction

Maternal psychological symptoms and behaviors relate to children's pain and anxiety. However, research in this area is limited by a lack of clarity in determining the specific parental variables of interest, and in understanding the nature of the relationships between parental behaviors and children's pain [1]. It is likely that such relationships are complex, involving multiple levels of parental influence, but the specific mechanisms involved in parental transmission of anxiety and pain to children are largely unknown.

Parental influences in children's pain have been studied in a variety of settings, including children's dental pain and fear [2], chronic pain [3,4], health-care utilization associated with pain [5] and post-operative pain and distress [6]. The aggregate of these findings points to the coexistence of maternal psychological distress and children's pain-related distress and pain sensitivity. Even subtle displays of parental fear and anxiety can transmit powerful messages to children regarding the meaning of pain. The mere presence of a parent can cause distress in the child undergoing painful procedures [7]. A mother's heart rate variability, a marker of stress and autonomic function, two hours preceding their child's surgery has been found to significantly predict children's post-anesthetic agitation [8]. In addition, when a parent displays overt symptoms of distress, the impact upon children's pain and distress may be even more pronounced. For example, children of mothers who were instructed to exaggerate pain during a child observed-cold pressor task had lower pain thresholds compared to no instruction controls [9].

Additional research links specific parenting behaviors to increased children's pain and anxiety. Solicitous or protective parenting behaviors, which involve positive reinforcement for child pain behaviors such as exempting the child from chores or providing special privileges or attention [10], is one construct that has been studied in the context of child acute and chronic pain. When parents are overly protective, their children show higher distress and report higher bodily pain intensity [11,12]. Children with recurrent abdominal pain are more likely to endorse their parents as using solicitous strategies than are healthy children [13]. One explanation for findings linking parental protective attempts and the subsequent increase in children's pain is that parental protection may act as a signal to the child that the caregiver is anxious, thus exacerbating the child's distress [14].

As yet, limited research has mapped out the relationships between maternal anxiety, solicitous behaviors, and children's pain and pain-related anxiety. Recently, a model found support for the role of parental anxiety and solicitousness in pediatric cancer patients' pain and quality of life. In this study, parent trait anxiety was a significant predictor of parent solicitous behaviors, as well as a range of parent-reported child pain and quality of life variables in a large sample of children treated for cancer [15]. Although postulated, a meditational model was not examined. An additional study that tested the mediating role of solicitousness in children's chronic pain reported that parent solicitousness mediated the relationship between parent distress and child functional disability [16]. However, child pain variables were not examined. Thus, few studies reveal how parental variables such as anxiety and solicitousness work together to impact children's pain or pain-related anxiety.

For parents high in trait anxiety, observing their child's pain may elicit an aversive state of increased self-oriented distress, leading them to engage in solicitous responses. In a sequential analysis of mothers' reassurance and children's postoperative distress, mothers with higher anxiety were more likely to engage in child distress-promoting reassurance behaviors than were mothers lower in anxiety [6]. Relationships between maternal anxiety, solicitousness and child distress and pain may become generalized, and observable in the laboratory. Laboratory paradigms offer the opportunity to test the direct and indirect pathways among these variables in a controlled setting where the intensity and type of pain stimulus can be standardized. An important step is to examine the nature of the relationship between parental distress, solicitousness and child pain outcomes in the laboratory.

We sought to test a conceptual model (Figure 1) in children with chronic pain undertaking a series of laboratory pain tasks. It was anticipated that higher maternal anxiety would predict increased maternal solicitous behaviors as perceived by children, in turn predicting increased child laboratory-based anticipatory anxiety and pain intensity in children. We also aimed to test sex differences to understand whether boys and girls with chronic pain responded to maternal influences in dissimilar ways. It was hypothesized that the model would explain the relationship between maternal anxiety and solicitousness for girls, and we wished to explore whether this was the case for boys too. Sex differences seem to exist in the relationship between parent factors and children's pain, with particular relationships evident between maternal behavior and girls' pain [17]. In an examination of parental reinforcement of child laboratory-pain, girls whose mothers interacted with them in a pain-promoting manner reported more cold-pressor pain than girls of mothers who received no training. Girls of mothers who received pain-reducing training reported the least amount of pain. No relationships were evident for boys. [18]. An additional study showed that the effect of maternal attention was greater on daughters' gastrointestinal symptoms than on sons' symptoms [19].

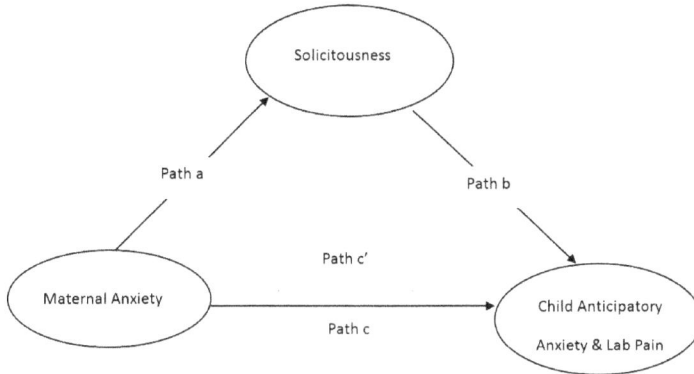

Figure 1. Conceptual model of maternal anxiety, responses to child pain, and dependent child laboratory pain variables.

2. Methods

2.1. Participants

The sample for this study was part of a larger study examining sex and pubertal relationships to pain in healthy children and those with chronic pain. Participants in the present study included 80 children and adolescents (ages 8–18) with chronic pain and their mothers, recruited through a multidisciplinary, tertiary clinic specializing in pediatric chronic pain (approximately 10% of the sample were recruited though craigslist postings). Inclusion criteria followed the commonly accepted definition of pain persisting for three months or longer [20]. Each diagnosis of a chronic pain condition was confirmed by a pediatrician specializing in chronic pain (Dr. Lonnie Zeltzer.).

Eligibility was confirmed by telephone. Parents were asked whether their child met any of the following exclusionary criteria: acute illness/injury that may impact laboratory performance (e.g., fever) or that affects sensitivity of the extremities (e.g., Raynaud's disease); daily use of opioids; recent traumatic experiences; developmental delay; autism; or significant anatomic impairment that could preclude participation in pain induction. Three hundred and sixty-four families were screened for eligibility by telephone: eight families (five control, three pain) were excluded as a result of acute injury/illness, recent traumatic experiences, or developmental delay/autism. Of the 138 families of children with pain who called to participate, 58 declined to participate due to lack of interest or scheduling difficulties.

The average age of children in the final sample was 13 years and 8 months (52 girls and 28 boys), and the average age of mothers was 45 years. The majority of mothers possessed some college qualifications, and the majority of children were non-Hispanic white (see Table 1).

Written informed consent forms were completed by parents, while children and adolescents completed written assent. The study was approved by the University of California, Los Angeles (UCLA, Los Angeles, CA, USA) institutional review board. Each family member received $50 cash for participating.

Table 1. Demographic information.

	Pain Boys (*n* = 28)	Pain Girls (*n* = 52)
Child Age (mean (SD))	12.72 (2.35)	14.92 * (2.45)
Pain Group Diagnoses (*n* (%))		
Headaches	16 (57.1)	33 (63.5)
Neurovisceral	12 (42.9)	25 (48.1)
Myofascial (non headache)	10 (35.7)	17 (32.7)
Fibromyalgia	4 (14.3)	17 (32.7)
CRPS	3 (10.7)	5 (9.6)
Joint pain	3 (10.7)	5 (9.6)
Child Ethnicity (*n* (% of subgroup))		
Non-Hispanic/Latino	21 (75.0)	36 (69.2)
Hispanic/Latino	7 (25.0)	16 (30.8)
Child Race (*n* (% of subgroup))		
White	17 (60.7)	37 (71.2)
African-American	6 (21.4)	5 (9.6)
Asian	1 (3.6)	1 (1.9)
American Indian/Alaska Native	0 (0.0)	0 (0.0)
Multi-Racial	4 (14.3)	9 (17.3)
Mother age [mean (SD)]	44.70 (5.29)	45.62 (6.63)
Mother Education Level (*n* (% of subgroup))		
High school graduate or below	4 (14.3)	8 (15.4)
Some college/AA degree	8 (28.6)	12 (23.1)
College graduate (BA/BS)	8 (28.6)	15 (28.8)
Post-graduate degree	8 (28.6)	17 (32.7)

Note: * indicates significant difference from other groups, $p < 0.05$.

2.2. Procedures

The study protocol and laboratory pain tasks have been described in previous reports relating to the larger study [21–23]. Briefly, children and their mothers were escorted to separate rooms to complete questionnaires using an online survey system; there was no contact between children and their mothers during the entire laboratory session. Children were then escorted to the laboratory where they were instructed on the use of the 0–10 Numerical Rating Scale (NRS, described in the measures section), and completed four laboratory pain tasks: an evoked pressure task, a cold pressor tolerance task, a focal pressure tolerance task, and a conditioned pain modulation (CPM) task (see task descriptions below). Tasks were completed in the same order since previous research showed no order effects [24]. The laboratory session took 30–45 min.

2.2.1. Evoked Pressure (EP) Task

To assess pressure pain sensitivity, we used the Gracely procedure [25], in which discrete 5 s pressure stimuli were applied to the fixated thumbnail of the left hand with a 1×1 cm hard rubber probe. The rubber probe was attached to a hydraulic piston, which was controlled by a computer-activated pump to provide repeatable pressure-pain stimuli of rectangular waveform. First, a series of stimuli was presented in a predictable, ascending manner, beginning at 0.066 kg/cm^2 and increasing in 0.132 kg/cm^2 intervals up to the participant's report of moderate pain (a 6 Numeric Ratings Scale (NRS) rating) or to a maximum of 1.12 kg/cm^2 (evoked pressure–ascending, EP ASC). Next, stimuli were delivered at 15 s intervals in random order using the multiple random staircase (evoked pressure–multiple random staircase, EP MRS) pressure-pain sensitivity method [26].

2.2.2. Cold Pressor Tolerance (CPT) Task

A single trial of the cold pressor was administered during which participants placed the right hand in a cold pressor unit comprising a Techne TE-10D Thermoregulator, B-8 Bath, and RU-200 Dip Cooler (Techne, Burlington, NJ, USA). The unit maintained the water at a temperature of 5 °C and kept the water circulating to prevent localized warming around the hand. Recent research has demonstrated 5 °C to be an appropriate temperature for use with children and adolescents in the age range of the current study [27], and a recent systematic review suggests that using a temperature of less than 10 °C in children older than eight years may reduce the likelihood of a ceiling effect [28]. Participants' hands were submerged up to approximately 2 inches above the wrist. Participants were instructed to keep their hand in the cold water for as long as they possibly could but that they could terminate the trial at any time. The task had an uninformed ceiling of 3 min.

2.2.3. Tonic Pressure Tolerance (TPT) Task

The Ugo Basile Analgesy-Meter 37215 (Ugo Basile Biological Research Apparatus, Comerio, Italy) was used to administer a single trial of focal pressure through a dull Lucite point approximately 1.5 mm in diameter to the second dorsal phalanx of the middle finger of the right hand. Participants were instructed to keep their finger under the pressure for as long as they possibly could, but that they could terminate the trial at any time. The task had an uninformed ceiling of 3 min.

2.2.4. Conditioned Pain Modulation (CPM) Task

The conditioned pain modulation task involved a test stimulus (TS) of phasic pressure stimuli delivered to the left thumbnail, and a conditioning stimulus (CS) of immersion of the right hand in 5 °C water [23]. The amount of pressure used as the TS was determined by averaging the final four pressure steps of the EP MRS high staircase. This value represents the amount of pressure that would reliably induce a rating of moderate pain in that participant. Participants were instructed to leave their hand in the water for 30 s and told that they would be informed by the research assistant when this time period had elapsed; participants were also told that they could remove their hand before the end of the 30 s if it became too uncomfortable/painful.

2.3. Measures

2.3.1. Pain Task Measures

Anticipatory anxiety: was assessed with a 0 (none) to 10 (worst or most possible) NRS after task instructions had been given, and before each task had commenced (*i.e.*, "now that you know what you will be doing, how nervous, afraid, or worried are you about the task").

Pain Intensity: was assessed using the same 0–10 NRS after each task. Participants were instructed that 0 meant "none" and 10 meant the "worst or most pain possible". The 11-point NRS has been demonstrated to be a reliable and valid method of assessing self-reported pain intensity in children as young as 8 years old [29].

2.3.2. Self-Reporting Questionnaires

The Anxiety subscale of the Brief Symptom Inventory-18-Item Version (BSI-18) [30] were used to assess mothers' anxiety. Mothers rated their own symptoms, with six items rated on a 5-point scale from "not at all" to "extremely". Responses are summed to obtain the total anxiety subscale score. The BSI-18 has demonstrated reliability and validity [30]. The cronbach's alpha for the present sample was 0.78.

Children's perceptions of their mother's solicitousness was assessed by the Protect subscale of the Adults' Responses to Children's Symptoms (ARCS) Child Report version [31,32]. The subscale is comprised of 15 items assessing the extent to which children perceive that their parents respond to their child's pain by placing the child in the "sick role" (e.g., limiting child's activities, granting special privileges, *etc.*) [31]. Responses are scored from 0 (never) to 4 (always); subscale scores are calculated by averaging the individual item responses. Higher scores indicate more of that behavior. Instructions were modified to inquire about parent behaviors when the child experienced pain as opposed to the original instructions which were focused on stomachaches. The child report version of the ARCS has a demonstrated alpha reliability of 0.86 and has shown to be correlated to the analogous parent report measure [32]. The cronbach's alpha for the present sample was 0.83.

2.4. Data Analysis

Analyses were conducted using SPSS 22. Data were screened to identify outliers and verify normality distribution. Descriptive analyses were conducted, including presentation of the sample, and differences between boys and girls were examined, using Chi squares, and *t*-tests where appropriate. Correlations were then performed between maternal and child variables separately for boys *versus* girls, followed by regression analyses.

Regression analyses were conducted to: (1) examine the relation between maternal anxiety and child anticipatory anxiety/pain intensity; (2) the relation between maternal anxiety and solicitousness; and (3) the relation between solicitousness and child anticipatory anxiety/pain intensity. Upon establishment of these conditions, bootstrapping analyses were then used to test the mediation hypotheses [33]. All analyses controlled for age. Bootstrapping involves repeatedly randomly sampling observations with replacement from the data set to compute the desired statistic in each resample. Indirect effects were analyzed based on 5000 bootstraps and were evaluated as significant if the 95% bias-corrected confidence interval of the indirect effect does not include zero. Consistent with recent views on mediation [34–36], we consider mediation analyses even in the absence of a direct effect. For example, Rucker and Preacher [34], argue that significant indirect effects can occur in the absence of significant total or direct effects.

3. Results

3.1. Descriptive Statistics

Demographic data, including sex, age, and race/ethnicity, are presented in Table 1. Presenting pain diagnoses were: 61.3% headaches (migraines and myofascial, vascular, tension, stress-related, or other type of headaches); 46.3% functional neurovisceral pain disorder (functional bowel, uterine, or bladder disorder); 33.8% myofascial pain (of any part of the body excluding headaches); 26.3% fibromyalgia; 10.0% complex regional pain syndrome; and 10.0% joint pain (note that percentages sum to more than 100% due to multiple pain diagnoses). Multiple pain diagnoses were present in 61.3% (n = 49) of the sample. Frequencies of each pain diagnosis by sex are presented in Table 1. Chi-squared analyses revealed no significant differences in diagnosis rate between sexes. The only significant group difference to emerge was for child age; girls with chronic pain were significantly older than boys.

Means and standard deviations for each of the maternal variables and child lab pain variables are displayed in Table 2. Maternal anxiety means were within population norms. There were no significant sex differences on the maternal or child questionnaire or laboratory variables.

As presented in Table 3, correlations between the maternal and child variables were performed for boys and girls on each of the laboratory pain task variables. For girls, maternal anxiety was significantly related to child anticipatory anxiety (for EP r = 0.45, p = 0.00; for CPT r = 0.45, p = 0.00; for TPT r = 0.42, p = 0.01; for conditioned pain modulation (CPM) r = 0.45, p = 0.00), while solicitousness was significantly associated with most child lab pain variables (for CPT r = 0.35, p = 0.01; for TPT r = 0.27, p = 0.049; for DNIC r = 0.32, p = 0.03). For boys, maternal anxiety was associated with child lab anxiety (for EP r = 0.38 p = 0.047; for DNIC r = 0.61, p = 0.00) and child lab pain (EP r = 0.41, p = 0.03; for CPT r = 0.57, p = 0.00; for TPT r = 0.53, p = 0.000; for DNIC r = 0.44, p = 0.03), whereas maternal solicitousness was not associated with any child variables. Age was not correlated with any of the maternal or child variables for girls with pain; however, since girls with pain were significantly older than the other sub-groups, age was included as a covariate in hypothesis testing. For boys with pain, age was significantly related to both maternal anxiety ($r = -0.40$, $p < 0.05$), and solicitousness ($r = -0.43$, $p < 0.05$), suggesting that, as they get older, boys perceive their mothers as using fewer solicitous responses, and mothers rate themselves as less anxious. Age was thus included as a covariate in all hypothesis testing.

Table 2. Means (standard deviation, SD) of maternal psychosocial variables and child laboratory pain variables for boys and girls.

	Pain Boys	Pain Girls
Mother BSI Anxiety Subscale	2.68 (3.14)	3.04 (3.11)
Child ARCS Protect Subscale	2.02 (0.71)	1.63 (0.58)
EP Ant Anx	3.07 (2.36)	2.92 (2.65)
EP Pain	6.04 (2.52)	6.51 (1.38)
CPT Ant Anx	1.61 (1.57)	1.98 (2.29)
CPT Pain	5.89 (2.56)	5.75 (2.90)
Pressure Ant Anx	4.07 (2.73)	3.18 (2.46)
Pressure Pain	5.78 (2.78)	6.02 (2.42)
CPM Ant Anx	3.68 (2.77)	3.21 (2.64)
CPM Pain	6.13 (2.85)	6.09 (2.90)

Note: BSI = Brief Symptom Inventory-18-Item Version; ARCS = Adults' Responses to Children's Symptoms; EP = Evoked Pressure task; CPT = Cold Pressor Tolerance task; CPM = Conditioned Pain Modulation task; Ant Anx = Anticipatory Anxiety.

Table 3. Correlations among maternal and child lab variables.

	Maternal Anxiety	Solicitousness
Girls with Pain		
Maternal Solicitousness	0.28 *	
Child Lab Pain		
EP- Anticipatory Anxiety	0.45 **	0.31 *
EP- Pain Intensity	0.02	0.20
CP- Anticipatory Anxiety	0.45 **	0.34 *
CP- Pain Intensity	0.12	0.35 *
TPT- Anticipatory Anxiety	0.35 *	0.30 *
TPT- Pain Intensity	0.01	0.27 *
CPM- Anticipatory Anxiety	0.45 **	0.40 *
CPM- Pain Intensity	0.20	0.33 *
Boys with Pain		
Maternal Solicitousness	-0.03	
Child Lab Pain		
EP- Anticipatory Anxiety	0.38 *	0.09
EP- Pain Intensity	0.41 *	-0.30
CP- Anticipatory Anxiety	0.17	0.03
CP- Pain Intensity	0.57 **	-0.12
TPT- Anticipatory Anxiety	0.27	0.29
TPT- Pain Intensity	0.53 **	0.23
CPM- Anticipatory Anxiety	0.61 **	-0.15
CPM- Pain Intensity	0.44 *	-0.11

EP: Evoked Pressure; CP: Cold Pressor; TPT: Tonic Pressure Tolerance; CPM: Conditioned Pain Modulation; * $p < 0.05$, ** $p < 0.01$

3.2. Hypothesis Testing

Average summary measures across all four laboratory tasks were created to produce a single score for each anticipatory anxiety and pain intensity. Hypothesis testing was performed on these summary measures controlling for child age.

Results for the regression analyses for girls with chronic pain are presented in Table 4. First, there was support for the relationship between maternal anxiety and girls' anticipatory anxiety ($\beta = 0.55$, $p = 0.00$). However, no significant direct effect of maternal anxiety on girls' lab pain intensity; Second, there was support for the relation between maternal anxiety and solicitousness, such that greater maternal anxiety was associated with greater use of mothers' solicitous responses for girls with chronic pain ($\beta = 0.28$, $p = 0.048$); Third, there was support for the relation between solicitous parenting and girls' anticipatory anxiety and pain intensity, such that greater use of solicitous responses was associated with greater anticipatory anxiety ($\beta = 0.39$, $p = 0.01$) and pain intensity in girls ($\beta = 0.36$, $p = 0.01$).

Table 4. Regression models for pre-conditions of mediation.

Maternal Predictors & Child Pain	Child Anticipatory Anxiety			Child Pain Intensity			Solicitousness		
	β	t	$R^2 \Delta$	β	t	$R^2 \Delta$	β	t	$R^2 \Delta$
Girls with Chronic Pain									
Child Age	−0.26	−10.79	0.07	0.02	0.14	0.00	0.04	0.301	0.001
Maternal Anxiety	0.55	4.60 **	0.30	0.15	10.0	0.02	0.28	2.03*	0.08
Solicitousness	0.39	2.95 **	0.15	0.36	2.6 *	0.13			
Boys with Chronic Pain									
Child Age	−0.27	−1.4	0.08	−0.17	−0.81	0.03	−0.43	−2.41 **	0.18
Maternal Anxiety	0.60	3.68 **	0.36	0.44	2.21 *	0.19	−0.23	−1.21	0.05
Solicitousness	0.03	0.12	0.01	−0.19	−0.73	0.03			

All models controlled for child age, * $p < 0.05$; ** $p < 0.01$, β denotes standardized beta coefficients.

For boys (as presented in Table 4), there was support for the relationship between maternal anxiety and boys' outcomes. Greater maternal anxiety was a significant predictor of boys' anticipatory anxiety ($\beta = 0.60$, $p = 0.00$) and pain intensity ($\beta = 0.44$, $p = 0.00$), explaining 36% and 19% of the variance respectively. However, there was no support for the relation between maternal anxiety and solicitousness. There was also no support for the relation between solicitous parenting and boys' pain outcomes. Thus, further mediation analyses for boys were not undertaken.

Bootstrapping analyses were conducted with solicitousness as a hypothesized mediator between maternal anxiety and anticipatory anxiety and pain intensity in girls only. Mothers' solicitousness mediated the relation between maternal anxiety and girls' anticipatory anxiety (see Figure 2). The direct effect of maternal anxiety on girls' anticipatory anxiety was reduced when solicitousness was included as a mediator. This result was supported by bootstrapping analyses, which showed the bootstrapped indirect effect was 0.05 (95% bootstrap confidence interval (BCI) = 0.01, 0.14) for girls' anticipatory anxiety. For girls' pain intensity, there was evidence of an indirect effect. When maternal anxiety and solicitousness were entered in the model together, they significantly predicted girls' pain intensity, yet maternal anxiety alone did not predict girls' pain intensity. Consistent with recent writings on mediation [34], significant indirect effects can occur in the absence of significant direct effects, often due to a suppression effect of a third variable, or a small sample size. The significance of the indirect effect of solicitousness on the relationship between maternal anxiety and girls' lab pain intensity was supported by bootstrapping analyses, which showed the bootstrapped indirect effect was 0.06 (95% BCI = 0.02, 0.13). Figures 2 and 3 summarize the significant mediating results.

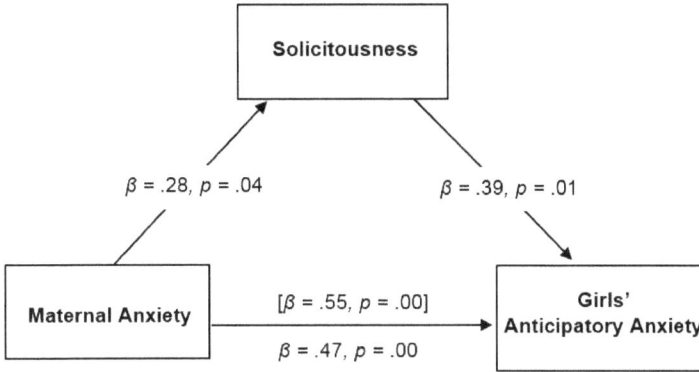

Figure 2. Mediating role of solicitousness in the relation of maternal anxiety with lab anticipatory anxiety for girls with chronic pain. Estimates of total effect of maternal anxiety on girls' pain outcomes are presented in brackets, with values representing estimates of the total indirect effect of maternal anxiety on girls' pain outcomes through maternal solicitousness presented below.

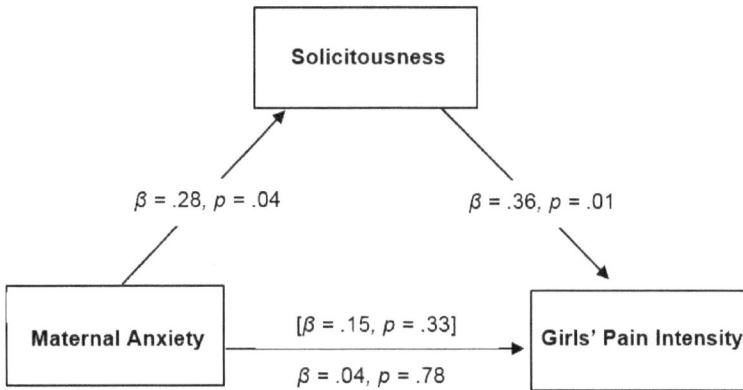

Figure 3. Mediating role of solicitousness in the relation of maternal anxiety with girls' lab pain intensity. Estimates of total effect of maternal anxiety on girls' pain outcomes are presented in brackets, with values representing estimates of the total indirect effect of maternal anxiety on girls' pain outcomes through maternal solicitousness presented below.

4. Discussion

This study sought to investigate the relationship between maternal anxiety and children's laboratory anticipatory anxiety and pain intensity in boys versus girls with chronic pain, and to test the hypothesis that these relationships were mediated by children's reports of maternal solicitous behavior. There were no sex differences in the degree to which children perceived their mothers as solicitous across the groups; mothers reported similar levels of anxiety; and maternal anxiety emerged as a significant predictor of both girls' and boys' laboratory pain and anxiety. However, there were differences in the relationships among these variables between the sexes. In particular, perceptions of mother's solicitous behavior mediated the relationship between maternal anxiety and child lab pain for girls only.

Our findings are consistent with the existing literature demonstrating links between parental distress and behaviors, and children's pain sensitivity and anxiety. For example, Logan and Scharff (2005) [37] found that maternal psychological distress was predictive of functional disability in children with chronic pain; moreover, mothers in the study were similar to the mothers in the present study in that they were not significantly more distressed than healthy populations. Other lab studies have reported that children of mothers that were instructed to exaggerate pain during a child observed-cold pressor task had lower pain thresholds compared to controls whose mothers were given no specific instructions [9]. The present study suggests that the relationship between maternal distress and child pain and pain-related anxiety may occur through maternal solicitousness for girls with chronic pain.

Our findings go beyond what is currently known about parental influences in children's pain and pain-related anxiety. Few studies have examined how parental variables interact in influencing children's pain. For example, in a recent study, parent trait anxiety emerged as a significant predictor of parent solicitous behaviors, parent-reported child pain, and child quality of life variables in children treated for cancer [15]; however, a model describing the nature of the relationships between the variables was not offered. In one mediation study, it was reported that parent protectiveness mediated the relationship between pain-specific parent distress and child functional disability [16]. The present study extends these findings to the laboratory, in which it is possible to measure the immediate effects of pain stimuli, including behavioral and emotional responding.

Overall, parental solicitousness has emerged as an important variable in understanding and treating the etiology and maintenance of chronic pain in children. For example, studies have shown that a brief cognitive behavioral therapy intervention, involving reducing parental solicitousness as one its components, resulted in pain reduction and decreased disability for children with chronic pain in both short- and long-term follow-up [4]. The present study is the first time that a meditational model for solicitousness has been demonstrated for the relationship between parental anxiety and child laboratory-based pain and anxiety.

This is also the first study where a meditation model has been examined in a sex specific manner. Consistent with our previous work, we report a greater influence of maternal symptoms on girls' pain outcomes than on boys' outcomes. In earlier studies, we demonstrated relationships between maternal symptoms (anxiety sensitivity, fear of pain, anxiety and bodily pain) and healthy girls' laboratory pain responses, but fewer relationships with boys' pain responses (Tsao, Lu, Myers *et al.*, 2006; Evans *et al.*, 2008; Evans *et al.*, 2010). For example, parent anxiety sensitivity was related to child laboratory pain intensity through its contribution to anxiety sensitivity in girls, but not in boys (Tsao, Lu *et al.*, 2006). Together, these findings highlight the particular influence of mothers on daughters' pain and the importance of examining sex differences in the context of pediatric pain.

A number of study limitations are worth noting. Our cross-sectional findings prohibit an understanding of the direction of the relationships. Does child pain elicit a solicitous parental reaction, or do certain parental styles elicit pain in children? Perhaps higher levels of negative affect in children with chronic pain drive the relationship. Other potential mediators, such as parental catastrophizing should be examined, especially given findings that catastrophizing may mediate the relationship between solicitous parenting and children's pain behaviors [38]. Future longitudinal analyses may reveal causal associations among a number of such constructs. In addition, since this study only included mothers, the impact of fathers both directly on daughters' and sons' anxiety and pain responses and indirectly through impact on the mother/child pain relationship was not explored. The lack of findings of mothers' solicitousness as a mediator of the relationship between maternal anxiety and child anxiety/pain relationships for sons, compared to that found for daughters, suggest that there may be other factors that mediate the mother/son pain relationship not explored in this study. It may also be the case that, since there were fewer boys in the study, the lack of mediation was due to lower power in the sample of boys. Possible moderators to examine in the future include duration and severity of the child's condition and whether the parent has chronic pain. While a strength of the sample is the blending of disease groups to allow for examination of psychological and family processes in a broad group of children chronic pain, it will be important in future research to explore the impact of specific disease-related factors such as duration of diagnosis on child and family outcomes. The present findings contribute to the literature on a broad population of children with chronic pain and reveal complex models of pain, maternal anxiety, parenting and laboratory based pain in families dealing with children who have chronic pain.

5. Conclusions

Children with chronic pain may benefit from a multifaceted intervention, including pain management strategies, treatment targeted to depressive or anxiety symptoms to improve coping skills, and parents and other family members may be taught adaptive, non-reinforcing responses to both distress and pain behaviors in their children to optimize child functioning (Sieberg *et al.*, 2011). Our findings highlight the importance of considering parental factors, and especially maternal anxiety when evaluating and treating children with chronic pain. Maternal anxiety appears to impact boys and girls through different mechanisms. Maternal solicitousness may be particularly important when understanding girls' anxiety and pain intensity, whereas maternal anxiety may affect boys' anxiety and pain through other, as yet untested, influences. It is possible that girls with chronic pain are highly sensitive to modeling of anxiety and reinforcing behaviors in their mothers, given findings that girls with pain tend to become heavily enmeshed and reliant on their mothers, whereas boys with pain may respond to maternal worries with increased efforts for independence [39]. Future studies should continue to focus on the impact of maternal emotional and behavioral contributors to boys' and girls' pain, as well as explore the role of fathers' emotional and behavioral functioning in boys and girls with chronic pain. Our findings relating to sex differences, if verified by further research, suggest that clinical efforts for girls with chronic pain should invest in mothers, and include strategies for reducing solicitous parenting that reinforces child pain behaviors.

Acknowledgments: This research was supported by a grant from the National Center for Complementary and Integrative Health (K01AT005093 Principal Investigator: Subhadra Evans), a grant from the National Institute of Dental and Craniofacial Research (5R01DE012754; PI: Lonnie K. Zeltzer), and UCLA General Clinical Research Center Grant M01-RR-00865 (PI: Lonnie K. Zeltzer).

Author Contributions: S.E. was responsible for the research concept, statistical analyses and writing up the findings; L.A.P made further advances to the research model, review and provided key concepts for the discussion; K.L and L.S contributed to data management and statistical analyses; J.C.I.T., and L. Z reviewed the article and updated the current literatures.

Conflicts of Interest: The authors declare no conflict of interest.

References

1. Palermo, T.M.; Chambers, C.T. Parent and family factors in pediatric chronic pain and disability: An integrative approach. *Pain* **2005**, *119*, 1–4. [CrossRef] [PubMed]
2. Coric, A.; Banozic, A.; Klaric, M.; Vukojevic, K.; Puljak, L. Dental fear and anxiety in older children: An association with parental dental anxiety and effective pain coping strategies. *J. Pain Res.* **2014**, *7*, 515–521. [PubMed]
3. Darlington, A.-S.E.; Verhulst, F.C.; De Winter, A.F.; Ormel, J.; Passchier, J.; Hunfeld, J.A.M. The influence of maternal vulnerability and parenting stress on chronic pain in adolescents in a general population sample: the TRAILS study. *Eur. J. Pain* **2012**, *16*, 150–159. [CrossRef] [PubMed]
4. Levy, R.L.; Langer, S.L.; Romano, J.M.; Labus, J.; Walker, L.S.; Murphy, T.B.; Tilburg, M.A.; Feld, L.D.; Christie, D.L.; Whitehead, W.E. Cognitive mediators of treatment outcomes in pediatric functional abdominal pain. *Clin. J. Pain* **2014**, *30*, 1033–1043. [CrossRef] [PubMed]
5. Lee, J.L.; Gilleland, J.; Campbell, R.M.; Simpson, P.; Johnson, G.L.; Dooley, K.J.; Blount, R.L. Health care utilization and psychosocial factors in pediatric noncardiac chest pain. *Health Psychol.* **2013**, *32*, 320–327. [CrossRef] [PubMed]
6. Martin, S.R.; Chorney, J.M.; Cohen, L.L.; Kain, Z.N. Sequential analysis of mothers' and fathers' reassurance and children's postoperative distress. *J. Pediatr. Psychol.* **2013**, *38*, 1121–1129. [CrossRef] [PubMed]
7. Tourigny, J. Emotional states of mothers and behavior of the child during minor surgery. *Can. J. Nurs. Res.* **1992**, *24*, 65–80. [PubMed]

8.   Arai, Y.C.; Ueda, W.; Ito, H.; Wakao, Y.; Matsura, M.; Komatsu, T. Maternal heart rate variability just before surgery significantly correlated with emergence behavior of children undergoing general anesthesia. *Paediatr. Anaesth.* **2008**, *18*, 167–171. [CrossRef] [PubMed]

9.   Goodman, J.E.; McGrath, P.J. Mothers' modeling influences children's pain during a cold pressor task. *Pain* **2003**, *104*, 559–565. [CrossRef]

10. Noel, M.; Palermo, T.M.; Essner, B.; Zhou, C.; Levy, R.L.; Langer, S.L.; Sherman, A.L.; Walker, L.S. A developmental analysis of the factorial validity of the parent-report version of the Adult Responses to Children's Symptoms in children versus adolescents with chronic pain or pain-related chronic illness. *J. Pain* **2015**, *16*, 31–41. [CrossRef] [PubMed]

11. Claar, R.L.; Simons, L.E.; Logan, D.E. Parental response to children's pain: the moderating impact of children's emotional distress on symptoms and disability. *Pain* **2008**, *138*, 172–179. [CrossRef] [PubMed]

12. Penner, L.A.; Cline, R.J.; Albrecht, T.L.; Harper, F.W.; Peterson, A.M.; Taub, J.M.; Ruckdeschel, J.C. Parents' Empathic Responses and Pain and Distress in Pediatric Patients. *Basic Appl. Soc. Psych.* **2008**, *30*, 102–113. [CrossRef] [PubMed]

13. Walker, L.S.; Garber, J.; Greene, J.W. Psychosocial correlates of recurrent childhood pain: A comparison of pediatric patients with recurrent abdominal pain, organic illness, and psychiatric disorders. *J. Abnorm. Psychol.* **1993**, *102*, 248–258. [CrossRef] [PubMed]

14. McMurtry, C.M.; McGrath, P.J.; Chambers, C.T. Reassurance can hurt: parental behavior and painful medical procedures. *J. Pediatr.* **2006**, *148*, 560–561. [CrossRef] [PubMed]

15. Link, C.J.; Fortier, M.A. The Relationship Between Parent Trait Anxiety and Parent-reported Pain, Solicitous Behaviors, and Quality of Life Impairment in Children With Cancer. *J. Pediatr. Hematol. Oncol.* **2015**, *1*, 58–62. [CrossRef] [PubMed]

16. Sieberg, C.B.; Williams, S.; Simons, L.E. Do parent protective responses mediate the relation between parent distress and child functional disability among children with chronic pain? *J. Pediatr. Psychol.* **2011**, *36*, 1043–1051. [CrossRef] [PubMed]

17. Tsao, J.C.; Lu, Q.; Myers, C.D.; Kim, S.C.; Turk, N.; Zeltzer, L.K. Parent and child anxiety sensitivity: Relationship to children's experimental pain responsivity. *J. Pain* **2006**, *7*, 319–326. [CrossRef] [PubMed]

18. Chambers, C.T.; Craig, K.D.; Bennett, S.M. The impact of maternal behavior on children's pain experiences: An experimental analysis. *J. Pediatr. Psychol.* **2002**, *27*, 293–301. [CrossRef] [PubMed]

19. Walker, L.S.; Williams, S.E.; Smith, C.A.; Garber, J.; Van Slyke, D.A.; Lipani, T.A. Parent attention versus distraction: impact on symptom complaints by children with and without chronic functional abdominal pain. *Pain* **2006**, *122*, 43–52. [CrossRef] [PubMed]

20. McGrath, P.J.; Walco, G.A.; Turk, D.C.; Dworkin, R.H.; Brown, M.T.; Davidson, K.; Eccleston, C.; Finley, G.A.; Goldschneider, K.; Haverkos, L.; *et al.* Core outcome domains and measures for pediatric acute and chronic/recurrent pain clinical trials: PedIMMPACT recommendations. *J. Pain* **2008**, *9*, 771–783. [CrossRef] [PubMed]

21. Payne, L.A.; Seidman, L.C.; Lung, K.C.; Zeltzer, L.K.; Tsao, J.C. Relationship of neuroticism and laboratory pain in healthy children: Does anxiety sensitivity play a role? *Pain* **2013**, *154*, 103–109. [CrossRef] [PubMed]

22. Tsao, J.C.; Li, N.; Parker, D.; Seidman, L.C.; Zeltzer, L.K. Pubertal status moderates the association between mother and child laboratory pain tolerance. *Pain Res. Manag.* **2014**, *19*, 23–29. [CrossRef] [PubMed]

23. Tsao, J.C.; Seidman, L.C.; Evans, S.; Lung, K.C.; Zeltzer, L.K.; Naliboff, B.D. Conditioned pain modulation in children and adolescents: Effects of sex and age. *J. Pain* **2013**, *14*, 558–567. [CrossRef] [PubMed]

24. Tsao, J.C.; Myers, C.D.; Craske, M.G.; Bursch, B.; Kim, S.C.; Zeltzer, L.K. Role of anticipatory anxiety and anxiety sensitivity in children's and adolescents' laboratory pain responses. *J. Pediatr. Psychol.* **2004**, *29*, 379–388. [CrossRef] [PubMed]

25. Gracely, R.H.; Grant, M.A.; Giesecke, T. Evoked pain measures in fibromyalgia. *Best. Pract. Res. Clin. Rheumatol.* **2003**, *17*, 593–609. [CrossRef]

26. Gracely, R.H.; Myers, C.D.; Craske, M.G.; Bursch, B.; Kim, S.C.; Zeltzer, L.K. A multiple random staircase method of psychophysical pain assessment. *Pain* **1988**, *32*, 55–63. [CrossRef]

27. Dufton, L.M.; Konik, B.; Colletti, R.; Stanger, C.; Boyer, M.; Morrow, S.; Compas, B.E. Effects of stress on pain threshold and tolerance in children with recurrent abdominal pain. *Pain* **2008**, *136*, 38–43. [CrossRef] [PubMed]

28. Birnie, K.A.; Petter, M.; Boerner, K.E.; Noel, M.; Chambers, C.T. Contemporary use of the cold pressor task in pediatric pain research: A systematic review of methods. *J. Pain* **2012**, *13*, 817–826. [CrossRef] [PubMed]
29. Von Baeyer, C.L.; Spagrud, L.J.; McCormick, J.C.; Choo, E.; Neville, K.; Connelly, M.A. Three new datasets supporting use of the Numerical Rating Scale (NRS-11) for children's self-reports of pain intensity. *Pain* **2009**, *143*, 223–227. [CrossRef] [PubMed]
30. Derogatis, L.R. Brief Symptom Inventory (BSI) 18. In *Administration, Scoring, and Procedures Manual*; NCS Pearson, Inc.: Minneapolis, MN, USA, 2001.
31. Van Slyke, D.A.; Walker, L.S. Mothers' responses to children's pain. *Clin. J. Pain.* **2006**, *22*, 387–391. [CrossRef] [PubMed]
32. Walker, L.S.; Levy, R.L.; Whitehead, W.E. Validation of a measure of protective parent responses to children's pain. *Clin. J. Pain* **2006**, *22*, 712–716. [CrossRef] [PubMed]
33. Preacher, K.J.; Hayes, A.F. Asymptotic and resampling strategies for assessing and comparing indirect effects in multiple mediator models. *Behav. Res. Methods* **2008**, *40*, 879–891. [CrossRef] [PubMed]
34. Rucker, D.D.; Preacher, K.J.; Tormala, Z.L.; Petty, R.E. Mediation analysis in social psychology: Current practices and new recommendations. *Soc. Personal. Psychol. Compass* **2011**, *5*, 359–371. [CrossRef]
35. MacKinnon, D.P.; Krull, J.L.; Lockwood, C.M. Equivalence of the mediation, confounding and suppression effect. *Prev. Sci.* **2000**, *1*, 173–181. [CrossRef] [PubMed]
36. Shrout, P.E.; Bolger, N. Mediation in experimental and nonexperimental studies: New procedures and recommendations. *Psychol. Methods.* **2002**, *7*, 422–445. [CrossRef] [PubMed]
37. Logan, D.E.; Scharff, L. Relationships between family and parent characteristics and functional abilities in children with recurrent pain syndromes: An investigation of moderating effects on the pathway from pain to disability. *J. Pediatr. Psychol.* **2005**, *30*, 698–707. [CrossRef] [PubMed]
38. Langer, S.L.; Romano, J.M.; Mancl, L.; Levy, R.L. Parental Catastrophizing Partially Mediates the Association between Parent-Reported Child Pain Behavior and Parental Protective Responses. *Pain Res. Treat.* **2014**, *2014*, 751097-05. [CrossRef] [PubMed]
39. Evans, S.; Taub, R.; Tsao, J.C.; Meldrum, M.; Zeltzer, L.K. Sociodemographic factors in a pediatric chronic pain clinic: The roles of age, sex and minority status in pain and health characteristics. *J. Pain Manag.* **2010**, *3*, 273–281. [PubMed]

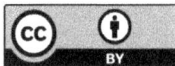

children

MDPI

Article

Parental Protectiveness Mediates the Association between Parent-Perceived Child Self-Efficacy and Health Outcomes in Pediatric Functional Abdominal Pain Disorder

Melissa M. DuPen [1],*, Miranda A. L. van Tilburg [2], Shelby L. Langer [3], Tasha B. Murphy [1], Joan M. Romano [4] and Rona L. Levy [1]

[1]   School of Social Work, University of Washington, Seattle, WA 98105, USA;
       tbmurphy@uw.edu (T.B.M.); rlevy@uw.edu (R.L.L.)
[2]   Center for Functional GI and Motility Disorders, University of North Carolina, Chapel Hill, NC 27599, USA;
       tilburg@med.unc.edu
[3]   College of Nursing and Health Innovation, Arizona State University, Phoenix, AZ 85004, USA;
       Shelby.Langer@asu.edu
[4]   Psychiatry and Behavioral Sciences, University of Washington, Seattle, WA 98105, USA; jromano@uw.edu
*   Correspondence: mmdupen@uw.edu; Tel.: +1-206-543-7138

Academic Editor: Sari Acra
Received: 16 August 2016; Accepted: 12 September 2016; Published: 19 September 2016

Abstract: Previous studies have shown that parental protectiveness is associated with increased pain and disability in Functional Abdominal Pain Disorder (FAPD) but the role that perceived child self-efficacy may play remains unclear. One reason why parents may react protectively towards their child's pain is that they perceive their child to be unable to cope or function normally while in pain (perceived low self-efficacy). This study sought to examine (a) the association between parent-perceived child pain self-efficacy and child health outcomes (symptom severity and disability); and (b) the role of parental protectiveness as a mediator of this association. Participants were 316 parents of children aged 7–12 years with FAPD. Parents completed measures of perceived child self-efficacy when in pain, their own protective responses to their child's pain, child gastrointestinal (GI) symptom severity, and child functional disability. Parent-perceived child self-efficacy was inversely associated with parent-reported child GI symptom severity and disability, and parental protectiveness mediated these associations. These results suggest that parents who perceive their child to have low self-efficacy to cope with pain respond more protectively when they believe he/she is in pain, and this, in turn, is associated with higher levels of GI symptoms and disability in their child. This finding suggests that directly addressing parent beliefs about their child's ability to manage pain should be included as a component of FAPD, and potentially other child treatment interventions.

Keywords: Functional Abdominal Pain Disorder; self-efficacy; somatic symptoms; disability; parenting; protectiveness; children; pain; coping

---

1. Introduction

One of the most common recurrent pain complaints of childhood is abdominal pain, which affects approximately 13.5% of children worldwide [1]. Many children with persistent abdominal pain meet criteria for Functional Abdominal Pain Disorder (FAPD), defined as episodic or continuous abdominal pain without evidence of physiological etiology [2]. FAPD accounts for approximately 3% of visits to pediatricians [3], more than 50% of the referrals to gastroenterology clinics [4], and is the main reason for gastrointestinal (GI) emergency room visits among children [5]. Children with FAPD not only experience frequent abdominal pain that interferes with normal activities, but also have higher rates of disability and other somatic complaints.

The cognitions, psychological state, and pain behaviors of parents have all been shown to be related to pain behaviors and functioning in children. Parental protective and solicitous responses to child pain behavior (parental protectiveness) are responses that tend to buffer the child from normal demands/activities or provide additional attention or rewards in response to child pain behaviors (e.g., giving the child special treats and/or keeping them home from school when in pain). Previous research has shown that parental protectiveness is associated with increased pain, disability, and somatic complaints in children with FAPD [6]. One logical hypothesis as to why parents react to their child's pain protectively is that they may believe that their child is unable to deal with and function normally while having pain (perceived low pain self-efficacy).

Self-efficacy was first conceptualized by Bandura as part of the Social Cognitive Theory [7–9]. Self-efficacy in a general context is a person's belief in his/her ability to perform a task or obtain a goal. Rosenstock [10], for example, suggested incorporating self-efficacy into the Health Belief Model, a model used to better understand individual health-related behaviors such as keeping preventive health appointments, adherence to treatment, and general confidence in medical care [11].

Relatedly, "pain self-efficacy" is a term defined as one's certainty or belief in one's ability to function normally when experiencing pain [12,13]. Studies have found that greater pain self-efficacy was associated with lower levels of disability in children with chronic headaches [14], and with lower levels of somatic symptoms in children with chronic pain [13]. However, the mechanisms by which pain self-efficacy might be related to symptoms and disability are unclear. Parental protectiveness is a plausible mechanism by which perceived self-efficacy may be related to health outcomes. Based on these considerations, this study sought to examine (a) the association between parent-perceived child pain self-efficacy and parent-reported child health outcomes (symptom severity and disability); and (b) the role of parental protectiveness as a mediator of these associations (Figures 1 and 2).

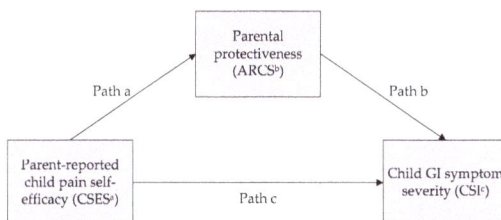

Figure 1. Mediation model 1—Parent-perceived child pain self-efficacy, parental protectiveness, and parent-reported child gastrointestinal (GI) symptom severity. [a] CSES: Child Self-Efficacy Scale; [b] ARCS: Adult Responses to Children's Symptoms—Protectiveness subscale; [c] CSI: Children's Somatization Inventory—GI subscale.

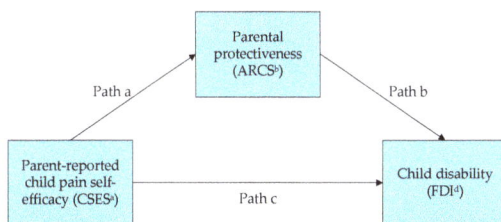

Figure 2. Mediation model 2—Parent-perceived child pain self-efficacy, parental protectiveness, and parent-reported child disability. [a] CSES: Child Self-Efficacy Scale; [b] ARCS: Adult Responses to Children's Symptoms—Protectiveness subscale; [d] FDI: Functional Disability Inventory.

2. Materials and Methods

2.1. Participants

Participants were 316 parents or caregivers of children enrolled in a large multi-site cognitive-behavioral intervention study for parents of children with FAPD [15]. Families were recruited from four pediatric gastroenterology clinics located in Seattle, WA, USA; Tacoma, WA, USA; Chapel Hill, NC, USA; and Bend, OR, USA. Children and parents were included in the study if the child was aged 7 to 12 years, lived with the parent or caregiver for at least the past three months, had a gastroenterologist-documented diagnosis of FAPD based on ROME III criteria [16], had abdominal pain at least once a week over the past two months, and spoke English. Families were excluded if the child had positive physical or laboratory findings that would explain the abdominal pain, any chronic disease, major surgery within the past year, or a developmental disability requiring full-time special education or that impaired their ability to participate.

The institutional review boards at each clinic location approved the study. Recruiters from each location screened potential participants based on the inclusion and exclusion criteria listed above and obtained verbal or written consent. 352 participants consented to be in the study; of those 316 completed baseline assessments and were randomized, and 36 did not complete baseline assessments and thus were not randomized (28 did not respond, five said they were too busy, and three did not complete for other reasons). Participants were randomly assigned to either a social learning and cognitive-behavioral therapy condition administered by phone or in-person; or an education and support condition administered by phone. Topics included teaching parents to model and reinforce wellness behaviors, decrease reinforcement of illness behaviors, reduce negative cognitions regarding FAPD; or education about the GI system, nutritional guidelines, and food safety.

2.2. Measures

All measures were completed by parents and collected online or by mail (over 90% completed online) at baseline, prior to randomization into the intervention component of the study. Measures are described in detail below.

2.2.1. Child Self-Efficacy Scale (parent-report) (CSES; [13])

The CSES assesses parent beliefs about their child's ability to function normally when in pain. The measure contains seven items rated on a 1–5 scale and was reverse-scored for ease of interpretation such that higher scores equal higher parent-perceived child pain self-efficacy. Example items are "How sure are you that your child can do well in school when in pain?" and "How sure are you that your child can do house chores when in pain?" This measure has demonstrated excellent reliability and validity for both parent and child-report versions and the developers reported an internal consistency (Cronbach's coefficient alpha) of 0.89 [13]. The internal consistency for this sample was 0.93.

2.2.2. Adult Responses to Children's Symptoms Scale (ARCS; [17–19])

The ARCS assesses parent responses to children's pain. We focused on the protectiveness subscale which has been recently revised to contain 13 items [19] rated on a 0–4 scale (higher scores indicate more protective and solicitous responses to pain behavior) and has been validated in a large sample of mothers [17]. Example items are "When your child has abdominal pain how often do you pay more attention to your child than usual?" and "When your child has abdominal pain how often do you keep your child inside the house?" Developers of the measure reported an internal consistency of 0.86. Internal consistency in the current sample was also found to be 0.86.

2.2.3. Children's Somatization Inventory (parent-report) (CSI; [20])

The CSI measures parent-report of their child's symptom severity during the past two weeks. We used the seven-item GI subscale (nausea or upset stomach; constipation; loose bowel movements or diarrhea; stomachaches; vomiting; feeling bloated or gassy, and food making child sick) which has been shown to be a valid and reliable measure of GI symptoms [21]. Items are rated on a 0–4 scale where higher scores indicate greater symptom severity. Internal consistency for a large sample of children with unexplained abdominal pain was 0.75 [22]; it was 0.68 for the current sample.

2.2.4. Functional Disability Inventory (parent-report) (FDI; [23])

The FDI asks parents to rate their child's difficulty doing regular activities such as "walking up stairs" and "being at school all day", over the past few days. This measure includes 15 items rated on a 0–4 scale, where higher scores indicate greater disability. Developers of the measure reported an internal consistency of 0.94 in a sample of mothers [23]. Internal consistency for this sample was also found to be 0.94.

2.3. Data Analysis

Analyses were conducted using IBM Statistical Package for the Social Sciences (version 19, Armonk, NY, USA). Descriptive analyses of demographic data for parents and children were conducted, followed by Pearson correlations to examine bivariate associations within parent-report measures. Two separate mediation analyses were then performed using the Hayes' PROCESS macro [24] to predict child GI symptom severity (Figure 1) and child disability (Figure 2). The Hayes' PROCESS macro is a regression-based path analytic framework [24] that calculates the regression of the outcome on the predictor, the regression of the mediator on the predictor, and the regression of the outcome on both the predictor and mediator. Bootstrap methods were used to test for an indirect effect and to compute bias-corrected confidence intervals for this effect, with 10,000 resamples. In both cases, parent-perceived child self-efficacy was treated as the predictor and parental protectiveness as the mediator.

3. Results

3.1. Descriptive Statistics

Demographic characteristics of the parents in the study were: mean (standard deviation, SD) age of 39.9 (7.4) years; 94.9% female; 84.8% White; 7.0% Hispanic or Latino; 47.2% with a 4-year college degree or higher; 57.3% employed at least part-time; and 79.4% married or cohabitating with a partner. Demographic characteristics of the children were: mean (SD) age of 9.4 (1.6) years; 64.6% female; 81.6% White; and 9.8% Hispanic or Latino.

Table 1 presents a correlation matrix, as well as descriptive statistics for study variables. Parent-perceived child self-efficacy was inversely correlated with parental protectiveness ($r = -0.55$, $p < 0.01$), parent-reported child GI symptom severity ($r = -0.25$, $p < 0.01$), and parent-reported child disability ($r = -0.43$, $p < 0.01$). These inverse relationships indicate that lower scores on the CSES (i.e., lower self-efficacy) were correlated with higher levels of parental protectiveness, child GI symptom severity, and child disability. Parental protectiveness was positively correlated with child GI symptom severity ($r = 0.25$, $p < 0.01$) and child disability ($r = 0.39$, $p < 0.01$); and child GI symptom severity was positively correlated with child disability ($r = 0.46$; $p < 0.01$).

Table 1. Correlations among study variables and descriptive statistics (*n* = 316).

	Protect (ARCS)	GI Symptoms (CSI-GI)	Disability (FDI)	M (SD)	Scale
CSES [a]	−0.55 **	−0.25 **	−0.43 **	3.30 (0.91)	1–5
ARCS [b]		0.25 **	0.39 **	1.17 (0.65)	0–4
CSI-GI [c]			0.46 **	1.42 (0.68)	0–4
FDI [d]				0.70 (0.73)	0–4

** *p* < 0.01; [a] CSES: Child Self-Efficacy Scale; [b] ARCS: Adult Responses to Children's Symptoms—Protectiveness subscale; [c] CSI: Children's Somatization Inventory—GI subscale; [d] FDI: Functional Disability Inventory. GI: gastrointestinal.

3.2. Mediation Analyses

Table 2 shows the results of the mediation analysis for Model 1 where parent-perceived child self-efficacy was the predictor, parental protectiveness was the mediator, and parent-reported child GI symptom severity was the outcome. Parent-perceived child self-efficacy was inversely associated with both child GI symptom severity (Path c, estimate (standard error—SE) = −0.19 (0.04), *p* < 0.001) and parental protectiveness (Path a, estimate (SE) = −0.39 (0.03), *p* < 0.001). Parental protectiveness was positively associated with child GI symptom severity (Path b, estimate (SE) = 0.18 (0.07), *p* = 0.011). Our mediation hypothesis was supported by a significant indirect effect (Path a × b, estimate (SE) = −0.07 (0.03), 95% CI with 10,000 resamples = −0.13, −0.01). The ratio of the indirect effect to the total effect, or the proportion of the total effects mediated for Model 1 was 37%.

Table 2. Results of mediation analysis for Model 1 (parent-reported child GI symptom severity).

	Estimate (SE)	*p*	95% CI
Path c (effect of predictor on outcome)	−0.19 (0.04)	<0.001	
Path a (effect of predictor on mediator)	−0.39 (0.03)	<0.001	
Path b (effect of mediator on outcome)	0.18 (0.07)	0.011	
Indirect effect: Path a × b	−0.07 (0.03)		−0.13, −0.01
Direct effect: Path c'	−0.12 (0.05)	0.016	
Ratio of indirect effect to total effect		37%	

SE: standard error; CI: confidence interval.

Table 3 shows the results of the mediation analysis for Model 2 where parent-perceived child self-efficacy was the predictor, parental protectiveness was the mediator, and parent-reported child disability was the outcome. This model showed similar results. Parent-perceived child self-efficacy was inversely associated with both child disability (Path c, estimate (SE) = −0.34 (0.04), *p* < 0.001) and parental protectiveness (Path a, estimate (SE) = −0.39 (0.03), *p* < 0.001). Parental protectiveness was positively associated with child disability (Path b, estimate (SE) = 0.24 (0.07), *p* < 0.001). Our mediation hypothesis was also supported here by a significant indirect effect (Path a × b, estimate (SE) = −0.10 (0.03), 95% CI with 10,000 resamples = −0.16, −0.04). The ratio of the indirect effect to the total effect for Model 2 was 28%.

Table 3. Results of mediation analysis for Model 2 (parent-reported child disability).

	Estimate (SE)	*p*	95% CI
Path c (effect of predictor on outcome)	−0.34 (0.04)	<0.001	
Path a (effect of predictor on mediator)	−0.39 (0.03)	<0.001	
Path b (effect of mediator on outcome)	0.24 (0.07)	<0.001	
Indirect effect: Path a × b	−0.10 (0.03)		−0.16, −0.04
Direct effect: Path c'	−0.25 (0.05)	<0.001	
Ratio of indirect effect to total effect		28%	

4. Discussion

The goal of this study was to examine whether parents respond with greater protectiveness if they perceive their child to have lower pain self-efficacy and whether this protectiveness is associated with more child GI symptoms and greater child disability. Results suggest support for this hypothesis. Parents who perceived their child's self-efficacy as low responded more protectively to their child when he/she was in pain and this was associated with higher levels of GI symptoms and disability in their child.

The role of self-efficacy in pediatric pain has been previously described with studies suggesting that lower self-efficacy is associated with more symptoms and greater disability [13,14]. Parent protectiveness has also been positively associated with symptoms and disability [6,25,26]. In the current study we not only replicated these findings, but our analyses further showed that parental perception of child pain self-efficacy may be driving parental protectiveness. Our findings suggest several areas for intervention. For example, cognitive interventions targeting parental perceptions of their child's pain may be effective in reducing child's symptoms and disability. In our own treatment trial, we have shown that reducing parental perception of the threat of child's pain mediated treatment outcomes [27] which lends support for parental intervention. Alternatively, as we do not know if parents wrongly assign low self-efficacy in their children or even if their judgment is correct, improving child self-efficacy may be a helpful target for treatment via self-management, relaxation training, or other methods to reduce the impact of FAPD.

Limitations of this study should be noted. All measures used in this study were parent-report, although developers of the self-efficacy measure used in this study found that parent and child-reports were significantly correlated with each other [13]. Nonetheless, the fact that parents were the only source of data increases the possibility of introducing single source bias, a type of common method variance, into the findings, potentially limiting their validity. Given that this is an inherent limitation of the study methods, it should be kept in mind when interpreting the findings. While evidence for mediation was found, the proportion of total effects accounted for was 28% and 37%, indicating that other factors besides parental protectiveness may play an important role in mediating the relationship between perceived child self-efficacy and outcomes. Further studies using multiple data sources and expanded mediational models are needed to address these limitations. It should also be noted that ninety-five percent of the parents were female, which could limit the generalizability of the findings. Studies including the effect of fathers' cognitions and behaviors are needed. The sample may also be biased by including parents who were willing to participate in a treatment trial for FAPD and therefore may not represent the entire population of FAPD children and their parents. Another study limitation is our cross-sectional design, which makes it difficult to determine cause and effect. We do not know if parental perceptions of child self-efficacy lead to parental protectiveness, if parental protectiveness affects parental perceptions of efficacy, or if there is a bidirectional relationship between the two. In addition, parents who perceive their child as more disabled or symptomatic may also respond more protectively and perceive their child as less effective in self-managing their pain. Longitudinal studies and treatment studies addressing parent cognitions and/or improving child self-efficacy are needed to address these questions of directionality.

5. Conclusions

Parents may respond protectively to their child (e.g., by keeping them home from school when in pain) if they perceive their child to be unable to deal with pain and function normally when in pain, and this is associated with higher child GI symptoms and disability. These findings suggest that directly addressing parent beliefs about their child's ability to manage his/her pain should be included as a component of FAPD, and potentially other child treatment interventions.

Acknowledgments: This study was supported by a grant from the National Institutes of Health (NIH)—National Institute of Child Health & Human Development. Grant #R01HD036069-0981 awarded to Rona L. Levy.

Author Contributions: M.M.D. analyzed the data and wrote the manuscript; M.A.L.v.T. conceptualized the mediation analysis and edited the manuscript; S.L.L. contributed to the statistical analysis, and reviewed and edited the manuscript; T.B.M. and J.M.R. reviewed and edited the manuscript; R.L.L. conceived and designed the intervention study and reviewed and edited the manuscript.

Conflicts of Interest: The authors declare no conflict of interest.

References

1. Korterink, J.J.; Diederen, K.; Benninga, M.A.; Tabbers, M.M. Epidemiology of pediatric functional abdominal pain disorders: A meta-analysis. *PLoS ONE* **2015**, *10*, e0126982. [CrossRef] [PubMed]
2. Hyams, J.S.; Di Lorenzo, C.; Saps, M.; Shulman, R.J.; Staiano, A.; van Tilburg, M. Functional disorders: Children and adolescents. *Gastroenterology* **2016**, *150*, 1456.e1452–1468.e1452. [CrossRef] [PubMed]
3. Starfield, B.; Gross, E.; Wood, M.; Pantell, R.; Allen, C.; Gordon, I.B.; Moffatt, P.; Drachman, R.; Katz, H. Psychosocial and psychosomatic diagnoses in primary care of children. *Pediatrics* **1980**, *66*, 159–167. [PubMed]
4. Rouster, A.S.; Karpinski, A.C.; Silver, D.; Monagas, J.; Hyman, P.E. Functional gastrointestinal disorders dominate pediatric gastroenterology outpatient practice. *J. Pediatr. Gastroenterol. Nutr.* **2015**, *62*, 847–851. [CrossRef] [PubMed]
5. Myer, P.A.; Mannalithara, A.; Singh, G.; Pasricha, P.J.; Ladabaum, U. Clinical and economic burden of emergency department visits due to gastrointestinal diseases in the united states. *Am. J. Gastroenterol.* **2013**, *108*, 1496–1507. [CrossRef] [PubMed]
6. Langer, S.L.; Romano, J.M.; Levy, R.L.; Walker, L.S.; Whitehead, W.E. Catastrophizing and parental response to child symptom complaints. *Child Health Care* **2009**, *38*, 169–184. [CrossRef] [PubMed]
7. Bandura, A. *Social Foundations of Thought and Action: A Social Cognitive Theory*; Prentice-Hall: New Jersey, NJ, USA, 1986.
8. Bandura, A. Human agency in social cognitive theory. *Am. Psychol.* **1989**, *44*, 1175–1184. [CrossRef] [PubMed]
9. Bandura, A. Self-efficacy: Toward a unifying theory of behavioral change. *Psychol. Rev.* **1977**, *84*, 191–215. [CrossRef] [PubMed]
10. Rosenstock, I.M.; Strecher, V.J.; Becker, M.H. Social learning theory and the health belief model. *Health Educ. Q.* **1988**, *15*, 175–183. [CrossRef] [PubMed]
11. Becker, M.H.; Rosenstock, I.M.; Drachman, R.H. Compliance with a medical regimen for asthma: A test of the health belief model. *Public Health Rep.* **1978**, *93*, 268–277. [PubMed]
12. Asghari, A.; Nicholas, M.K. Pain self-efficacy beliefs and pain behaviour. A prospective study. *Pain* **2001**, *94*, 85–100. [CrossRef]
13. Bursch, B.; Tsao, J.C.; Meldrum, M.; Zeltzer, L.K. Preliminary validation of a self-efficacy scale for child functioning despite chronic pain (child and parent versions). *Pain* **2006**, *125*, 35–42. [CrossRef] [PubMed]
14. Kalapurakkel, S.; Carpino, E.A.; Lebel, A.; Simons, L.E. "Pain can't stop me": Examining pain self-efficacy and acceptance as resilience processes among youth with chronic headache. *J. Pediatr. Psychol.* **2015**, *40*, 926–933. [CrossRef] [PubMed]
15. Levy, R.L.; van Tilburg, M.; Langer, S.L.; Romano, J.; Mancl, L.; Whitehead, W.E.; Feld, S.; Walker, L.S. Parent-only intervention reduces symptoms and disability in abdominal pain patients. *J. Pediatr. Gastroenterol. Nutr.* **2015**, *61*, S224. [CrossRef]
16. Drossman, D.A. *Rome III: The Functional Gastrointestinal Disorders*; Degnon Associates: McLean, VA, USA, 2006.
17. Walker, L.S.; Levy, R.L.; Whitehead, W.E. Validation of a measure of protective parent responses to children's pain. *Clin. J. Pain* **2006**, *22*, 712–716. [CrossRef] [PubMed]
18. Van Slyke, D.A.; Walker, L.S. Mothers' responses to children's pain. *Clin. J. Pain* **2006**, *22*, 387–391. [CrossRef] [PubMed]
19. Noel, M.; Palermo, T.M.; Essner, B.; Zhou, C.; Levy, R.L.; Langer, S.L.; Sherman, A.L.; Walker, L.S. A developmental analysis of the factorial validity of the parent-report version of the adult responses to children's symptoms in children versus adolescents with chronic pain or pain-related chronic illness. *J. Pain* **2015**, *16*, 31–41. [CrossRef] [PubMed]
20. Walker, L.S.; Beck, J.E.; Garber, J.; Lambert, W. Children's somatization inventory: Psychometric properties of the revised form (csi-24). *J. Pediatr. Psychol.* **2009**, *34*, 430–440. [CrossRef] [PubMed]

21. Dengler-Crish, C.M.; Horst, S.N.; Walker, L.S. Somatic complaints in childhood functional abdominal pain are associated with functional gastrointestinal disorders in adolescence and adulthood. *J. Pediatr. Gastroenterol. Nutr.* **2011**, *52*, 162–165. [CrossRef] [PubMed]

22. Anderson, J.L.; Acra, S.; Bruehl, S.; Walker, L.S. Relation between clinical symptoms and experimental visceral hypersensitivity in pediatric patients with functional abdominal pain. *J. Pediatr. Gastroenterol. Nutr.* **2008**, *47*, 309–315. [CrossRef] [PubMed]

23. Walker, L.S.; Greene, J.W. The functional disability inventory: Measuring a neglected dimension of child health status. *J. Pediatr. Psychol.* **1991**, *16*, 39–58. [CrossRef] [PubMed]

24. Hayes, A.F. *Introduction to Mediation, Moderation, and Conditional Process Analysis: A Regression-Based Approach*; The Guilford Press: New York, NY, USA, 2013.

25. Levy, R.L.; Whitehead, W.E.; Walker, L.S.; Von Korff, M.; Feld, A.; Garner, M.; Christie, D. Increased somatic complaints and health-care utilization in children: Effects of parent ibs status and parent response to gastrointestinal symptoms. *Am. J. Gastroenterol.* **2004**, *99*, 2442–2451. [CrossRef] [PubMed]

26. Claar, R.L.; Simons, L.E.; Logan, D.E. Parental response to children's pain: The moderating impact of children's emotional distress on symptoms and disability. *Pain* **2008**, *138*, 172–179. [CrossRef] [PubMed]

27. Levy, R.L.; Langer, S.L.; Romano, J.M.; Labus, J.; Walker, L.S.; Murphy, T.B.; Van Tilburg, M.; Feld, L.D.; Christie, D.L.; Whitehead, W.E. Cognitive mediators of treatment outcomes in pediatric functional abdominal pain. *Clin. J. Pain* **2014**, *30*, 1033–1043. [CrossRef] [PubMed]

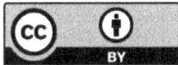

Article

"What Does Weight Have to Do with It?" Parent Perceptions of Weight and Pain in a Pediatric Chronic Pain Population

Keri R. Hainsworth [1,*], Kristen E. Jastrowski Mano [2], Alison M. Stoner [3], Kim Anderson Khan [1,4], Renee J. Ladwig [4], W. Hobart Davies [5], Ellen K. Defenderfer [5] and Steven J. Weisman [1,4]

[1] Department of Anesthesiology, Medical College of Wisconsin, Milwaukee, WI 53226, USA; kanderson@chw.org (K.A.K.); sweisman@chw.org (S.J.W.)

[2] Department of Psychology, University of Cincinnati, Cincinnati, OH 45221, USA; manokn@ucmail.uc.edu

[3] Department of Psychiatry, University of Massachusetts Medical School, Worcester, MA 01655; USA; alison.stoner@umassmemorial.org

[4] Jane B. Pettit Pain and Headache Center, Children's Hospital of Wisconsin, Milwaukee, WI 53226, USA; rladwig@chw.org

[5] Department of Psychology, University of Wisconsin-Milwaukee, Milwaukee, WI 53201, USA; hobart@uwm.edu (W.H.D.); defende2@uwm.edu (E.K.D.)

* Correspondence: khainswo@mcw.edu; Tel.: +1-414-266-6306

Academic Editor: Carl L. von Baeyer
Received: 31 August 2016; Accepted: 7 November 2016; Published: 14 November 2016

Abstract: Tailored pain management strategies are urgently needed for youth with co-occurring chronic pain and obesity; however, prior to developing such strategies, we need to understand parent perspectives on weight in the context of pediatric chronic pain. Participants in this study included 233 parents of patients presenting to a multidisciplinary pediatric chronic pain clinic. Parents completed a brief survey prior to their child's initial appointment; questions addressed parents' perceptions of their child's weight, and their perceptions of multiple aspects of the relationship between their child's weight and chronic pain. The majority (64%) of parents of youth with obesity accurately rated their child's weight; this group of parents was also more concerned ($p < 0.05$) about their child's weight than parents of youth with a healthy weight. However, the majority of parents of youth with obesity did not think their child's weight contributed to his/her pain, or that weight was relevant to their child's pain or pain treatment. Overall, only half of all parents saw discussions of weight, nutrition, and physical activity as important to treating their child's pain. Results support the need for addressing parents' perceptions of their child's weight status, and educating parents about the relationship between excessive weight and chronic pain.

Keywords: chronic pain; obesity; pediatrics; parents; attitudes

1. Introduction

Currently, 33% of youth in the U.S.A. are overweight or obese [1] and there is evidence to suggest that the prevalence of youth with elevated weight may be greater in chronic pain populations than in normative samples [2]. Additionally, there is increasing evidence that obesity exacerbates the impact of chronic pain in children. The first study to provide such evidence found that children and adolescents with co-occurring chronic pain and obesity reported lower health-related quality of life in all domains of functioning (i.e., physical, emotional, social, and school functioning) than youth who are overweight or those with healthy weight [3]. This study also showed that youth with chronic pain and obesity are 2.3 times more likely to report impaired physical functioning than youth with chronic pain alone and more than six times more likely than youth with obesity alone. Wilson and colleagues [2] found that in a sample of youth with chronic pain, body mass index (BMI) predicted functional disability for rigorous activities, based on parent reports. In a study focused on pediatric headache, Hershey et al. [4] found an association between obesity and both headache frequency and disability. This study also showed that for patients with weight concerns, weight loss was associated with reduced headache frequency at three- and six-month follow-up points. Most recently, Stoner et al. [5] found that obesity impedes improvement in functional disability, an important patient-reported outcome [6,7]. Among patients in active treatment for chronic pain, those with a healthy weight showed significant improvement in functional disability over time, in contrast to youth with both morbidities whose level of functional disability remained stagnant [5].

The studies above demonstrate the impact that obesity has on pediatric chronic pain. It is particularly concerning that obesity appears to impede improvement despite multidisciplinary pain treatment. However, to our knowledge, no tailored interventions exist to meet the needs of youth with these dual conditions. Therefore, it is critical that we go beyond the initial call to simply screen for obesity in pediatric chronic pain [3] and begin to develop tailored treatment approaches to meet the needs of this population. If we do *not* address weight in youth suffering from chronic pain in childhood, it is likely that these children may face a lifetime of suffering. In a qualitative study focused on adults with chronic pain and obesity, participants poignantly describe the cycle of pain and disability that ensues from the co-morbid state. In contrast, pediatric chronic pain patients may experience several important benefits if we *do* address their weight in addition to their chronic pain. For example, by increasing physical activity, we may reduce pain through decreased levels of systemic inflammation, elevations of mood, and decreased biomechanical forces on the back and lower extremities [8].

Before such approaches can be developed and implemented, however, we need to know more about factors that may potentially hinder the acceptance of treatment strategies that target both pain and weight. Looking to the pediatric obesity literature, one likely example is parents' perceptions of their child's weight; parents commonly misperceive their child's weight [9–13], which in turn has important clinical implications. Taveras et al. [14] found that parents who misperceived their child's elevated weight were more likely to refuse their child's participation in a weight management program than parents who accurately rated their child's weight. If parents of youth with chronic pain misperceive their child's weight, they may be less likely to adhere to treatment recommendations that involve physical activity or other strategies that might be construed as weight-related recommendations.

This study sought to characterize parents' perceptions of and attitudes around weight in the context of pediatric chronic pain. The primary aims of this study were to determine whether parents of youth presenting to a multidisciplinary pain clinic with co-occurring chronic pain and weight concerns (1) are accurate in their assessment of their child's weight; and (2) saw their child's weight as contributing to his/her pain. We also aimed to (3) assess whether parents of children in all weight groups thought that discussions of weight, nutrition and physical activity might be important to treating chronic pain, particularly among parents of youth with co-morbid weight concerns. Secondary aims were to assess parents' level of concern about their child's weight, as well as factors that may influence adherence to integrated pain and weight interventions.

2. Methods

2.1. Participants

This study was part of a quality improvement (QI) project aimed at developing pain treatment approaches for our patients with co-morbid obesity. The convenience sample included consecutive parents of patients seen in a multidisciplinary pediatric pain clinic, over a designated 4.5 month timeframe.

2.2. Procedures

Upon arrival for their child's initial appointment, parents were asked to complete a brief survey along with other paperwork. The hospital Institutional Review Board approved a retrospective chart review and use of the data for study purposes.

2.3. Measures

2.3.1. Demographic Data

Demographic data were obtained from the electronic medical record (EMR), and included patient age, gender, race, ethnicity, weight, height, BMI and BMI percentile. Height and weight are measured by nurses at the time of the initial appointment, and directly entered into the EMR. Both BMI and BMI percentile are calculated within the EMR by the software program (EPIC), and are based on the Centers for Disease Control and Prevention (CDC) profiles for gender and age adjusted weight scales [15]. The American Academy of Pediatrics [16] criteria were used to categorize patients' weight status: <5th percentile = underweight; ≥5th percentile to <85th percentile = healthy weight; ≥85th percentile to <95th percentile = overweight; ≥95th percentile = obese.

2.3.2. Survey Questions

The survey used in this study was created for the QI project by a panel of experts in pediatric chronic pain. To minimize completion time in the waiting room, the survey was intentionally designed to be brief, consisting of only five items. Survey questions are listed here.

1. Question 1, *"Do you consider your child to be"* was presented with the response options "Overweight," "Underweight," "Just about the right weight," and "Don't know." This question was adopted and modified slightly from a study aimed at examining the accuracy of maternal perceptions of their child's weight status, in a group of Hispanic WIC (a nutritional program for Women, Infants, and Children) participants [10].
2. Question 2, *"On a scale of 1–5, how concerned are you about your child's present weight or body size?"* was adopted verbatim from a study by Campbell et al. [9]. Response options ranged from "Not Concerned" (1) to "Very Concerned" (5). This question was chosen to address the first of three primary aims.
3. Question 3, *"Do you think that your child's weight contributes to your child's pain?"* was created to address the second of three primary aims. Response options were "yes" or "no."
4. Question 4, *"Do you believe that discussions of weight, nutrition and physical activity might be important to treating pain?"* was created to address the third of three primary aims. Response options were "yes" or "no."
5. Item 5, which asked parents to *"Check all that apply"*, was designed to capture factors that may affect adherence to integrated chronic pain and weight interventions. The five response options included (a) "I do not think weight is relevant to his/her pain treatment"; (b) "Weight has been discussed with healthcare providers several times"; (c) "We have tried to address weight in the past without success"; (d) "I have little hope he/she will be able to lose weight"; and (e) "My child's pain prevents him/her from losing weight". Reponses were treated as endorsed or not endorsed. Item b specified "several times," in an attempt to get at more than just a cursory mention of weight by any provider in the past.

2.4. Data Analysis

Descriptive statistics were used to characterize the children of the participants (i.e., the pediatric pain patients) and parental responses to survey questions. Parametric (Student's *t*-tests, and analysis of variance (ANOVA)) statistics were used for continuous variables and non-parametric (chi-square) statistics were used for categorical variables. To determine accuracy of parental estimates of their child's weight, any response (including "I don't know") that did not match the child's measured weight status was categorized as inaccurate.

3. Results

3.1. Patient Population

A total of 239 parents completed surveys. No information is known about parents who did not complete surveys or were missed. Only six of the participants' children were underweight, and therefore these surveys were excluded from analyses, yielding a final sample size of 233 parents. Patients (their children) were primarily adolescent females (64%, mean (M) = 13 ± 3.3 years; 4 to 18 years). Patients were also primarily Caucasian (n = 179, 78%), with 15% (n = 35) African American, and were primarily non-Hispanic (n = 197, 86%). The majority of patients were classified as having a healthy weight (57% of the sample), with 18% classified as overweight, and 25% as obese. The vast majority of the sample (n = 169, 73%) was being treated for a primary pain location of the head, followed equally by back (n = 19, 8%), abdomen (n = 19, 8%), and extremity pain (n = 19, 8%). Demographics are presented in Table 1. No differences across weight groups were found for any of the demographic variables (including pain location; data not shown).

Table 1. Patient demographics. Categorical variables are listed as n (%); continuous variables are listed as mean (standard deviation, SD).

		Total Sample (233)	Healthy Weight (133, 57.1%)	Overweight (42, 18.0%)	Obese (58, 24.9%)
Gender [1]	Male	83 (35.6)	46 (34.6)	16 (38.1)	21 (36.2)
	Female	149 (63.9)	87 (65.4)	26 (61.9)	36 (62.1)
Age		13.00 (3.30)	12.57 (3.35)	13.57 (2.81)	13.59 (3.38)
Race [1]	African American	35 (15.6)	23 (18.0)	4 (9.8)	8 (14.5)
	Caucasian	174 (77.7)	98 (76.6)	35 (85.4)	41 (74.5)
	Multi-racial	6 (2.7)	1 (0.8)	1 (2.4)	4 (7.3)
	Other	9 (4.0)	6 (4.7)	1 (2.4)	2 (3.6)
Ethnicity [1]	Hispanic	33 (14.3)	18 (13.7)	3 (7.1)	12 (21.1)
	Non-Hispanic	197 (85.7)	113 (86.3)	39 (92.9)	45 (78.9)

[1] Missing cases = one gender, nine race, three ethnicity; no differences across weight groups for any variable (all p > 0.05).

3.2. Parents' Assessment of Their Child's Weight Status

The data from question 1, addressing the accuracy of parental perceptions of their child's weight, are shown in Table 2. As indicated, any response (including "I don't know") that did not match the child's measured weight status was categorized as inaccurate. Results suggest that the majority (64%) of parents whose children are obese accurately rate their child's weight status, with about one-quarter (27%) rating the child's weight as "just about the right weight". This pattern reflects greater accuracy than reports by parents from other populations [10,11]. In contrast, the majority (90.5%) of parents whose children are overweight misperceive their child's weight status, which is very similar to reports of parents in the pediatric obesity literature [10].

3.3. Parental Concern about Their Child's Present Weight or Body Size

Parents of obese chronic pain patients were significantly (p < 0.001) more concerned (M = 2.7 ± 1.4) about their child's weight than parents of youth with overweight status (M = 1.4 ± 0.8) or parents of youth with healthy weight (M = 1.4 ± 0.9). However, the average rating from parents of youth with obesity showed only moderate concern, and was only slightly higher than the average rating from the latter two subgroups. Further examination of responses by parents of obese youth shows that while approximately one-third (33%, n = 18/55) indicated that they were very concerned (endorsement of response options 4 or 5) about their child's weight, the majority, about one half (47%, $n = 26/55$), were not concerned (endorsement of response options 1 or 2). Using the same question, Campbell reported that the majority of parents whose overweight and obese children (3 to 17 years old) were referred to a multidisciplinary weight management clinic were very concerned about their child's weight, with 77% rating their concern as a "5" (very concerned). In the current sample, only 12.7% ($n = 5$) of the parents with obese children rated their concern as a "5". A single-sample t-test using Campbell's data [9] indicates that parents of youth with both chronic pain and obesity ($M = 2.7 \pm 1.4$) are less concerned ($p < 0.05$) about their child's weight than parents whose children have obesity alone ($M = 4.7 \pm 0.7$).

Table 2. Parental responses to question 1 shown in relation to the patient's measured weight status [10].

Parent Perceptions [1]	Measured Weight Status			
	Healthy Weight	Overweight	Obese	Total
Overweight	1 (0.8)	**4 (9.5)**	**36 (64.3)**	41 (18.0)
Underweight	11 (8.5)	1 (2.4)	0 (0)	12 (5.3)
Just about the right weight	**117 (90)**	35 (83.3)	15 (26.8)	167 (73.2)
Don't know	1 (0.8)	2 (4.8)	5 (8.9)	8 (3.5)

[1] $n = 228$ (five missing cases). Boldface values indicate accuracy in parental perceptions of their child's weight.

3.4. Parental Perception of a Weight-Pain Association

In response to question 3 (data for questions 3 and 4 are shown in Table 3), asking whether their child's weight contributed to their child's pain, the vast majority of the whole sample responded "no". However, significant ($p < 0.001$) weight-based differences were found in the responses to this question. All (100%) parents of overweight children and 76% (40/53) of parents with obese children, thought that their child's weight did not contribute to the child's pain. In fact, only 24.5% of the parents with obese children responded "yes" to this question. To examine these responses more closely, we conducted a second chi-square analysis to determine if parents' responses to this question were related to the accuracy of the estimate of their child's weight. The analysis showed that parents who accurately rated their obese child as overweight were more likely to respond "yes" to this question ($\chi^2 = 16.88$ (2), $p < 0.001$; *Standardized Residual [Std. Resid]* 2.9). This subset was approximately one-third of the parents who accurately rated their obese child's weight ($n = 12$).

Table 3. Parental responses to questions 3 and 4 shown in relation to the patient's measured weight status. Data reflect n (%) of "no" responses.

Survey Question	Total Sample	Healthy Weight	Overweight	Obese	*p*-Value
Q3. Do you think that your child's weight contributes to your child's pain?	196 (89.1)	115 (91.3)	41 (100) [1]	40 (75.5) [2]	<0.001
Q4. Do you believe that discussions of weight, nutrition and physical activity might be important to treating pain? [3]	116 (55.5)	73 (60.3)	19 (50.0)	24 (48.0)	>0.05

[1] Parents of overweight youth were under-represented in the group responding yes to this question (*Std. Resid.* -2.1); [2] Parents of obese youth were over-represented in the group responding yes to this question (*Std. Resid.* 3.0); [3] Four parents who wrote in "maybe" were excluded from this analysis.

3.5. Parental Responses to the Question "Do You Believe That Discussions of Weight, Nutrition and Physical Activity Might Be Important to Treating Pain?"

Just over half (56%) of the entire sample (i.e., parents of youth in all weight categories) endorsed "no" in response to question 4. In fact, there were no weight group differences in response to this question ($p > 0.05$), with approximately half of the parents in each weight group indicating that these discussions are not important to treating pain. Four parents wrote in "maybe" in response to this question (responses not included in analysis). Two of the children represented by these latter responses were obese, one was overweight, and one was a healthy weight.

3.6. Parents' Endorsement of Factors That May Act as Barriers to Integrated Chronic Pain and Weight Interventions

3.6.1. I Do Not Think Weight Is Relevant to His/Her Pain or Pain Treatment.

The majority of the sample (83%) endorsed this item, indicating their perception that weight is not relevant to their child's pain treatment (data for question 5a–e are shown in Table 4). Consistent with this pattern of results, approximately 88% of parents of overweight youth and 68% of parents of obese youth endorsed this item. Parents of obese youth were over-represented in the unendorsed group ($p < 0.001$; *Std. Resid.* 2.7), suggesting that a small subset of parents with obese children may think that weight is relevant to their child's pain.

Table 4. Parental responses to question 5a–e shown in relation to the patient's measured weight status. Data reflect *n* (%) of parents who endorsed each option.

Survey Question	Total Sample	Healthy Weight	Overweight	Obese	*p*-Value
Q5a. I do not think weight is relevant to his/her pain or pain treatment	189 (82.9)	115 (87.8)	36 (87.8)	38 (67.9) [1]	<0.001
Q5b. Weight has been discussed with healthcare providers several times	29 (12.7)	14 (10.7)	3 (7.3)	12 (21.4)	>0.05
Q5c. We have tried to address weight in the past without success	14 (6.1)	4 (3.1)	1 (2.4)	9 (16.1) [2]	<0.01
Q5d. I have little hope he/she will be able to lose weight	4 (1.8)	1 (0.8)	0 (0)	3 (5.4)	>0.05
Q5e. Child's pain prevents him/her from losing weight	11 (4.8)	2 (1.5)	0 (0)	9 (16.1) [3]	<0.001

[1] Parents of obese youth were over-represented in the unendorsed group (*Std. Resid.* 2.7); [2] Parents of obese youth were over-represented in the endorsed group (*Std. Resid.* 3.0); [3] Parent of obese youth were over-represented in the endorsed group (*Std. Resid.* 3.8).

3.6.2. Weight Has Been Discussed with Healthcare Providers Several Times

Across the entire sample, only 13% of parents endorsed the item "weight has been discussed with healthcare providers several times". Though plausible that parents of obese youth would endorse this option more frequently than parents of overweight or healthy-weight youth, this was not the case ($p > 0.05$). Of parents with obese children, only 21% indicated that weight had been discussed several times with healthcare providers.

3.6.3. We Have Tried to Address Weight in the Past without Success

Across the sample, only 6% of parents indicated that they had tried to address their child's weight without success. The weight-based analysis showed that significantly more parents of obese youth endorsed previous, unsuccessful attempts to address weight ($p < 0.01$); however, this only represented 16% (9/56) of the obese subgroup.

3.6.4. I Have Little Hope He/She Will Be Able to Lose Weight

No weight group differences were found for this item ($p > 0.05$), as only a few parents endorsed it: one parent of a child with a healthy weight (0.8%), and three parents of children with obesity (5.4%) indicated that they have little hope that their child will be able to lose weight.

3.6.5. My Child's Pain Prevents Him/Her from Losing Weight

Across the entire sample, only 5% of parents endorsed this item. Despite the small number overall, the analysis of weight-based differences showed that significantly more ($p < 0.001$) parents of obese youth (16%) endorsed this item compared to parents of either overweight or healthy-weight youth.

4. Discussion

The goal of this study was to better understand parents' attitudes and perceptions about weight in the context of pediatric chronic pain. The results showed that among parents whose children have both chronic pain and obesity, more than half accurately rate their child's weight status. However, as a group, the majority were not concerned about their child's weight, did not see a relationship between their child's pain and weight, did not see weight as relevant to their child's pain, and did not see discussions of weight, nutrition and physical activity as important to treating pain. In short, for most parents whose children have co-occurring chronic pain and obesity, there is little foundation upon which to build a case to treat both weight and pain simultaneously.

We hypothesized that having a child with a medical condition (i.e., chronic pain) might improve the accuracy of parents' perceptions of their child's weight. It is common for youth with chronic pain to be seen by multiple practitioners prior to being seen in a pain clinic [17]. Therefore, it is plausible that having repeated weight/height measurements increases awareness of their child's weight status, and in turn, the accuracy of their estimates. The fact that 64% of parents of obese youth accurately estimated their child's weight status, a rate that is higher than reports by parents of youth with obesity alone, provides support for this hypothesis. Nonetheless, it is concerning that 36% of parents of obese children and 91% of parents of overweight children inaccurately estimated their child's weight status. Taveras et al. [14] found that a parent's misperception of their child's weight status was associated with not allowing their child to participate in a weight management program. Given that almost half of the children represented in this sample were overweight/obese, it is particularly concerning that collectively, 59% of their parents inaccurately rated their weight status. Furthermore, we found that when parents of chronic pain patients with obesity accurately estimated their child's weight status, they were also more likely to say that their child's weight contributes to the child's pain. Although speculative, if the results of Taveras et al. translate to the pediatric pain population, patients who would benefit from tailored interventions could miss out on attempts to treat weight in the context of pediatric pain, and/or may be less likely to adhere to treatment recommendations that involve physical activity or what might be perceived as weight-related recommendations. Based on the influential role of parents' attitudes and behaviors on their child's own health behaviors, Duncan [12] has called for interventions to correct parents' misperceptions of their child's weight. This type of parent education could certainly be part of tailored interventions for chronic pain and weight, and could be as simple as pain practitioners pointing out that the child is overweight/obese and providing some examples of the ways in which weight and pain are related. Based on the fact that nearly all parents of youth with overweight status inaccurately rated their child's weight, interventions must include parents of children with overweight, as well as those whose children have obesity.

Other results from this study suggest that parents lack awareness of the relationship between weight and chronic pain. In their review of the literature on pain and obesity, Narouze and Souzdalnitski [18] indicate that the relationship between obesity and chronic pain has been a focus of attention since the late 1990s, and that the evidence points to a strong association between these chronic conditions. The evidence provided in their review of high-quality studies demonstrates a relationship between obesity and pain in weight-bearing joints, but also between obesity and headache/migraine pain, upper extremity pain, chronic widespread pain and fibromyalgia, abdominal/pelvic pain and chronic neuropathic pain. Despite this evidence, as well as a worldwide focus on obesity in adults and children, our data suggests that parents of both overweight and obese children are not aware that these conditions are related. Parents of overweight and obese children did not think that their child's weight contributes to their child's pain, nor did they think that weight was relevant to the child's pain treatment or that discussions of weight, nutrition and physical activity might be important in treating pain. Several factors may shed light on these results. First, these results may be explained in part by the fact that only 7% of parents with overweight children and 21% of parents with obese children reported discussing weight with healthcare providers. This may suggest that providers lack an awareness of the relationship between obesity and chronic pain, and/or that they lack training in counseling patients with both conditions. Patients may have had up to 15 office visits for their chronic pain in the year prior to being seen in a pain center [17]; therefore, it is surprising that so few had been discussing weight concerns with providers. To the degree that providers are not talking to patients and their families about these concerns, we can understand why parents may not be aware of the relationship. It is noteworthy that multidisciplinary chronic pain management programs commonly include approaches to increase activity [19]. Additionally, it is not uncommon for weight gain to follow injury and pain in childhood [20], and some pain medications (e.g., pregabalin and gabapentin) are associated with weight gain [18]. Therefore, educating parents about the importance of weight, nutrition and physical activity is important, regardless of the weight status of the patient at the time of intake. Additionally, these results may be explained in part by the type and location of patient pain complaints. It is important to note that almost 73% of the children represented in this study reported a primary pain location of the head. While it may/may not be more intuitive for parents to be aware of a link between obesity and, for example, lower back pain, it would be less intuitive to be aware of a link between obesity and chronic headache or migraine pain. Studies involving adults (e.g., [21,22]) and children [4] have provided strong evidence of a link between these two conditions, which underscores the necessity for further parent education.

This study also aimed to better understand factors that may act as barriers to the acceptance of future tailored interventions for children with co-occurring chronic pain and weight concerns. Overall, very few parents of overweight or obese patients indicated that they had previous unsuccessful attempts to lose weight, had little hope that their child would lose weight, or that their child's weight prevented him/her from losing weight. This pattern of responses is consistent with a lack of awareness of a chronic pain/obesity relationship, and suggests that these may not actually be common barriers affecting the acceptance of integrated chronic pain and weight interventions in this population. However, it is plausible that attempts to increase awareness of the child's overweight/obesity status may alter parents' responses to these questions, and/or may increase worry over their child's weight, in turn affecting adherence to treatment recommendations and/or readiness to change. If parents of youth with chronic pain do not expect their child's pain provider to address their child's weight concerns, what seemed like a simple matter of educating parents to raise awareness may escalate into a need for additional treatment components to assuage worry. In this regard, the sensitivity of the provider's approach may be particularly important in tailored interventions. Furthermore, it is well known that having a child with a chronic pain condition is stressful, and is associated with reduced parental health-related quality of life [23] and numerous direct and indirect burdens, such as high financial costs, time spent in appointments and missed time at work [24,25]. It is plausible that parents are compartmentalizing their child's chronic pain and weight conditions, and therefore pointing out that they should be concerned about their child's weight in addition to his/her chronic pain might increase worry, and in turn decrease acceptance and adherence to integrated weight and chronic pain interventions. If this is the case, pain providers can play a critical role by helping to shift parents' perspective from seeing chronic pain and obesity as two separate issues into understanding how pain and weight are inherently intertwined.

Based on the current and previous [2,3,5] findings, it is critical that we go beyond the initial call to simply screen for obesity in pediatric chronic pain [3], and begin to develop tailored treatment approaches to meet the needs of this population. *Not addressing* [26] weight in children with chronic pain may have devastating lifetime consequences, while *addressing* [8] weight in this population has the potential to reduce pain and improve functioning. In fact, Narouze and Souzdalnitski [18,27] suggest that the infrastructure to treat both chronic pain and obesity already exists in pain medicine, including medications, physical and psychological rehabilitation, and interventional management. Although these authors provide potentially effective options for the co-management of both conditions, as well as nuances that require consideration for each individual condition, the majority of the research upon which these recommendations have been based has involved adults with co-occurring chronic pain and obesity. These recommendations should be empirically evaluated in a pediatric population. However, we do agree that "further research should focus on comparing existing, and developing new, evidence-based strategies for the treatment of these complex patients, and exploring the advantages of simultaneously managing obesity and chronic pain" [27] (p. 219).

There are several limitations to this study. Similar to the limitations outlined by Connelly et al. [28], parents in the current study completed the surveys in a naturalistic setting, which may have affected data completion and the response rate, and the question set was minimized in order to limit interruption to the clinical flow. While this method allows for broad characterizations, it precludes the depth of inquiry required to fully understand parent perceptions and attitudes. Questions 2 and 3 were taken from studies for which no psychometric data are available. Related to this limitation, it is possible that the pattern of responses was affected by the forced choice response options and/or the phrasing of the questions. For example, responses to questions 3 and 4 may have been affected by the yes/no response choices. Additionally, responses to the question regarding discussions of weight, pain, and physical activity may have been different if the three options had been presented in separate questions. While this is improbable, based on the overall pattern of responses, without follow-up questions, it is not possible to determine whether responses would have been different. In addition, the sample was comprised of parents of primarily adolescent, Caucasian female patients. While this is common for most pediatric chronic pain samples [19], the demographic make-up limits the generalizability of the findings. Finally, it is clear that acceptance and adherence to future tailored interventions will be affected by a number of factors, including individual and contextual factors (see Simons et al. [19]). Among such factors are the patient's own perceptions and attitudes about weight in the context of chronic pain. Future studies should not only examine parental attitudes in greater depth, but should also examine patient attitudes. Such studies should examine if and to what extent attitudes and perceptions interact with other factors to affect parent and patient acceptance of chronic pain interventions that also target weight.

Overall, the results of this study suggest that two salient factors characterize parental perceptions and attitudes about weight in the context of pediatric chronic pain. First, accurate estimates of weight status do not translate into an appreciation of the complex role that weight may play in an overweight or obese child's chronic pain condition. Second, parents of children with chronic pain and overweight/obesity did not report expected barriers to acceptance of, or adherence to, tailored interventions. Specifically, most did not endorse failed attempts to reduce their child's weight, a sense of hopelessness about their child losing weight, or the belief that their child's pain prevents him/her from losing weight. Based on our findings, we offer two primary recommendations prior to implementing tailored interventions in the context of pediatric chronic pain and obesity: (1) pain providers should address parental misperceptions of their child's weight; and (2) the integration of weight management into chronic pain interventions should begin with educating parents about the relationships between weight and pain.

Acknowledgments: The authors thank Patricia Madrid, Karley Wentz, and Ratka Galijot for their help with data entry. We thank Laura Pettineo for her helpful review and comments on earlier drafts of this manuscript.

Author Contributions: K.R.H., K.A.K., W.H.D., R.J.L. and S.J.W. conceived and designed the study; K.R.H. and E.K.D. analyzed the data; K.R.H. wrote the manuscript; K.J.M., A.M.S., K.A.K., W.H.D., R.J.L, E.K.D. and S.J.W. reviewed and make significant contributions to the manuscript.

Conflicts of Interest: The authors declare no conflict of interest.

References

1. Ogden, C.L.; Carroll, M.D.; Lawman, H.G.; Fryar, C.D.; Kruszon-Moran, D.; Kit, B.K.; Flegal, K.M. Trends in Obesity Prevalence among Children and Adolescents in the United States, 1988–1994 through 2013–2014. *JAMA* **2016**, *315*, 2292–2299. [CrossRef] [PubMed]
2. Wilson, A.C.; Samuelson, B.; Palermo, T.M. Obesity in children and adolescents with chronic pain: Associations with pain and activity limitations. *Clin. J. Pain* **2010**, *26*, 705–711. [CrossRef] [PubMed]
3. Hainsworth, K.R.; Davies, W.H.; Khan, K.A.; Weisman, S.J. Co-occurring Chronic Pain and Obesity in Children and Adolescents: The Impact on Health-related Quality of Life. *Clin. J. Pain* **2009**, *25*, 715–721. [CrossRef] [PubMed]
4. Hershey, A.D.; Powers, S.W.; Nelson, T.D.; Kabbouche, M.A.; Winner, P.; Yonker, M.; Linder, S.L.; Bicknese, A.; Sowel, M.K.; McClintock, W. American Headache Society Pediatric Adolescent Section Obesity in the Pediatric Headache Population: A Multicenter Study. *Headache* **2009**, *49*, 170–177. [CrossRef] [PubMed]
5. Stoner, A.M.; Jastrowski Mano, K.; Weisman, S.J.; Hainsworth, K.R. Impact of obesity on improvements in functional disability over time in a pediatric chronic pain population. Under review.
6. Palermo, T.M.; Law, E.F.; Zhou, C.; Holley, A.L.; Logan, D.; Tai, G. Trajectories of Change During a Randomized Controlled Trial of Internet-delivered Psychological Treatment for Adolescent Chronic Pain: How does Change in Pain and Function Relate? *Pain* **2015**, *156*, 626–634. [CrossRef] [PubMed]
7. Lynch-Jordan, A.M.; Sil, S.; Peugh, J.; Cunningham, N.; Kashikar-Zuck, S.; Goldschneider, K.R. Differential changes in functional disability and pain intensity over the course of psychological treatment for children with chronic pain. *Pain* **2014**, *155*, 1955–1961. [CrossRef] [PubMed]
8. Paley, C.; Johnson, M.I. Chronic pain in the obese population: Is exercise the key? *Pain Manag.* **2016**, *6*, 121–123. [CrossRef] [PubMed]
9. Campbell, M.; Benton, J.M.; Werk, L.N. Parent perceptions to promote a healthier lifestyle for their obese child. *Soc. Work Health Care* **2011**, *50*, 787–800. [CrossRef] [PubMed]
10. Chaparro, M.P.; Langellier, B.A.; Kim, L.P.; Whaley, S.E. Predictors of accurate maternal perception of their preschool child's weight status among Hispanic WIC participants. *Obesity (Silver Spring)* **2011**, *19*, 2026–2030. [CrossRef] [PubMed]
11. Bradford, K.; Kihlstrom, M.; Pointer, I.; Skinner, A.C.; Slivka, P.; Perrin, E.M. Parental attitudes toward obesity and overweight screening and communication for hospitalized children. *Hosp. Pediatr.* **2012**, *2*, 126–132. [CrossRef] [PubMed]
12. Duncan, D.T. Parental misperception of their child's weight status: Clinical implications for obesity prevention and control. *Obesity (Silver Spring)* **2011**, *19*, 2293. [CrossRef] [PubMed]
13. Lundahl, A.; Kidwell, K.M.; Nelson, T.D. Parental Underestimates of Child Weight: A Meta-analysis. *Pediatrics* **2014**, *133*, e689–e703. [CrossRef] [PubMed]
14. Taveras, E.M.; Hohman, K.H.; Price, S.N.; Rifas-Shiman, S.L.; Mitchell, K.; Gortmaker, S.L.; Gillman, M.W. Correlates of participation in a pediatric primary care-based obesity prevention intervention. *Obesity (Silver Spring)* **2011**, *19*, 449–452. [CrossRef] [PubMed]
15. Kuczmarski, R.J.; Ogden, C.L.; Grummer-Strawn, L.M.; Flegal, K.M.; Guo, S.S.; Wei, R.; Mei, Z.; Curtin, L.R.; Roche, A.F.; Johnson, C.L. CDC growth charts: United States. *Adv. data.* **2000**, *314*, 1–27.
16. Krebs, N.F.; Himes, J.H.; Jacobson, D.; Nicklas, T.A.; Guilday, P.; Styne, D. Assessment of child and adolescent overweight and obesity. *Pediatrics* **2007**, *120* (Suppl. 4), S193–S228. [CrossRef] [PubMed]
17. Guite, J.W.; Kim, S.; Chen, C.P.; Sherker, J.L.; Sherry, D.D.; Rose, J.B.; Hwang, W.T. Treatment expectations among adolescents with chronic musculoskeletal pain and their parents before an initial pain clinic evaluation. *Clin. J. Pain* **2014**, *30*, 17–26. [CrossRef] [PubMed]
18. Narouze, S.; Souzdalnitski, D. Obesity and chronic pain: Systematic review of prevalence and implications for pain practice. *Reg. Anesth. Pain Med.* **2015**, *40*, 91–111. [CrossRef] [PubMed]
19. Simons, L.E.; Logan, D.E.; Chastain, L.; Cerullo, M. Engagement in Multidisciplinary Interventions for Pediatric Chronic Pain: Parental Expectations, Barriers, and Child Outcomes. *Clin. J. Pain* **2010**, *26*, 291–299. [CrossRef] [PubMed]
20. Myer, G.D.; Faigenbaum, A.D.; Foss, K.B.; Xu, Y.; Khoury, J.; Dolan, L.M.; McCambridge, T.M.; Hewett, T.E. Injury initiates unfavourable weight gain and obesity markers in youth. *Br. J. Sports Med.* **2014**, *48*, 1477–1481. [CrossRef] [PubMed]

21. Peterlin, B.L.; Rapoport, A.M.; Kurth, T. Migraine and Obesity: Epidemiology, Mechanisms, and Implications. *Headache* **2010**, *50*, 631–648. [CrossRef] [PubMed]

22. Recober, A.; Peterlin, B.L. Migraine and obesity: moving beyond BMI. *Future Neurol.* **2014**, *9*, 37–40. [CrossRef] [PubMed]

23. Jastrowski Mano, K.E.; Khan, K.A.; Ladwig, R.J.; Weisman, S.J. The Impact of Pediatric Chronic Pain on Parents' Health-Related Quality of Life and Family Functioning: Reliability and Validity of the PedsQL 4.0 Family Impact Module. *J. Pediatr. Psychol.* **2011**, *36*, 517–527. [CrossRef] [PubMed]

24. Ho, I.K.; Goldschneider, K.R.; Kashikar-Zuck, S. Healthcare utilization and indirect burden among families of pediatric patiens with chronic pain. *J. Musculoskelet. Pain* **2008**, *16*, 155–164. [CrossRef]

25. Sleed, M.; Eccleston, C.; Beecham, J.; Knapp, M.; Jordan, A. The economic impact of chronic pain in adolescence: Methodological considerations and a preliminary costs-of-illness study. *Pain* **2005**, *119*, 183–190. [CrossRef] [PubMed]

26. Amy Janke, E.; Kozak, A.T. "The More Pain I Have, the More I Want to Eat": Obesity in the Context of Chronic Pain. *Obesity (Silver Spring)* **2012**, *20*, 2027–2034. [CrossRef] [PubMed]

27. Narouze, S.; Souzdalnitski, D. Obesity and chronic pain: opportunities for better patient care. *Pain Manag.* **2015**, *5*, 217–219. [CrossRef] [PubMed]

28. Connelly, M.; Wallace, D.P.; Williams, K.; Parker, J.; Schurman, J.V. Parent Attitudes toward Pain Management for Childhood Immunizations. *Clin. J. Pain* **2016**, *32*, 654–658. [CrossRef] [PubMed]

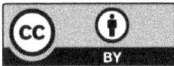

children

MDPI

Article

Parent and Child Report of Pain and Fatigue in JIA: Does Disagreement between Parent and Child Predict Functional Outcomes?

Amy C. Gaultney [1],*, Maggie H. Bromberg [2], Mark Connelly [3], Tracy Spears [4] and Laura E. Schanberg [5]

[1]   Duke Children's Hospital and Health Center, 2301 Erwin Road, Durham, NC 27710, USA
[2]   Seattle Children's Research Institute, Center for Child Health, Behavior, and Development, M/S CW8-6, Seattle, WA 98145, USA; bromberg.maggie@gmail.com
[3]   Children's Mercy Hospital Kansas City, 2401 Gillham Road, Kansas City, MO 64108, USA; mconnelly1@cmh.edu
[4]   Duke Clinical Research Institute, 2400 Pratt Street, Durham, NC 27705, USA; tracy.g.spears@duke.edu
[5]   Duke Children's Hospital and Health Center, 2301 Erwin Road, Durham, NC 27710, USA; laura.schanberg@dm.duke.edu
*   Correspondence: amy.gaultney@duke.edu; Tel.: +619-247-4059

Academic Editor: Lynn S. Walker
Received: 15 September 2016; Accepted: 23 January 2017; Published: 30 January 2017

Abstract: While previous research in juvenile idiopathic arthritis (JIA) has identified discrepancy between parent and child perception of disease-related symptoms such as pain, the significance and impact of this disagreement has not been characterized. We examined the extent to which parent-child discordance in JIA symptom ratings are associated with child functional outcomes. Linear regression and mixed effects models were used to test the effects of discrepancy in pain and fatigue ratings on functional outcomes in 65 dyads, consisting of youth with JIA and one parent. Results suggested that children reported increased activity limitations and negative mood when parent and child pain ratings were discrepant, with parent rated child pain much lower. Greater discrepancy in fatigue ratings was also associated with more negative mood, whereas children whose parent rated child fatigue as moderately lower than the child experienced decreased activity limitations relative to dyads who agreed closely on fatigue level. Implications of these results for the quality of life and treatment of children with JIA are discussed.

Keywords: pain; JIA; activity limitation

1. Introduction

Juvenile idiopathic arthritis (JIA) is a common chronic childhood illness often characterized by episodes of musculoskeletal pain and fatigue, which may contribute to problems with social and physical functioning [1,2]. Parents play an important role in the experience and treatment of pain and other symptoms in youth with chronic health issues [3]. Previous work has focused on the agreement between physicians and parents on the child's global disease severity [4]; however, there has been limited research on whether discrepancies in ratings of pain and fatigue between parents and children with JIA influence social and physical activity participation and mood. In one study of children with JIA, Garcia-Munitis et al. demonstrated moderate to poor agreement on pain intensity ratings between parents and children, but did not identify predictors or outcomes of the reported discrepancy [5]. A longitudinal study by Palermo et al. examining parent-child discrepancy in pain reporting found that parents and children with JIA often disagreed on pain and functional disability ratings: the authors suggested a link between increased disagreement on pain ratings and increased child depression, but did not assess fatigue [6]. Their prior work is also limited in that it relied on one-time assessments or intermittent clinic based assessments, both subject to recall bias. Given the daily fluctuations in pain and fatigue typical of JIA, discrepancies in parent-child reports may be stable or dynamic over time. Intensive repeated measurement is ideal for assessing dynamic variables and characterizing reporting patterns [7]. This study employs an ecological data-gathering model to capture day-to-day variability in pain and fatigue reporting and interrogates whether the parent-child discrepancies themselves are associated with outcomes of interest.

The current study investigated discrepancies between parent and child reports of common JIA symptoms (pain and fatigue), expanding on the work of Garcia-Munitis et al. and Palermo et al. in describing discrepancies between parent report of child pain and fatigue and child self-reported fatigue in the setting of a daily electronic diary study. We also examined whether the direction of discrepancy affected the key outcomes of child negative mood and activity limitations. We expected to find that children whose parents over reported child pain and fatigue intensity would have poorer outcomes. This hypothesis is consistent with published literature suggesting that children whose parents use protective strategies, which might result in over reporting pain relative to the child, experience greater functional disability and negative mood [8–10].

2. Methods

The institutional review board at the study site approved study procedures (IRB Study ID: Pro00007325). Full study procedures were included in past publications using the larger dataset, which described child-reported daily symptom ratings and child sleep [11–13]. A pilot study performed with a smaller sample of patients examined parent responses to child pain [14]. The current study uniquely focused on the discordance between parent and child reports of pain and fatigue, not previously examined in this dataset. As part of the larger study, 74 dyads of children and their caregivers where initially recruited from the outpatient rheumatology clinic of an academic pediatric center. As the caregivers were predominantly biological mothers and fathers, with few other types of caregivers (stepparents, unspecified), we refer to the caregivers as "parents" for the remainder of the article. All children had a diagnosis of polyarticular JIA. Children were ineligible to participate if they had a current psychiatric diagnosis (specifically, mood disorders, fibromyalgia and pervasive developmental delay). The excluded disorders are known to affect pain and functioning and could confound experimental results. Children were also excluded if they were not attending school since school attendance was an outcome measure in the original study, physically incapable of completing the diary entries, non-English speaking, or if either they or the parent were illiterate. The sample analyzed for the current study includes 65 of the dyads; 9 dyads failed to complete the larger study or were missing data required for this analysis [15]. Of the included 65 dyads, 2537 fatigue reports (60.3% of all fatigue score reports) had both a parent and a child pain score, and 2411 pain reports had both a child and a parent pain score (57.3% of all pain score reports).

The dyads completed a battery of baseline questionnaires, including demographics reported by the parent. Each parent and child was provided with a T-Mobile Dash smartphone (T-Mobile, Bonn, Germany) and a study-specific instruction manual. Research staff trained each parent and child in use of the device. Each parent and child were instructed to complete thrice daily ratings of pain, fatigue, mood, and activity limitations at predetermined times selected by the family and programmed by the research staff. Diary data was collected for a total of 28 days.

2.1. Electronic Diary Variables

2.1.1. Pain Intensity

Children and parents rated pain intensity three times per day using a visual analogue scale (VAS) ranging from 0 to 100 mm based on a validated pain assessment for children [15]. Figure 1 shows the pain intensity VAS used.

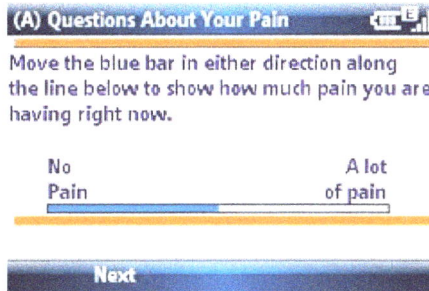

Figure 1. Pain Intensity Screen.

2.1.2. Fatigue Intensity

Children and parents were asked to rate the intensity of fatigue three times a day using a validated visual analogue scale (VAS) ranging from 0 to 100 mm [16].

2.1.3. Activity Limitations

Items from the Activity Scale for Kids and the Child Activity Limitations Questionnaire were combined to assess physical, academic and social limitations in study participants. Children were asked to rate on a 4-point scale how difficult it was to complete each of eight different activities due to pain [17,18]. The list of activities differed depending on time of day. For example, the question "How difficult was it to put your clothes on this morning?" (See Figure 2) was asked only during the morning assessment. Other topics addressed in this scale included questions about difficulties with bathing, walking up stairs and staying seated in school. A total functional limitations score was calculated for each e-diary report by averaging the child's responses.

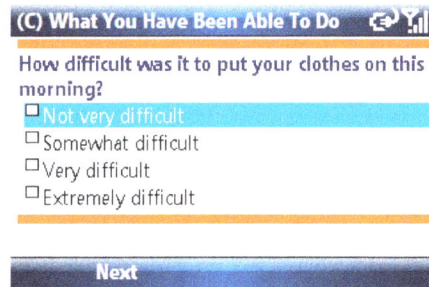

Figure 2. Activity Limitations Screen.

2.1.4. Negative Mood

Child self-reported negative mood was measured by 5 items taken from the Positive and Negative Affect Scale for children (PANAS-C), which was initially validated in a general population of school-aged children [19]. Responses to the negative affect items were averaged to provide a mean negative mood score on each e-diary report. Research in adults and the school-aged population has demonstrated that negative affect scores are significantly correlated with symptoms of both anxiety and depression [19,20]. The initial scale validators argue that the negative mood score is best seen as a measure of psychological distress [20].

2.2. Data Analysis Plan

Statistical analyses were performed using version 9.4 of Statistical Analysis Software (SAS) (Cary, NC, USA). Descriptive statistics (means, standard deviations, frequencies) were used to summarize demographics and primary study variables, as applicable. To address our primary aim, mixed effect models were constructed to evaluate the extent to which parent-child discordance in symptom ratings (pain and fatigue) were associated with the two outcomes of interest (activity limitations and mean negative mood score). To derive the predictor variable for these analyses, we first calculated simple difference scores (parent minus child report) on ratings of pain and fatigue. The resulting discrepancy scores then were classified into five groups for analyses, as follows: −100 to −51 mm (high discrepancy, parent < child), −51 to −11 mm (moderate discrepancy, parent < child), −10 to 9 mm (low discrepancy), 10–49 mm (moderate discrepancy, parent > child), and 50–100 mm (high discrepancy, parent > child). The decision to group the scores was made to facilitate data interpretation and presentation as well as to clearly delineate whether the extent and direction of disagreement were correlated with functional outcomes. The cut points for the groups were selected on the basis of the data distribution shown in Figures 3 and 4. The parent-child discrepancy groups were treated as fixed effects, and the parent-child dyad was specified as a random effect to allow clustering of repeated measures by dyad. The low discrepancy group (score discrepancies of −10 to 9 mm) was used as the reference group in all analyses. Reference cell coding was used for the discrepancy groups. Analyses were adjusted for days since study onset (fixed effect), since it was associated with our outcomes of interest (activity limitations and mean negative mood score).

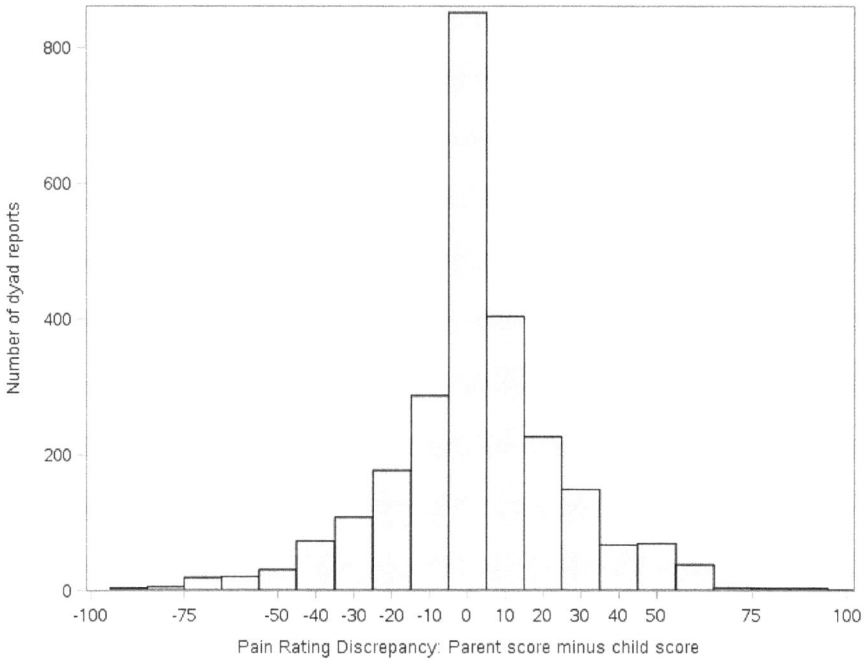

Figure 3. Discrepancy between child and parent ratings of child pain (parent score minus child score). Positive values indicate that the parent scored pain higher than the child. Negative numbers indicate that the child scored pain higher than the parent.

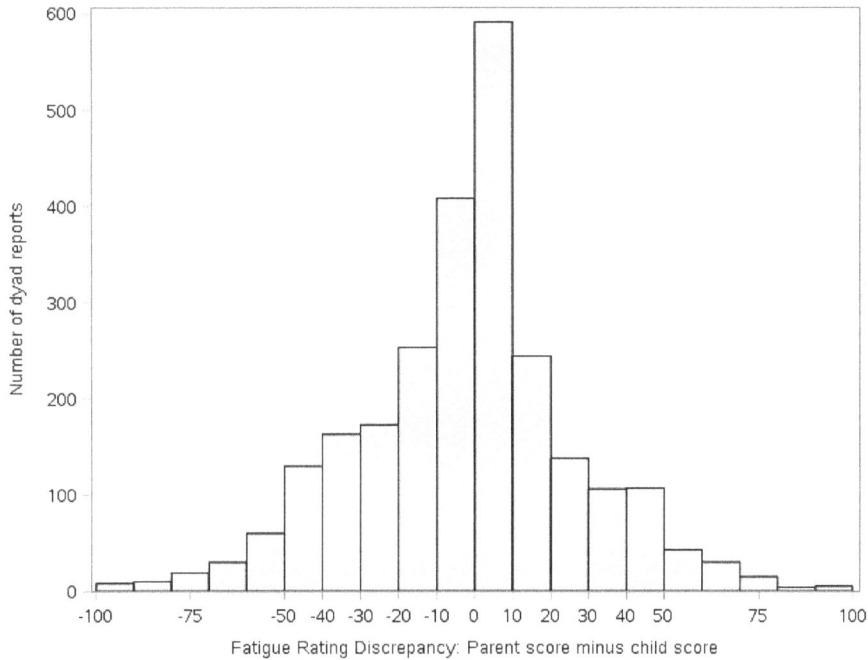

Figure 4. Discrepancy between child and parent rating of child fatigue (parent score minus child score). Positive values indicate that the parent scored the fatigue higher than the child. Negative numbers indicate that the child scored the fatigue higher than the parent.

3. Results

3.1. Descriptive Statistics

3.1.1. Demographics

Our sample was predominantly female (72% female) and Caucasian (75% Caucasian, 19% African American, 5% unanswered and 1.5% Pacific Islander). The mean age of children in our sample was 12.7 years, with a standard deviation of 2.8 years.

3.1.2. Discrepancies between Child and Parent Report of Pain and Fatigue

Figure 3 illustrates the distribution of the simple difference between parent and child pain scores, while Figure 4 illustrates the distribution of simple difference between parent and child fatigue score at all study time points. "Simple difference" refers to parent score minus child score. For example, if a parent rates the child's pain at 50 mm and the child rates their pain at 75 mm, the simple difference is −25 mm. For Figures 3 and 4, when $x = 0$, there is no difference between parent and child score. The y axis represents the number of dyad reports in each group over the course of the study.

Tables 1 and 2 provide the distribution of simple difference between parent and child pain and fatigue scores, respectively, for all time points in the study. The percent recorded in the second column represents the percentage of all observations in the study that fall into each discrepancy group, where N = total study observations.

Table 1. Groups of Pain Score Discrepancy.

Discrepancy Group (Parent Score-Child Score)	Dyad Reports *n* (%) (*N* [1] = 2537)
High Discrepancy (−100 to −51, child rated higher)	177 (7.0%)
Moderate Discrepancy (−50 to −11, child rated higher)	467 (18.4%)
Low Discrepancy (−10 to 9, parent and child rated similarly) [2]	1172 (46.2%)
Moderate Discrepancy (10 to 49, parent rated higher)	640 (25.2%)
High Discrepancy (50 to 100, parent rated higher)	81 (3.2%)

[1] *N* represents the total number of fatigue reports for the entire study. Percentages represent the number of individual reports in each group; [2] Reference group in mixed model analysis.

Table 2. Groups of Fatigue Score Discrepancy.

Discrepancy Group (Parent Score-Child Score)	Dyad Reports *n* (%) (*N* [1] = 2411)
High Discrepancy (−100 to −51, child rated higher) [2]	0
Moderate Discrepancy (−50 to −11, child rated higher)	719 (29.8%)
Low Discrepancy (−10 to 9, parent and child rated similarly) [3]	1000 (41.5%)
Moderate Discrepancy (10 to 49, parent rated higher)	595 (24.7%)
High Discrepancy (50 to 100, parent rated higher)	97 (4.0%)

[1] There were no dyads reports in the −100 to −49 range (parent fatigue score was much lower than child score); [2] *N* represents the total number of fatigue reports for the entire study. Percentages represent the number of individual reports in each group; [3] Reference group in mixed model analysis.

3.2. Hypothesis Testing

3.2.1. Parent-Child Discrepancies in Pain Intensity and Fatigue Reports as a Predictor of Mood

Compared to the low discrepancy reference group, children whose parents over reported their child's pain by 50–100 mms had a higher mean negative mood score (*p* value = 0.0136), as shown in Table 3. Children whose parents either over reported the child's fatigue by 50–100 mms or under reported their child's pain by 11–50 mms also had higher negative mean scores (*p* value = 0.003 and 0.002, respectively), as shown in Table 4.

Table 3. Relationship between simple difference of pain score and mean negative mood score.

Predictor variable: Discrepancy Group [1] (Parent Score-Child Score, Pain)	Estimate	Standard Error	*p*-Value
High Discrepancy (−100 to −51, child rated higher)	0.074	0.030	0.014
Moderate Discrepancy (−50 to −11, child rated higher)	0.001	0.020	0.964
Moderate Discrepancy (10 to 49, parent rated higher)	0.017	0.019	0.373
High Discrepancy (50 to 100, parent rated higher)	0.011	0.045	0.813

[1] The reference group in mixed model analyses (not shown) is the low discrepancy group.

Table 4. Relationship between simple difference of fatigue scores and mean negative mood scores.

Predictor Variable: Discrepancy Group [1] (Parent Score-Child Score, Fatigue)	Estimate	Standard Error	*p*-Value
High Discrepancy (−100 to −51, child rated higher) [2]	-	-	-
Moderate Discrepancy (−50 to −11, child rated higher)	0.056	0.017	0.002
Moderate Discrepancy (10 to 49, parent rated higher)	0.016	0.019	0.397
High Discrepancy (50 to 100, parent rated higher)	0.113	0.038	0.003

[1] The reference group in mixed model analyses (not shown) is the low discrepancy group; [2] There were no dyads in the −100 to −49 range (parent fatigue score was much lower than child score).

3.2.2. Parent-Child Discrepancy in Pain Intensity and Fatigue Reports as a Predictor of Activity Limitation

Children whose parents under reported their pain by 49 to 100 mms had a higher activity limitation score ($p = 0.043$) compared to the low discrepancy group, as shown in Table 5. Conversely, children whose parents under reported their fatigue by 11 to 50 mms had fewer activity limitations ($p = 0.016$), as shown in Table 6.

Table 5. Relationship between simple difference of pain scores and activity limitation.

Predictor Variable: Discrepancy Group [1] (Parent Score-Child Score, Pain)	Estimate	Standard Error	*p*-Value
High Discrepancy (−100 to −51, child rated higher)	1.097	0.538	0.043
Moderate Discrepancy (−50 to −11, child rated higher)	0.277	0.368	0.452
Moderate Discrepancy (10 to 49, parent rated higher)	−0.037	0.354	0.916
High Discrepancy (50 to 100, parent rated higher)	−1.471	0.820	0.075

[1] The reference group in mixed model analyses (not shown) is the low discrepancy group.

Table 6. Relationship between simple difference of fatigue scores activity limitation.

Predictor Variable: Discrepancy Group [1] (Parent Score-Child Score, Fatigue)	Estimate	Standard Error	*p*-Value
High Discrepancy (−100 to −51, child rated higher) [2]	-	-	-
Moderate Discrepancy (−50 to −11, child rated higher)	−0.796	0.328	0.016
Moderate Discrepancy (10 to 49, parent rated higher)	−0.230	0.350	0.512
High Discrepancy (50 to 100, parent rated higher)	−1.179	0.704	0.096

[1] The reference group in mixed model analyses (not shown) is the low discrepancy group; [2] There were no dyads in the −100 to −49 range (parent fatigue score was much lower than child score).

4. Discussion

This study examined associations between degree of discordance in parent and child ratings of child symptoms, functioning, and mood. Our data suggest that parent reports of child pain and fatigue often closely match those of the child, as evidenced by the center clustering in Figures 3 and 4. However, we also found that parents and children at times disagreed markedly on these measures and that discrepancies in reports, when present, were correlated with functional outcomes.

In contrast with what was expected, we found that children whose parents highly underreported their pain experienced higher rates of negative mood and greater activity limitation. We hypothesized that children whose parents overreported their pain would have greater activity limitations and negative mood based on previous research regarding parental overprotectiveness and its impact on activity and mood. However, we did not find a relationship between parental over reporting of child pain and increased negative mood or activity limitations.

It is possible that parents under report their child's pain as a minimizing response. Children may then respond by experiencing and recording an exaggerated pain level in an attempt to legitimize their experience, which would further exacerbate parent-child discordance. Previous work in children with chronic pain has demonstrated that minimizing parental responses can contribute to increased somatic symptoms, particularly in anxious children [21]. Additionally, previous work has demonstrated that depression in JIA patients is associated with higher activity limitation and higher disease severity [22]. Although negative mood is not synonymous with depression, as a marker of general psychological distress, it may be that negative mood plays a synergistic role with parental discordance in driving activity limitations [19].

We also found that children whose parents moderately overreported or highly underreported their fatigue had increased negative mood. Children whose parents underreported their fatigue had lower levels of activity limitation, but we again did not find that parental overreporting of fatigue correlated with greater activity limitation in the child. Our data regarding fatigue and negative mood suggest that child-parental discordance itself regarding perception of fatigue is correlated with greater negative mood in the child. It is unclear from our study why discrepancy in fatigue reporting generally, rather than discrepancy in a particular direction (e.g., parental over- or under reporting), was correlated with increased activity limitation. It may be that our measurement of discrepancies in parent and child fatigue report is confounded by a lack of family cohesiveness or poor communication, which drives both bidirectional disagreement on fatigue level and increased negative mood in the child. Previous research has demonstrated an association between a negative family environment and depressive symptoms in healthy children [23]. Our findings regarding parent-child discrepancy in fatigue report contributes to a gap in knowledge regarding fatigue in JIA. Although we know that fatigue is common in JIA, there is significantly less published work on fatigue in this disease relative to pain, and the existing evidence is somewhat conflicting [14,24,25].

Future work should explore whether particular family behavioral patterns are associated with increased disagreement between parent and child reports of symptoms and functional outcomes, data which was not available to us in this cohort. The current findings could be further characterized by future research exploring whether different caregiver characteristics predict discordance with child symptom report and whether different caregivers of the same child show agreement on child pain and fatigue ratings. Caregivers participating in this study were not diverse enough to explore inter-rater agreement between children and different types of caregivers, such as grandparents, mothers and fathers. Garcia-Munitis et al. demonstrated that certain caregivers, namely mothers, are more likely than others to agree closely with the child [5]. Additional family factors such as communication quality and style and level of parental monitoring may also be related to discordant reporting; future work should evaluate the role of these factors. It would also be worthwhile to explore whether informing the parent and child of the difference in their perception of the child's pain and fatigue would improve agreement between their ratings, and ultimately, the child's pain, mood, and ability to participate in social and physical activities.

Our results should be interpreted in light of several limitations. While the results discussed were statistically significant, we cannot infer causation. We view this work as preliminary and as a starting point for further research. A type one error is always a possibility given that we ran several statistical analyses. The sample was obtained from a single center and was a sample of convenience, limiting generalizability. All measures of pain and fatigue were self-reported, and some children may be poor or inaccurate reporters. In addition, unaccounted for confounders may have influenced the results.

In spite of these limitations, these results suggest that discrepancy often exists between parent and child ratings of pain and fatigue, raising questions about how clinicians respond to parent and child report of symptoms when there is considerable discrepancy, especially considering treatment decisions. There are objective measures of disease activity in JIA, such as inflammatory markers, joint exam, X-rays, but subjective patient and parent reported symptoms also guide therapy. This study reaffirms the need for clinicians to assess perception of disease severity from the perspective of both parent and child when making treatment decisions. Additionally, because the results suggest that the discrepancies are associated with functional outcomes, healthcare providers may preemptively wish to refer parents and children who demonstrate disagreement on levels of pain and fatigue to mental health professionals such as social workers and psychologists, as these children may be at risk for suboptimal functional and emotional outcomes.

Acknowledgments: Sources of funding include an R01 grant (R01AR53845, PI: Laura E. Schanberg) from the National Institute of Arthritis and Musculoskeletal and Skin Diseases for original data collection and a Duke Institute of Pediatric Research Resident Research Grant (Awardee: Amy Gaultney) in support of the publication of this article.

Author Contributions: Mark Connelly, Laura E. Schanberg and Maggie H. Bromberg participated in the study design for this article, manuscript editing, and original data collection as a part of R01 grant. Tracy Spears conducted the statistical analysis and participated in manuscript editing. Amy Gaultney wrote the manuscript and participated in study design and planning of the statistical analysis.

Conflicts of Interest: The authors declare no conflict of interest.

References

1. Schanberg, L.E.; Sandstrom, M.J. Causes of pain in children with arthritis. *Rheum. Dis. Clin. N. Am.* **1999**, *1*, 31–53. [CrossRef]
2. Gutierrez-Suarez, R.; Pistorio, A.; Cespedes, C.; Norambuena, X.; Flato, B.; Rumba, I.; Harjacek, M.; Nielsen, S.; Susic, G.; Mihaylova, D.; et al. For Pediatric Rheumatology International Trials Organisation (PRINTO). Health-related quality of life of patients with juvenile idiopathic arthritis coming from 3 different geographic areas. The PRINTO multinational quality of life cohort study. *Rheumatology* **2007**, *46*, 314–320. [CrossRef] [PubMed]
3. Palermo, T.M.; Chambers, C.T. Parent and family factors in pediatric chronic pain and disability: An integrative approach. *Pain* **2005**, *119*, 1–4. [CrossRef] [PubMed]
4. Sztajnbok, F.; Coronel-Martinez, D.L.; Diaz-Maldonado, A.; Novarini, C.; Pistorio, A.; Viola, S.; Ruperto, N.; Buoncompagni, A.; Martini, A.; Ravelli, A. Discordance between physician's and parent's global assessments in juvenile idiopathic arthritis. *Rheumatology* **2007**, *46*, 141–145. [CrossRef] [PubMed]
5. Garcia-Munitis, P.I.; Bandeira, M.; Pistorio, A.; Magni-Manzoni, S.; Ruperto, N.; Schivo, A.; Martini, A.; Ravelli, A. Level of agreement between children, parents, and physicians in rating pain intensity in juvenile idiopathic arthritis. *Arthritis Rheum.* **2006**, *55*, 177–183. [CrossRef] [PubMed]
6. Palermo, T.M.; Zebracki, K.; Cox, S.; Newman, A.J.; Singer, N.G. Juvenile idiopathic arthritis: Parent-child discrepancy on reports of pain and disability. *J. Rheumatol.* **2004**, *31*, 1840–1846. [PubMed]
7. Stone, A.A.; Shiffman, S. Ecological momentary assessment: Measuring real world processes in behavioral medicine. *Ann. Behav. Med.* **1994**, *16*, 199–202.
8. Claar, R.L.; Guite, J.W.; Kaczynski, K.J.; Logan, D.E. Factor structure of the Adult Responses to Children's Symptoms: Validation in children and adolescents with diverse chronic pain conditions. *Clin. J. Pain* **2010**, *26*, 410–417. [CrossRef] [PubMed]
9. Guite, J.W.; McCue, R.L.; Sherker, J.L.; Sherry, D.D.; Rose, J.B. Relationships among pain, protective parental responses, and disability for adolescents with chronic musculoskeletal pain: The mediating role of pain catastrophizing. *Clin. J. Pain* **2011**, *27*, 775–781. [CrossRef] [PubMed]
10. Simons, L.E.; Claar, R.L.; Logan, D.L. Chronic pain in adolescence: Parental responses, adolescent coping, and their impact on adolescent's pain behaviors. *J. Pediatr. Psychol.* **2008**, *33*, 894–904. [CrossRef] [PubMed]
11. Bromberg, M.H.; Connelly, M.; Anthony, K.K.; Gil, K.M.; Schanberg, L.E. Prospective mediation models of sleep, pain, and daily function in children with arthritis using ecological momentary assessment. *Clin. J. Pain* **2016**, *32*, 471–477. [CrossRef] [PubMed]
12. Connelly, M.; Bromberg, M.H.; Anthony, K.K.; Gill, K.M.; Franks, L.; Schanberg, L.E. Emotion regulation predicts pain and functioning in children with juvenile idiopathic arthritis: An electronic diary study. *J. Pediatr. Psychol.* **2012**, *37*, 43–52. [CrossRef] [PubMed]
13. Bromberg, M.H.; Connelly, M.; Anthony, K.K.; Gil, K.M.; Schanberg, L.E. Self-reported pain and disease symptoms persist in juvenile idiopathic arthritis despite treatment advances: An electronic diary study. *Arthritis Rheumatol.* **2014**, *66*, 462–469. [CrossRef] [PubMed]
14. Connelly, M.; Anthony, K.K.; Sarniak, R.; Bromberg, M.H.; Gil, K.M.; Schanberg, L.E. Parent pain responses as predictors of daily activities and mood in children with juvenile idiopathic arthritis: The utility of electronic diaries. *J. Pain Symptom Manag.* **2010**, *39*, 579–590. [CrossRef] [PubMed]
15. Stinson, J.N.; Stevens, B.J.; Feldman, B.M.; Streiner, D.L.; McGrath, P.J.; Dupuis, A. Using an electronic pain diary to better understand pain in children and adolescents with arthritis. *Pain Manag.* **2011**, *1*, 127–137. [CrossRef] [PubMed]
16. Lee, K.A.; Hicks, G.; Nino-Murcia, G. Validity and reliability of a scale to assess fatigue. *Psychiatry Res.* **1991**, *36*, 291–298. [CrossRef]
17. Palermo, T.M.; Witherspoon, D.; Valenzuela, D.; Drotar, D.D. Development and validation of the Child Activity Limitations Interview: A measure of pain-related functional impairment in school-age children and adolescents. *Pain* **2004**, *109*, 461–470. [CrossRef] [PubMed]

18. Young, N.L.; Williams, J.I.; Yoshida, K.K.; Wright, J.G. Measurement properties of the activities scale for kids. *J. Clin. Epidemiol.* **2000**, *53*, 125–137. [CrossRef]
19. Laurent, J.; Salvatore, J.; Catanzaro, T.E.; Joiner, K.D.; Rudolph, K.I.; Potter, S.L.; Osborne, L.; Gathright, T. A measure of positive and negative affect for children: Scale development and preliminary validation. *Psychol. Assess.* **1999**, *11*, 326–338. [CrossRef]
20. Watson, W.; Lee, A.C.; Carey, G. Positive and negative affectivity and their relation to anxiety and depressive disorders. *J. Abnorm. Psychol.* **1998**, *97*, 346–353. [CrossRef]
21. Claar, R.L.; Simons, L.E.; Logan, D. Parental response to children's pain: The moderating impact of children's emotional distress on symptoms and disability. *Pain* **2008**, *138*, 172–179. [CrossRef] [PubMed]
22. El-Najjar, A.R.; Negm, M.G.; El-Sayed, W.M. The relationship between depression, disease activity and physical function in juvenile idiopathic arthritis patients in Zagazig University Hospitals—Egypt. *Egypt. Rheumatol.* **2014**, *36*, 145–150. [CrossRef]
23. Normura, Y.; Wickramaratne, P.J.; Warner, V.; Weissman, M. Family discord, parental depression and psychopathology in offspring: Ten-year follow-up. *J. Am. Acad. Child Adolesc. Psychiatry* **2002**, *41*, 402–409. [CrossRef] [PubMed]
24. Östlie, I.L.; Aasland, A.; Johansson, I.; Flatö, B.; Möller, A. A longitudinal follow-up study of physical and psychosocial health in young adults with chronic childhood arthritis. *Clin. Exp. Rheumatol.* **2009**, *27*, 1039–1046. [PubMed]
25. Schanberg, L.E.; Anthony, K.K.; Gil, K.M.; Maurin, E.C. Daily Pain and Symptoms in Children with Polyarticular Arthritis. *Arthritis Rheum.* **2003**, *48*, 1390–1397. [CrossRef] [PubMed]

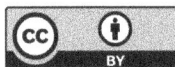

— *children*

MDPI

Article

Pain in School: Patterns of Pain-Related School Impairment among Adolescents with Primary Pain Conditions, Juvenile Idiopathic Arthritis Pain, and Pain-Free Peers

Anna Monica Agoston [1,2], Laura S. Gray [3,4] and Deirdre E. Logan [1,2,*]

1   Division of Perioperative and Pain Medicine, Department of Anesthesia, Boston Children's Hospital, Pain Treatment Service, 333 Longwood Ave., Boston, MA 02115, USA; monicaagost@gmail.com
2   Department of Psychiatry, Harvard Medical School, Boston, MA 02115, USA
3   Division of Anesthesiology, Sedation and Perioperative Medicine, Children's National Health System, Washington, DC 20010, USA; deirdre.logan@childrens.harvard.edu
4   The George Washington University School of Medicine, Washington, DC 20037, USA
*   Correspondence: Deirdre.logan@childrens.harvard.edu; Tel.: +1-617-355-7040; Fax: +1-617-730-0199

Academic Editor: Carl L. von Baeyer
Received: 16 September 2016; Accepted: 21 November 2016; Published: 30 November 2016

Abstract: Children with chronic pain frequently experience impairment in the school setting, but we do not yet understand how unique these struggles are to children with primary pain conditions compared to peers with disease-related pain or those without chronic pain symptoms. The objective of this study is to examine school functioning, defined as school attendance rates, overall quality of life in the school setting, and school nurse visits among adolescents with primary pain conditions, those with juvenile idiopathic arthritis (JIA)-related pain, and healthy peers. Two hundred and sixty adolescents participated in the study, including 129 with primary pain conditions, 61 with JIA, and 70 healthy comparison adolescents. They completed self- and parent-reported measures of school function. Findings show that as a group, youth with primary pain conditions reported more school absences, lower quality of life in the school setting, and more frequent school nurse visits compared to both adolescents with JIA-related pain and healthy peers. We conclude that compared to those who experience pain specific to a disease process, adolescents with primary pain conditions may face unique challenges in the school setting and may require more support to help them succeed in school in spite of pain.

Keywords: chronic pain; child and adolescent; school functioning

1. Introduction

School functioning is known to be impaired in adolescents with chronic pain [1–7]. A 2008 study by Logan and colleagues [4] demonstrated that adolescents with chronic pain without clear etiology, or "primary pain conditions" [8], missed significant amounts of school, with close to half of those sampled missing at least a quarter of school days. Other areas of school function including academic performance, engagement, attention to classwork, and keeping up with activities may be affected as well. Few studies have examined utilization of medical resources at school such as frequency of nurse visits; this is also important to understand, as it is both an indicator of health service use and of time spent disengaged from the classroom.

Although rates of school absences in pediatric primary pain conditions have been shown to be higher than rates for most other chronic illnesses [2,9], few direct comparisons have been made with chronic diseases that include a significant pain component. Previous studies suggest that teachers and school administrators lack an understanding of primary pain conditions and of the biopsychosocial framework that explains such pain experiences [10,11]. In vignette-based studies, the absence of a clear, organic explanation for pain symptoms has been linked to more negative responses to pain complaints and less willingness to provide classroom accommodations [12]. Such attributions may be a perpetuating factor in the pain-related school impairment of youth with primary conditions. Peer reactions may also differ to these varied types of pain experience, which could further affect the child's ability to cope with pain in school. In addition, children's own self-perceptions around their pain and their attributions of its causes may also differ by the type of pain experience and may in turn affect their school functioning. However, the current literature does not adequately explore differences in youth with primary pain compared to those with disease-related pain symptoms, whose pain may be more easily understood by school personnel due to its more straightforward biomedical nature.

To date, the existing literature is contradictory. One study comparing youth with headache to those with disease-related pain (i.e., juvenile idiopathic arthritis (JIA), sickle cell disease) found no differences in rates of school attendance [13]. Another study comparing youth with JIA to youth with primary musculoskeletal pain found that patients with non-disease-related pain reported more school impairment as indicated by more worries about school and the presence of learning disabilities [14]. Additional studies are needed to clarify the relationship between school functioning and chronic pain in children with primary pain vs. pain due to a specific etiology and to expand the definition of school functioning beyond simply school attendance rates. There is also a dearth of research directly comparing school functioning in children with chronic pain with their healthy peers. The lack of available normative rates of school absence, nurse visits, and other indicators of school functioning makes it difficult to interpret reports of these issues in youth with chronic pain. Comparing these youth to healthy peers of a similar age and sex is critical for understanding the extent and implications of impaired school functioning in children with primary pain conditions.

Our study investigated whether children with chronic pain of an unknown origin differed in reports of school functioning compared to children with pain due to a specific disease process, in this case JIA, and to pain-free peers. Clarifying the picture of school functioning with regard to absences, quality of life in the school setting, and utilization of health care services (e.g., number of nurse visits in children with primary pain conditions) compared to other populations will improve our understanding of risk and protective factors for school outcomes in children with primary chronic pain.

2. Material and Methods

2.1. Participants

Three groups of adolescents aged 12–19 years were recruited, a primary chronic pain ("PCP") group, a group diagnosed with juvenile idiopathic arthritis ("JIA"), and a comparison group of healthy adolescents ("Healthy").

The PCP group was made up of adolescent patients who underwent a multidisciplinary pain evaluation at tertiary pain clinic in a large, urban northeast pediatric hospital (Boston Children's Hospital, Boston, MA, US). These patients included adolescents with physician-assigned diagnosis of functional gastrointestinal disorders (FGID), headache, or diffuse/localized musculoskeletal/ neuropathic pain syndrome without clear disease etiology. Patients for the JIA group were recruited from pediatric rheumatology outpatient clinics at Boston Children's Hospital Boston, MA, US. JIA was selected as the disease-based pain comparison group because it has been included in numerous other studies of pain-related functioning, including a few studies specifically examining school impairment and contrasting this condition to primary pain conditions [13–15]. Additionally, JIA is more prevalent in girls, which is a similar profile to most types of primary pain conditions. Girls were over-sampled for the Healthy group to align with the characteristics of the PCP and JIA groups.

Eligibility criteria for participants in the PCP and JIA groups included a current pain frequency of at least once a week or five days per month. JIA patients were excluded if they had any medical condition or separate chronic pain syndrome (e.g., migraine headache, functional abdominal pain disorder). Healthy participants were excluded if they had any current chronic pain problem that occurred at least once a week or five days per month, or any current chronic medical condition. Across all groups, participants were excluded if they were not in the 12–19 year age range, were unable to speak sufficient English, had any cognitive impairment or severe psychiatric disorder, or were not enrolled in a structured school setting. Mental health conditions such as anxiety or depression were not exclusionary. Youth receiving temporary homebound tutoring because of pain problems were included.

2.2. Procedures

Data presented herein are drawn from a larger longitudinal study on school functioning and self-image in adolescents with pain. Institutional Review Board approval (IRB-P00000729) was obtained prior to the start of the study. All data collection occurred during the school months so that current school-year data could be collected for all participants. Adolescents in the PCP and JIA groups were identified in advance of scheduled clinic appointments and sent information about the study by mail. Participants who did not wish to be approached about the study during their clinic visit were asked to send back a stamped postcard indicating this. Those who did not opt out were approached when arriving for their clinic visit and the study was explained to them in detail. Adolescents recruited during hospital clinic visits were given the option of completing measures on paper immediately or receiving a link to complete them electronically. Healthy adolescent participants contacted the study team through information provided in advertisements for a study about health and school functioning. These advertisements were posted on the hospital website (accessed by staff and families) and on notices throughout the community. Girls were over-sampled by posting advertisements recruiting only for girls once sufficient numbers of boys were enrolled. Healthy participants completed all measures electronically. Assent was obtained from all participants under 18 in the PCP and JIA groups. Informed written consent was obtained from the participant's parent and directly from the participant if over 18. Permission was received by the Institutional Review Board to provide healthy participants with an information form in lieu of formal written consent, since these participants were not recruited in person. All available data were included for analyses, thus some analyses differed in sample size due to missing data.

2.3. Measures

2.3.1. Demographic and Medical Information

Age, sex, grade, and ethnicity were provided by parents of all participants. Diagnoses were obtained from medical records based on the evaluations at the clinical visit concurrent with study enrollment. Pain characteristics included "typical" pain intensity, assessed with a numeric rating scale, frequency of pain (measured on an eight-point scale from "Never" to "Daily or Almost Daily") and time since pain onset.

2.3.2. Self-Report of School Functioning

The Pediatric Quality of Life inventory (Peds-QL) [16] school functioning subscale is a five-item child/adolescent rating scale assessing subjective impressions of the extent to which pain interferes with school attendance and performance (e.g., "In the past 3 months, how much of a problem have you had with keeping up with school activities?"). The Peds-QL is a well-validated instrument for use with children with a variety of chronic medical conditions and demonstrates high reliability across items ($\alpha = 0.80$).

2.3.3. School Attendance

Parents reported the number of days that their adolescent missed school in the previous three months, a time frame that has been used in our previous studies of school function, showing good reliability. If participants arrived at school late or left early on a given day due to pain, these days were counted as 0.5 of a missed day, consistent with previous research [4,17]. Past studies have demonstrated close correlations between official school absence records and parent reports of school attendance, which tends to be more accessible information in the context of a research study [4].

2.3.4. Frequency of Nurse'S Visits

Adolescents estimated the frequency of use of school medical services (e.g., visits to the nurse's office) in the previous month. The time frame for reporting nurse visits was limited to one month in hopes of maintaining a reliable time frame for retrospective recall.

2.4. Data Analytic Plan

The statistical analysis program SPSS version 23 (IBM Corp., Armonk, NY, USA) was used for all data analyses. Group differences in school functioning across diagnoses were examined using one-way analysis of variance (ANOVA), analysis of covariance (ANCOVA), and Student's *t*-tests.

3. Results

3.1. Descriptive Findings

One hundred and twenty-nine patients with primary pain, 61 with JIA, and 70 healthy comparison adolescents were recruited for a total of 260 participants. Participant ages ranged from 12 to 19 years (Mean (M) age = 15.25, standard deviation (SD) = 1.67), with no significant differences between groups in age ($F(2,252) = 0.91$, $p = 0.41$). The grade in school ranged from 6th to 12th grade. Further, 85.8% of respondents were Caucasian. In all three groups the majority of adolescent participants were female (70.5%), but a higher proportion of the PCP group were female (81.4%) compared to the JIA (62.3%) and Healthy (65.7%) comparison groups despite efforts to recruit comparable samples. Mothers were the parent responders for 86% of the sample. Families tended to report relatively high socio-economic status, with a mean Hollingshead score of 5.2 (5 = Clerical and Sales Worker) for mothers and 6.2 (6 = Technicians, Semiprofessionals) for fathers. Mothers had a mean of 5.9 education (6 = Standard College) and fathers had a mean of 5.6 education (5 = Partial College). Across the sample, 76.7% of parents were married, but this differed across groups (72% for the PCP group, 85.5% for the JIA group, and 78.4% for the Healthy group).

Table 1 displays the frequency of specific primary diagnoses within each of the two pain groups. Compared to the JIA group, the primary pain group reported higher typical pain intensity ratings (PCP group typical pain M = 5.73, SD = 2.10; JIA group typical pain M = 2.47, SD = 2.16; $t = 9.45$, $p < 0.001$) and greater pain frequency (PCP group M = 5.88 where 6 = several times per week, SD = 2.00; JIA group M = 4.28 where 4 = several times per month, SD = 2.43; $t = 8.74$, $p < 0.001$). On the contrary, participants with JIA report a significantly longer time since pain onset compared to the primary pain group (mean time since pain onset in JIA group = 77.0 months, SD = 50.9 months; $t = 6.4$, $p < 0.001$). Given the significant between-group differences in pain characteristics, these variables were incorporated into subsequent group comparisons.

Table 1. Frequency of primary diagnoses in primary pain (PCP) and juvenile idiopathic arthritis (JIA) groups.

PCP Group (*n* = 129)	*n* (%)
Neuropathic pain	31 (24%)
Back or neck pain	20 (15.5%)

Table 1. *Cont.*

PCP Group (*n* = 129)	*n* (%)
Other myofascial/musculoskeletal pain	15 (11.6%)
Joint pain [1]	15 (11.6%)
Functional abdominal pain	12 (9.3%)
Pelvic pain/Endometriosis [2]	7 (5.4%)
Headache (migraine and/or tension)	5 (3.8%)
Chest pain	4 (3.1%)
Other (e.g., TMJ, coccydynia)	20 (15.5%)
JIA Group (*n* = 61)	***n* (%)**
Polyarticular arthritis	18 (29.5%)
Pauciarticular arthritis	9 (14.8%)
Spondyloarthropathy	16 (26.2%)
Psoriatic arthritis	12 (19.7%)
Systemic arthritis	2 (3.3%)
Enthesitis-related	2 (3.3%)
Osteomyelitis	2 (3.3%)

[1] Of participants with joint pain as a major complaint, five had a diagnosis (current or historical) of Ehlers–Danlos syndrome but were found to have pain that was not accounted for by this diagnosis, and therefore were viewed as having a primary pain condition; [2] Of participants with pelvic pain as a major complaint, six had a diagnosis (current or historical) of endometriosis but were found to have pain that was not accounted for by this diagnosis, and therefore were viewed as having a primary pain condition; TMJ: temporomandibular joint disorders.

3.2. Quality of Life in the School Setting.

The PCP group (M = 46.32, SD = 23.42) had lower school functioning scores on the Peds-QL compared to both the JIA group (M = 66.59, SD = 20.99; $p < 0.001$) and the Healthy group (M = 73.91, SD = 16.32; $p < 0.001$) (Figure 1). Significant differences were found between groups for Peds-QL school functioning ($F_{(2, 241)} = 41.21$, $p < 0.001$), with Tukey's post hoc tests revealing significantly lower scores in the PCP group compared to the JIA and Healthy groups. The JIA and Healthy group means did not differ statistically. ANCOVA analyses incorporating pain characteristics revealed that group differences in Peds-QL school function scores were not accounted for by pain intensity, pain frequency, or time since pain onset. However, pain intensity did emerge as a predictor of school-related quality of life in ANCOVAs focused on the two pain groups ($F_{(1,157)} = 13.17$, $p < 0.001$). Neither pain frequency nor time since pain onset were significant predictors of Peds-QL scores.

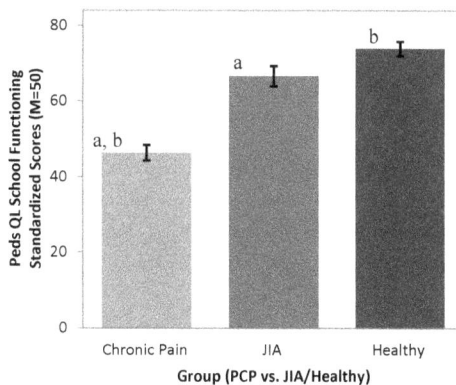

Figure 1. Pediatric Quality of Life inventory (Peds-QL) school function scores in Chronic Pain (PCP), juvenile idiopathic arthritis (JIA) and Healthy groups. Groups marked "a" differ from one another at $p < 0.001$; Groups marked "b" differ from one another at $p < 0.001$.

3.3. Attendance

The PCP group (M = 8.95, SD = 12.22) had significantly higher numbers of school days missed in the past three months compared to both the JIA group (M = 1.69, SD = 3.76; $p < 0.001$) and the Healthy group (M = 0.33, SD = 0.93; $p < 0.001$) (Figure 2). There were significant between-group differences between the number of school days missed ($F(2,245) = 26.21$, $p < 0.001$). Tukey's post hoc tests revealed a significantly higher number of days missed in the PCP group compared to the JIA and Healthy groups. The JIA and Healthy group means did not differ statistically. ANCOVA analyses incorporating pain characteristics revealed that group differences in school attendance rates were not accounted for by pain intensity, pain frequency, or time since pain onset. No pain characteristics emerged as significant predictors of school attendance rates in these analyses.

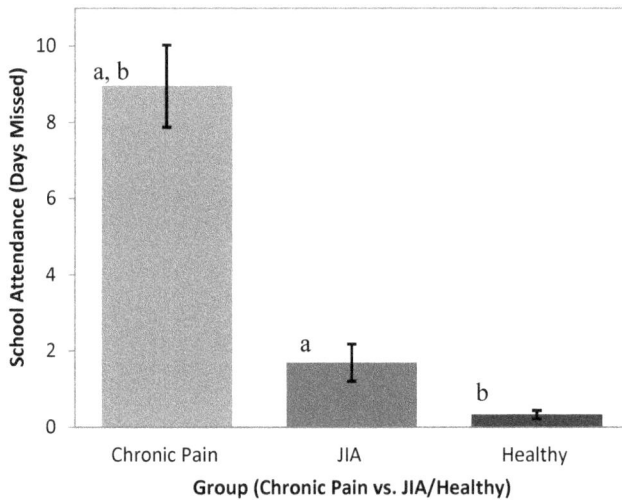

Figure 2. School absences in previous three months in youth in PCP, JIA, and Healthy groups. Groups marked "a" differ from one another at $p < 0.001$; Groups marked "b" differ from one another at $p < 0.001$.

3.4. Nurse's Office Visits

The PCP group was found to utilize school nurse visits more often (M = 5.71, SD = 7.81) than the JIA group (M = 1.07, SD = 1.67) (see Figure 3). A Student's *t*-test revealed a significant between-group difference between school nurse visits for the PCP vs. JIA groups (this variable was not collected for the Healthy group): $t(170) = 4.43$, $p < 0.001$. ANCOVA analyses incorporating pain characteristics revealed that group differences in the frequency of school nurse visits could be explained by differences in pain intensity between groups ($F(1,154) = 1.65$, $p = 0.201$). Pain intensity was a significant independent predictor of the frequency of nurse office visits ($F(1,154) = 6.57$, $p < 0.05$). Neither pain frequency nor time since pain onset accounted for group variation in nurse office visits.

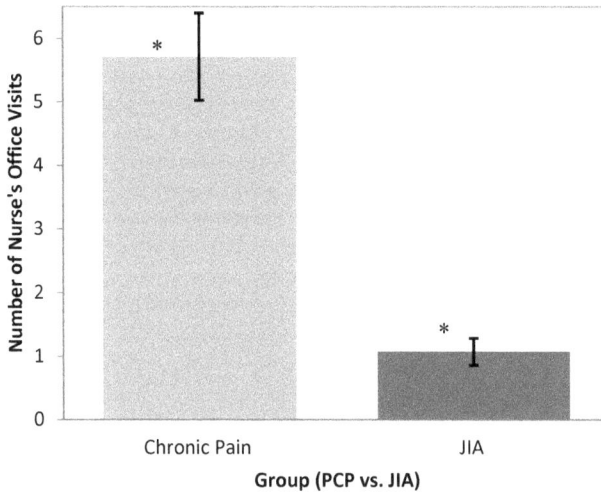

Figure 3. Frequency of school nurse visits in past month in PCP and JIA groups. * Groups differ significantly at $p < 0.001$.

4. Discussion

Our study suggests that school functioning among youth with primary pain conditions differed significantly from that of youth with chronic pain related to JIA. Specifically, adolescents with primary pain conditions had poorer school functioning/quality of life, missed an average of nine days of school in three months compared to 1.7 days missed on average in the JIA group, and reported more nurse visits than adolescents with chronic pain due to JIA. Our results also demonstrated that youth with primary pain conditions had a lower school quality of life and missed more school than participants in a comparison group of peers without chronic pain.

To date, studies reporting school-related outcomes in adolescents with chronic pain have suffered from a lack of context to understand the extent of school impairment among this group.

The findings of the current study add to our knowledge regarding school functioning in adolescents with primary pain conditions by highlighting ways in which this group may experience greater levels of impairment compared to adolescents with pain due to a specific disease process and to healthy adolescents. Importantly, although pain characteristics were dissimilar across the groups in several ways, the results show that factors such as pain intensity or frequency did not fully explain group differences in school functioning, suggesting a more qualitative difference in the school experiences of youth with different types of pain conditions.

Integrating the current findings with previous research allows us to speculate on some possible explanations for these differences. Prior studies have demonstrated that school personnel express a limited understanding of primary pain disorders and more difficulty responding in a supportive manner to pain when symptoms are not tied to a specific disease etiology [10,11]. Adolescents with primary pain conditions may consequently feel less accepted and supported at school by both peers and school staff. Other studies have indicated that these adolescents report more difficulty with peer relationships than healthy peers and are more isolated and withdrawn, less well liked, and have fewer reciprocal friendships [18]. It is possible that peers and school staff alike have difficulty understanding and acknowledging pain that does not have a straightforward familiar cause. Youth with primary pain conditions may feel invalidated in their interactions with peers and school staff and may avoid these situations, resulting in greater school absences.

In addition to differences in school attendance and overall school functioning, youth with primary pain conditions were found to utilize school health resources more often when at school compared to youth with JIA-related pain. On average, the PCP group reported visiting the nurse close to six times in the past month, compared to the one visit average reported in the JIA group. More research is needed to understand how youth are utilizing these resources and whether these resources are supporting their school functioning. For example, youth with primary chronic pain may be visiting the school nurse for an opportunity to practice active coping strategies for pain management, to obtain medication, or to avoid class time due to feeling unprepared during class or unsupported by teachers. Importantly, one must be present at school to visit the school nurse, so in some ways this behavior represents less impaired function compared to complete school absence. Future studies may explore the clinical implications of nurse visits and whether these visits are detrimental or supportive toward improving school functioning. Finally, considering our results are mixed with regard to consistency with prior studies [14,15], additional studies are needed to replicate our findings.

A major challenge to this line of research is the significant role of individual differences in efforts to foster school success among youth with chronic pain. The unique strengths and needs of each child, coupled with vast differences across school environments, require tailored school planning and make it difficult to establish uniform "best practices" regarding school accommodations for youth with primary pain conditions [19]. Nonetheless, continued research in this area plays an important role in establishing recommended approaches to addressing the needs of adolescents whose pain has led to school impairment.

Several limitations to the study bear noting. Recruitment approaches and referral patterns in the clinic settings where the study took place may have resulted in some selection bias to the sample, limiting the comparability of the groups. Firstly, our JIA sample was recruited from rheumatology clinics where such patients are typically seen on a regular basis for ongoing monitoring, whereas the primary chronic pain patients recruited from a tertiary chronic pain clinic may have been more likely to schedule visits due to current levels of symptom distress and/or disability. Thus, our clinically-referred primary chronic pain group may represent a more severely symptomatic and/or disabled subgroup than our clinically-referred JIA group. Secondly, the Healthy group was recruited through advertisements for a study on "health and school functioning", which may have yielded a response bias toward individuals with an interest in reporting on their school functioning, possibly due to more positive self-perception in this realm. Furthermore, the tracking of study refusals or consent without completed surveys was inconsistent across groups (i.e., better tracking occurred for the clinical samples than the healthy sample) and thus cannot be reliably reported. Another study limitation is the failure to collect data on nurse visits from the Healthy group. This was a flaw in the survey design, as such data would have informed our understanding of normal rates of this behavior.

This study helps elucidate the relationship between school functioning and chronic pain in children with primary pain conditions compared to JIA-related pain, with possible implications for disease-related pain more broadly. By directly comparing school functioning in children with chronic pain with their healthy peers, the study also fosters increased understanding of the extent and implications of impaired school functioning in children with primary chronic pain conditions. Future studies may expand from this set of findings to advance our knowledge of risk and protective factors for school outcomes in children with chronic pain.

Acknowledgments: The study was conducted with support from the Sara Page Mayo Endowment for Pediatric Pain Research and Treatment (to Charles B. Berde M.D., Ph.D.) and the Department of Anesthesiology, Perioperative and Pain Medicine.

Author Contributions: A.M.A. analyzed the data and wrote the manuscript. D.L. conceived and designed the study and edited the manuscript. L.G. contributed to data collection, management and analyses as well as study design.

Conflicts of Interest: All authors have been surveyed and have declared no conflict of interest affecting this manuscript.

References

1. Chann, E.; Piira, T.; Betts, G. The school functioning of children with chronic and recurrent pain. *Pediatr. Pain Lett.* **2005**, *7*, 11–14.
2. Hunfeld, J.A.; Perquin, C.; Duivenvoorden, H.J.; Hazebroek-Kampschreur, A.; Passchier, J.; van Suijlekom-Smit, L.; van der Wouden, J. Chronic pain and its impact on quality of life in adolescents and their families. *J. Pediatr. Psychol.* **2001**, *26*, 145–153. [CrossRef] [PubMed]
3. Konijnenberg, A.Y.; Uiterwaal, C.S.; Kimpen, J.L.; van der Hoeven, J.; Buitelaar, J.K.; de Graeff-Meeder, E.R. Children with unexplained chronic pain: Substantial impairment in everyday life. *Arch. Dis. Child* **2005**, *90*, 680–686. [CrossRef] [PubMed]
4. Logan, D.E.; Simons, L.E.; Stein, M.J.; Chastain, L. School impairment in adolescents with chronic pain. *J. Pain* **2008**, *9*, 407–416. [CrossRef] [PubMed]
5. Merlijn, V.P.; Hunfeld, J.A.; van der Wouden, J.C.; Hazebroek-Kampschreur, A.A.; Passchier, J.; Koes, B.W. Factors related to the quality of life in adolescents with chronic pain. *Clin. J. Pain* **2006**, *22*, 306–315. [CrossRef] [PubMed]
6. Roth-Isigkeit, A.; Thyen, U.; Stoven, H.; Schwarzenberger, J.; Schmucker, P. Pain among children and adolescents: Restrictions in daily living and triggering factors. *Pediatrics* **2005**, *115*, e152–e162. [CrossRef] [PubMed]
7. Sato, A.F.; Hainsworth, K.R.; Khan, K.A.; Ladwig, R.J.; Weisman, S.J.; Davies, W.H. School absenteeism in pediatric chronic pain: Identifying lessons learned from the general school absenteeism literature. *Child. Health Care* **2007**, *36*, 355–372. [CrossRef]
8. Schechter, N.L. Functional pain: Time for a new name. *JAMA Pediatr.* **2014**, *168*, 693–694. [CrossRef] [PubMed]
9. Newacheck, P.W.; Taylor, W.R. Childhood chronic illness: Prevalence, severity, and impact. *Am. J. Public Health* **1992**, *82*, 364–371. [CrossRef] [PubMed]
10. Logan, D.E.; Curran, J.A. Adolescent chronic pain problems in the school setting: Exploring the experiences and beliefs of selected school personnel through focus group methodology. *J. Adolesc. Health* **2005**, *37*, 281–288. [CrossRef] [PubMed]
11. Logan, D.E.; Catanese, S.P.; Coakley, R.M.; Scharff, L. Chronic pain in the classroom: Teachers' attributions about the causes of chronic pain. *J. Sch. Health* **2007**, *77*, 248–256. [CrossRef] [PubMed]
12. Logan, D.E.; Coakley, R.M.; Scharff, L. Teachers' perceptions of and responses to adolescents with chronic pain syndromes. *J. Pediatr. Psychol.* **2007**, *32*, 139–149. [PubMed]
13. Lewandowski, A.S.; Palermo, T.M.; Kirchner, H.L.; Drotar, D. Comparing diary and retrospective reports of pain and activity restriction in children and adolescents with chronic pain conditions. *Clin. J. Pain* **2009**, *25*, 299–306. [CrossRef] [PubMed]
14. Aasland, A.; Flato, B.; Vandvik, I.H. Psychosocial factors in children with idiopathic musculoskeletal pain: A prospective, longitudinal study. *Acta Paediatr.* **1997**, *86*, 740–746. [CrossRef] [PubMed]
15. Sturge, C.; Garralda, M.E.; Boissin, M.; Dore, C.J.; Woo, P. School attendance and juvenile chronic arthritis. *Br. J. Rheumatol.* **1997**, *36*, 1218–1223. [CrossRef] [PubMed]
16. Varni, J.W.; Seid, M.; Rode, C.A. The PedsQL: Measurement model for the pediatric quality of life inventory. *Med. Care* **1999**, *37*, 126–139. [CrossRef] [PubMed]
17. Logan, D.E.; Simons, L.E.; Kaczynski, K. School functioning in adolescents with chronic pain: The role of depressive symptoms in school impairment. *J. Pediatr. Psychol.* **2009**, *34*, 882–892. [PubMed]
18. Kashikar-Zuck, S.; Lynch, A.M.; Graham, T.B.; Swain, N.F.; Mullen, S.M.; Noll, R.B. Social functioning and peer relationships of adolescents with juvenile fibromyalgia syndrome. *Arthritis Rheum.* **2007**, *57*, 474–480. [CrossRef] [PubMed]
19. Walker, L.S. Helping the child with recurrent abdominal pain return to school. *Pediatr. Ann.* **2004**, *33*, 128–136. [CrossRef] [PubMed]

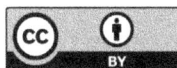

Article

Neighborhood Characteristics: Influences on Pain and Physical Function in Youth at Risk for Chronic Pain

Cathleen Schild [1], Emily A. Reed [2], Tessa Hingston [3], Catlin H. Dennis [4] and Anna C. Wilson [4],*

[1] Pacific University, Department of Clinical Psychology, Forest Grove, OR 97116, USA; schi6727@pacificu.edu
[2] Oregon State University, Department of Psychological Science, Corvallis, OR 97331, USA; emilyreed9394@gmail.com
[3] George Fox University, Department of Psychology, Newberg, OR 97132, USA; hingstot@ohsu.edu
[4] Oregon Health & Science University, Institute on Development and Disability, Department of Pediatrics, Portland, OR 97239, USA; dennica@ohsu.edu
* Correspondence: longann@ohsu.edu; Tel.: +1-503-494-0333

Academic Editor: Carl L. von Baeyer
Received: 1 September 2016; Accepted: 9 November 2016; Published: 19 November 2016

Abstract: Neighborhood features such as community socioeconomic status, recreational facilities, and parks have been correlated to the health outcomes of the residents living within those neighborhoods, especially with regard to health-related quality of life, body mass index, and physical activity. The interplay between one's built environment and one's perceptions may affect physical health, well-being, and pain experiences. In the current study, neighborhood characteristics and attitudes about physical activity were examined in a high-risk (youths with a parent with chronic pain) and low-risk (youths without a parent with chronic pain) adolescent sample. There were significant differences in neighborhood characteristics between the high-risk ($n = 62$) and low-risk ($n = 77$) samples (ages 11–15), with low-risk participants living in residences with more walkability, closer proximity to parks, and higher proportion of neighborhood residents having college degrees. Results indicate that neighborhood features (e.g., walkability and proximity to parks), as well as positive attitudes about physical activity were correlated with lower levels of pain and pain-related disability, and higher performance in physical functioning tests. These findings suggest that the built environment may contribute to pain outcomes in youth, above and beyond the influence of family history of pain.

Keywords: walkability; attitudes about physical activity; chronic pain; adolescents

1. Introduction

Neighborhood characteristics have an impact on the health outcomes of residents, in terms of health-related quality of life (HRQOL), body mass index (BMI) and the experience of chronic pain [1–3]. The accessibility of neighborhood amenities (e.g., being able to walk to the grocery store) is thought to be related to physical activity level among residents, leading to changes in health outcomes. To quantify the accessibility of neighborhood amenities, such as schools, grocery stores, and restaurants, walkability scores can be assigned to each physical address based on ease of access without a car.

Adolescents may be especially vulnerable to the effects of a neighborhood with low walkability [4]. Low walkability indicates that places of interest, including parks, schools, and stores, are not easily accessed on foot. Prior to receiving a driver's license or having other autonomous transportation options, young adults have limited access to amenities outside their neighborhood. By living in a walkable neighborhood, adolescents have more autonomy compared to those living in a less walkable neighborhood. Therefore, the accessibility of the neighborhood in which adolescents live is vital for promoting and providing outlets for adolescent physical activity.

Research exploring socioeconomic status (SES), with respect to both family and the neighborhood, has found that SES has a large effect on the resources available to lead healthy lives. Neighborhoods with a higher median SES are associated with a higher density of recreational facilities, parks and walkable pathways, and are believed to promote healthy lifestyles more than neighborhoods with a lower median SES [5]. Families with higher SES are better able to afford living in neighborhoods where there is a more developed built environment (e.g., developed sidewalks and landscaping) and more amenities. Neighborhoods that are associated with a lower socioeconomic status feature a less developed built environment (e.g., undeveloped sidewalks and fewer trees) [6], which can lead to lower activity rates, higher rates of disability and higher BMI trends over time [2]. Children and adolescents raised in underdeveloped neighborhoods are more likely to be inactive or to be overweight than those living in highly developed neighborhoods [7].

Additionally, there is a direct relationship between the experience of chronic illness and SES in the United States; people of lower SES experience more chronic illness than their more affluent counterparts [8–10]. In particular, chronic pain conditions are experienced disproportionately by people in the lowest income bracket (i.e., people that are unemployed and receiving disability) [11,12]. Therefore, because SES is related to both neighborhood amenities and to conditions such as chronic pain, it is necessary to explore the associations between the neighborhoods people live in and their risk for experiencing chronic pain.

Previously held beliefs about physical activity have also been shown to influence the activity level of adolescents. Positive attitudes about physical activity, as well as the intention to perform physical activity, were found to be consistent indicators of physical activity among adolescents [13]. The perception of having available physical activity resources is nearly as important as the resources themselves [5]. Additionally, when a neighborhood features a variety of physical activity amenities, such as parks or sport facilities, adult and adolescent residents are more likely to meet physical activity guidelines [4,5]. Having access to at least one recreational facility within walking distance significantly decreases the odds of being overweight, compared to a similar population with no access to recreational facilities [14]. Overweight and obese weight status has been associated with increased risk for a variety of chronic pain conditions, as well as increased pain and pain-related disability [15–18].

Chronic pain conditions have been found to negatively impact a child's physical activity level. Children with chronic pain exhibit a lower peak activity level, and are sedentary for more minutes a day than their healthy counterparts [19]. Lower activity levels have been associated with more perceived physical limitations among participants [19], indicating a connection between physical activity and perceived barriers to activity. Limited research has examined neighborhood level contributions to pain and related outcomes in pediatric chronic pain samples. Among youth with sickle cell disease, living in a distressed neighborhood was found to be associated with diminished physical HRQOL and increased reports of pain [1]. Thus, neighborhood level characteristics may be associated with chronic pain and related disability, particularly in high-risk samples, or in individuals who are at increased risk for pain due to the presence of comorbidities or other risk factors (e.g., low physical activity, or high BMI).

The current study has three primary aims. The first is to compare neighborhood characteristics between two parent-child samples: those in which the parent had a chronic pain condition (high-risk group) and those not impacted by parental chronic pain (low-risk group). It is well-established that youth who have a parent with pain are at increased risk for developing pain problems [20]. Differences in neighborhood characteristics associated with parental pain may confer additional risk for pain, disability, and poor physical function outcomes. It was hypothesized that high-risk youth would live in neighborhoods with lower walkability and more restricted access to recreation compared to low-risk youth. The second aim is to examine whether neighborhood level sociodemographic factors (median income, population education) contribute to child pain and disability above and beyond family socioeconomic factors (i.e., family income and parental education). The third aim is to examine the contribution of neighborhood built environment (e.g., walkability and access to recreation) and youth's attitudes about physical activity to youth pain, activity limitations, and physical function outcomes. Physical function outcomes included laboratory-based tests of physical function, and self-report of physical activity. It was hypothesized that both neighborhood-level factors and individual attitudes would contribute to outcomes, above and beyond risk group membership and BMI.

2. Materials and Methods

2.1. Participants

The data used was taken from a larger prospective study examining the impact of parental chronic pain on youth. Data from the baseline time point of the larger study was used in the current analysis. Children of parents without a chronic pain condition—the low-risk study group—was made up of parent–child dyads ($n = 77$) and children of parents with a chronic pain condition—the high-risk study group—also consisted of parent–child dyads ($n = 62$). All study procedures were approved by the institutional review board (No. IRB#00005973) at Oregon Health & Science University in Portland, Oregon.

All participants were recruited from a major metropolitan area in the Pacific Northwest of the United States. Flyers explaining the study purpose were posted in clinics that specialized in multidisciplinary chronic pain services. Potentially eligible participants were identified through the clinic medical records and then sent a flyer that advertised the current study. Healthy parents and guardians were recruited through study flyers posted in the community and the university's research website.

Inclusion criteria specified that participating parents in both groups had to have a biological child between the ages of 11 and 15 who was willing to participate. Inclusion in the chronic pain group required that parents must have had pain for a period of three months or longer, and had to be receiving specialty medical care for their pain. Parents in the healthy group were excluded if they reported historical or current chronic pain that persisted for a period of three months or longer. Parents in the healthy group were also deemed ineligible if they stated that the child's other parent (biological or a co-habiting parent, such as a step-parent) had a history of chronic pain. Additional exclusionary criteria for both groups included the presence of chronic or serious illness (e.g., cancer, or arthritis), non-fluency in English, or cognitive impairment of either the parent or child.

2.2. Procedure

Potential participants called the study phone number or provided their contact information on the study website. A telephone interview was conducted with potential participants to evaluate both inclusion and exclusion criteria, verbal consent was attained, and a study visit was scheduled for data collection. Of the families who completed phone screens, three failed the screen because the child in the target age range was not a biological child (adopted or other biological relation). Two families were excluded from the healthy sample due to a biological parent having a history of chronic pain. During the phone screens, no participants declined participation; however, three families were not enrolled post-phone screen due to scheduling conflicts and illness. During the study visit written consent was attained from parents and assent was attained from child participants. Parents and children completed pain and physical activity questionnaires via REDCap (Research Electronic Data Capture), a secure web-based computerized survey system used for collecting and managing study data [21]. Children participated in standardized tests of physical function and had their height and weight taken during the study visit. Parent and child participants were compensated for participation in the form of a gift card to a local store.

2.3. Measures

2.3.1. Sociodemographic Characteristics

Parent participants reported on individual items assessing sociodemographic characteristics, including parent and child ethnicity and racial background, parent education level, parent marital status, and family income. Parents also reported on their child's sex and date of birth, and on their own sex and date of birth, as well as residential address. Birth dates were used to calculate ages of participants on the date of visit.

2.3.2. Pain Characteristics

Adolescents were asked to describe pain characteristics of the last three months using a pain questionnaire. Children reported on pain location(s), frequency, and usual pain intensity. Pain location was marked on a validated body outline and pain location followed the nine standardized body regions identified by Lester and colleagues [22]. Pain frequency items are based on questionnaire items used in the World Health Organization's survey on health behaviors in school-age children [23], which have been used to assess pain frequency in this age group [24]. Adolescents were asked to report pain frequency in the past three months with close-ended response options ranging from 0 (never) to 6 (daily). Adolescents were asked to report how much pain they usually have from aches and pains; usual pain intensity was reported using a 10-point Numeric Rating Scale (NRS; 0–10), ranging from 0 (No Pain) to 10 (Worst Pain Possible) [25,26].

2.3.3. Pain-Related Activity Limitations

Adolescents reported on pain-related activity limitations using the Children's Activity Limitation Interview (CALI-21), a 21-item inventory of perceived difficulty with activities of daily living because of pain. Each activity was rated on a 5-point scale (0–4), where 0 represented no difficulty and 4 represented extreme difficulty. Higher scores indicate a greater perceived impairment. The CALI-21 has excellent internal consistency, and moderate test–retest and cross–informant reliability [27,28].

2.3.4. Self-Report of Physical Activity

Adolescent self-reports of physical activity were assessed using the International Physical Activity Questionnaire (IPAQ-7). Adolescents reported on physical activity undertaken across various domains including moderate and vigorous exercise, walking and sitting, and transport-related activity in the last seven days. The IPAQ-7 provides time spent in physical activity of different intensities. This time is then multiplied by multiples of the resting metabolic rate (METS), which measure typical energy expenditure at the various physical activity intensity levels. This 7-item questionnaire has adequate reliability and has been validated with objective measures of energy expenditure in adolescents [29,30]. The total MET-minutes per week score was used in the current analyses.

2.3.5. Attitudes about Physical Activity

Adolescent self-reports of attitudes about physical activity were assessed using the Attitudes about Physical Activity-Child Report (APA-C). The APA-C is a 14-item questionnaire that assesses negative and positive attitudes toward activity. Each item was rated on a 5-point scale (1–5), where 1 represented disagree a lot and 5 represented agree a lot. This questionnaire has good reliability and validity [31].

2.3.6. Body Mass Index (BMI)

Child height (centimeters) and weight (kilograms) were taken by trained research assistants at the study visit. BMI percentile for exact age was calculated using height, weight, date of birth and date of measurement via the Center for Disease Control's online pediatric BMI calculator [32]. BMI percentile was used in the current study.

2.3.7. Tests of Physical Function

Trained research assistants administered tests of physical function. A standardized, scripted set of instructions was given to each participant. Adolescents were asked to complete a sit-to-stand test that requires sitting in a chair with feet on the ground and knees at approximately a 90 degree angle. From a seated position, participants stood up and sat back down as quickly as possible for a 1-minute period. A trained research assistant recorded how many times each participant completed a full sit-to-stand motion. The sit-to-stand task is a commonly used test of physical function and is associated with exercise capacity, functional balance, and physical health-related quality of life [33–35].

Each participant also completed a timed 10-meter walk. They were instructed to walk a distance of 10 meters as quickly as possible. A trained research assistant timed how long it took for the walk to be completed in minutes and seconds. Timed fast walk performance tests are used frequently for assessing walk speed and other gait characteristics in children and adults, and norms based on age are available [36–38].

2.3.8. Neighborhood Characteristics

Walkability

Individual residential street addresses were used to obtain a Walk Score (Walk Score, Seattle, WA, USA) for each participating dyad. Walk Score is a patented methodology that uses data from a variety of sources, including online map systems, USA Census data, and information from educational databases to analyze walking routes to a variety of amenities from a given street address. Scores are assigned into five categories based on their position in a hierarchy, ranging from very car dependent (scores from 0 to 24) to walker's paradise (scores from 90 to 100) on a continuous 0–100 scale. In the lower-scored categories, transportation is needed to complete most or all errands outside the home. In the higher-scored categories, most errand locations (e.g., stores, schools, or recreation facilities) are within walking distance. Increasing Walk Score indicates that the corresponding location is closer to amenities [39]. This methodology has been validated in a number of metropolitan areas [40]. The continuous Walk Score was used in the current analyses.

Proximity to Parks

The Walk Score program also provides an exact distance (in miles) from each participant's street address to the nearest park or public greenspace. For the purposes of this study, this distance was coded into a Park Score ranging from 0 to 2, with higher scores indicating closer proximity to parks, as follows: an address with a park within 0.5 miles was assigned a Park Score of 2, an address with a park between 0.5 miles and 1 mile away was assigned a Park Score of 1, and if the nearest park or recreational facility was located more than 1 mile away from a participant's address it was assigned a Park Score of 0.

Census Neighborhood Data

The United States Census database (i.e., Census-Explorer, maintained by the USA Census Bureau, USA Department of Commerce, Economics & Statistics Administration, Suitland, MD, USA) was used to obtain demographic information about participants' neighborhoods. Using Census-Explorer, participant addresses were entered and neighborhood level demographic information (percent of residents below poverty level, median income, percent college graduates) was extracted. This census tract-level information was obtained for each participant's primary residential address to characterize the sociodemographic characteristics of the adolescent's neighborhood.

2.4. Analyses

All analyses were conducted using IBM SPSS Statistics version 22.0 (IBM Corporation, Armonk, NY, USA). All data were screened for normality, appropriate ranges, and univariate outliers prior to performing analyses. Descriptive statistics were performed to characterize the sample. Independent samples *t*-tests were performed to examine potential group differences in neighborhood characteristics between the high-risk and low-risk groups. Multiple linear regressions were used to test whether median income and percent college graduates (neighborhood level sociodemographic factors) contribute to child pain and disability, above and beyond family income and parental education (family socioeconomic factors) and risk group. Multiple linear regressions were then performed to examine the contribution of neighborhood built environment (e.g., park proximity and Walk Score) and youth's positive and negative attitudes about physical activity to pain, disability, and physical function outcomes, after controlling for risk group and BMI. Physical function outcomes included lab-based tests of physical function and self-report of physical activity.

3. Results

3.1. Descriptive Statistics

The sample consisted of adolescents from the high-risk group ($n = 77$) and low-risk group ($n = 62$). Mean age of the adolescent participants was 13.44 years (Standard deviation (SD) = 1.47), and 59.7% of the sample was female. The majority of participating adolescents reported Caucasian racial background (82.7%), with others reporting mixed race (10.8%), African American (3.6%), Asian (2.1%), and American Indian/Alaska Native (0.7%) racial background. A minority of the sample reported Hispanic ethnicity (7.2%). The high-risk and low-risk groups did not differ from each other on age, sex, ethnicity, or race.

3.2. Neighborhood Characteristics between High-Risk and Low-Risk Adolescents

Independent sample *t*-tests were used to compare the high-risk group to the low-risk group on the following neighborhood characteristics: Walk Score, percent below poverty level, median household income, and percent college graduates (see Table 1). There was a difference in the park scores between the groups, with the low-risk group having a significantly higher park score; $t(134) = 2.43$, $p = 0.016$. Additionally, there was a difference in the Walk Score for the groups, with the low-risk group having significantly higher scores; $t(134) = 3.70$, $p < 0.001$. There was also a significant difference found in the neighborhood percentage of college degrees, with the high-risk group having a lower percentage of college degrees than the low-risk group; $t(135) = 2.51$, $p = 0.013$. The percentage of the neighborhood population in poverty and neighborhood median income was not significantly different between study groups.

3.3. Contribution of Neighborhood Sociodemographic Factors to Child Pain and Disability

A multiple regression analysis was performed to evaluate the extent to which neighborhood level sociodemographic factors (i.e., median income, or percent college graduates) contributed to child pain and disability above and beyond family level sociodemographic factors (e.g., family income and parental education). Contrary to hypotheses, the analyses showed that after accounting for the significant effect of risk group, no family or neighborhood level income or education variables contributed significantly to adolescent pain intensity, pain frequency, or pain-related activity limitations. The study risk group was a significant predictor of pain intensity ($\beta = 0.28$, $p = 0.006$), pain frequency ($\beta = 0.29$, $p = 0.003$), and pain-related activity limitations ($\beta = 0.40$, $p < 0.001$), with high-risk group status being associated with increased pain and activity limitations.

3.4. Contribution of Walkability, Distance to Parks, and Attitudes about Physical Activity

Models of these adolescent outcomes included the same three steps. The first step included study risk group and BMI percentile, the second step included neighborhood walkability and proximity to parks, and the third step included adolescent positive and negative attitudes about physical activity. In a multiple regression model predicting adolescent's usual pain intensity, negative attitudes about physical activity contributed significantly to higher usual pain intensity scores after controlling for study group, which also made a significant contribution. Overall, this model accounted for 20.2% of the variance in pain intensity scores (see Table 2). In a model predicting adolescent's usual pain frequency, study group contributed significantly with the high-risk group having more frequent pain at entry in the model. Proximity to parks was also associated with pain frequency, such that closer proximity to parks (as assessed by park score) was related to lower pain frequency scores. In the final step of the model, higher negative attitudes about physical activity were significantly associated with increased pain frequency. Overall, this model accounted for 31.3% of the variance in pain frequency (see Table 3).

In a model predicting pain-related activity limitations, study group made a significant contribution with the high risk group reporting higher activity limitations. After controlling for group status and BMI percentile, proximity to parks also contributed significantly to activity limitations. Closer proximity to parks was associated with decreased activity limitations. Negative attitudes about physical activity also made a significant contribution to activity limitations in the final step of the model, such that increasing negative attitudes were associated with increasing activity limitations. Overall, this model accounted for 39.9% of the variance in activity limitations scores (see Table 4).

Results from a model predicting adolescents' sit-to-stand performance scores showed that study group was associated with performance in the first two steps of the model, such that the high risk group completed fewer sit-to-stand motions during the task. BMI percentile was also associated with task performance such that youth with higher BMI percentile completed fewer sit-to-stand movements. Neighborhood walkability and proximity to parks did not contribute to performance on this task. However, in the final step of the model, negative attitudes about physical activity were associated with performance such that more negative attitudes were related to poorer sit-to-stand task performance. Overall, this model accounted for 21.5% of the variance in sit-to-stand performance (see Table 5).

In a model predicting timed 10 m walk performance, the high-risk group demonstrated significantly slower walk times. Additionally, neighborhood walkability contributed to walk times such that higher neighborhood walkability was associated with better performance in this task. In the final step of the model, positive attitudes about physical activity were significantly associated with shorter walk times, while negative attitudes about physical activity were significantly associated with longer walk times. Overall, this model accounted for 18.0% of the variance in 10 m walk time (see Table 6).

Contrary to hypotheses, none of the variables entered in the regression model predicting total MET minutes were associated with this self-report measure of physical activity.

Table 1. Neighborhood characteristics: Comparison between high-risk and low-risk adolescents.

	High-Risk		Low-Risk		Mean Difference	95% Confidence Interval	d	t	p Value
	Mean	Standard Deviation	Mean	Standard Deviation					
Walk Score	34.27	23.4	49.61	24.54	15.34	7.13, 23.55	0.64	3.694 **	<0.001
Park Score	1.49	0.77	1.76	0.52	0.27	0.50, 0.49	0.41	2.430 *	0.016
Percent Below Poverty Level	15.86	7.27	15.94	7.78	0.08	−2.49, 2.65	0.01	0.063	0.950
Median Household Income ($)	73,446.74	21,643.12	73,103.51	18,152.98	−343.23	−7092.41, 6405.95	0.02	−0.101	0.920
Percent College Graduates	21.74	9.01	25.24	7.31	3.50	0.74, 6.26	0.43	2.511 *	0.013

* $p < 0.05$, ** $p < 0.001$.

Table 2. Multiple regression model of adolescent usual pain intensity.

Variable	Step 1			Step 2			Step 3		
	Unstandardized		Standardized	Unstandardized		Standardized	Unstandardized		Standardized
	B	SE B	β	B	SE B	β	B	SE B	β
Group [a]	0.888	0.301	0.259 *	1.0006	0.319	0.293 *	0.818	0.309	0.239 *
Body Mass Index (BMI)	0.006	0.005	0.104	0.007	0.005	0.112	0.005	0.005	0.089
Park Score				−0.252	0.247	−0.097	−0.098	0.240	−0.038
Walk Score				0.011	0.007	0.160	0.010	0.006	0.154
Positive PA Attitudes							0.007	0.037	0.016
Negative PA Attitudes							0.097	0.026	0.322 *
R^2	0.084			0.106			0.202		
F change for R^2	5.498 **			1.439			6.997 ***		
Total Model F							4.89 ***		

* $p < 0.05$, ** $p < 0.01$, *** $p < 0.001$; [a] Coded as 0 = low risk, 1 = high risk; PA: physical activity.

Table 3. Multiple regression model of child usual pain frequency.

Variable	Step 1			Step 2			Step 3		
	Unstandardized		Standardized	Unstandardized		Standardized	Unstandardized		Standardized
	B	SE B	β	B	SE B	β	B	SE B	β
Group [a]	0.759	0.255	0.260 *	0.662	0.264	0.226 *	0.475	0.244	0.162 *
BMI	0.007	0.004	0.145	0.008	0.004	0.158	0.006	0.004	0.128
Park Score				−0.599	0.204	−0.269 *	−0.467	0.190	−0.210 *
Walk Score				0.003	0.005	0.059	0.002	0.005	0.038
Positive PA Attitudes							0.049	0.029	0.130
Negative PA Attitudes							0.097	0.021	0.379 ***
R^2	0.097			0.159			0.313		
F change for R^2	6.444 **			4.380 *			12.937 ***		
Total Model F							8.796 ***		

* $p < 0.05$, ** $p < 0.01$, *** $p < 0.001$; [a] Coded as 0 = low risk, 1 = high risk.

Table 4. Multiple regression model of child activity limitations.

Variable	Step 1			Step 2			Step 3		
	Unstandardized		Standardized	Unstandardized		Standardized	Unstandardized		Standardized
	B	SE B	β	B	SE B	β	B	SE B	β
Group [a]	7.218	1.583	0.385 ***	7.292	1.630	0.389 ***	5.896	1.462	0.315 ***
BMI	0.013	0.027	0.039	0.018	0.026	0.055	0.008	0.023	0.024
Park Score				−3.822	1.260	−0.268 *	−2.693	1.138	−0.189 *
Walk Score				0.063	0.034	0.171	0.059	0.030	0.162
Positive PA Attitudes							0.075	0.176	0.031
Negative PA Attitudes							0.719	0.123	0.439 ***
R^2	0.154			0.219			0.399		
F change for R^2	10.887 ***			4.972 **			17.326 ***		
Total Model F							12.831 ***		

* $p < 0.05$, ** $p < 0.01$, *** $p < 0.001$; [a] Coded as 0 = low risk, 1 = high risk.

Table 5. Multiple regression model of sit-to-stand test.

Variable	Step 1			Step 2			Step 3		
	Unstandardized		Standardized	Unstandardized		Standardized	Unstandardized		Standardized
	B	SE B	β	B	SE B	β	B	SE B	β
Group [a]	−3.933	1.572	−0.209 *	−4.164	1.678	−0.222 *	−3.058	1.623	−0.163
BMI	−0.080	0.027	−0.246 *	−0.080	0.027	−0.247 *	−0.078	0.026	−0.240 *
Park Score				0.488	1.333	0.034	−0.345	1.287	−0.024
Walk Score				−0.024	0.035	−0.064	−0.034	0.033	−0.091
Positive PA Attitudes							0.352	0.190	0.150
Negative PA Attitudes							−0.452	0.132	−0.284 **
R^2	0.116			0.119			0.215		
F change for R^2	8.407 **			0.242			7.561 **		
Total Model F							5.667 **		

* $p < 0.05$, ** $p < 0.001$; [a] Coded as 0 = low-risk, 1 = high-risk.

Table 6. Multiple regression of 10-meter walk time.

Variable	Step 1			Step 2			Step 3		
	Unstandardized		Standardized	Unstandardized		Standardized	Unstandardized		Standardized
	B	SE B	β	B	SE B	β	B	SE B	β
Group [a]	0.427	0.162	0.225 *	0.496	0.171	0.261 *	0.412	0.168	0.217 *
BMI	0.005	0.003	0.152	0.005	0.003	0.155	0.005	0.003	0.154
Park Score				−0.139	0.136	−0.095	−0.074	0.133	−0.050
Walk Score				0.007	0.004	0.186	0.008	0.003	0.218 *
Positive PA Attitudes							−0.048	0.020	−0.201 *
Negative PA Attitudes							0.030	0.014	0.186 *
R^2	0.081			0.110			0.180		
F change for R^2	5.675 **			2.005			5.317 **		
Total Model F							4.539		

* $p < 0.05$, ** $p < 0.01$; [a] Coded as 0 = low-risk, 1 = high-risk.

4. Discussion

The current study found some support for the hypothesis that youth at increased risk for chronic pain, due to family history, experience different neighborhood characteristics. Low-risk adolescents were more likely than their high-risk counterparts to live in walkable neighborhoods, have nearby parks, and have a larger proportion of college graduates in their neighborhood. This supports the idea that having a parent with a chronic pain condition likely represents a complex set of risk factors. A recently published model of the intergenerational transmission of pain proposes genetic, neurobiological, psychological, behavioral, stress, and health mechanisms of risk for chronic pain in the offspring of youth [41]. The results of the current study provide some initial support for neighborhood characteristics differing in high-risk youth, suggesting that factors outside of the immediate family environment may also play a role, or further contribute to children's stress or poor health.

Additionally, these neighborhood level characteristics, specifically proximity to parks and walkability, contributed to pain frequency, pain-related activity limitations and a lab-based test of physical function, above the effect of study group status and BMI percentile. This suggests that the built environment may contribute additional unique variance to these outcomes. This could be related to increased or decreased levels of physical activity based on available outlets. Higher neighborhood walkability was associated with elevated performance on the timed 10 m walk test, such that adolescents living in more walkable neighborhoods walked at a quicker pace in the laboratory. This was above and beyond the contribution of study group and BMI. Previous research on neighborhood walkability has demonstrated that increased walkability of the neighborhood is associated with individual's likelihood to walk for daily transportation, and reduces risk for individuals being overweight or obese [42]. Additionally, moving to a neighborhood with a 10-point increase in walkability leads to increased walking and decreased BMI [43], suggesting that these neighborhood characteristics have the potential to change important health behaviors and health indicators. Regular exercise or lack thereof may contribute directly to pain symptoms, perceived activity limitations, and physical function. For instance, recent research has demonstrated that aerobic exercise prior to surgery is associated with reduced pain after surgery [44], suggesting that regular exercise may be protective against the development of chronic pain. Among adolescents, the regular exercise that is associated with the built environment might also be associated with reduced pain. In the current study, closer proximity to parks was associated with lower pain frequency and lower pain-related activity limitations, indicating that there may be a relationship between the availability of parks or greenspace and the perceived limitations that an adolescent experiences due to pain. In addition to the exercise opportunities provided by parks and green spaces, access to green space has been associated with reduced psychological distress [45]. Psychological distress (e.g., depression, anxiety) plays an important role in pain persistence and pain-related disability among children and adolescents [46–48], and proximity to parks may make additional contributions to psychological function.

Negative attitudes about physical activity were associated with both physical functioning tests and experience of pain in the current study. Participants with more negative attitudes about physical activity scored lower on the physical functioning tests, and higher on perceived activity limitations (CALI-21). Negative attitudes about physical activity were correlated with longer timed 10 m walks, and poorer performance in the sit-to-stand test. Inversely, positivity about physical activity is correlated with a shorter timed 10 m walk. These results are consistent with past research that activity level is predicted by attitudes toward activity [13]. It appears that attitudes about physical activity influence the pace or eagerness of engaging in physical activity, even in a laboratory setting. The correlation between CALI-21 scores and negative attitudes about physical activity suggests that negative attitudes about physical activity may lead adolescents to perceive themselves as more limited in their ability to do activities because of pain. Participants with negative attitudes about physical activity were more likely to have more frequent and more intense pain. An individual that experiences frequent and intense pain is likely to have negative feelings about physical activity in the event that such activity exacerbates the pain. Contrary to prior research with youth with chronic pain [15], BMI was not a significant predictor of perceived activity limitations; however, higher BMI was associated with decreased ability to perform activity tasks. The discrepancy with prior literature could be explained by the difference in sample, with previous literature focusing primarily on children with chronic pain conditions and the current study examining a non-clinical sample of children.

Overall, group membership was strongly associated with the majority of the dependent variables that were analyzed in this study. This finding provides further support for past literature indicating that there is a strong relationship between parental chronic pain and chronic pain in adolescent offspring [20]. Being a member of the low-risk group alone was associated with decreased pain intensity, frequency, and perceived activity limitations in this sample. This study adds to the literature in terms of our understanding of the impact of parental chronic pain on offspring physical functioning, as the high-risk group in the current sample demonstrated poorer physical function on performance tests.

Contrary to hypotheses, neither family nor neighborhood-level SES variables were significantly associated with pain or activity limitations after accounting for study group. This finding may indicate that having a parent with chronic pain represents a significant risk factor in itself, and this risk may account for or include SES factors. The study also did not find support for parental chronic pain or any neighborhood characteristics predicting youth self-report of physical activity. Assessment of physical activity via self-report may be problematic in this age group, or this measure may be systematically biased in the high-risk group. Future studies might include objective measures of physical activity such as actigraphy [19,49].

The current study adds to our understanding of the potential role that the neighborhood and built environment might play in increasing or decreasing risk for pain, activity limitations, and physical function. Overall, the models tested in the current study accounted for approximately 18% to 40% of the variance in outcomes, with the built environment variables being significant in a number of models. Findings of this study support the upstream public health concept that built environments can play a pivotal role in the health of its residents [50]. Additionally, this study provides information about how specific environmental characteristics are associated with functioning, which can better inform caregivers and medical providers in facilitating achievement of optimal success in pain-reduction and pain-management [50]. Findings from this study suggest that increasing accessibility to parks and greenspaces and shifting attitudes surrounding physical activity may result in decreased pain and reduced psychological distress, which should be examined in future longitudinal studies. The study had several strengths, including the use of individual address-based data about neighborhood walkability and proximity to parks (vs. relying on participant self-report of neighborhood features). The use of objective measures of physical function is also a strength.

Future research should focus on further delineating how patients' built environments around their homes can affect their recovery and ability to strive for optimal health. Additionally, longitudinal research would increase knowledge of temporal relationships and changes over time. It will also be important to test more complex models of associations among predictors and outcomes in longitudinal data sets, including mediation models. For instance, it is possible that the built environment influences attitudes, which in turn impact health behaviors and pain outcomes. Future studies might examine these kinds of complex models over time.

There are several limitations that should be kept in mind when interpreting these results. First and foremost, the data is cross-sectional, and as such no inference about directionality or causality of the observed associations can be made. Studies examining this topic have not been longitudinal, which precludes research in this area from commenting on pain development. Additionally, the relatively small sample size likely limited the statistical power and ability to detect smaller effect sizes.

5. Conclusions

The current study adds to our understanding of the role that neighborhood features may play in adolescent pain and related functioning. Neighborhood characteristics appear to influence increasing or decreasing risk for pain, activity limitations, and physical function. Adolescents at a lower risk for developing chronic pain were more likely to live in walkable neighborhoods, have nearby parks, and have a larger proportion of college graduates in their neighborhood. These neighborhood level characteristics relate to pain frequency, pain-related activity limitations, and a laboratory-based test of physical function, above the effect of study group status and BMI percentile, suggesting that the built environment may contribute additional unique variance to these outcomes. Negative attitudes about physical activity also made important contributions to pain characteristics and other outcomes. Future studies of risk for chronic pain should consider including assessment of neighborhood characteristics.

Acknowledgments: This study was funded by the National Institute of Health and the Eunice Kennedy Shriver National Institute of Child Health and Human Development (No. K23HD064705); the principal investigator of the project was Dr. Anna C. Wilson.

Author Contributions: C.S. contributed to the conceptualization of the project, data analysis, and writing of the manuscript; E.A.R. and T.H. contributed to data extraction, data analysis, and writing of the manuscript; C.H.D. contributed to data extraction and writing and editing of the manuscript; A.C.W. contributed to conceptualization of the project, data analysis, writing and editing of the manuscript.

Conflicts of Interest: The authors declare no conflict of interest. The founding sponsors had no role in the design of the study; in the collection, analyses, and interpretation of data; in the writing of the manuscript, nor in the decision to publish the results.

References

1. Palermo, T.M.; Riley, C.A.; Mitchell, B.A. Daily functioning and quality of life in children with sickle cell disease pain: Relationship with family and neighborhood socioeconomic distress. *J. Pain* **2008**, *9*, 833–840. [CrossRef] [PubMed]
2. Duncan, D.T.; Sharifi, M.; Melly, S.J.; Marshall, R.; Sequist, T.D.; Rifas-Shiman, S.L.; Taveras, E.M. Characteristics of walkable built environments and BMI z-scores in children: evidence from a large electronic health record database. *Environ. Health Perspect.* **2014**, *122*, 1359–1365. [CrossRef] [PubMed]
3. Roth-Isigkeit, A.; Thyen, U.; Stoven, H.; Schwarzenberger, J.; Schmucker, P. Pain among children and adolescents: Restrictions in daily living and triggering factors. *Pediatrics* **2005**, *115*, e152–e162. [CrossRef] [PubMed]
4. De Meester, F.; Van Dyck, D.; De Bourdeaudhuij, I.; Deforche, B.; Sallis, J.F.; Cardon, G. Active living neighborhoods: Is neighborhood walkability a key element for Belgian adolescents? *BMC Public Health* **2012**, *12*, 7. [CrossRef] [PubMed]
5. Sallis, J.F.; Floyd, M.F.; Rodriguez, D.A.; Saelens, B.E. Role of built environments in physical activity, obesity, and cardiovascular disease. *Circulation* **2012**, *125*, 729–737. [CrossRef] [PubMed]
6. Beard, J.R.; Blaney, S.; Cerda, M.; Frye, V.; Lovasi, G.S.; Ompad, D.; Rundle, A.; Vlahov, D. Neighborhood characteristics and disability in older adults. *J. Gerontol. B Psychol. Sci. Soc. Sci.* **2009**, *64*, 252–257. [CrossRef] [PubMed]
7. Singh, G.K.; Siahpush, M.; Kogan, M.D. Neighborhood socioeconomic conditions, built environments, and childhood obesity. *Health Aff. (Project Hope)* **2010**, *29*, 503–512. [CrossRef] [PubMed]
8. Andersson, H.I.; Ejlertsson, G.; Leden, I.; Rosenberg, C. Chronic pain in a geographically defined general population: Studies of differences in age, gender, social class, and pain localization. *Clin. J. Pain* **1993**, *9*, 174–182. [CrossRef] [PubMed]
9. Spilsbury, J.C.; Storfer-Isser, A.; Kirchner, H.L.; Nelson, L.; Rosen, C.L.; Drotar, D.; Redline, S. Neighborhood disadvantage as a risk factor for pediatric obstructive sleep apnea. *J. Pediatr.* **2006**, *149*, 342–347. [CrossRef] [PubMed]
10. Diez Roux, A.V.; Merkin, S.S.; Arnett, D.; Chambless, L.; Massing, M.; Nieto, F.J.; Sorlie, P.; Szklo, M.; Tyroler, H.A.; Watson, R.L. Neighborhood of residence and incidence of coronary heart disease. *N. Engl. J. Med.* **2001**, *345*, 99–106. [CrossRef] [PubMed]
11. Johannes, C.B.; Le, T.K.; Zhou, X.; Johnston, J.A.; Dworkin, R.H. The prevalence of chronic pain in United States adults: Results of an Internet-based survey. *J. Pain* **2010**, *11*, 1230–1239. [CrossRef] [PubMed]
12. Fuentes, M.; Hart-Johnson, T.; Green, C.R. The association among neighborhood socioeconomic status, race and chronic pain in black and white older adults. *J. Natl. Med. Assoc.* **2007**, *99*, 1160–1169. [PubMed]

13. Sallis, J.F.; Prochaska, J.J.; Taylor, W.C. A review of correlates of physical activity of children and adolescents. *Med. Sci. Sports Exerc.* **2000**, *32*, 963–975. [CrossRef] [PubMed]
14. Gordon-Larsen, P.; Nelson, M.C.; Page, P.; Popkin, B.M. Inequality in the built environment underlies key health disparities in physical activity and obesity. *Pediatrics* **2006**, *117*, 417–424. [CrossRef] [PubMed]
15. Wilson, A.C.; Samuelson, B.; Palermo, T.M. Obesity in children and adolescents with chronic pain: Associations with pain and activity limitations. *Clin. J. Pain* **2010**, *26*, 705–711. [CrossRef] [PubMed]
16. Hainsworth, K.R.; Davies, W.H.; Khan, K.A.; Weisman, S.J. Co-occurring chronic pain and obesity in children and adolescents: The impact on health-related quality of life. *Clin. J. Pain* **2009**, *25*, 715–721. [CrossRef] [PubMed]
17. Hershey, A.D.; Powers, S.W.; Nelson, T.D.; Kabbouche, M.A.; Winner, P.; Yonker, M.; Linder, S.L.; Bicknese, A.; Sowel, M.K.; McClintock, W. Obesity in the pediatric headache population: A multicenter study. *Headache* **2009**, *49*, 170–177. [CrossRef] [PubMed]
18. Smith, S.M.; Sumar, B.; Dixon, K.A. Musculoskeletal pain in overweight and obese children. *Int. J. Obes. (Lond.)* **2014**, *38*, 11–15. [CrossRef] [PubMed]
19. Wilson, A.C.; Palermo, T.M. Physical activity and function in adolescents with chronic pain: A controlled study using actigraphy. *J. Pain* **2012**, *13*, 121–130. [CrossRef] [PubMed]
20. Higgins, K.S.; Birnie, K.A.; Chambers, C.T.; Wilson, A.C.; Caes, L.; Clark, A.J.; Lynch, M.; Stinson, J.; Campbell-Yeo, M. Offspring of parents with chronic pain: A systematic review and meta-analysis of pain, health, psychological, and family outcomes. *Pain* **2015**, *156*, 2256–2266. [CrossRef] [PubMed]
21. Harris, P.A.; Taylor, R.; Thielke, R.; Payne, J.; Gonzalez, N.; Conde, J.G. Research electronic data capture (REDCap)—A metadata-driven methodology and workflow process for providing translational research informatics support. *J. Biomed. Inform.* **2009**, *42*, 377–381. [CrossRef] [PubMed]
22. Lester, N.; Lefebvre, J.C.; Keefe, F.J. Pain in young adults: I. Relationship to gender and family pain history. *Clin. J. Pain* **1994**, *10*, 282–289. [CrossRef] [PubMed]
23. Currie, C.; Samdal, O.; Boyce, W.; Smith, R. *Health Behaviour in School-Aged Children: A WHO Cross-National Study (HBSC): Research Protocol for the 2001/2002 Survey*; Child and Adolescent Research Unit, University of Edinburgh: Edinburgh, UK, 2001.
24. Stanford, E.A.; Chambers, C.T.; Biesanz, J.C.; Chen, E. The frequency, trajectories and predictors of adolescent recurrent pain: A population-based approach. *Pain* **2008**, *138*, 11–21. [CrossRef] [PubMed]
25. Palermo, T.M.; Valenzuela, D.; Stork, P.P. A randomized trial of electronic versus paper pain diaries in children: Impact on compliance, accuracy, and acceptability. *Pain* **2004**, *107*, 213–219. [CrossRef] [PubMed]
26. Peterson, C.C.; Palermo, T.M. Parental reinforcement of recurrent pain: The moderating impact of child depression and anxiety on functional disability. *J. Pediatr. Psychol.* **2004**, *29*, 331–341. [CrossRef] [PubMed]
27. Palermo, T.M.; Lewandowski, A.S.; Long, A.C.; Burant, C.J. Validation of a self-report questionnaire version of the Child Activity Limitations Interview (CALI): The CALI-21. *Pain* **2008**, *139*, 644–652. [CrossRef] [PubMed]
28. Palermo, T.M.; Witherspoon, D.; Valenzuela, D.; Drotar, D. Development and validation of the Child Activity Limitations Interview: A measure of pain-related functional impairment in school-age children and adolescents. *Pain* **2004**, *109*, 461–470. [CrossRef] [PubMed]
29. Arvidsson, D.; Slinde, F.; Hulthen, L. Physical activity questionnaire for adolescents validated against doubly labelled water. *Eur. J. Clin. Nutr.* **2005**, *59*, 376–383. [CrossRef] [PubMed]
30. Craig, C.L.; Marshall, A.L.; Sjostrom, M.; Bauman, A.E.; Booth, M.L.; Ainsworth, B.E.; Pratt, M.; Ekelund, U.; Yngve, A.; Sallis, J.F.; et al. International physical activity questionnaire: 12-country reliability and validity. *Med. Sci. Sports Exerc.* **2003**, *35*, 1381–1395. [CrossRef] [PubMed]
31. Nelson, T.D.; Benson, E.R.; Jensen, C.D. Negative attitudes toward physical activity: Measurement and role in predicting physical activity levels among preadolescents. *J. Pediatr. Psychol.* **2010**, *35*, 89–98. [CrossRef] [PubMed]
32. Control, C.F.D. BMI Calculator for Child and teen: English Version. Available online: http://apps.nccd.cdc.gove/dnpabmi/calculator.aspx (accessed on 1 February 2008).
33. Radtke, T.; Puhan, M.A.; Hebestreit, H.; Kriemler, S. The 1-min sit-to-stand test—A simple functional capacity test in cystic fibrosis? *J. Cyst. Fibros.* **2016**, *15*, 223–226. [CrossRef] [PubMed]
34. Kumban, W.; Amatachaya, S.; Emasithi, A.; Siritaratiwat, W. Five-times-sit-to-stand test in children with cerebral palsy: Reliability and concurrent validity. *NeuroRehabilitation* **2013**, *32*, 9–15. [PubMed]

35. Jones, C.J.; Rikli, R.E.; Beam, W.C. A 30-s chair-stand test as a measure of lower body strength in community-residing older adults. *Res. Q. Exerc. Sport* **1999**, *70*, 113–119. [CrossRef] [PubMed]

36. Lythgo, N.; Wilson, C.; Galea, M. Basic gait and symmetry measures for primary school-aged children and young adults. II: Walking at slow, free and fast speed. *Gait Posture* **2011**, *33*, 29–35. [CrossRef] [PubMed]

37. Thompson, P.; Beath, T.; Bell, J.; Jacobson, G.; Phair, T.; Salbach, N.M.; Wright, F.V. Test-retest reliability of the 10-metre fast walk test and 6-minute walk test in ambulatory school-aged children with cerebral palsy. *Dev. Med. Child. Neurol.* **2008**, *50*, 370–376. [CrossRef] [PubMed]

38. Graham, J.E.; Ostir, G.V.; Fisher, S.R.; Ottenbacher, K.J. Assessing walking speed in clinical research: A systematic review. *J. Eval. Clin. Pract.* **2008**, *14*, 552–562. [CrossRef] [PubMed]

39. Tuckel, P.; Milczarski, W. Walk Score (TM), Perceived Neighborhood Walkability, and walking in the US. *Am. J. Health Behav.* **2015**, *39*, 242–256. [CrossRef] [PubMed]

40. Duncan, D.T.; Aldstadt, J.; Whalen, J.; Melly, S.J.; Gortmaker, S.L. Validation of Walk Score® for estimating neighborhood walkability: An analysis of four US metropolitan areas. *Int. J. Environ. Res. Public Health* **2011**, *8*, 4160–4179. [CrossRef] [PubMed]

41. Stone, A.L.; Wilson, A.C. Transmission of risk from parents with chronic pain to offspring: An integrative conceptual model. *Pain* **2016**, *157*, 2628–2639. [CrossRef] [PubMed]

42. Smith, K.R.; Brown, B.B.; Yamada, I.; Kowaleski-Jones, L.; Zick, C.D.; Fan, J.X. Walkability and body mass index. *Am. J. Prev. Med.* **2008**, *35*, 237–244. [CrossRef] [PubMed]

43. Hirsch, J.A.; Diez Roux, A.V.; Moore, K.A.; Evenson, K.R.; Rodriguez, D.A. Change in walking and body mass index following residential relocation: The multi-ethnic study of atherosclerosis. *Am. J. Public Health* **2014**, *104*, e49–e56. [CrossRef] [PubMed]

44. Vaegter, H.B.; Handberg, G.; Emmeluth, C.; Graven-Nielsen, T. Preoperative hypoalgesia after cold pressor test and aerobic exercise is associated with pain relief six months after total knee replacement. *Clin. J. Pain* **2016**, in press. [CrossRef] [PubMed]

45. Pope, D.; Tisdall, R.; Middleton, J.; Verma, A.; van Ameijden, E.; Birt, C.; Macherianakis, A.; Bruce, N.G. Quality of and access to green space in relation to psychological distress: Results from a population-based cross-sectional study as part of the EURO-URHIS 2 project. *Eur. J. Public Health* **2015**. [CrossRef] [PubMed]

46. Tran, S.T.; Jastrowski Mano, K.E.; Hainsworth, K.R.; Medrano, G.R.; Anderson Khan, K.; Weisman, S.J.; Davies, W.H. Distinct influences of anxiety and pain catastrophizing on functional outcomes in children and adolescents with chronic pain. *J. Pediatr. Psychol.* **2015**, *40*, 744–755. [CrossRef] [PubMed]

47. Huguet, A.; Tougas, M.E.; Hayden, J.; McGrath, P.J.; Chambers, C.T.; Stinson, J.N.; Wozney, L. Systematic review of childhood and adolescent risk and prognostic factors for recurrent headaches. *J. Pain* **2016**, *17*, 855–873. [CrossRef] [PubMed]

48. Kashikar-Zuck, S.; Goldschneider, K.R.; Powers, S.W.; Vaught, M.H.; Hershey, A.D. Depression and functional disability in chronic pediatric pain. *Clin. J. Pain* **2001**, *17*, 341–349. [CrossRef] [PubMed]

49. Kashikar-Zuck, S.; Flowers, S.R.; Verkamp, E.; Ting, T.V.; Lynch-Jordan, A.M.; Graham, T.B.; Passo, M.; Schikler, K.N.; Hashkes, P.J.; Spalding, S.; et al. Actigraphy-based physical activity monitoring in adolescents with juvenile primary fibromyalgia syndrome. *J. Pain* **2010**, *11*, 885–893. [CrossRef] [PubMed]

50. Frank, L.D.; Engelke, P.O. The built environment and human activity patterns: Exploring the impacts of urban form on public health. *J. Plan. Lit.* **2001**, *16*, 202–218. [CrossRef]

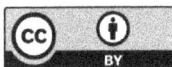

Section 4:
Assessment and Treatment

children

MDPI

Review

Pain Neuroscience Education: State of the Art and Application in Pediatrics

Hannah Robins [1], Victoria Perron [1], Lauren C. Heathcote [2] and Laura E. Simons [2,*]

[1]   Division of Pain Medicine, Department of Anesthesiology, Perioperative and Pain Medicine,
      Boston Children's Hospital, MA 02115, USA; hrobins4@binghamton.edu (H.R.); perronv@bc.edu (V.P.)
[2]   Department of Anesthesiology, Perioperative and Pain Medicine, Stanford University School of Medicine,
      1070 Arastradero Road, Palo Alto, CA 94304, USA; lcheath@stanford.edu
*   Correspondence: lesimons@stanford.edu; Tel.: +1-(650)-736-0838

Academic Editor: Carl L. von Baeyer
Received: 19 August 2016; Accepted: 12 December 2016; Published: 21 December 2016

Abstract: Chronic pain is a widespread problem in the field of pediatrics. Many interventions to ameliorate pain-related dysfunction have a biobehavioral focus. As treatments for chronic pain (e.g., increased movement) often stand in stark contrast to treatments for an acute injury (e.g., rest), providing a solid rationale for treatment is necessary to gain patient and parent buy-in. Most pain treatment interventions incorporate psychoeducation, or pain neuroscience education (PNE), as an essential component, and in some cases, as a stand-alone approach. The current topical review focuses on the state of pain neuroscience education and its application to pediatric chronic pain. As very little research has examined pain neuroscience education in pediatrics, we aim to describe this emerging area and catalyze further work on this important topic. As the present literature has generally focused on adults with chronic pain, pain neuroscience education merits further attention in the realm of pediatric pain in order to be tailored and implemented in this population.

Keywords: pain neuroscience education; psychoeducation; cognitive intervention; biopsychosocial model; pediatric chronic pain

1. Introduction

Pediatric chronic pain has reached epidemic proportions with an estimated 1.7 million children in the USA alone suffering from moderate to severe persistent pain [1]. With the high number of children affected, it is of extreme importance to discover new, innovative methods of treatment for the pediatric population. One approach that has been researched and implemented in adult populations over the past several decades is psychoeducation, either as one element of a comprehensive treatment program or as a stand-alone intervention. By explaining the scientific concepts that are central to the pathogenesis and perpetuation of chronic pain, clinical providers hope to create lasting change in the patient's beliefs about pain, and in turn, increase their engagement in the biobehavioral recommendations made for pain management and reduction. Pain education addresses patient misconceptions about physiological phenomena and helps shift their perspective to the idea that pain is dependent on biological, psychological, and social processes. One common message is that pain is dependent on meaning [2], and that how the patient perceives their pain is key to how a patient's brain processes pain signaling [3]. Taken together, pain education programs center on an explanatory model that understanding pain can modify pain itself.

Several terms have been coined in relation to pain education with each aiming to convey the central idea of a given approach. They include psychoeducation, pain neuroscience education (PNE), pain biology education, therapeutic neuroscience education, and Explain Pain (EP). For simplicity, we will refer to these approaches broadly as pain neuroscience education (PNE) [4], unless describing a study where a specific approach was empirically tested. PNE can be taught as an intervention on its own, as well as in combination with another form of therapy (such as cognitive-behavioral or physical) [5]. Although it is likely that all patients suffering with chronic pain can benefit from a shift in mindset provided via PNE, it might be critical for patients who suffer from a centralized pain problem and/or struggle with maladaptive perceptions about their pain [6]. This paper reviews the current state of the art in pediatric PNE. As most PNE research has been conducted in adult populations to date, we discuss both adult and pediatric studies within each section, considering how adult studies can inform future pediatric research, and presenting next steps for the pediatric pain field.

2. Why Pain Neuroscience Education?

2.1. Contextual Information about Pain Influences Pain Perception

When examining the concept of PNE, it is helpful to look to experimental research to determine the theoretical efficacy of education in altering pain outcomes. When we educate patients about pain, this new information alters the context in which they perceive their pain. In adult non-patient populations, research has demonstrated that manipulation of information and context regarding a stimulus can modulate pain. In one adult study using a cold pressor test (CPT), stimulus information was manipulated by having one group read a threatening passage about frostbite, while another read a passage about the safety of the test and how pain can be unrelated to tissue damage [7]. They found that the group that read the threatening passage had a lower mean pain tolerance time. In another adult study, investigators examined the idea that heat can be perceived to be more tissue-damaging than cold [8]. A $-25\,^\circ$C metal stick was placed on participants' necks after telling them that it was either hot or cold. Those who were told that the metal bar was hot rated both the painfulness and the damaging properties of the stimulus higher than participants who were told the metal bar was cold. In a third adult study, it was shown that using the colors red and blue as visual cues before presentation of a stimulus modulated pain intensity [9]. A red visual cue indicating heat resulted in higher pain ratings than a blue visual cue indicating cold.

In pediatrics, the manipulation of information and context has also been shown to modulate pain expectations and emotional response to pain. In one study [10], non-patient children completing a CPT received either threatening CPT information (CPT described as very painful, high pain expressions depicted) or non-threatening CPT information (standard CPT instructions provided, low pain expressions depicted). Children in the high-threat condition expected more pain, perceived the pain as more threatening, and catastrophized more about the pain. Parents of children in the high threat condition also expected their child to experience more pain. In another, parent-focused study [11], parents received either threatening information (stimulus described as painful and barely tolerable, high pain expressions depicted) or non-threatening information (stimulus described as slightly unpleasant, low pain expressions depicted) about a heat stimulus their child would receive. Parents who received the threatening information showed stronger negative physiological responses (EMG corrugator activity and fear-potentiated startle reflex) to cues of upcoming child pain. This was particularly the case when the child's pain facial expression was high, suggesting that parent beliefs are impacted by information from the environment and from the child.

With regards to patient populations, many individuals suffering from chronic pain can develop irrational beliefs and fears (including catastrophizing) about their pain. Many patients believe that their pain is harmful to their bodies and associate it with danger, despite the absence of tissue damage. These associations, similar to a red light visual cue or a passage about the dangers of frostbite, may worsen their pain. In adult patient populations, it has been shown that exposing patients to inaccurate information regarding illness may harm health outcomes and care [12]. Moreover, adult patients who are unsure of the diagnosis of their pain problem or perceive their pain as enduring and mysterious display higher levels of catastrophizing and are less likely to use coping strategies to deal with their pain [13,14].

In pediatrics, qualitative research also indicates a negative impact of diagnostic uncertainty and inaccurate information provision on child and parent pain and medical experiences. Children who are better informed about a forthcoming medical procedure are generally shown to have better outcomes (lower distress and better adjustment) during and after the procedure [15]. For parents, feeling uncertain with regards to their child's chronic pain condition and prognosis is shown to relate to parental feelings of helplessness and distress [16]. Studies are now needed to directly examine the effects of information provision in pediatric clinical populations. Due to the important role of child and parent beliefs and fears, it is crucial that healthcare professionals assess and appreciate these beliefs in order to determine if PNE would be an appropriate and worthwhile intervention within the context of pediatric pain.

2.2. Pain Neuroscience Education Provides a Common Language between Provider and Patient

A gap in understanding and communication between the patient and doctor can be a barrier in the treatment of chronic pain. PNE may provide a common language to aid communication and understanding. However, doctors' expectations of patient understanding and actual patient ability to understand must align for patients to receive helpful information about pain. A study with adults used the Neurophysiology of Pain Test to assess the ability of patients and healthcare professionals to accurately understand the neurophysiology of pain, as well as healthcare professionals' perceptions of the ability of patients to understand the concepts [17]. The results showed that after an education session, both groups were able to understand the information, but healthcare professionals significantly underestimated the ability of patients to do well on the Neurophysiology of Pain Test.

In pediatrics, discrepancies between doctors' expectations of patient understanding and actual patient ability to understand may be particularly pertinent, as patients' cognitive capacity changes across development, and does not always align with child age. The effect of age and cognitive capacity on PNE efficacy is currently unknown. However, a 2007 review acknowledged the importance of cognitive-developmental considerations within the provision of information regarding pediatric medical procedures [15]. Research has also indicated communication issues between child chronic pain patients and doctors, as well as discrepancies between doctor information provision and patient needs. The oral testimonies of patients at the Pediatric Pain Clinic at UCLA revealed patient frustration regarding the doctor's lack of interest in their experience [18]. The testimonies suggested a fundamental difference in the language and orientation of patients and doctors in regards to pain. While the child's orientation was experiential and emotional, the doctor's was instructive and diagnostic. This suggests that changes are needed in the communication models employed in treating pediatric chronic pain so that information being exchanged between treatment providers and patients begins to resonate. In addition, if providers assume their patients will not understand pain neuroscience information, they will not attempt to include it in appointments or treatment sessions. Thus, it is necessary for providers to be well-versed in PNE and to feel comfortable delivering that information in a developmentally appropriate way.

3. Overview of Pain Neuroscience Education

3.1. Explanatory Models

There are several theoretical models that have emerged to explain chronic pain, many of which have already been applied to a pediatric population. These models outline the concepts that are the foundation of PNE, provide physicians with a way to conceptualize different aspects of the patient's pain (including the obstacles that patients must overcome), and offer scaffolding for researchers formulating new research questions. As more information is learned over time about pain, the components of these theoretical models have evolved. Here we describe each model in turn, before presenting their pediatric application, where evident.

Originally, pain was viewed within a biomedical model. This model assumes a one-to-one correspondence between tissue damage, nociceptive input, and pain sensation. Thus, pain was thought to be a direct response to injury, and psychological or behavioural issues were thought to arise as a consequence of pain but not to influence the pain itself [19]. However, by the late 20th century, scientists began to shift away from this idea and moved towards the concept that motivational, affective, and cognitive processes can modulate pain, and can in some cases be the initial factor in pain etiology [20]. This is especially relevant to those suffering from chronic pain, as the pain often emerges despite seemingly normal biological functioning. The biomedical model has now largely been replaced with a biopsychosocial model, which incorporates all of the aspects in a patient's life that converge and potentially maintain a cycle of pain [21]. This has been determined to be a more effective conceptual and theoretical stance as it is suggested that pain cognitions are not only associated pain intensity, but may also be barriers to effective treatment if left unaddressed [22].

The biopsychosocial model puts an emphasis on the fact that 'pain itself is modulated by beliefs ... and can therefore be improved by modifying inaccurate beliefs' [2]. In order for this model to be successful, health-care providers need to convey the multi-dimensional causes of pain that are to be tackled in the intervention. The biological component of the biopsychosocial model largely revolves around the complex interplay of several cortical and subcortical brain regions involved in sensory, motor, cognitive, affective, and motivational functions [23]; with recent data suggestive of global brain connectivity reorganization among chronic pain patients [24]. This bombardment of neural input is a key mechanism that leads to chronic pain, as the brain keeps sending pain signals even in the absence of tissue damage. One theory that centers on the psychological aspect of the biopsychosocial model, entitled The "Common Sense Model of Self-Regulation" [25] highlights health beliefs and builds a hierarchical framework of patient cognition [26]. The model details the individual's representation of a health threat and the factors that contribute to this representation. It describes the way in which a person responds to any given health threat, including cognitive and emotional processes. Five dimensions of these cognitions have been identified and include: (1) identity (the effort to evaluate symptoms and label the illness); (2) cause (the subjectively formulated belief of what is causing the symptoms); (3) time-line (the patient's perception of how long the problem will last); (4) consequences (the patient's predictions of how the illness will affect them in different areas of their life); and (5) controllability (the patient's belief regarding their outcome and personal ability to change it) [2,3,27]. PNE, being closely tied to cognitive-behavioral treatments, shares significant ideology with the Common Sense Model of Self-Regulation. PNE aims to help patients reevaluate their pain problem, to target beliefs in order to develop more effective coping skills, and to ultimately change each of the five cognitive dimensions to achieve a positive outcome. The Common Sense Model has been said to be instrumental in the foundation of many cognitive treatments [26], and has been used in a randomized controlled trial of pain education in adults with cancer [28].

In addition to the comprehensive biopsychosocial model, additional theoretical models have emerged that highlight and attempt to explain in greater detail the different aspects of this larger framework. John D. Loeser has described pain as an onion consisting of four layered components: nociception, pain, suffering, and pain behavior [29] (Figure 1). The lower layers of suffering, pain, and nociception are not visible on the outside, being private experiences that only the patient is subjected to. The exterior of the onion is pain behavior, which is how the individual expresses his/her pain to the public. This could be through words, actions, or expressions. The onion model illustrates that in order to deliver effective treatment, the patient's hidden layers must be acknowledged and understood.

Among several cognitive-affective processes at work in the context of chronic pain, none have received greater research [30] and clinical attention [31] than pain-related fear. This is likely due to the inherently adaptive nature of fear in response to a noxious stimulus. The Fear-Avoidance Model (FAM) [30,32] details the cycle of pain-related fear and activity avoidance that ultimately leads to functional disability. As we adopt a biopsychosocial stance on the persistence of chronic pain, fear is argued to influence patient motivations, decisions, and well-being. For some individuals, breaking a vicious cycle of fear and avoidance will necessitate an extensive and thorough PNE. Through learning new information about the biology of pain, patients may be able to rework their relationship to their pain and change their maladaptive and fearful response to an adaptive and flexible one, eventually leading to a better quality of life [33].

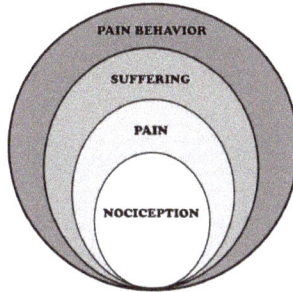

Figure 1. Loeser's onion model displaying the four components of pain phenomena. Reprinted from Loeser, J.D. Pain as a Disease [29].

Application of Explanatory Models to Pediatrics

The models described above are often used in pediatric clinical settings [34], although there is little published research presenting adaptations of these models for pediatric delivery. The importance of the biopsychosocial model was highlighted in a recent case study of a nine-year-old girl with functional abdominal pain [35]. In this case, it was explained to the patient that pain does not necessarily require a noxious stimulus and can be modulated by experience and context. By using diagrams and age-appropriate metaphors (Figure 2), the complex scientific topics were put into simpler terms and provided the patient and her family concrete reasoning for her persistent pain state.

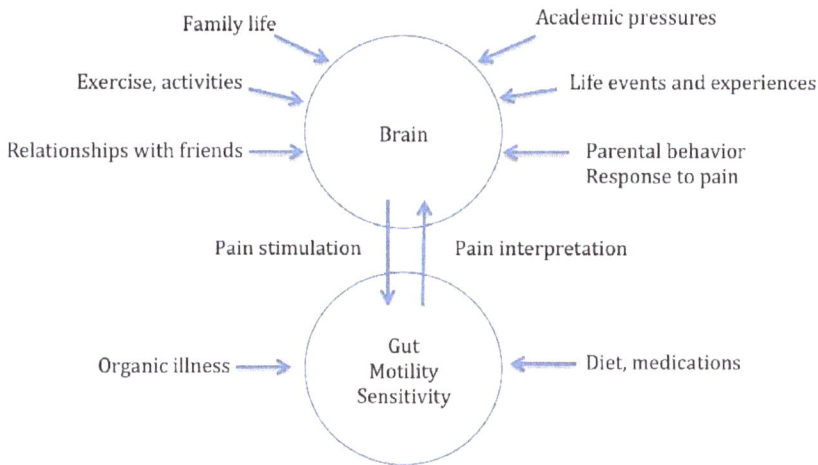

Figure 2. Visual representation of the biopsychosocial model in the context of pediatric functional abdominal pain. Adapted from Brown, L.K.; Beattie, R.M.; Tighe, M.P. Practical management of functional abdominal pain in children [35].

The Common Sense Model has also been explored in youth with type 1 diabetes and sickle cell disease, conditions which are often accompanied by frequent pain [36]. However, it has yet to be well applied to other pediatric chronic pain populations. Perhaps the most well-adapted model for pediatric populations is the Fear Avoidance Model (FAM), which has been adapted [37] and validated [38] for youth with chronic pain (Figure 3). In particular, the pediatric FAM considers the important influence of parents for the child pain experience, including parental cognitions, affective responding, and coping behaviors. In a first empirical study, child FA factors were shown to be a good predictor of functional disability in youth with chronic pain [39]. Interestingly, duration of pain contributed to the model for younger children, whereas pain-related fears were more influential for adolescent patients, highlighting the importance of developmental factors in the application of explanatory models to pediatric populations.

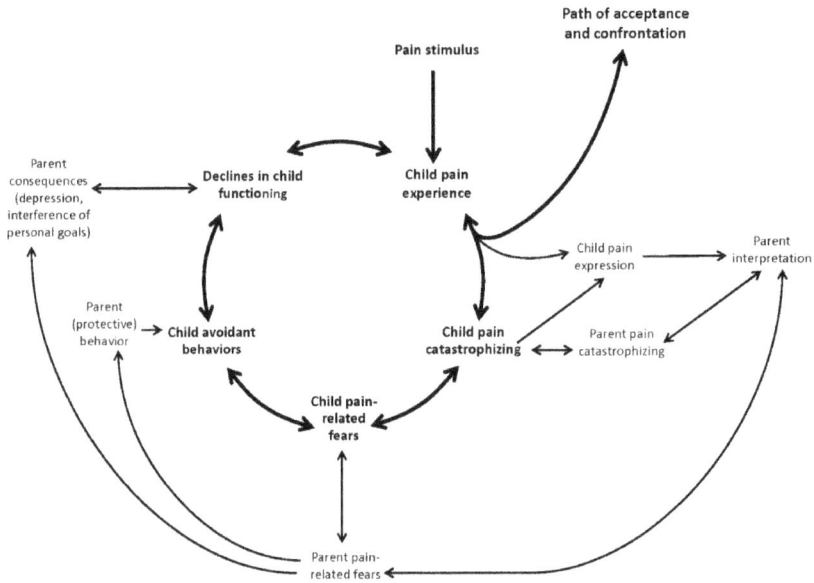

Figure 3. The interpersonal fear-avoidance model of chronic pain. Reprinted from Simons, L.; Smith, A.; Kaczynski, K.; Basch, M. Living in fear of your child's pain: The parent fear of pain questionnaire [38].

3.2. Current Evidence for PNE among Adults

There have been several systematic reviews conducted for adult PNE research that point to potential areas for growth in the field. For example, in 2011 Clarke and colleagues [40] reviewed studies of PNE specifically for chronic low back pain, for which they included only two randomized controlled trials (RCTs). The review revealed very low quality evidence that PNE is beneficial for pain, physical functioning, psychological functioning, and social functioning in this population, although the authors acknowledge that the review was limited by the small number of studies. More recently, Louw and colleagues [41] conducted an additional systematic review with a broader scope. Specifically, they included 13 RCTs that examined the influence of PNE on chronic musculoskeletal pain conditions. Five trials demonstrated positive effects in decreasing pain ratings, while three trials showed no effectiveness. Interestingly, of the three studies that were identified to increase pain knowledge, two of them showed an increase in pain knowledge, as well as a positive effect on pain catastrophization. However, an increase in pain knowledge is yet to be shown to correlate with decreased pain and disability [41].

Overall, the evidence for the effectiveness of PNE in adult patient populations is modest, particularly for long-term outcomes. However, the field is rapidly gaining momentum with additional studies being done each year. Moreover, it may be that the impact of PNE is better measured via its influence on mediators (e.g., pain catastrophizing, fear of pain) that ultimately influence outcomes. Perhaps PNE does not demonstrate a direct impact on pain-related function, but rather exerts its influence via these key mechanisms of change that have a demonstrated impact on outcomes in the literature.

Current Evidence for Pain Neuroscience Education in Pediatrics

To date, there are few studies that examine the utility of PNE in pediatric populations. There is preliminary evidence that psychoeducation may be efficacious for improving pediatric outcomes, however, most studies have investigated educational programs focused on pain management rather than explaining the biology and neuroscience of pain. In 2007, Abram and colleagues [42] randomized pediatric headache patients to receive either a traditional neurological examination only, or the examination alongside a group educational session. The education session comprised information regarding stressors contributing to pain, pharmaceutical and behavioral treatments, and guided relaxation skills practice. Patients receiving the additional educational session demonstrated greater gains in headache knowledge and required slightly less physician face-to-face time. Both groups experienced a sustained decline in headache-related disability. Whilst this study provides preliminary evidence that psychoeducation can increase knowledge about pain management, the study did not examine PNE specifically.

Perhaps unsurprisingly, many Cognitive-Behavioral Therapy (CBT) programs for pediatric chronic pain are delivered within a psychoeducational frame. Interestingly, a small number of RCTs for psychological therapies in pediatric chronic pain have used psychoeducation as a control intervention (see [43]). These studies have typically revealed superiority of psychological therapies (CBT and internet-based self-help training) over education for primary outcomes of functional disability and pain symptoms. However, where information regarding education content was provided [44,45], it is clear that education again focused on pain management rather than PNE specifically. Studies of primary PNE interventions for pediatric populations, particularly with randomized controlled designs, are greatly needed to advance understanding of the efficacy of PNE for pediatric populations.

3.3. New Applications of PNE: Preoperative Preparation and Cancer Pain Treatment

Adult PNE research has rapidly expanded over the past decade, and has branched into new areas such as preoperative preparation and cancer treatment. For example, the Preoperative Neuroscience Education Tool (PNET) targets adult patients undergoing lumbar radiculopathy [46]. The goal of PNET is to reduce post-operative pain levels, catastrophizing, and disability, as well as increase physical performance. Since postoperative rehabilitation is often ineffective in reducing pain levels, preoperative education that addresses pain physiology by using illustrations (Figure 4), metaphors, and explanatory examples has been of recent interest.

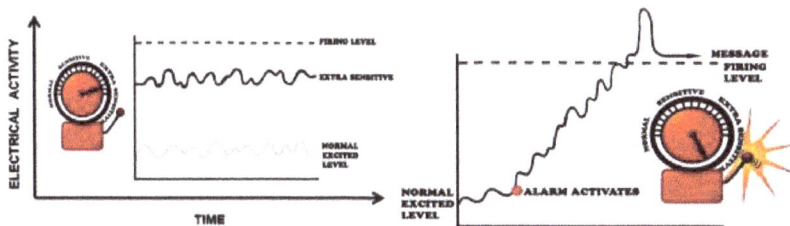

Figure 4. Example of illustration used in the PNET program to explain nervous system processes related to persistent pain. Reprinted from Louw, A.; Puentedura, E.J.; Diener, I.; Peoples, R.R. Preoperative therapeutic neuroscience education for lumbar radiculopathy: A single-case fMRI report [47].

Similar to PNET is the program RIDcancerPain (The Representational Intervention to Decrease Cancer Pain), that has been used as part of an RCT among adults with cancer pain [28]. RIDcancerPain aims to address the patient's current beliefs about pain before changing their perceptions through a one-time educational program that introduces new concepts surrounding pain physiology and coping strategies. Results showed that patients receiving RIDcancerPAIN reported greater decreases in barriers to pain control and greater decreases in pain severity than those in the control group. This study is similar to a previous program on cancer pain management, which showed a moderately positive effect on pain intensity after patients watched an educational video and had an informal discussion with a nurse [48]. Although some elements diverge between palliative care and chronic pain management, the emphasis on doctor interaction and education on pain physiology highlighted in these studies demonstrates where PNE converges across patient populations.

In pediatrics, Chambers and colleagues [49] conducted a randomized trial of a pain education booklet for parents of children undergoing surgery. Parents receiving the pain education booklet, in comparison to those receiving a pain assessment control or no pain education, had fewer concerns about the use of analgesics for children, but there were no group differences in parents' pain symptom assessments on any of the three days following surgery. Again, the pain education booklet focused on pain management strategies rather than explaining the neuroscience of pain. More recently, Tabrizi and colleagues [50] investigated the use of an anesthesia education booklet to alleviate preoperative anxiety in children ages 8–10 and their parents. Whilst parents and children receiving the education intervention reported reduced preoperative anxiety, similar reductions were seen in a control group receiving routine preoperative preparation without education.

3.4. A Combined Approach of Pain Neuroscience Education and Physiotherapy

It has been suggested that PNE sessions alone may not be sufficient to reach efficacious outcomes. Multiple studies have thus examined the success of combining PNE with physical therapy and exercise [51]. In a recent adult study [52], patients with chronic low back pain (CLBP) ($n = 30$) underwent two sessions of PNE followed by 12 sessions of aquatic exercise, all in a small group setting. The combination of both approaches resulted in statistically and clinically significant reductions in pain and functional disability when compared to the control group ($n = 32$) that received only the aquatic exercise sessions. This extends the results of a similar study in adult patients with fibromyalgia ($n = 58$) where the combination of pool exercise and PNE was found to be more effective than physiotherapy alone [53].

This combined approach is not limited to aquatic exercises. Land-based physiotherapy programs have also been successful. This integrated approach has lowered pain and disability in a recent RCT among adults with CLBP when compared to a control group [54]. While the control group ($n = 28$) only received advice from their general practitioners, the experimental group ($n = 29$) had a four-week PNE course that incorporated trunk muscle training and a standardized home-exercise program. Another study ($n = 41$) was completed shortly after, and investigated the use of group or individual education when used in combination with motor control training [55]. The individual education group showed larger decreases in pain and disability than the control group. A similar program was implemented in Brazil, where patients ($n = 79$) received one hour of stretching alongside a physiotherapist and one hour of CBT-focused psychoeducation with a nurse and psychologist, weekly for eight weeks [56]. Over the eight weeks, patients' pain intensity and disability levels significantly decreased. Although the latter study did not contain a control group and should thus be evaluated with caution, these studies highlight that PNE within the realm of a multidisciplinary cognitive-behavioral pain management program may enhance patient treatment in the future.

Not all trials have indicated better results when combining PNE with other treatments compared with PNE alone. For example, one recent study among adult patients with LBP found greater decreases in pain and increases in pain self-efficacy in patients who only received pain biology education ($n = 18$), compared to those who also received group exercise classes ($n = 20$) [51]. Although this was an unanticipated finding, the authors suggested that an exercise-only group would be important to tease apart findings in a future study.

Again, pediatric research on the combined effects of PNE and physiotherapy is lacking. However, given promising findings from adult studies, and growing support for the effectiveness of physiotherapy within an interdisciplinary program for treating children with chronic pain [57], research in this area is warranted.

4. Delivery Methods

The way that pain education is delivered and presented to patients may be as important as the content itself. Evaluating patients' individual needs and capacities for understanding PNE is important for PNE success. This may be especially pertinent in a pediatric setting, where PNE must be adapted to match patients' cognitive capacities. There are many modalities already in use in both adult and pediatric clinical populations, giving healthcare professionals options in how to engage their patients, and giving patients resources they can utilize outside of a doctor's office. Below we examine common PNE delivery methods, particularly considering their use in pediatric populations.

4.1. Metaphor

When educating patients about pain, creative ways of explaining biological processes are necessary. This is especially relevant to the pediatric population, where traditional lectures or scientific models may be ineffective. Metaphor or story-telling as a way of discussing pain phenomena can be a helpful tool in PNE. A 2013 randomized controlled trial [58] found that adult chronic pain patients given a book of metaphors and stories to explain pain biology, Painful Yarns [59], had a larger increase in knowledge about pain biology and a larger decrease in pain catastrophizing compared to patients who were given a book about pain management. Interestingly, patients in the metaphor group reported reading an average of 82% of their book, as opposed to 47% for the control group, suggesting that metaphor not only has the potential to alter perceptions, but it is also more engaging than more traditional methods of delivery [58].

One metaphor proposed as a way of conceptualizing the pain problem for both patients and healthcare professionals is the pain puzzle (Figure 5); a visual and conceptual metaphor that identifies the multitude of factors that play into pain (nociception, affect/feelings, cognition/thoughts, and behavior). It can be explained that different individuals may have different pieces of varying sizes that make up their 'personal pain puzzle'. The pain puzzle has been utilized in pediatric clinical settings for patients with rheumatic disease [60].

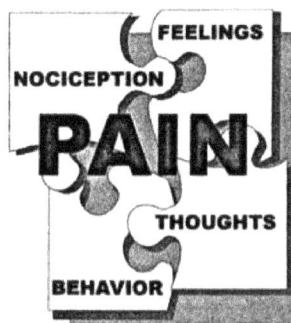

Figure 5. The pain puzzle visual metaphor. Reprinted from Rapoff, M.A.; Lindsley, C.B. The pain puzzle: A visual and conceptual metaphor for understanding and treating pain in pediatric rheumatic disease [59].

A recent commentary detailed an extensive collection of metaphors and analogies that have been used by clinicians in multiple pediatric settings (Figure 6) [34]. They focus on four explanatory categories: (1) the difference between acute and chronic pain; (2) pain transmission/spreading; (3) factors that impact pain perception; and (4) pain rehabilitation. These metaphors have been used by numerous professionals to explain pain biology, outline treatment goals, and to help patients reconceptualize the pain problem.

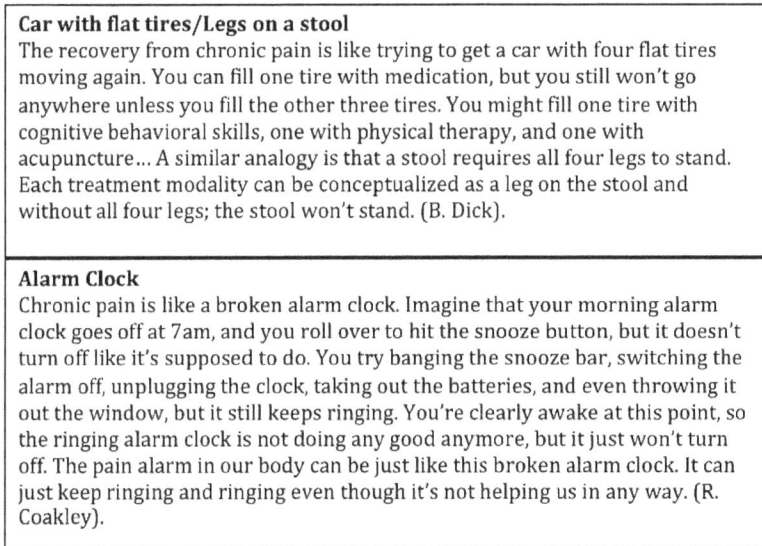

Car with flat tires/Legs on a stool
The recovery from chronic pain is like trying to get a car with four flat tires moving again. You can fill one tire with medication, but you still won't go anywhere unless you fill the other three tires. You might fill one tire with cognitive behavioral skills, one with physical therapy, and one with acupuncture... A similar analogy is that a stool requires all four legs to stand. Each treatment modality can be conceptualized as a leg on the stool and without all four legs; the stool won't stand. (B. Dick).

Alarm Clock
Chronic pain is like a broken alarm clock. Imagine that your morning alarm clock goes off at 7am, and you roll over to hit the snooze button, but it doesn't turn off like it's supposed to do. You try banging the snooze bar, switching the alarm off, unplugging the clock, taking out the batteries, and even throwing it out the window, but it still keeps ringing. You're clearly awake at this point, so the ringing alarm clock is not doing any good anymore, but it just won't turn off. The pain alarm in our body can be just like this broken alarm clock. It can just keep ringing and ringing even though it's not helping us in any way. (R. Coakley).

Figure 6. Example metaphors for explaining chronic pain to children. Adapted from Coakley, R.; Schechter, N.L. Chronic pain is like . . . the clinical use of analogy and metaphor in the treatment of pain in children [34].

4.2. Books

Providing patients with written resources that they can utilize outside of the clinical setting can be an instrumental factor in consolidating their reconceptualization of pain.

4.2.1. Adult Pain Books

Explain Pain and Protectometer: The book *Explain Pain* [61] is being recognized as an invaluable resource for chronic pain patients and for professionals delivering PNE to patients. The book, written by David Butler and Lorimer Moseley, details many facets of pain biology and pain management. It is written in an approachable and engaging format, and includes illustrations throughout [61]. An education program based on the book was shown to result in lower pain scores at a three-month follow up in a group of fibromyalgia patients compared to patients who received education about activity management [62]. A pilot study also utilized the book in a session treating patients with chronic whiplash, and revealed a significant decrease in disability and an increase in pain thresholds at follow-up [63].

A recently published follow-up book, *The Explain Pain Handbook: Protectometer* [64], is a patient-targeted handbook with updated information which includes an interactive pain treatment tool. The 'Protectometer' is a tool that allows patients to map out their pain on a day-to-day basis and identify stressors and what the authors call 'DIMS' (Danger(s) In Me) and 'SIMS' (Safety(s) In Me).

There is also a 'Protectometer' iOS APP available (Figure 7) to build upon the activity in the handbook and to provide patients with a user-friendly way to define their 'personal pain formula' [64].

Why Do I Hurt: Another recent series of patient education books was written by physical therapist and clinical neuroscientist, Adrianne Louw. *Why Do I Hurt?* [65] is a basic patient pain neuroscience manual for chronic pain, covering pain biology and nervous system phenomena. The material is accessible for readers not already versed in the science, and includes illustrations, metaphors, and examples. Other books in his PNE series are focused on specific chronic pain problems including *Why Pelvic Pain Hurts* [66], *Your Headache Isn't All In Your Head* [67], *Whiplash: An Alarming Message From Your Nerves* [68], and more [69,70]. There is also a workbook in the series specifically for PNE providers, *Therapeutic Neuroscience Education: Teaching Patients About Pain* [71]. This book is unique in that it is geared towards clinicians and focuses on the best ways to explain pain and demonstrate pain biology concepts. Louw has also developed the "*Why You Hurt: Therapeutic Neuroscience Education System*", a clinical tool including colorful educational flashcards, teaching cues, pain questionnaire cards, and homework cards, all aimed at facilitating PNE [72]. The system provides an innovative way to help providers execute PNE in clinical settings. Although not written for a pediatric audience, these interactive resources hold great potential for engaging younger patients.

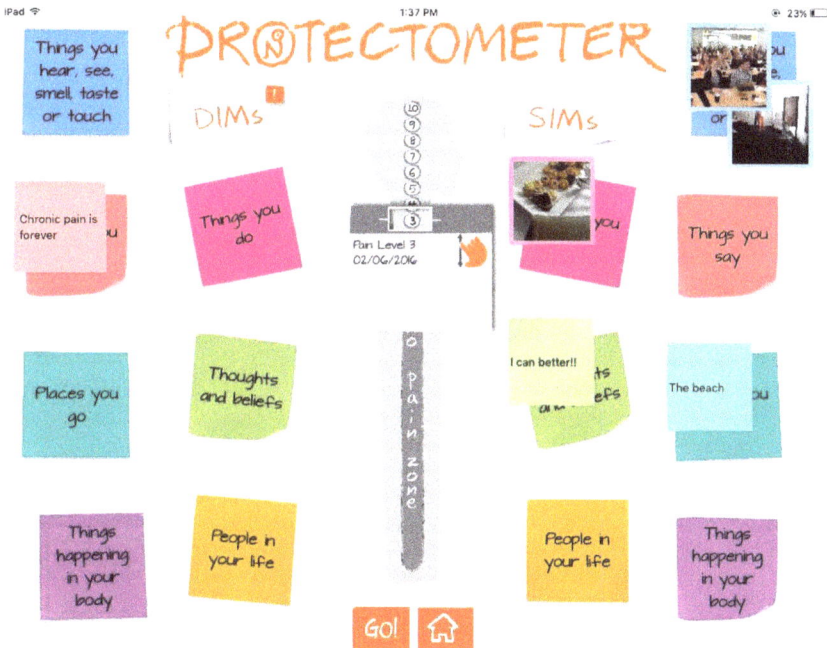

Figure 7. Example diagram of the 'Protectometer' tool provided in the available iOS app. Adapted from Protectometer: iOS Application in *Appliquette*. Available online [73].

Despite the potential value of these materials to patients, they may not be sufficient to replace in-person PNE. In a group of adult fibromyalgia patients, written education alone did not significantly impact pain catastrophizing or functioning during daily tasks [74]. Even if patients may appreciate receiving written PNE, for it to truly be an agent of change, it may need to be delivered in person to provide an engaging, interactive format, or incorporated into a larger treatment plan that targets multiple elements of the biopsychosocial model [75].

4.2.2. Pediatric Pain Books

There is no book that exclusively focuses on PNE in pediatric pain. However, there are several published books from the past decade that have been directed toward parents of youth with chronic pain, a key audience for PNE. These books comprise multiple sections that often include: PNE, education on treatment options, and an introduction to pain management skills (e.g., relaxation, behavioral activation) that parents can foster in their children. For example, "*Conquering Your Child's Chronic Pain*" [76] introduces parents to valuable PNE topics and helpful relaxation and visualization techniques. "*Relieve Your Child's Pain*" [77] details ways that parents can reduce stress in the home and properly evaluate their child's pain, and addresses fears parents may have about their child's pain problem. More recent contributions include "*Managing Your Child's Chronic Pain*" [78], which provides parents with insight on CBT strategies as well as vignettes and stories of patient and family experiences, and "*When your child hurts,*" [34], which provides extensive PNE (over 30 pages dedicated to "Understanding What Pain is (and is Not)") along with specific strategies geared toward breaking the cycle of the child's pain problem. The goal of these books is to provide valuable insight and relief as parents struggle to help their child manage chronic pain. Despite the growth in these resources, there are no published studies that examine their impact on parent and child function in the context of child pain.

4.3. Group Education Models

When considering practical and efficient methods of delivering PNE to patients, group education is a viable option. Group models allow for a more time- and cost-efficient platform to educate patients with similar needs. The RCT by Abram and colleagues [42] described above delivered psychoeducation within a group setting, and revealed some positive effects. A group model of education may be a more efficient way to deliver information to patients instead of incorporating it into individual appointments [42]. In addition to increasing efficiency, group PNE sessions may be advantageous in that they give patients an opportunity to connect with other patients and even learn from others' experiences. However, it has also been shown that a group model, as opposed to a one-on-one session, may suffer in efficacy [51]. The group model has the potential to prevent patients from asking questions or voicing concerns, and the one-on-one patient-clinician model may be vital for clinicians to assist in a patients' individual reconceptualization of pain. Moreover, there are several issues to consider in relation to group composition that can potentially impact outcomes, such as size of the group, homogeneity/heterogeneity, and age (see recent review [79]). It is likely that a combination of group and one-on-one sessions may provide increased efficiency in a manner that does not sacrifice the individually tailored care that may be essential for effective pediatric pain treatment.

4.4. Video

When presenting PNE to patients, especially in pediatrics, it is likely important to engage them using multiple modalities to facilitate processing complex and novel information. One approach is the use of short video clips. These videos are likely a familiar platform for patients to explore PNE in their own time and in comfortable home environments. One video, created by the German Pediatric Pain Center (Figure 8), explains pain for patients with migraines. Cartoons are used to explain why some people have migraines, what they mean, and how one can manage them [80]. Another video entitled "*Understanding pain in less than 5 min*" [81] uses active illustrations to present chronic pain from a biopsychosocial perspective. It is available on YouTube in over ten different languages.

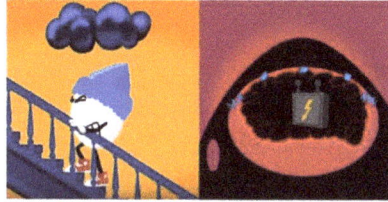

Figure 8. Image obtained from the online video, 'Migraine: how it works and how to get it under control' [80].

5. Developmental Considerations and Next Steps

Research examining PNE for pediatric chronic pain is somewhat uncharted territory. Despite the clear relevance of PNE to children and young people, RCTs of PNE programs have typically been conducted with adults, and most RTCs employing psychoeduation in pediatric populations have examined psychoeducation only as part of a broader psychological treatment package and in many cases focus on pain management versus pain neurophysiology. As described above, educational resources that are appropriate for pediatric populations are currently available, such as *Explain Pain*, *The Protectometer* [64], and online animated videos. However, given that the neuroscience of pain is complex, resources that align with the child's current state of cognitive and psychosocial development will be essential. Of particular importance for pediatrics, children who are unwell or highly stressed may also be functioning at lower cognitive levels than they otherwise would [15]. Materials must, therefore, be tailored according to both the child's cognitive-developmental stage and his/her physical and affective state. Consideration of Piaget's developmental stages may provide insight into the appropriate adaptation for PNE materials and delivery across early and middle childhood. The review by Jaaniste and colleagues [15] provides an excellent example of how to consider these conceptual stages when providing children with information about forthcoming medical procedures, and these examples could be usefully applied to PNE development. In order to appeal to youth at different developmental stages, resources could also be available in multiple modalities. These may be in the format of written resources, in-person dialogue models, or online animated videos and apps. Metaphors and stories should be further utilized to create specific pediatric educational tools as they provide a format for making complex concepts concrete and accessible. It is also important to consider the changing parent-child relationship across development, and recognition of the impact of parents on child learning and beliefs [82]. Most of the pain books developed for pediatric populations described above are targeted at parents, and this may indeed be an ideal method of PNE transmission for younger patients who frequently look to parents for learning opportunities.

6. Conclusions

PNE is receiving growing interest as an intervention in the field of chronic pain. Its potential application is vast, ranging from preoperative prevention programs to cross-disciplinary chronic pain management programs. Since PNE can be applied to multiple treatment scenarios and delivered by a variety of health professionals, its potential influence on patients is broad. Pain neuroscience education is in the midst of finding its place among a plethora of cognitive-behavioral treatments for chronic pain. A necessary next step is the inclusion of pediatric populations. Rationale for PNE, such as the detriment of irrational beliefs and maintenance of fear-avoidance, are equally relevant for younger patients. Given existing evidence for PNE in adults, this topic deserves more attention in the pediatric realm.

Acknowledgments: This work was supported by a National Institutes of Health grant (R01 HD083270) awarded to L.E.S.

Conflicts of Interest: The authors declare no conflicts of interest.

References

1. Groenewald, C.B.; Essner, B.S.; Wright, D.; Fesinmeyer, M.D.; Palermo, T.M. The Economic Costs of Chronic Pain Among a Cohort of Treatment-Seeking Adolescents in the United States. *J. Pain* **2014**, *15*, 925–933. [CrossRef] [PubMed]
2. Moseley, G.L.; Butler, D.S. Fifteen Years of Explaining Pain: The Past, Present, and Future. *J. Pain* **2015**, *16*, 807–813. [CrossRef] [PubMed]
3. Moseley, G.L. A pain neuromatrix approach to patients with chronic pain. *Man. Ther.* **2003**, *8*, 130–140. [CrossRef]
4. Louw, A.; Puentedura, E.L.; Zimney, K. Teaching patients about pain: It works, but what should we call it? *Physiother. Theory Pract.* **2016**, *32*, 328–331. [CrossRef] [PubMed]
5. Louw, A.; Puentedura, E.J.; Zimney, K.; Schmidt, S. Know Pain, Know Gain? A Perspective on Pain Neuroscience Education in Physical Therapy. *J. Orthop. Sports Phys. Ther.* **2016**, *46*, 131–134. [CrossRef] [PubMed]
6. Nijs, J.; Paul van Wilgen, C.; Van Oosterwijck, J.; van Ittersum, M.; Meeus, M. How to explain central sensitization to patients with 'unexplained' chronic musculoskeletal pain: Practice guidelines. *Man. Ther.* **2011**, *16*, 413–418. [CrossRef] [PubMed]
7. Jackson, T.; Pope, L.; Nagasaka, T.; Fritch, A.; Iezzi, T.; Chen, H. The impact of threatening information about pain on coping and pain tolerance. *Br. J. Health Psychol.* **2005**, *10*, 441–451. [CrossRef] [PubMed]
8. Arntz, A.; Claassens, L. The meaning of pain influences its experienced intensity. *Pain* **2004**, *109*, 20–25. [CrossRef] [PubMed]
9. Moseley, G.L.; Arntz, A. The context of a noxious stimulus affects the pain it evokes. *Pain* **2007**, *133*, 64–71. [CrossRef] [PubMed]
10. Boerner, K.E.; Noel, M.; Birnie, K.A.; Caes, L.; Petter, M.; Chambers, C.T. Impact of Threat Level, Task Instruction, and Individual Characteristics on Cold Pressor Pain and Fear among Children and Their Parents. *Pain Pract.* **2016**, *16*, 657–668. [CrossRef] [PubMed]
11. Caes, L.; Vervoort, T.; Trost, Z.; Goubert, L. Impact of parental catastrophizing and contextual threat on parents' emotional and behavioral responses to their child's pain. *Pain* **2012**, *153*, 687–695. [CrossRef] [PubMed]
12. Murray, E.; Lo, B.; Pollack, L.; Donelan, K.; Catania, J.; Lee, K.; Zapert, K.; Turner, R. The impact of health information on the Internet on health care and the physician-patient relationship: National U.S. survey among 1.050 U.S. physicians. *J. Med. Internet Res.* **2003**, *5*, e17. [CrossRef] [PubMed]
13. Geisser, M.E.; Roth, R.S. Knowledge of and agreement with chronic pain diagnosis: Relation to affective distress, pain beliefs and coping, pain intensity, and disability. *J. Occup. Rehabil.* **1998**, *8*, 73–88. [CrossRef]
14. Williams, D.A.; Keefe, F.J. Pain beliefs and the use of cognitive-behavioral coping strategies. *Pain* **1991**, *46*, 185–190. [PubMed]
15. Jaaniste, T.; Hayes, B.; von Baeyer, C.L. Providing Children with Information about Forthcoming Medical Procedures: A Review and Synthesis. *Clin. Psychol. Sci. Pract.* **2007**, *14*, 124–143. [CrossRef]
16. Jordan, A.L.; Eccleston, C.; Osborne, M. Being a parent of the adolescent with complex chronic pain: An interpretative phenomenological analysis. *Eur. J. Pain* **2007**, *11*, 49–56. [CrossRef] [PubMed]
17. Moseley, L. Unraveling the barriers to reconceptualization of the problem in chronic pain: The actual and perceived ability of patients and health professionals to understand the neurophysiology. *J. Pain* **2003**, *4*, 184–189. [CrossRef]
18. Nutkiewicz, M. Diagnosis versus dialogue: Oral testimony and the study of pediatric pain. *Oral. Hist. Rev.* **2008**, *35*, 11–21. [CrossRef] [PubMed]
19. Chorney, J.M.; Crofton, K.; McClain, B.C. Theories on Common Adolescent Pain Syndromes. In *Handbook of Pediatric Chronic Pain*; McClain, B.C., Suresh, S., Eds.; Springer: New York, NY, USA, 2011; pp. 27–44.
20. Kenshalo, D.R.; Florida State University. *The Skin Senses; Proceedings*; Thomas: Springfield, IL, USA, 1968.
21. Basch, M.C.; Chow, E.T.; Logan, D.E.; Schechter, N.L.; Simons, L.E. Perspectives on the clinical significance of functional pain syndromes in children. *J. Pain Res.* **2015**, *8*, 675–686. [PubMed]

22. Meeus, M.; Nijs, J.; Van Oosterwijck, J.; Van Alsenoy, V.; Truijen, S. Pain physiology education improves pain beliefs in patients with chronic fatigue syndrome compared with pacing and self-management education: A double-blind randomized controlled trial. *Arch. Phys. Med. Rehabil.* **2010**, *91*, 1153–1159. [CrossRef] [PubMed]

23. Bushnell, M.C.; Ceko, M.; Low, L.A. Cognitive and emotional control of pain and its disruption in chronic pain. *Nat. Rev. Neurosci.* **2013**, *14*, 502–511. [CrossRef] [PubMed]

24. Mansour, A.; Baria, A.T.; Tetreault, P.; Vachon-Presseau, E.; Chang, P.C.; Huang, L.; Apkarian, A.V.; Baliki, M.N. Global disruption of degree rank order: A hallmark of chronic pain. *Sci. Rep.* **2016**, *6*, 34853. [CrossRef] [PubMed]

25. Leventhal, H.; Brisette, I.; Leventhal, E.A. The common-sense model of self-regulation of health and illness. In *the Self-Regulation of Health and Illness Behavior*; Cameron, L.D., Leventhal, H., Eds.; Routledge: London, UK, 2003; pp. 42–65.

26. Hale, E.D.; Treharne, G.J.; Kitas, G.D. The common-sense model of self-regulation of health and illness: How can we use it to understand and respond to our patients' needs? *Rheumatology (Oxford)* **2007**, *46*, 904–906. [CrossRef] [PubMed]

27. Siemonsma, P.C.; Schroder, C.D.; Dekker, J.H.; Lettinga, A.T. The benefits of theory for clinical practice: Cognitive treatment for chronic low back pain patients as an illustrative example. *Disabil. Rehabil.* **2008**, *30*, 1309–1317. [CrossRef] [PubMed]

28. Ward, S.; Donovan, H.; Gunnarsdottir, S.; Serlin, R.C.; Shapiro, G.R.; Hughes, S. A randomized trial of a representational intervention to decrease cancer pain (RIDcancerPain). *Health Psychol.* **2008**, *27*, 59–67. [CrossRef] [PubMed]

29. Loeser, J.D. Chapter 2 Pain as a disease. *Handb. Clin. Neurol.* **2006**, *81*, 11–20. [PubMed]

30. Vlaeyen, J.W.; Linton, S.J. Fear-Avoidance model of chronic musculoskeletal pain: 12 years on. *Pain* **2012**, *153*, 1144–1147. [CrossRef] [PubMed]

31. De Jong, J.R.; Vlaeyen, J.W.; van Eijsden, M.; Loo, C.; Onghena, P. Reduction of pain-related fear and increased function and participation in work-related upper extremity pain (WRUEP): Effects of exposure in vivo. *Pain* **2012**, *153*, 2109–2118. [CrossRef] [PubMed]

32. Vlaeyen, J.W.; Linton, S.J. Fear-Avoidance and its consequences in chronic musculoskeletal pain: A state of the art. *Pain* **2000**, *85*, 317–332. [CrossRef]

33. Den Hollander, M.; Goossens, M.; de Jong, J.; Ruijgrok, J.; Oosterhof, J.; Onghena, P.; Smeets, R.; Vlaeyen, J.W. Expose or protect? A randomized controlled trial of exposure in vivo vs pain-contingent treatment as usual in patients with complex regional pain syndrome type 1. *Pain* **2016**, *157*, 2318–2329. [CrossRef] [PubMed]

34. Coakley, R.; Schechter, N. Chronic pain is like... The clinical use of analogy and metaphor in the treatment of chronic pain in children. *Pediatr. Pain Lett.* **2013**, *15*, 1–8.

35. Brown, L.K.; Beattie, R.M.; Tighe, M.P. Practical management of functional abdominal pain in children. *Arch. Dis. Child.* **2016**, *101*, 677–683. [CrossRef] [PubMed]

36. Huston, S.A.; Houk, C.P. Common sense model of illness in youth with type 1 diabetes or sickle cell disease. *J. Pediatr. Pharmacol. Ther.* **2011**, *16*, 270–280. [PubMed]

37. McGrath, P.J.; Stevens, B.J.; Walker, S.M.; Zempsky, W.T. *Oxford Textbook of Paediatric Pain*; Oxford University Press: Oxford, UK; New York, NY, USA, 2014.

38. Simons, L.E.; Smith, A.; Kaczynski, K.; Basch, M. Living in fear of your child's pain: The Parent Fear of Pain Questionnaire. *Pain* **2015**, *156*, 694–702. [CrossRef] [PubMed]

39. Simons, L.E.; Kaczynski, K.J. The Fear Avoidance model of chronic pain: Examination for pediatric application. *J. Pain* **2012**, *13*, 827–835. [CrossRef] [PubMed]

40. Clarke, C.L.; Ryan, C.G.; Martin, D.J. Pain neurophysiology education for the management of individuals with chronic low back pain: Systematic review and meta-analysis. *Man. Ther.* **2011**, *16*, 544–549. [CrossRef] [PubMed]

41. Louw, A.; Zimney, K.; Puentedura, E.J.; Diener, I. The efficacy of pain neuroscience education on musculoskeletal pain: A systematic review of the literature. *Physiother. Theory Pract.* **2016**, *32*, 332–355. [CrossRef] [PubMed]

42. Abram, H.S.; Buckloh, L.M.; Schilling, L.M.; Wiltrout, S.A.; Ramirez-Garnica, G.; Turk, W.R. A randomized, controlled trial of a neurological and psychoeducational group appointment model for pediatric headaches. *Child. Health Care* **2007**, *36*, 249–265. [CrossRef]

43. Fisher, E.; Heathcote, L.; Palermo, T.M.; de C Williams, A.C.; Lau, J.; Eccleston, C. Systematic review and meta-analysis of psychological therapies for children with chronic pain. *J. Pediatr. Psychol.* **2014**, *39*, 763–782. [CrossRef] [PubMed]

44. Kashikar-Zuck, S.; Ting, T.V.; Arnold, L.M.; Bean, J.; Powers, S.W.; Graham, T.B.; Passo, M.H.; Schikler, K.N.; Hashkes, P.J.; Spalding, S.; et al. Cognitive behavioral therapy for the treatment of juvenile fibromyalgia: A multisite, single-blind, randomized, controlled clinical trial. *Arthritis. Rheum.* **2012**, *64*, 297–305. [CrossRef] [PubMed]

45. Levy, R.L.; Langer, S.L.; Walker, L.S.; Romano, J.M.; Christie, D.L.; Youssef, N.; DuPen, M.M.; Feld, A.D.; Ballard, S.A.; Welsh, E.M.; et al. Cognitive-Behavioral Therapy for Children With Functional Abdominal Pain and Their Parents Decreases Pain and Other Symptoms. *Am. J. Gastroenterol.* **2010**, *105*, 946–956. [CrossRef] [PubMed]

46. Louw, A.; Butler, D.S.; Diener, I.; Puentedura, E.J. Development of a preoperative neuroscience educational program for patients with lumbar radiculopathy. *Am. J. Phys. Med. Rehabil.* **2013**, *92*, 446–452. [CrossRef] [PubMed]

47. Louw, A.; Puentedura, E.J.; Diener, I.; Peoples, R.R. Preoperative therapeutic neuroscience education for lumbar radiculopathy: A single-case fMRI report. *Physiother. Theory Pract.* **2015**, *31*, 496–508. [CrossRef] [PubMed]

48. Aubin, M.; Vezina, L.; Parent, R.; Fillion, L.; Allard, P.; Bergeron, R.; Dumont, S.; Giguère, A. Impact of an educational program on pain management in patients with cancer living at home. *Oncol. Nurs. Forum* **2006**, *33*, 1183–1188. [CrossRef] [PubMed]

49. Chambers, C.T.; Reid, G.J.; McGrath, P.J.; Finley, G.A.; Ellerton, M.L. A randomized trial of a pain education booklet: Effects on parents' attitudes and postoperative pain management. *Child. Health Care* **1997**, *26*, 1–13. [CrossRef]

50. Sadegh Tabrizi, J.; Seyedhejazi, M.; Fakhari, A.; Ghadimi, F.; Hamidi, M.; Taghizadieh, N. Preoperative Education and Decreasing Preoperative Anxiety Among Children Aged 8–10 Years Old and Their Mothers. *Anesth. Pain Med.* **2015**, *5*, e25036. [CrossRef] [PubMed]

51. Ryan, C.G.; Gray, H.G.; Newton, M.; Granat, M.H. Pain biology education and exercise classes compared to pain biology education alone for individuals with chronic low back pain: A pilot randomised controlled trial. *Man. Ther.* **2010**, *15*, 382–387. [CrossRef] [PubMed]

52. Pires, D.; Cruz, E.B.; Caeiro, C. Aquatic exercise and pain neurophysiology education versus aquatic exercise alone for patients with chronic low back pain: A randomized controlled trial. *Clin. Rehabil.* **2015**, *29*, 538–547. [CrossRef] [PubMed]

53. Mannerkorpi, K.; Nyberg, B.; Ahlmen, M.; Ekdahl, C. Pool exercise combined with an education program for patients with fibromyalgia syndrome. A prospective, randomized study. *J. Rheumatol.* **2000**, *27*, 2473–2481. [PubMed]

54. Moseley, L. Combined physiotherapy and education is efficacious for chronic low back pain. *Aust. J. Physiother.* **2002**, *48*, 297–302. [CrossRef]

55. Moseley, G.L. Joining forces—Combining cognition-targeted motor control training with group or individual pain physiology education: A successful treatment for chronic low back pain. *J. Man. Manip. Ther.* **2003**, *11*, 88–94. [CrossRef]

56. Salvetti Mde, G.; Cobelo, A.; Vernalha Pde, M.; Vianna, C.I.; Canarezi, L.C.; Calegare, R.G. Effects of a psychoeducational program for chronic pain management. *Rev. Lat. Am. Enfermagem.* **2012**, *20*, 896–902. [CrossRef] [PubMed]

57. Campos, A.A.; Amaria, K.; Campbell, F.; McGrath, P.A. Clinical Impact and Evidence Base for Physiotherapy in Treating Childhood Chronic Pain. *Physiother. Can.* **2011**, *63*, 21–33. [CrossRef] [PubMed]

58. Gallagher, L.; McAuley, J.; Moseley, G.L. A randomized-controlled trial of using a book of metaphors to reconceptualize pain and decrease catastrophizing in people with chronic pain. *Clin. J. Pain* **2013**, *29*, 20–25. [CrossRef] [PubMed]

59. Moseley, G.L. *Painful Yarns: Metaphors and Stories to Help Understand the Biology of Pain*; Dancing Giraffe Press: Minneapolis, MN, USA, 2007.

60. Rapoff, M.A.; Lindsley, C.B. The pain puzzle: A visual and conceptual metaphor for understanding and treating pain in pediatric rheumatic disease. *J. Rheumatol. Suppl.* **2000**, *58*, 29–33. [PubMed]

61. Butler, D.S.; Moseley, G. *Explain Pain*; Noigroup Publications: Adelaide, Australia, 2013.

62. Van Oosterwijck, J.; Meeus, M.; Paul, L.; De Schryver, M.; Pascal, A.; Lambrecht, L.; Nijs, J. Pain physiology education improves health status and endogenous pain inhibition in fibromyalgia: A double-blind randomized controlled trial. *Clin. J. Pain* **2013**, *29*, 873–882. [CrossRef] [PubMed]

63. Van Oosterwijck, J.; Nijs, J.; Meeus, M.; Truijen, S.; Craps, J.; Van den Keybus, N.; Paul, L. Pain neurophysiology education improves cognitions, pain thresholds, and movement performance in people with chronic whiplash: A pilot study. *J. Rehabil. Res. Dev.* **2011**, *48*, 43–58. [CrossRef] [PubMed]

64. Moseley, G.L.; Butler, D.S. *The Explain Pain Handbook: Protectometer*; Noigroup Publications: Adelaide, Australia, 2015.

65. Louw, A. *Why do I hurt?: A Patient Book about the Neuroscience of Pain*, 1st ed.; International Spine and Pain Institute: Story City, IA, USA, 2013.

66. Louw, A.; Hilton, S.; Vandyken, C. *Why Pelvic Pain Hurts*, 1st ed.; International Spine And Pain Institute: Story City, IA, USA, 2014.

67. Louw, A.; Diener, I. *Your Headache Isn't all in Your Head: Neuroscience Education for Patients with Headache Pain*, 1st ed.; International Spine and Pain Institute: Story City, IA, USA, 2014.

68. Louw, A. *Whiplash: An Alarming Message from Your Nerves*; International Spine and Pain Institute: Story City, IA, USA, 2012.

69. Louw, A. *Your Nerves Are Having Back Surgery*, 1st ed.; International Spine and Pain Institute: Story City, IA, USA, 2012.

70. Louw, A.; Flynn, T.; Puentedura, E.J. *Everyone Has Back Pain*, 1st ed.; International Spine and Pain Institute: Story City, IA, USA, 2015.

71. Louw, A.; Puentedura, E.J. *Therapeutic Neuroscience Education: Teaching Patients about Pain*, 1st ed.; International Spine and Pain Institute: Story City, IA, USA, 2013.

72. Louw, A. *Why You Hurt: Therapeutic Neuroscience Education System*; International Spine and Pain Institute: Story City, IA, USA, 2014.

73. Appliquette. Protectometer. Appliquette. 2016. Available online: http://www.appliquette.com.au/project/protectometer/ (accessed on 30 July 2016).

74. Van Ittersum, M.W.; van Wilgen, C.P.; van der Schans, C.P.; Lambrecht, L.; Groothoff, J.W.; Nijs, J. Written pain neuroscience education in fibromyalgia: A multicenter randomized controlled trial. *Pain Pract.* **2014**, *14*, 689–700. [CrossRef] [PubMed]

75. Van Ittersum, M.W.; van Wilgen, C.P.; Groothoff, J.W.; van der Schans, C.P. Is appreciation of written education about pain neurophysiology related to changes in illness perceptions and health status in patients with fibromyalgia? *Patient Educ. Couns.* **2011**, *85*, 269–274. [CrossRef] [PubMed]

76. Zeltzer, L.; Schlank, C.B. *Conquering Your Child's Chronic Pain: A Pediatrician's Guide for Reclaiming a Normal Childhood*; HarperCollins: New York, NY, USA, 2005.

77. Krane, E.J.; Mitchell, D. *Relieve Your Child's Chronic Pain: A Doctor's Program for Easing Headaches, Abdominal Pain, Fibromyalgia, Juvenile Rheumatoid Arthritis, and More*; Simon & Schuster: New York, NY, USA, 2005.

78. Palermo, T.M.; Law, E.F. *Managing Your Child's Chronic Pain*; Oxford University Press: Oxford, UK, 2015.

79. Wilson, D.; Mackintosh, S.; Nicholas, M.K.; Moseley, G.L. Harnessing group composition-related effects in pain management programs: A review and recommendations. *Pain Manag.* **2016**, *6*, 161–173. [CrossRef] [PubMed]

80. Migraine: How it works and how to get it under control. Deutsches Kinderschmerzzentrum; Center, G.P.P. Available online: https://www.youtube.com/watch?v=JrCdyuDsg6c (accessed on 30 July 2016).

81. Hunter Integrated Pain Service. *Understanding Pain and What to Do about it in Less Than Five Minutes*; HIPS: New Lambton, Australia, 2014.

82. Noel, M.; Palermo, T.M.; Chambers, C.T.; Taddio, A.; Hermann, C. Remembering the pain of childhood: Applying a developmental perspective to the study of pain memories. *Pain* **2015**, *156*, 31–34. [CrossRef] [PubMed]

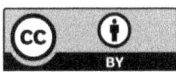

Review

Chronic Pain in Children and Adolescents: Diagnosis and Treatment of Primary Pain Disorders in Head, Abdomen, Muscles and Joints

Stefan J. Friedrichsdorf [1,2,*], James Giordano [3], Kavita Desai Dakoji [1], Andrew Warmuth [1], Cyndee Daughtry [1] and Craig A. Schulz [1,4]

[1] Children's Hospitals and Clinics of Minnesota, Minneapolis, MN 55404, USA; Kavita.DesaiDakoji@childrensMN.org (K.D.D.); Andrew.Warmuth@childrensMN.org (A.W.); Cyndee.Daughtry@childrensMN.org (C.D.); Craig.Schulz@childrensMN.org (C.S.)
[2] Department of Pediatrics, University of Minnesota Medical School, Minneapolis, MN 55455, USA
[3] Georgetown University Medical Center, Washington, DC 20057, USA; james.giordano@georgetown.edu
[4] Center for Spirituality & Healing, University of Minnesota, Minneapolis, MN 55455, USA
* Correspondence: Stefan.Friedrichsdorf@childrensMN.org; Tel.: +1-612-813-6450

Academic Editor: Carl L. von Baeyer
Received: 31 August 2016; Accepted: 1 December 2016; Published: 10 December 2016

Abstract: Primary pain disorders (formerly "functional pain syndromes") are common, under-diagnosed and under-treated in children and teenagers. This manuscript reviews key aspects which support understanding the development of pediatric chronic pain, points to the current pediatric chronic pain terminology, addresses effective treatment strategies, and discusses the evidence-based use of pharmacology. Common symptoms of an underlying pain vulnerability present in the three most common chronic pain disorders in pediatrics: primary headaches, centrally mediated abdominal pain syndromes, and/or chronic/recurrent musculoskeletal and joint pain. A significant number of children with repeated acute nociceptive pain episodes develop chronic pain in addition to or as a result of their underlying medical condition "chronic-on-acute pain." We provide description of the structure and process of our interdisciplinary, rehabilitative pain clinic in Minneapolis, Minnesota, USA with accompanying data in the treatment of chronic pain symptoms that persist beyond the expected time of healing. An interdisciplinary approach combining (1) rehabilitation; (2) integrative medicine/active mind-body techniques; (3) psychology; and (4) normalizing daily school attendance, sports, social life and sleep will be presented. As a result of restored function, pain improves and commonly resolves. Opioids are not indicated for primary pain disorders, and other medications, with few exceptions, are usually not first-line therapy.

Keywords: chronic pain; interdisciplinary treatment; children; adolescents; biopsychosocial; primary pain disorder; pediatric pain clinic

1. Introduction

Pediatric chronic pain is a significant problem with conservative estimates that posit 20% to 35% of children and adolescents affected by it worldwide [1–3]. Pain experienced in children's hospitals is known to be common, under-recognized, and under-treated, with more than 10% of hospitalized children showing features of chronic pain [4–7]. Although the majority of children reporting chronic pain are not greatly disabled by it [8], about 3% of pediatric chronic pain patients require intensive rehabilitation [9]. The total costs to society incurred by care for children and adolescents with moderate to severe chronic pain has been extrapolated to $19.5 billion annually in the USA [10]. For a recent systematic review of the etiology of chronic and recurrent pediatric pain not associated with disease, see King et al., 2011 [2].

The underlying pathophysiology of pain in children includes acute nociceptive pain (i.e., pain arising from the activation of peripheral nerve endings, including somatic and visceral pain), neuropathic pain (i.e., resulting from injury to, or dysfunction of, the somatosensory system), psycho-social-spiritual-emotional pain, total pain and/or the topic of this paper, chronic pain. Pain may originate from one, but more commonly involves a combination of these pathophysiologies. Commonly accepted definitions of chronic pain describe pain that persists for three months; however, the Rome IV criteria for functional abdominal pain disorders, for instance, typically require symptoms to be present and persist for at least two months [11]. Like many pediatric pain programs, we define chronic pain not necessarily by using arbitrary temporal parameters, but rather employ a more functional definition such as "pain that extends beyond the expected period of healing" and "hence lacks the acute warning function of physiological nociception" [12,13]. Simply put, pain lasting two months and 29 days does not necessarily change from "acute" to "chronic" once it merely extends to a period of three months in duration.

The 2012 American Pain Society Position Statement, "Assessment and Management of Children with Chronic Pain", indicates that chronic pain in children is the result of a dynamic integration of biological processes, psychological factors, and sociocultural variables, considered within a developmental trajectory [14]. Chronic pain includes persistent (ongoing) and recurrent (episodic) pain in children with underlying health conditions (e.g., inflammatory bowel disease, sickle cell disease, rheumatoid arthritis), and pain that is the disorder itself (e.g., primary headaches, centrally mediated abdominal pain syndrome, musculoskeletal pain, complex regional pain syndrome), with a significant number of children experiencing both entities, i.e., "chronic-on-acute" pain. Chronic pain affects the entire nervous system, and the term central sensitization, which is an increased central neural responsiveness to painful and non-painful stimuli, has been used to describe any central nervous system dysfunction or pathology that may contribute to the development or maintenance of many types of chronic pain [14,15].

Chronic childhood and adolescent pain is not only an issue of importance for the clinical care of pediatric patients, but also is a condition that exerts considerable bearing upon the medical, social and economic sectors. We believe that an improved understanding, definition and approach to treating chronic childhood and adolescent pain represent important steps toward both optimizing the clinical care of pediatric pain patients, and in this way, diminishing the overall negative impact of chronic pain on patients, medicine and society. In this light, and as an introduction to the Special Issue "Chronic and Recurrent Pain" in *Children* edited by L.S. Walker and C.L. von Baeyer [16], the aim of this paper is to highlight important key aspects in support of a fortified understanding of the development and expression of chronic pain in children and adolescents, such as pain catastrophizing and fear of pain. In addition, we aim to review the current pediatric chronic pain terminology and provide a brief description of the approach to assessing and treating chronic pain as practiced in our interdisciplinary pediatric pain clinic.

2. Children with Chronic Pain

2.1. Trajectory

Untreated chronic pain in children incurs a high risk for the subsequent development of pain and psychological disorders later in life. Seventeen percent of adult chronic pain patients reported a history of chronic pain in childhood or adolescence, with close to 80% indicating that the pain in childhood continued and persisted until adulthood [17]. In the USA, adults with chronic pain have a lower household income and higher risk of unemployment [18]. Studies of two birth cohorts from 1946 and 1958 showed that children with persistent abdominal pain and headaches go on to suffer more physical symptoms, anxiety and depression in adult life than healthy children [19–22]. A prospective study by Mulvaney and colleagues of 132 children with abdominal pain indicated long-term, high level risk of (adult) symptoms and impairment for a cluster of patients who did not have the most severe pain, but who had significantly more anxiety, depression, lower perceived self-worth, and more negative life events at baseline [23].

In another three-year prospective cohort study [24] involving 1336 children and teens in pain aged 11–14 years, Dunn et al. showed that 44% displayed a developmental trajectory for increased pain disorders and conditions, primarily presenting as headaches, back pain, abdominal pain and facial pain, and 12% presented with persistent pain. Individuals at highest risk to develop persistent pain were predominantly female, demonstrated the highest level of somatization and depression at both the start and end of the study period, and were least likely to be satisfied with their life. As well, research has shown that extra-intestinal somatic and depressive symptoms at the initial pediatric evaluation for functional abdominal pain were significant predictors of functional gastrointestinal disorders in adulthood [25]. Pediatric patients with functional abdominal pain exhibit long-term vulnerability to anxiety that begins in childhood and persists into late adolescence and early adulthood, even if abdominal pain resolves [26]. The National Longitudinal Study of Adolescent to Adult Health included more than 14,000 study participants and has shown that chronic pain in adolescence is associated with higher rates of mental health disorders reported in adulthood with anxiety (21.1% vs. 12.4% pain-free adolescents) and depressive disorders (24.5% vs. 14.1%) being most common [27]. Van Tilburg and colleagues analyzed data from a longitudinal study of a nationally representative sample of 9970 adolescents in the USA to show that adolescents with chronic pain and depression are at increased risk for both suicidal ideation and suicide attempt [28].

2.2. Pain Catastrophizing and Fear of Pain

The fear avoidance model of pain with an emphasis on the maladaptive behaviors that lead to activity avoidance has guided pediatric chronic pain research and clinical practice [29]. Certainly most, if not all, people seek to avoid pain. Fear of pain and subsequent exacerbation of its effects is common in both adults and children. Catastrophizing (or "Awfulizing") is a key mechanism by which the experience of pain can be exacerbated in children and adolescents. Catastrophizing represents a set of negative cognitive/emotional processes that include magnification (amplification of the significance of pain), rumination (anxious preoccupation with pain) and pessimism about pain sensations and feelings of helplessness when in pain. There is a significant body of research showing a correlation of children's pain behaviors and their (as well as their parents') extent of catastrophizing [30–32]. Pain reduction through distraction is delayed by catastrophizing [33], is associated with greater pain in children when either child or parent displays high pain catastrophizing [34]. Negative pain memory bias is advanced by parental (more than children's) pain catastrophizing and, in addition, expectations as well as cognitions of parents influence child pain memory formation [35].

Both physical and psychological dysfunction in pediatric chronic pain is modulated and upregulated by fear of pain [36]. Diminishing the fear of pain strongly correlates with positive functional outcomes in children with primary pain disorders [36]. Further, there is a robust positive association between pain-related fear and disability [37]. Consistent with the fear-avoidance model of chronic pain, these findings suggest that pain-related fear may be an important therapeutic target for approaches aimed at reducing pain-related disability.

2.3. Time for a New Name: "Primary Pain Disorder"

Many different chronic and recurrent pain syndromes in both adult and pediatric populations are now considered to be manifestations of an underlying vulnerability or pain spectrum condition, rather than being viewed as separate disorders [38]. Considerable evidence, especially from twin studies, points to a role of shared biological sensitivity, "pain vulnerability," "pain sensitivity," or "central sensitivity syndrome" [38–42]. Thus, conditions such as primary headaches (including tension headaches), centrally mediated abdominal pain syndromes, localized or widespread musculoskeletal pain (including "pain amplification syndrome," "non-cardiac chest pain," "costochondritis," "temporomandibular joint disorder," "juvenile fibromyalgia," etc.) are no longer regarded as separate entities with differing underlying pathophysiologies in need of different treatments. Instead, these conditions are now generally regarded as pain manifestations of the same underlying condition that present at varied locations.

The term primary pain disorder (formerly: functional pain syndrome) was first employed by Schechter in 2014 [43]. It describes a chronic pain disorder that cannot be explained by appropriate medical assessment(s) in terms of conventionally defined medical disease, as based on biochemical or structural abnormalities. A primary pain disorder is associated with significant disruption of everyday life and often leads to incapacitation. This disorder is not typically responsive to unimodal medical therapy, and attempts at such management can consume significant time, medical resources and finances. Persistent treatment failures can lead to pejorative implications such as patients perceiving that their pain is not organic and therefore not real or serious, and/or stigmatization (i.e., patients' symptoms may be characterized as fictitious or as evidence of malingering).

Toward advancing an improved understanding of primary pain disorder and its relation to chronic pain in children and adolescents, the following section presents a review of the three most prevalent symptoms, manifestations, and locations of a primary pain disorder (headaches, abdominal pain, and/or musculoskeletal pain).

3. Pain Manifestations and Locations of a Primary Pain Disorder

3.1. Primary Headache: Tension Headaches and Migraines

Traditionally, headaches were classified using a bimodal construct: tension headaches (infrequent episodic, frequent episodic, or chronic) versus migraines (with or without aura) [44]. In 2013 the International Headache Society (IHS) [45] classified "primary headaches" as migraines, tension-type headaches, trigeminal autonomic cephalalgias and "secondary headaches," e.g., a headache attributed to trauma or injury to the head, cranial or cervical vascular disorders, etc. Pediatric data supports the notion that childhood headaches are a continuum, rather than discrete entities [46,47]. Recent findings [48] suggest that "migraine" and "tension-type" headaches might not be separate diagnostic/disease entities, but rather represent a severity continuum for young adults 18–24 years of age who experience chronic headaches more than 3–4 days per week. Two cross-sectional studies [48] with more than 3400 headache patients revealed that those who are experiencing headaches at a younger age (18–24 years old) and with higher frequency (more than 15 headache days/month) displayed a unimodal distribution, suggesting the dimensional construct of a primary headache. Conversely, patients who experienced a lower frequency of headaches and were of older age showed bimodal headache distributions, which could be differentiated into "migraine" versus "tension-type" headache. In addition, pressure pain thresholds over the temporalis, masseter, and frontalis muscles in patients with headaches do not exhibit strong differences between migraine and tension headaches [49]. In other words, for pediatric patients who are headache-free most of the time and (only) experience episodic headaches, the "bimodal" classification of "tension-type" versus "migraines" continues to be clinically appropriate, as migraines (as opposed to tension-type) might be alleviated by a medication regimen [50–52] (see Section 5). On the other hand, for patients who present with chronic, daily headaches (or headaches that occur and persist more than 50% of the time) separation into "tension-type headaches" and "migraines" appears to be a less helpful distinction. For clinical signs that may require further workup of headache, see Table 1.

Medication overuse headaches (MOH) are not uncommon among pediatric patients with chronic headaches and usually occur when patients are taking analgesics (including acetaminophen, non-steroidal anti-inflammatory drugs (NSAIDs), or opioids), triptans, and/or ergotamine for more than 10–15 days/month (depending on medication class) [53–55]. Effective treatment requires a rapid discontinuation of medication [56]. In a case study of children and adolescents with daily or almost-daily headache concomitant with daily or almost-daily analgesic intake, Hering-Hanit et al. reported that a successful wean from analgesics was achieved without hospitalization or significant interference with daily life, and resulted in complete cessation of chronic daily headache in 25 of 26 patients [57].

Table 1. Headache warning signals requiring further workup, including neuroimaging.

- Focal or abnormal neurological signs, ataxia
- Papilledema (including rule out pseudotumor cerebri)
- Age < 3 years
- "Worst headache of my life"
- Progressive worsening headaches
- Ventriculoperitoneal-shunt
- Neurocutaneous syndrome
- Immunocompromised → Cerebrospinal fluid? (check with Infectious disease, oncology or transplant clinician)

Rule out: carbon monoxide toxicity; Obstructive sleep apnea.

3.2. Centrally Mediated Abdominal Pain Syndrome

In the 2016 revision of the Rome Criteria (now in its 4th iteration), the term "functional abdominal pain" has been replaced by "centrally mediated abdominal pain syndrome" (CAPS), which occurs as a result of central sensitization with disinhibition of pain signals, rather than increased peripheral afferent excitability [58]. For example, when compared to healthy peers, pre-adolescent girls with irritable bowel syndrome display impaired endogenous inhibition of somatic pain [59]. Adolescents with irritable bowel syndrome (IBS) symptoms are also more likely to experience widespread hyperalgesia [60]. CAPS in childhood and adolescence increases the risk for chronic primary pain disorder (abdominal pain, migraine/tension headache, and chronic musculoskeletal pain) in adulthood [61,62], and women with a pediatric history of functional abdominal pain display long-term vulnerability to pain [63]. For clinical warning signs that may require further workup of abdominal pain, see Table 2.

Table 2. Abdominal pain warning signals requiring further workup.

- Persistent right upper or right lower quadrant pain
- Pain that wakes child from sleep
- Dysphagia
- Arthritis
- Persistent vomiting
- Perirectal disease
- Gastrointestinal blood loss
- Involuntary weight loss
- Nocturnal diarrhea
- Deceleration of linear growth
- Unexplained fever

3.3. Musculoskeletal and Joint Pain

A systematic review by King et al. [2] reported that back pain is common in children and adolescents, with one-month prevalence rates ranging from 18% to 24% in samples of English and Swedish children [64,65]. Weekly or "at least weekly" back pain was reported in 9%–25% of patients [3,64,66].

Stanford et al. have shown that parent- and youth-reported anxiety/depression were predictive of start and end points of back pain trajectories [3]. Four studies reported a 9%–39% prevalence of musculoskeletal and/or limb pain in 3842 children and adolescents, depending on time period of reporting [67–70]. The relation between musculoskeletal/limb pain and athletic participation confounds findings in this area, as many participants reported that their pain was the result of a sports injury. The majority of the studies reported that musculoskeletal pain is more common in girls than in boys [2].

Diagnostic criteria for "fibromyalgia" are not validated in children and teenagers, and the term "widespread musculoskeletal pain" is more commonly used instead. For clinical warning signs that may require further workup in children presenting with musculoskeletal and/or joint pain, see Table 3.

Table 3. Musculoskeletal/joint pain warning signals requiring further workup.

- Arthralgia: Rubor, calor, edema
- Pain/stiffness in the morning
- Abnormal radiographic findings
- Pain at rest, relieved by activity
- Pain at night: Worsened by massage, analgesics ineffective
- Bony tenderness
- Poor growth
- Weight loss
- Abnormal blood results: Including complete blood count (CBC), C-reactive protein (CRP), erythrocyte sedimentation rate (ESR)

3.4. Orthostatic Dysfunction as Part of the Chronic Pain Picture: From "POTS" and "Autonomic Dysfunction", to "Chronic Lyme Disease"

During initial intake, more than 50% of our chronic pain patients reveal in their medical history that they experienced episodes of enigmatic symptoms of dizziness, fatigue, low energy, blurry vision, "blacking out," and/or tachycardia, which we usually interpret as a result of deconditioning; these symptoms are frequently exacerbated by anxiety. We nearly always see this as a result of fear of pain and deconditioning, and not as a unifying diagnosis of a medical condition.

In short, like the vast majority of pediatric pain centers, we do not support the notion that "post-orthostatic tachycardia syndrome" (POTS), "autonomic dysfunction," and/or "chronic Lyme disease" (i.e., diagnosis of persistent infection with *Borrelia burgdorferi* despite negative titers calling for long-term antibiotic treatment) [71] are either the underlying pathophysiology or a significant contributor of a primary pain disorder. In fact, in nearly all of our patients, the clinical symptoms of orthostatic dysfunction and other co-existing, enigmatic symptoms (following a reasonable negative workup) disappear during our rehabilitative pain program.

3.5. Conversion Disorder

An estimated 5%–10% of patients referred to our pain clinic display clinical signs of a conversion disorder, either singularly or more commonly in conjunction with a primary pain disorder. Conversion disorder is a condition, in which the patient may present with numbness, paralysis, blindness, inability to speak, and/or other neurologic symptoms that cannot be explained by medical evaluation and for which diagnostic testing does not reveal any physical cause [72,73]. Often, the patient presents with a debilitating symptom that begins suddenly, has a history of a psychological problem(s) that gets better after the symptom appears, and shows lack of concern that would usually occur with symptoms of such severity (e.g., a 12-year-old boy seen in our clinic who was not concerned by the fact that he could not bear any weight on his limb and had been in a wheelchair for eight months).

3.6. Children with Acute and Chronic Pain: Co-Existing Pain Entities Requiring Advanced Treatment Strategies

Primary pain disorders also co-exist, or can even be triggered by underlying organic disease, and pain symptoms do not necessarily represent inadequate treatment, flare-up, or recurrence. As previously mentioned, approximately 5% of children and teenagers in the general population have significant pain-related dysfunction [2]. As a result, we can expect that at least the same percentage of children with recurrent painful episodes, such as that occurring in sickle cell disease, inflammatory bowel disease, rheumatoid arthritis, congenital heart disease, or cancer, will display chronic pain features in addition (i.e., co-existance) to their underlying somatic pain episodes, and that pain is not necessarily caused by the organic disease itself.

The realization that a significant number of children with recurrent organic painful episodes whose pain proves to be complicated to treat, have what is known as "chronic-on-acute" disease, which may be potentially complicated even further by neuropathic and/or psycho-social-spiritual pain. Such pain is important, and we believe it has beneficial, clinical implications. Namely, it reduces over-investigation of the underlying organic disease, and over-treatment of pain (e.g., inappropriate long-term opioid administration). Clearly, repeated acute pain episodes increase the risk of significant pain-related dysfunction. For instance, chronic pain is significantly higher in survivors of childhood cancer than in their healthy siblings [74]. Chronic post-surgical pain (CPSP), potentially a transition from acute to chronic pain, has recently been described to occur in 12%–22% of children [75–77], and is possibly associated with parental catastrophizing [78].

In practical terms, for treatment of acute tissue injuries (such as new vaso-occlusive sickle cell disease or a flare-up of Crohn's disease with bloody diarrhea), short-term administration of opioids titrated to effect are in fact usually required for adequate analgesia as part of an advanced multimodal analgesic strategy [79,80]. However, as discussed below (in Section 5.3), in patients with chronic daily sickle-cell pain or chronic daily abdominal pain due to Crohn's disease that is in clinical remission, long-term daily administration of opioids would not be indicated.

4. Interdisciplinary Rehabilitative Pediatric Pain Program: Our Approach

Since 2006, our interdisciplinary rehabilitative pain clinic at Children's Hospitals and Clinics of Minnesota in Minneapolis, MN, USA, has been dedicated to the care of children and teenagers in pain. A multidisciplinary bio-psycho-social rehabilitation and functional restoration approach has been shown to effectively and efficiently improve function both in adults [81] and children/teenagers [82–86]. However, it remains unclear how long we can wait to send a child to a pain program, and it is also unknown at what point clinical deterioration begins. Adult meta-data show that wait times for chronic pain treatment of six months or longer are medically unacceptable and result in significant decreases in both health-related quality of life and psychological well-being [87]. Two-thirds of USA pediatricians felt it was not their primary responsibility to treat chronic pain [88]. The Pediatric Pain Screening Tool (PPST) was recently validated to assist clinicians stratifying their pediatric pain patients to appropriate interventions [89].

The three most commonly seen manifestations of a primary pain disorder in our pain clinic are (1) primary headache (tension headaches/migraines); (2) centrally mediated abdominal pain syndrome; and (3) chronic and recurrent musculoskeletal/joint pain, with the majority of patients having at least two of those symptoms. The frequency of these conditions is followed closely by the prevalence of Complex regional pain syndrome (CRPS) Type 1, with 11% of our patients presenting with this condition (See Table 6).

Consistent with the treatment approach of the majority of pediatric pain clinics in the USA and Canada [90], our clinic offers an interdisciplinary rehabilitative approach aiming at returning to normal function.

4.1. From Clinic Intake to the Exit Interview

In our clinic, children whose daily functioning is disrupted due to pain (e.g., are missing school, displaying poor sleep, withdrawing from social life and/or having been assessed with anxiety or depression) will be offered a 90-minute multidisciplinary intake (in the same room at the same time) with the patient/parents and a physical therapist, psychologist, social worker/family therapist and a pain physician or advanced nurse practitioner. Following this, the patient undergoes three individual evaluations: clinical examination, a physical therapy evaluation, and a psychological evaluation. Parents/caregivers meet separately with the social worker/family therapist for an evaluation of family factors that may impact the child's pain, including beliefs about pain and response to pain. Afterwards, the clinical team meets to discuss findings and suggest recommendations, while the family is given a short rest period/hiatus. Following the clinical team meeting, either the MD or NP meets with the patient and his or her family for a 60-minute exit interview to present and explain recommendations and treatment plan.

We found it most effective for a child with a primary pain disorder to return to normal function first, and as a result of such functional reintegration, to then subsequently focus upon decreasing pain subsequently. During the exit interview we reveal that we believe the child's pain to be "real," and establish the expectation that as a first step we work toward "life gets back to normal," and then as a result—"the pain gets better"—and not the other way around. For patients with a primary pain disorder, we set the expectation of becoming pain-free or mostly pain-free. We have found that this positive expectation represents something of a self-fulfilling prophecy, and data support that expectations predict chronic pain treatment outcomes [91]. In our clinic, only 16% of children at intake reported that they believed they could ever be pain-free. Upon exit interview at the end of the first visit, which represents the first formal intervention, 92% of children expressed the belief that they could, in fact, become pain-free.

We put great importance on demystifying the problem: pain has lost its warning signal, and using the affected body part does not result in greater harm. During the exit interview, we explain in age-appropriate language how the pain "is real," but "has lost its warning function". Using drawings on a flip-chart and age-appropriate examples, we then go into greater detail about the concept of pain transmission and important modalities to down-modulate pain (so-called "OFF-Switch" modulation) through activation of descending inhibiting pathways (DIP) from the "control-center" periaqueductal grey (PAG), which are engaged by (1) physical therapy/exercise and (2) integrative medicine/distraction. We also discuss up-regulation (so called "ON-switch" activation induced by the prefrontal cortex which worsens pain through stress, negative mood, anxiety, depression, school absenteeism, social withdrawal, insomnia, etc.) and which is mitigated by (3) psychological counseling; and (4) normalizing activities of daily life. We then discuss the need to target both shutting off the "ON-switch" and turning on the "OFF-switch" at the same time, explaining why all four modalities are offered concurrently in our clinic, and why these modalities might not have worked in the past, if and when administered separately.

4.2. Rehabilitative Pain Program Modalities

In order to enroll in our rehabilitative pain program, we expect children and their parents to participate in all (i.e., not just some) of the following five modalities.

4.2.1. Physical Therapy

Physical therapy and exercise are key modalities in the treatment of pediatric patients with primary pain disorder and/or CRPS [82,84–86,92–95]. Adolescents with chronic pain usually have a lower physical activity level [96] and physical activity has been shown to reduce the risk for depression in female adolescents [97]. In children and adolescents participating in a rehabilitative pain program, the rate of improvement in function was significantly more rapid than the decrease in pain [92].

In our clinic, a physical therapist (PT) facilitates restoration of movement and the reduction of pain. PTs develop an individualized treatment plan that is based on each patient's functional goals (e.g., returning to a sport or age-appropriate play activity). PTs who work with children with chronic pain utilize traditional therapeutic techniques (e.g., normalizing lost range of motion, strength, balance, etc.) along with more pain-specific interventions (e.g., graded motor imagery [98], pain-physiology education, etc.). The majority of chronic pain patients entering our clinic are found to be de-conditioned upon physical therapy evaluation. Clinically, many of our chronic pain patients place a high value on athletics, with the majority of patients participating in some form of sport. If pain disrupts physical activity, it likely also impacts patients' coping strategies as well as their socialization. Reasons we assert to be important to refer pediatric/adolescent pain patients to physical therapy are provided in Table 4.

The treatment goal we establish for and with our patients is to first return to function, and then to secondarily attempt to decrease pain as a result of this functional restoration.

The initial assessment goals include determining if any neuro-musculoskeletal factors contribute to pain, if any, and defining the patient's movement goals. Treatment goals are aimed at normalizing a patient's environmental interactions and engagements, and addressing and mitigating those neuro-musculoskeletal variables contributing to pain.

Table 4. Reasons to refer a pediatric chronic pain patient to physical therapy.

- Goals of returning to sport or activities
- Not participating in gym class
- Signs of weakness, poor balance, poor endurance, abnormal movement patterns, or poor posture, etc.
- Diagnoses associated with abnormal movement patterns or weakness: e.g., Ehlers–Danlos syndrome, complex regional pain syndrome (CRPS), centrally mediated abdominal pain syndrome (CAPS), chronic musculoskeletal pain, chronic headaches, etc.

4.2.2. Integrative Medicine: Active Mind-Body Techniques

Integrative modalities (sometimes referred to as complementary and alternative medicine) that have been described as effective in the management of pediatric pain include hypnosis, yoga, acupuncture, and massage [99–107]. Active mind-body techniques, such as guided imagery, hypnosis, biofeedback, yoga, and distraction each and all evoke pain modulation by engaging a number of mechanisms within the analgesic neuraxis. Techniques such as distraction and guided imagery appear to modulate the release of endogenous opioids from the periaqueductal and periventricular grey regions to disinhibit descending inhibitory pathways of the brainstem to suppress pain transmission in the dorsal horn of the spinal cord [108–112]. As well, distraction has been shown to increase activity of the orbitofrontal and perigenual anterior cingulate cortex, as well as periaqueductal grey and the posterior thalamus to modulate pain at the supraspinal level [113,114].

In our clinic, integrative and active mind-body techniques are taught to patients, or to the parents, when children are younger than school age, or cognitively impaired. Mind-body techniques focus on intervention strategies that integrate cognitive and emotional processes with physiological functions and experience in order to promote health. We expect all our patients (who are older than five years, and cognitively capable) to learn at least one active integrative medicine technique and incorporate this into their daily routine. Parents are offered training in the same techniques so that they can be aware of what their child is learning, and can reinforce practice as needed. We also expect our patients to learn in our clinic and practice daily at home or school at least one age-appropriate mind-body technique of relaxation and self-regulation. Modalities our patients have reported to be helpful include breathing strategies (e.g., diaphragmatic breathing, square breathing, and "snake"/slow exhale breathing), aromatherapy, biofeedback, progressive muscle relaxation, autogenic training, mindfulness, yoga, and/or self-hypnosis. In addition, we support and offer passive integrative modalities such as acupressure, acupuncture, and/or massage (as supplemental to, but not in place of, self-directed techniques).

4.2.3. Psychological Intervention

Anxiety, depressive, and behavioral disorders are early risk factors of chronic pain (rather than vice versa) [115]. At low levels of anxiety, higher pain is predictive of greater disability; however, highly anxious adolescents tend to function poorly regardless of level of pain [116]. Psychological treatments significantly reduce pain intensity that is reported by children and adolescents with headache, abdominal pain, and musculoskeletal/joint pain [117,118]. Cognitive behavioral therapy (CBT) led to significant improvements in pain coping, catastrophizing, and efficacy that were sustained over time in adolescents with chronic pain [119]. CBT has been shown to increase grey matter in the prefrontal cortex of patients with chronic pain, and this increase in prefrontal cortical grey matter has been associated with reduced pain catastrophizing [120].

In our clinic, psychological intervention is a routine part of our treatment approach, and serves to teach patients general coping skills and integrative medicine strategies, as well as help incorporate these into a daily routine to promote consistent practice, and to promote normalization of a patient's daily life. Most patients in our clinic experience psychological distress due to disrupted functioning, as secondary to pain, and not as a primary presenting concern. As such, our psychologists' role is to promote restoration of baseline functioning by teaching appropriate coping strategies and by targeting pain-related fears and catastrophizing that may disrupt normal cognitive and behavioral functions.

4.2.4. Normalizing Life: "The 4 S's": Sports, Social, Sleep and School

As previously discussed, we explain to our patients that "first your life gets back to normal, then your pain decreases—unfortunately it's not the other way around." We go on to explain "sometimes, pain may even increase, before it gets better." We explain that the "4 S's": sports, socialization, sleep and school need to return to normal parameters before pain resolution could or should be expected.

- Sports: As mentioned in the previous section addressing physical therapy, we place strong emphasis on restoring activity and returning patients to their normal regimen of physical activity, exercise and/or sports.
- Social: When adolescents with chronic pain do not perceive their friends as providing support, they tend to avoid social situations [121]. The social lives of the chronic pain patients in our clinic are commonly disrupted for a variety of reasons, including inability to keep up with peers, disruptions to sports/extra-curricular activities where social contacts occur, experience or fear of being teased because of pain ("you are faking it") or disability. In our clinic, the family therapist and psychologist work with the patient and his or her family to develop strategies and tactics to regain a balanced social life, provide validation of feeling misunderstood, and continuous medical reassurance that pain is physiologically mediated or "real".
- Sleep: The majority of children with chronic pain have sleep difficulties, including problems with sleep initiation, sleep maintenance, and/or early morning awakening [122]. These sleep problems tend to be persistent and are associated with negative impact for youths with chronic pain [123]. Treatment of insomnia in youths with chronic pain may lead to improvements in quality of life and reduction in healthcare cost. In our practice, the majority of patients' parents are successfully coached to assist their children in waking in the morning, having breakfast, attending to personal hygiene, and leaving the house in time to attend the first class at school. We encourage a "no nap" policy, and allow patients to "sleep in" one to two hours later (but no longer) on weekends. We expect that illuminated screens (e.g., television, computer monitors, smart phones, tablets, etc.) will not be used starting one hour before bedtime (or after bedtime), as studies have shown that the blue light emitted by such screens can interfere with melatonin production and/or release [124,125].

- School: Parental catastrophizing and protective responses to their child's pain predict school attendance rates and overall school performance [126]. Long-term scholastic impairment results in reduced occupational achievement, increased educational costs, and increased risk of developing psychiatric disorders (e.g., anxiety, depression) [127–129]. In our clinic, the child's social worker and psychologist work closely with the patient, parent, and school (if and when permission is granted) to develop a personalized school re-entry plan. Factors considered in developing a re-entry plan include possible learning concerns, stigmatization, teasing and/or bullying by peers, and secondary gain/special attention due to pain and/or disability behavior(s). We have found that with close communication, most schools are supportive of having students take time-limited breaks to practice integrative medicine strategies before returning to the classroom. We typically work with schools for informal accommodations, instead of pursuing an Individualized Education Plan (IEP) or a 504 plan (Section 504 of the USA Rehabilitation Act was developed to guarantee that a child with a disability as identified under the law who is attending an elementary or secondary educational institution will receive accommodations that insure equal capacity to access the learning environment and achieve academic success) to underscore our expectation that the student will return to baseline functioning without accommodation(s).

Parents are asked if they can consistently and successfully get their child/teenager to school regardless of the patient's report of their inability to go (due to chronic pain). The social worker helps the parent to develop a plan to insure their child's school attendance, inclusive of conjoining other family members to such tasks, if and as necessary to assist parents.

We usually do not support online school or home schooling for children who have attended a physical facility school prior to their pain.

4.2.5. Parent Coaching

Children with chronic pain often have a negative influence in and upon their family life, can pose a financial burden, both in direct and indirect costs incurred from healthcare utilization and lost wages due to parents taking time off work to care for the child, and the child in pain can exert considerable emotional toll on family members. Families of children with chronic pain generally have poorer family functioning, and pain-related disability is more consistently related to family functioning than pain intensity [130]. Studies have shown that mothers of children with chronic abdominal pain show pain bias when interpreting ambiguous emotional expressions, and such bias might possibly contribute to parenting behaviors that maintain or enhance the child's pain [131]. Children of parents with chronic pain have been shown to display poorer outcomes in health, as well as psychological and familial functioning [132], and show increased risk of developing anxiety and depression as teenagers [133].

Parents in our clinic tend to be hypervigilant and pay increased attention to their children's pain reports/behaviors, given that they commonly are asked to report on pain specifics and details during routine medical consults. As such, parents may accidentally reinforce their child's pain behaviors. It is our clinical experience that parents are often defensive about their role in (maintaining) their child's pain. Normalizing parental protectiveness is a helpful first step toward shifting parents' focus to attend to healthy, adaptive behaviors, and decreasing their attention to their child's pain behaviors. We often ask parents to focus on their child's functioning and ask about specific daily activities, instead of attending to pain-related disruptions of their child's functioning. Depending on the child's age and developmental level, we may encourage parents to actively model mind-body and integrative medicine strategies to help their child engage in active and appropriate coping.

Parents' experiences of/with chronic pain and disability can influence their children's pain beliefs and behaviors. Parents' pain experiences are openly addressed and discussed with both the child and parent(s). The social worker discusses how the patient's pain is different from the parent's disability and pain, and the expectation that the child can become pain-free. The message we seek to communicate is that there is no reason to believe that they will be disabled like their parent.

Parents are often taught some of the same skills that are taught to their child/teenager by the psychologist. The social worker does this in order to teach the parents how to calm themselves when their child is having a pain flare. The parent is encouraged to use such skills to avoid incurring emotional escalations when dealing with their child. We believe that the parent is in an ideal position to emotionally anchor their child and support the use of calming skills to reduce pain levels. It is also important to teach parents to gently remind their child that normalization of daily functioning must come first before pain starts to decrease, and that progress is measured initially by the patient's return to a normalized daily life for sports, social life, sleep and school. Indeed it is easy for both the patient and parent to lose sight of this when the child continues to experience and present with pain. While active engagement of the parent(s) is advocated when working with younger children, a different approach is used when the patient is a teenager. Teenagers are taught and encouraged to acquire, develop and employ such skills more independently, and to foster greater capabilities for independence in activities of daily living. It has been our experience that parents are usually motivated to change any maladaptive or deleterious behavior. Clearly, they are very distressed by both seeing their child in pain and not knowing how to help them. The skills provided by our approach give the parent focus and a set of tasks, which can reduce their sense of helplessness and decrease their catastrophizing, while concomitantly helping their child.

5. Medications

In our pediatric pain practice we commonly find medications as a sole therapy for primary pain disorders to be ineffective, especially if they are not accompanied by the aforementioned modalities of our rehabilitative pain program. Still, it is important to consider the validity and value of pharmacological interventions as part of an integrative approach to pediatric pain care. In this regards some pharmacological considerations are included below.

5.1. Basic Analgesics: Acetaminophen and Ibuprofen

For mild, acute pain (i.e., associated with tissue injury), acetaminophen and ibuprofen are the agents of choice [80]. No other NSAID has been sufficiently studied for efficacy and safety in the pediatric population so as to be recommended as an alternative to ibuprofen. Although there is evidence for the superior analgesic properties of ibuprofen versus acetaminophen, it is considered to be of limited value because the studies were mostly performed in acute pain settings and lack long-term safety data. Both acetaminophen and ibuprofen have potential toxicities. There are concerns about renal and gastrointestinal toxicity, and bleeding with ibuprofen and other NSAIDs, and risks of hepatotoxicity and acute overdose are associated with acetaminophen [80]. Celecoxib (a cyclooxygenase-2 (COX-2) enzyme inhibitor) might be considered, if classical NSAIDs are contraindicated (e.g., owing to bleeding risks, or gastrointestinal side effects). Celecoxib does not display less renal toxicity as compared to classic NSAIDs. Safety and efficacy have been established only in children two years of age or older with juvenile rheumatoid arthritis, and for a maximum of six months of treatment.

With the exception of ibuprofen's proven efficacy in reducing pain at the onset of a migraine episode [50–52], basic analgesics generally are not used to treat primary pain disorders in the absence of new tissue injury. As discussed earlier, daily use of analgesics in headache patients incurs significant risk of leading to medication overuse headaches ("rebound headaches").

Fast-Acting NSAID: Ibuprofen-Sodium

Data have shown that when compared to ibuprofen, ibuprofen-sodium produced significantly greater analgesia over 6 h, and required fewer re-medications than standard formulations [134]. In addition, 200 mg fast-acting ibuprofen (Numbers-needed-to-treat (NNT) 2.1; 95% confidence interval (CI) 1.9–2.4) was as effective as 400 mg standard ibuprofen (NNT 2.4; 95% CI 2.2–2.5), and produced a faster onset of analgesia. Meta-analysis showed that NSAID-salts display more rapid absorption, faster initial pain reduction, good overall analgesia in more patients at the same dose, and probably evoke longer-lasting analgesia, without reports of adverse events [135]. For example, in our practice, we suggest fast-acting ibuprofen plus acetaminophen as a first step, followed by a triptan, if ineffective, be utilized within 10 min of onset of a migraine attack. In the USA, ibuprofen-sodium is available over the counter for about $8–$10 for 80 tablets (containing 266 mg of ibuprofen sodium, which is the equivalent to 200 mg of standard ibuprofen).

5.2. Opioids

The Center for Disease Control and Prevention's recently published 2016 Guidelines for Prescribing Opioids for Chronic Pain [136] do not apply to children and teenagers [137] and encompass only "patients aged ≥18 years with chronic pain outside of palliative and end-of-life care." The guidelines state further that the "recommendations do not address the use of opioid pain medication in children or adolescents aged <18 years".

Opioids administered for primary pain disorders have low long-term efficacy, a poor safety profile, and commonly a worse clinical outcome [133–139]. Thus, opioids should not be administered to pediatric patients with primary pain disorders [43], i.e., chronic pain defined that extends beyond the expected time of healing and hence lacks the acute warning function of physiological nociception. Opioids may be more likely to cause more harm than benefit in the treatment of primary pain disorders, which include conditions such as tension-type/migraines headaches, chronic musculoskeletal pain, "chronic sickle cell pain" (pain that extends beyond the expected time of acute vaso-occlusive crisis) and centrally mediated abdominal pain syndrome. In our practice, we do not prescribe opioids for primary pain disorders in children or teenagers, as we consider them to be contraindicated. On the other hand, in persistent pain conditions (i.e., long-lasting and/or repetitive nociceptive pain caused by tissue injury, such as in children with junctional epidermolysis bullosa, osteogenesis imperfecta, or advanced metastasized bone tumors (e.g., Ewing sarcoma)) opioids are important and effective for long-term analgesic management.

5.3. Adjuvant Analgesics

Adjuvant analgesics (e.g., low-dose tricyclic antidepressants, gabapentinoids, α-agonists, melatonin, etc.) may serve as valuable adjuncts. Although commonly used for primary pain disorders, there is little evidence to support their use against pediatric pain. Most pediatric data for this heterogeneous class of medications is derived from neuropathic and acute pain conditions [138–144]. The most commonly prescribed adjuvant analgesics in our pain clinic are melatonin, lidocaine 5% patch, gabapentin, and low-dose amitriptyline (See Table 5).

For migraines, only ibuprofen and triptans are supported by sufficient evidence to engender use in pediatrics [50–52]. Medication to treat migraines in adolescents have a strong placebo effect, with pain relief at 2 h in the placebo arms of seven randomized controlled trials ranging from 53% to 57.5%. A meta-analysis of 21 randomized controlled trials (RCTs) of pediatric headache management [145] revealed that placebo decreased headache frequency from 5.6 to 2.9 headaches/month, and also most commonly used drugs had little to no evidence to support their use in children and adolescents. Drugs shown to be ineffective included clonidine, flunarizine, pizotifen, propranolol, valproate, and fluoxetine [145].

Table 5. Adjuvant analgesics used in pediatric pain management (Pain Medicine and Palliative Care, Children's Hospitals and Clinics of Minnesota) [79].

Class	Medication	Dose	Route of Administration	Comments/Side Effects (See Text for Further Details)
Tricyclic Antidepressants (TCA)	Amitriptyline	Starting dose 0.1 mg/kg QHS, usually slowly titrated up to 0.5 mg/kg (max. 20-25 mg)	PO	Tertiary amine TCA; stronger anticholinergic side effects (including sedation) than nortriptyline
	Nortriptyline	Starting dose 0.1 mg/kg QHS, usually titrated up to 0.5 mg/kg (max. 20-25 mg)	PO	Secondary amine TCA; anticholinergic side effects
Gabapentenoids	Gabapentin	Starting dose 2 mg/kg QHS, usually slowly titrated up to initial target dose of 6 mg/kg/dose TID (max. 300 mg/dose TID). Max. dose escalation to 24 mg/kg/dose TID (max. 1200 mg/dose TID)	PO	Slow dose increase required; side effects: ataxia, nystagmus, myalgia, hallucination, dizziness, somnolence, aggressive behaviors, hyperactivity, thought disorder, peripheral edema
	Pregabaline	Starting dose 0.3 mg/kg QHS, usually slowly titrated up to initial target dose of 1.5 mg/kg/dose BID (max. 75 mg/dose BID). Max. dose escalation to 6 mg/kg/dose BID (max. 300 mg/dose BID)	PO	Switch from gabapentin, if distressing side effects or inadequate analgesia. Side effects: ataxia, nystagmus, myalgia, hallucination, dizziness, somnolence, aggressive behaviors, hyperactivity, thought disorder, peripheral edema; Associated with weight gain
Sodium Channel Blocker/Local anesthetic	Lidocaine 5%	Max. of 4 patches (in patients > 50 kg) 12 h on/12 h off	Transdermal patch	Not for severe hepatic dysfunction
Alpha-Agonist	Clonidine	1–3 mcg/kg QHS to Q6h	PO/transdermal	
	Dexmedetomidine	Infusion: 0.3 mcg/kg/h; titrate to max. 2 mcg/kg/h	IV	
Hormone	Melatonin	0.06–0.2 mg/kg (max. 3–10 mg) QHS	PO	Sleep induction, use extended-release, if interrupted sleep, possible analgesic effect

QHS: every night at bedtime; PO: per os, oral administration; IV: intravenous administration; BID: bis in die, twice a day; TID: ter in die, three times a day; Q6h: every 6h.

5.4. Selective Serotonin Re-Uptake Inhibitors (SSRI)/Serotonin and Norepinephrine Reuptake Inhibitors (SNRI)

There is little evidence to support the use of SSRIs or SNRIs in children/teenagers with primary pain disorders. An over-quoted, uncontrolled open-label case series for example has claimed that 21 of 25 children with recurrent abdominal pain improved following SSRI treatment [146]. However, placebo effects were large with pediatric antidepressant trials in other settings, regression to the mean must be expected, and there might be inherent bias at play. Efficacy studies for duloxetine in pediatric pain patients are lacking. In our clinic practice, we add an SSRI (such as citalopram, sertraline, escitalopram) in addition to (not in substitution for) individual psychotherapy to the treatment regimen of some patients who present with an underlying mental health diagnosis of anxiety and/or depression.

5.5. Laxatives

Constipation is the most common diagnosis in children presenting with abdominal pain in the emergency room [147], and in our practice, we see a surprisingly large number of children with long-standing abdominal pain, who have constipation and/or overflow diarrhea despite having been seen by many clinicians and reports that they have tried many laxatives. In our practice, we nearly always employ a scheduled (not "as needed" or pro re nate "prn")) regimen of (1) "Mush" (stool softener such as lactulose or polyethylenglycol 3350); (2) "Push" (stimulant such as senna) and (3) "Uncorking" (glycerin suppository for children <4 years, and bisodacyl suppository for older children) if no stool has been evacuated in the previous 24 h. This regimen has proven to be highly effective in resolving constipation, thereby decreasing or resolving abdominal pain [148].

5.6. Multimodal ("Opioid-Sparing") Analgesia

Multimodal analgesia is an approach used to prevent and treat pain in children: multiple agents, interventions, rehabilitation, and psychological and integrative therapies often act synergistically to elicit more effective pediatric pain control with fewer side effects than a single analgesic or modality [149]. Multimodal analgesic therapy (versus opioids alone) has been shown to reduce the length of hospitalization in patients undergoing surgery [150].

Evidence-based, safe multimodal (i.e., opioid-sparing) analgesia may include one, several or all of the following approaches: pharmacology (e.g., simple analgesia and/or opioids and/or adjuvant analgesia), anesthetic interventions (e.g., neuroaxial analgesia, nerve blocks), rehabilitation (e.g., physical therapy, occupational therapy, sleep hygiene), psychological counseling (e.g., cognitive behavioral therapy), and age-appropriate positioning and integrative (non-pharmacological) therapies, such as breathing techniques, self-hypnosis, and distraction.

6. From Mechanism and Classifications to Practice: Obligations for Care

Taken together, the use of these approaches has been shown to be highly effective in treating primary pain disorder in our clinical experience. Our approach is based and built upon a growing body of information that is both revising extant concepts of pain and pain modulation, and exploring new approaches to the assessment and treatment of pain. To be sure, new insights and perspectives about mechanisms and categorizations of pain in general, and pediatric pain in particular, are indubitably important to provide better understanding of pathology and more precise nosology [151,152]. Large-scale initiatives, such as the ongoing, federally directed Brain Research through Advancing Innovative Neurotechnologies (BRAIN) [153], and precision medicine initiatives, are developing more finely grained approaches to research, which seek to better define the neurobiology and psychosocial aspects of pediatric pain. Such knowledge must be appreciated and employed for its practical utility toward improving diagnosis and treatment of the pain patient [154].

As we have stated previously, and reaffirm here: " . . . we . . . study pain so that we may unravel its mysteries and develop more and better ways of relieving pain...to restore and sustain . . . living a life unencumbered by suffering" [155]. Understanding the bio-psychosocial dimensions of pain—as symptom, pathology and manifest illness—compels providing a more comprehensive and integrative approach to both assessment and treatment [156,157]. Such an approach entails the coordinated use of multiple disciplines, and engages both "high tech" and "low tech" means [158]. This enables both a more thorough evaluation of each patient's needs (in physiological, psychological and social dimensions), and more personalized, evidence-based intervention(s) to lessen or eradicate pain, and its manifest effects.

7. From Concepts to Practice: Our Experience at a Glimpse

Our interdisciplinary, rehabilitative pediatric pain clinic at Children's Minnesota has been seeing pediatric patients since 2006. Based on a 2007–2009 three-year prospective study (n = 145) and two chart reviews (2010 and 2014, n = 135) by Desai et al. [159,160] the majority (74%) of our new patients are female with an average age of 14 years (range ten-day-old infant to 17 years). The most common presenting conditions are listed in Table 6.

Table 6. Presenting or accompanying pain conditions: Initial intake at interdisciplinary pediatric pain clinic at Children's Minnesota.

- 74% Chronic or recurrent musculoskeletal pain
- 61% Primary headaches (tension-type/migraines)
- 38% CAPS
- 11% CRPS type I
- 26% Additional or accompanying underlying conditions, including

  Avascular necrosis
  Caffe's disease
  Cerebral palsy/spasticity
  Chiari-I-malformation with ventricular-peritoneal (VP) shunt
  Chronic postsurgical pain
  Conversion disorder
  CRPS type 2
  Erythromelalgi
  Inflammatory bowel disease (Crohn's disease, ulcerative colitis)
  Irritable bowel syndrome
  Juvenile rheumatoid/idiopathic arthritis (JRA/JIA)
  Malignancy
  Muscular dystrophy
  Penilodynia
  Phantom limb pain
  Progressive neurodegenerative/metabolic conditions incl. mitochondriopathies
  Sickle cell disease
  Vulvodynia

On average, our patients' pain began 2.4 years prior to intake and 57% of our patients had an immediate family member with chronic pain. On a pain scale 0–10, with 10 being the worst, our patients' average daily pain was rated 5.6/10 (worst: 8.8/10, least bad 3/10). A total of 75% of our pain patients also received a mental health diagnosis; 67% presented with anxiety (including general anxiety disorder, panic episodes, anxiety disorder not otherwise specified (NOS)), and 30% presented with depression (including major depression, and depressive disorder NOS) [160].

In reviewing our data from 2007 to 2009, 2010, and 2014, it appears that between 83% and 92% of new patients chose to follow-up with the rehabilitative treatment recommendations provided by our clinic after the initial intake. Of those, the majority (67%–79%) graduated successfully, (i.e., are pain-free or pain-free most of the time). Of the remaining, up to 26% were referred to additional and/or separate services (e.g., inpatient or outpatient psychiatry, eating disorder program, physical therapy/mental health provider closer to home) and of our most recent data review, 13% were still in treatment 6–12 months later [159]. The patients who successfully graduated had seen the physical therapist eight (mean; range 1–25) times, psychologist ten times (range 1–34), parents the family therapist/social four times (range 1–16), and the physician/nurse practitioner 2.5 times (range 1–7).

As previously noted, in our clinic at the first visit only 16% of children reported that they believed they could ever become pain-free. However, at the exit interview following the first visit, 92% of children asserted that they believed being pain-free was possible. The rehabilitative interdisciplinary treatment approach does not only seem to be effective for patients with primary pain disorders and CRPS, but also, in addition to other multimodal analgesia strategies, for the treatment of chronic-on-acute pain or chronic-on-neuropathic pain patients (see Section 3.6), indicating the significant overlap these conditions may have.

The work of our interdisciplinary team can be seen in a short movie, "Little Stars—Treating Chronic Pain in Children [161]."

8. Conclusions

Primary pain disorder (what was formerly known as "functional pain syndrome") is a common, under-diagnosed and under-treated condition in pediatric patients. Primary pain disorder occurs as a mechanistic vulnerability to multi-focal pain that can occur and be expressed at a number of bodily sites. Common symptoms of this underlying pain vulnerability include primary headache, centrally mediated abdominal pain syndrome, and chronic/recurrent musculoskeletal pain. A significant number of children with repeated acute nociceptive pain episodes develop chronic pain in addition to or as a result of their condition. Untreated chronic pediatric pain can increase the risk of pain, as well as physical and psychiatric disorders in adulthood. These findings reinforce the importance, if not obligation, to effectively address and treat pain in children and adolescents.

In our interdisciplinary pediatric pain management practice, we have shown that an integrative, multidisciplinary approach combining rehabilitation, complementary therapies (e.g., distraction, hypnosis, etc.), psychological counseling, and normalization of physical/sports activity, sleep, socialization, and school attendance—together with the prudent use of pharmacological agents—effectively mitigates and/or commonly resolves our patients' pain. Of note, however, is that opioids are not indicated for primary pain disorders, and other medications do not usually represent first-line therapy.

Further Resources for Clinicians and Patients

(1) Pediatric Pain Clinics in USA and Canada (American Pain Society): http://americanpainsociety. org/uploads/get-involved/PainClinicList_12_2015.pdf [162].
(2) Short Movie: Meet the Interdisciplinary Chronic Pain Clinic Team at Children's Minnesota: LittleStars TV https://www.youtube.com/watch?t=13&v=Bb1fHxfjdWI [161].
(3) Pain Bytes (Australia) [163].
(4) Persistent (Chronic) Pain 5-min video [164].
(5) Kiran Stordalen and Horst Rechelbacher Pediatric Pain, Palliative and Integrative Medicine Clinic Tour [165].
(6) Elliot Krane (TED-Talk) The mystery of chronic pain [166].
(7) The Department of Pain Medicine, Palliative Care, and Integrative Medicine, Children's Hospitals and Clinics of Minnesota [167].

Author Contributions: S.F. is primarily responsible for this review's conception, design and drafting of the text. All authors provided evaluation and revision of the manuscript, and have given final approval of the manuscript.

Conflicts of Interest: S.F. is supported, in part, by the The Mayday Fund, National Institutes of Health/National Cancer Institute, Children's Hospitals and Clinics of Minnesota Research Grant Program, National Institutes of Health/National Institute of Nursing Research, and the Canadian Partnership against Cancer. J.G. is supported, in part, by the Children's Hospitals and Clinics of Minneapolis Foundation, the William H. and Ruth Crane Schaefer Endowment, and the Clark Family Foundation. Other authors declare no conflict of interest.

References

1. Goodman, J.E.; McGrath, P.J. The epidemiology of pain in children and adolescents: A review. *Pain* **1991**, *46*, 247–264. [CrossRef]
2. King, S.; Chambers, C.T.; Huguet, A.; MacNevin, R.C.; McGrath, P.J.; Parker, L.; MacDonald, A.J. The epidemiology of chronic pain in children and adolescents revisited: A systematic review. *Pain* **2011**, *152*, 2729–2738. [CrossRef] [PubMed]
3. Stanford, E.A.; Chambers, C.T.; Biesanz, J.C.; Chen, E. The frequency, trajectories and predictors of adolescent recurrent pain: A population-based approach. *Pain* **2008**, *138*, 11–21. [CrossRef] [PubMed]
4. Friedrichsdorf, S.J.; Postier, A.; Eull, D.; Weidner, C.; Foster, L.; Gilbert, M.; Campbell, F. Pain outcomes in a US children's hospital: A prospective cross-sectional survey. *Hosp. Pediatr.* **2015**, *5*, 18–26. [CrossRef] [PubMed]
5. Taylor, E.M.; Boyer, K.; Campbell, F.A. Pain in hospitalized children: A prospective cross-sectional survey of pain prevalence, intensity, assessment and management in a Canadian pediatric teaching hospital. *Pain Res. Manag.* **2008**, *13*, 25–32. [CrossRef] [PubMed]
6. Zhu, L.M.; Stinson, J.; Palozzi, L.; Weingarten, K.; Hogan, M.E.; Duong, S.; Carbajal, R.; Campbell, F.A.; Taddio, A. Improvements in pain outcomes in a Canadian pediatric teaching hospital following implementation of a multifaceted knowledge translation initiative. *Pain Res. Manag. J. Can. Pain Soc.* **2012**, *17*, 173–179. [CrossRef]
7. Stevens, B.J.; Harrison, D.; Rashotte, J.; Yamada, J.; Abbott, L.K.; Coburn, G.; Stinson, J.; Le May, S. Pain assessment and intensity in hospitalized children in canada. *J. Pain* **2012**, *13*, 857–865. [CrossRef] [PubMed]
8. Huguet, A.; Miro, J. The severity of chronic pediatric pain: An epidemiological study. *J. Pain* **2008**, *9*, 226–236. [CrossRef] [PubMed]
9. Hechler, T.; Dobe, M.; Zernikow, B. Commentary: A worldwide call for multimodal inpatient treatment for children and adolescents suffering from chronic pain and pain-related disability. *J. Pediatr. Psychol.* **2010**, *35*, 138–140. [CrossRef] [PubMed]
10. Groenewald, C.B.; Essner, B.S.; Wright, D.; Fesinmeyer, M.D.; Palermo, T.M. The economic costs of chronic pain among a cohort of treatment-seeking adolescents in the United States. *J. Pain* **2014**, *15*, 925–933. [CrossRef] [PubMed]
11. Hyams, J.S.; di Lorenzo, C.; Saps, M.; Shulman, R.J.; Staiano, A.; van Tilburg, M. Functional disorders: Children and adolescents. *Gastroenterology* **2016**. [CrossRef]
12. Turk, D.; Okifuji, A. Pain terms and taxonomies of pain. In *Bonica's Management of Pain*; Bonica, J., Loeser, J., Chapman, C., Turk, D., Butler, S., Eds.; Lippincott Williams & Wilkins: Philadelphia, PA, USA, 2001.
13. Treede, R.D.; Rief, W.; Barke, A.; Aziz, Q.; Bennett, M.I.; Benoliel, R.; Cohen, M.; Evers, S.; Finnerup, N.B.; First, M.B.; et al. A classification of chronic pain for ICD-11. *Pain* **2015**, *156*, 1003–1007. [CrossRef] [PubMed]
14. Force, A.P.S.P.C.P.T. Assessment and Management of Children with Chronic Pain. A Position Statement from the American Pain Society. Available online: http://americanpainsociety.org/uploads/get-involved/pediatric-chronic-pain-statement.pdf (accessed on 7 December 2016).
15. Woolf, C.J. Central sensitization: Implications for the diagnosis and treatment of pain. *Pain* **2011**, *152*, S2–S15. [CrossRef] [PubMed]
16. Special Issue "Chronic and Recurrent Pain". Available online: http://www.mdpi.com/journal/children/special_issues/chronic_pain (accessed on 7 December 2016).
17. Hassett, A.L.; Hilliard, P.E.; Goesling, J.; Clauw, D.J.; Harte, S.E.; Brummett, C.M. Reports of chronic pain in childhood and adolescence among patients at a tertiary care pain clinic. *J. Pain* **2013**, *14*, 1390–1397. [CrossRef] [PubMed]
18. Johannes, C.B.; Le, T.K.; Zhou, X.; Johnston, J.A.; Dworkin, R.H. The prevalence of chronic pain in United States adults: Results of an internet-based survey. *J. Pain* **2010**, *11*, 1230–1239. [CrossRef] [PubMed]

19. Hotopf, M.; Mayou, R.; Wadsworth, M.; Wessely, S. Psychosocial and developmental antecedents of chest pain in young adults. *Psychosom. Med.* **1999**, *61*, 861–867. [CrossRef] [PubMed]
20. Hotopf, M.; Carr, S.; Mayou, R.; Wadsworth, M.; Wessely, S. Why do children have chronic abdominal pain, and what happens to them when they grow up? Population based cohort study. *BMJ* **1998**, *316*, 1196–1200. [CrossRef] [PubMed]
21. Jones, G.T.; Silman, A.J.; Power, C.; Macfarlane, G.J. Are common symptoms in childhood associated with chronic widespread body pain in adulthood? Results from the 1958 British birth cohort study. *Arthritis Rheum.* **2007**, *56*, 1669–1675. [CrossRef] [PubMed]
22. Power, C.; Elliott, J. Cohort profile: 1958 British birth cohort (National Child Development Study). *Int. J. Epidemiol.* **2006**, *35*, 34–41. [CrossRef] [PubMed]
23. Mulvaney, S.; Lambert, E.W.; Garber, J.; Walker, L.S. Trajectories of symptoms and impairment for pediatric patients with functional abdominal pain: A 5-year longitudinal study. *J. Am. Acad. Child Adolesc. Psychiatry* **2006**, *45*, 737–744. [CrossRef] [PubMed]
24. Dunn, K.M.; Jordan, K.P.; Mancl, L.; Drangsholt, M.T.; Le Resche, L. Trajectories of pain in adolescents: A prospective cohort study. *Pain* **2011**, *152*, 66–73. [CrossRef] [PubMed]
25. Horst, S.; Shelby, G.; Anderson, J.; Acra, S.; Polk, D.B.; Saville, B.R.; Garber, J.; Walker, L.S. Predicting persistence of functional abdominal pain from childhood into young adulthood. *Clin. Gastroenterol. Hepatol.* **2014**, *12*, 2026–2032. [CrossRef] [PubMed]
26. Shelby, G.D.; Shirkey, K.C.; Sherman, A.L.; Beck, J.E.; Haman, K.; Shears, A.R.; Horst, S.N.; Smith, C.A.; Garber, J.; Walker, L.S. Functional abdominal pain in childhood and long-term vulnerability to anxiety disorders. *Pediatrics* **2013**, *132*, 475–482. [CrossRef] [PubMed]
27. Noel, M.; Groenewald, C.B.; Beals-Erickson, S.E.; Gebert, J.T.; Palermo, T.M. Chronic pain in adolescence and internalizing mental health disorders: A nationally representative study. *Pain* **2016**, *157*, 1333–1338. [CrossRef] [PubMed]
28. Van Tilburg, M.A.; Spence, N.J.; Whitehead, W.E.; Bangdiwala, S.; Goldston, D.B. Chronic pain in adolescents is associated with suicidal thoughts and behaviors. *J. Pain* **2011**, *12*, 1032–1039. [CrossRef] [PubMed]
29. Fisher, E.; Palermo, T.M. Goal pursuit in youth with chronic pain. *Children* **2016**, *3*, 36. [CrossRef] [PubMed]
30. Cunningham, N.R.; Lynch-Jordan, A.; Barnett, K.; Peugh, J.; Sil, S.; Goldschneider, K.; Kashikar-Zuck, S. Child pain catastrophizing mediates the relation between parent responses to pain and disability in youth with functional abdominal pain. *J. Pediatr. Gastroenterol. Nutr.* **2014**, *59*, 732–738. [CrossRef] [PubMed]
31. Lynch-Jordan, A.M.; Kashikar-Zuck, S.; Szabova, A.; Goldschneider, K.R. The interplay of parent and adolescent catastrophizing and its impact on adolescents' pain, functioning, and pain behavior. *Clin. J. Pain* **2013**, *29*, 681–688. [CrossRef] [PubMed]
32. Williams, S.E.; Blount, R.L.; Walker, L.S. Children's pain threat appraisal and catastrophizing moderate the impact of parent verbal behavior on children's symptom complaints. *J. Pediatr. Psychol.* **2011**, *36*, 55–63. [CrossRef] [PubMed]
33. Campbell, C.M.; Witmer, K.; Simango, M.; Carteret, A.; Loggia, M.L.; Campbell, J.N.; Haythornthwaite, J.A.; Edwards, R.R. Catastrophizing delays the analgesic effect of distraction. *Pain* **2010**, *149*, 202–207. [CrossRef] [PubMed]
34. Birnie, K.A.; Chambers, C.T.; Chorney, J.; Fernandez, C.V.; McGrath, P.J. Dyadic analysis of child and parent trait and state pain catastrophizing in the process of Children's Pain Communication. *Pain* **2016**, *157*, 938–948. [CrossRef] [PubMed]
35. Noel, M.; Rabbitts, J.A.; Tai, G.G.; Palermo, T.M. Remembering pain after surgery: A longitudinal examination of the role of pain catastrophizing in children's and parents' recall. *Pain* **2015**, *156*, 800–808. [CrossRef] [PubMed]
36. Simons, L.E.; Kaczynski, K.J.; Conroy, C.; Logan, D.E. Fear of pain in the context of intensive pain rehabilitation among children and adolescents with neuropathic pain: Associations with treatment response. *J. Pain* **2012**, *13*, 1151–1161. [CrossRef] [PubMed]
37. Zale, E.L.; Lange, K.L.; Fields, S.A.; Ditre, J.W. The relation between pain-related fear and disability: A meta-analysis. *J. Pain* **2013**, *14*, 1019–1030. [CrossRef] [PubMed]
38. Von Baeyer, C.L.; Champion, G.D. Commentary: Multiple pains as functional pain syndromes. *J. Pediatr. Psychol.* **2011**, *36*, 433–437. [CrossRef] [PubMed]

39. Kindler, L.L.; Bennett, R.M.; Jones, K.D. Central sensitivity syndromes: Mounting pathophysiologic evidence to link fibromyalgia with other common chronic pain disorders. *Pain Manag. Nurs.* **2011**, *12*, 15–24. [CrossRef] [PubMed]
40. Williams, F.M.; Spector, T.D.; MacGregor, A.J. Pain reporting at different body sites is explained by a single underlying genetic factor. *Rheumatology* **2010**, *49*, 1753–1755. [CrossRef] [PubMed]
41. Mayer, E.A.; Bushnell, M.C. *Functional Pain Syndromes: Presentation and Pathophysiology*; IASP Press: Seattle, WA, USA, 2009.
42. Burri, A.; Ogata, S.; Vehof, J.; Williams, F. Chronic widespread pain: Clinical comorbidities and psychological correlates. *Pain* **2015**, *156*, 1458–1464. [CrossRef] [PubMed]
43. Schechter, N.L. Functional pain: Time for a new name. *JAMA Pediatr.* **2014**, *168*, 693–694. [CrossRef] [PubMed]
44. McAbee, G.N.; Morse, A.M.; Assadi, M. Pediatric aspects of headache classification in the international classification of headache disorders-3 (ichd-3 beta version). *Curr. Pain Headache Rep.* **2016**, *20*, 7. [CrossRef] [PubMed]
45. Headache Classification Committee of the International Headache Society. The International Classification of Headache Disorders, 3rd Edition (Beta Version). *Cephalalgia Int. J. Headache* **2013**, *33*, 629–808.
46. Viswanathan, V.; Bridges, S.J.; Whitehouse, W.; Newton, R.W. Childhood headaches: Discrete entities or continuum? *Dev. Med. Child Neurol.* **1998**, *40*, 544–550. [CrossRef] [PubMed]
47. Zebenholzer, K.; Wober, C.; Kienbacher, C.; Wober-Bingol, C. Migrainous disorder and headache of the tension-type not fulfilling the criteria: A follow-up study in children and adolescents. *Cephalalgia Int. J. Headache* **2000**, *20*, 611–616. [CrossRef]
48. Turner, D.P.; Smitherman, T.A.; Black, A.K.; Penzien, D.B.; Porter, J.A.; Lofland, K.R.; Houle, T.T. Are migraine and tension-type headache diagnostic types or points on a severity continuum? An exploration of the latent taxometric structure of headache. *Pain* **2015**, *156*, 1200–1207. [CrossRef] [PubMed]
49. Andersen, S.; Petersen, M.W.; Svendsen, A.S.; Gazerani, P. Pressure pain thresholds assessed over temporalis, masseter, and frontalis muscles in healthy individuals, patients with tension-type headache, and those with migraine—A systematic review. *Pain* **2015**, *156*, 1409–1423. [CrossRef] [PubMed]
50. Sun, H.; Bastings, E.; Temeck, J.; Smith, P.B.; Men, A.; Tandon, V.; Murphy, D.; Rodriguez, W. Migraine therapeutics in adolescents: A systematic analysis and historic perspectives of triptan trials in adolescents. *JAMA Pediatr.* **2013**, *167*, 243–249. [CrossRef] [PubMed]
51. Silver, S.; Gano, D.; Gerretsen, P. Acute treatment of paediatric migraine: A meta-analysis of efficacy. *J. Paediatr. Child Health* **2008**, *44*, 3–9. [CrossRef] [PubMed]
52. Damen, L.; Bruijn, J.K.; Verhagen, A.P.; Berger, M.Y.; Passchier, J.; Koes, B.W. Symptomatic treatment of migraine in children: A systematic review of medication trials. *Pediatrics* **2005**, *116*, e295–e302. [CrossRef] [PubMed]
53. Sun-Edelstein, C.; Bigal, M.E.; Rapoport, A.M. Chronic migraine and medication overuse headache: Clarifying the current international headache society classification criteria. *Cephalalgia Int. J. Headache* **2009**, *29*, 445–452. [CrossRef] [PubMed]
54. Bigal, M.E.; Tepper, S.J.; Sheftell, F.D.; Rapoport, A.M.; Lipton, R.B. Chronic daily headache: Correlation between the 2004 and the 1988 international headache society diagnostic criteria. *Headache* **2004**, *44*, 684–691. [CrossRef] [PubMed]
55. Limmroth, V.; Katsarava, Z.; Fritsche, G.; Przywara, S.; Diener, H.C. Features of medication overuse headache following overuse of different acute headache drugs. *Neurology* **2002**, *59*, 1011–1014. [CrossRef] [PubMed]
56. MacGregor, E.A.; Steiner, T.J.; Davies, P.T.G. *Guidelines for All Healthcare Professionals in the Diagnosis and Management of Migraine, Tension-Type, Cluster and Medication-Overuse Headache*, 3rd ed. (1st revision). Available online: http://www.nhsgrampian.org/neurology/files/2010_BASH_Guidelines.pdf (accessed on 7 December 2016).
57. Hering-Hanit, R.; Gadoth, N.; Cohen, A.; Horev, Z. Successful withdrawal from analgesic abuse in a group of youngsters with chronic daily headache. *J. Child Neurol.* **2001**, *16*, 448–449. [CrossRef] [PubMed]
58. Keefer, L.; Drossman, D.A.; Guthrie, E.; Simren, M.; Tillisch, K.; Olden, K.; Whorwell, P.J. Centrally mediated disorders of gastrointestinal pain. *Gastroenterology* **2016**. [CrossRef] [PubMed]

59. Williams, A.E.; Heitkemper, M.; Self, M.M.; Czyzewski, D.I.; Shulman, R.J. Endogenous inhibition of somatic pain is impaired in girls with irritable bowel syndrome compared with healthy girls. *J. Pain* **2013**, *14*, 921–930. [CrossRef] [PubMed]
60. Stabell, N.; Stubhaug, A.; Flaegstad, T.; Mayer, E.; Naliboff, B.D.; Nielsen, C.S. Widespread hyperalgesia in adolescents with symptoms of irritable bowel syndrome: Results from a large population-based study. *J. Pain* **2014**, *15*, 898–906. [CrossRef] [PubMed]
61. Walker, L.S.; Dengler-Crish, C.M.; Rippel, S.; Bruehl, S. Functional abdominal pain in childhood and adolescence increases risk for chronic pain in adulthood. *Pain* **2010**, *150*, 568–572. [CrossRef] [PubMed]
62. Dengler-Crish, C.M.; Horst, S.N.; Walker, L.S. Somatic complaints in childhood functional abdominal pain are associated with functional gastrointestinal disorders in adolescence and adulthood. *J. Pediatr. Gastroenterol. Nutr.* **2011**, *52*, 162–165. [CrossRef] [PubMed]
63. Dengler-Crish, C.M.; Bruehl, S.; Walker, L.S. Increased wind-up to heat pain in women with a childhood history of functional abdominal pain. *Pain* **2011**, *152*, 802–808. [CrossRef] [PubMed]
64. Petersen, S.; Bergstrom, E.; Brulin, C. High prevalence of tiredness and pain in young schoolchildren. *Scand. J. Public Health* **2003**, *31*, 367–374. [CrossRef] [PubMed]
65. Watson, K.D.; Papageorgiou, A.C.; Jones, G.T.; Taylor, S.; Symmons, D.P.; Silman, A.J.; Macfarlane, G.J. Low back pain in schoolchildren: Occurrence and characteristics. *Pain* **2002**, *97*, 87–92. [CrossRef]
66. Kristjansdottir, G. Prevalence of self-reported back pain in school children: A study of sociodemographic differences. *Eur. J. Pediatr.* **1996**, *155*, 984–986. [CrossRef] [PubMed]
67. Smedbraten, B.K.; Natvig, B.; Rutle, O.; Bruusgaard, D. Self-reported bodily pain in schoolchildren. *Scand. J. Rheumatol.* **1998**, *27*, 273–276. [PubMed]
68. Brun Sundblad, G.M.; Saartok, T.; Engstrom, L.M. Prevalence and co-occurrence of self-rated pain and perceived health in school-children: Age and gender differences. *Eur. J. Pain* **2007**, *11*, 171–180. [CrossRef] [PubMed]
69. Vahasarja, V. Prevalence of chronic knee pain in children and adolescents in Northern Finland. *Acta Paediatr.* **1995**, *84*, 803–805. [CrossRef] [PubMed]
70. Mikkelsson, M.; Salminen, J.J.; Kautiainen, H. Non-specific musculoskeletal pain in preadolescents. Prevalence and 1-year persistence. *Pain* **1997**, *73*, 29–35. [CrossRef]
71. Centers for Disease Control and Prevention. Post-Treatment Lyme Disease Syndrome. Available online: http://www.cdc.gov/lyme/postlds/ (accessed on 7 December 2016).
72. U.S. National Library of Medicine. Conversion Disorder. Available online: https://medlineplus.gov/ency/article/000954.htm (accessed on 7 December 2016).
73. Cottencin, O. Conversion disorders: Psychiatric and psychotherapeutic aspects. *Neurophysiol. Clin.* **2014**, *44*, 405–410. [CrossRef] [PubMed]
74. Lu, Q.; Krull, K.R.; Leisenring, W.; Owen, J.E.; Kawashima, T.; Tsao, J.C.; Zebrack, B.; Mertens, A.; Armstrong, G.T.; Stovall, M.; et al. Pain in long-term adult survivors of childhood cancers and their siblings: A report from the childhood cancer survivor study. *Pain* **2011**, *152*, 2616–2624. [CrossRef] [PubMed]
75. Fortier, M.A.; Chou, J.; Maurer, E.L.; Kain, Z.N. Acute to chronic postoperative pain in children: Preliminary findings. *J. Pediatr. Surg.* **2011**, *46*, 1700–1705. [CrossRef] [PubMed]
76. Page, M.G.; Stinson, J.; Campbell, F.; Isaac, L.; Katz, J. Identification of pain-related psychological risk factors for the development and maintenance of pediatric chronic postsurgical pain. *J. Pain Res.* **2013**, *6*, 167–180. [CrossRef] [PubMed]
77. Sieberg, C.B.; Simons, L.E.; Edelstein, M.R.; DeAngelis, M.R.; Pielech, M.; Sethna, N.; Hresko, M.T. Pain prevalence and trajectories following pediatric spinal fusion surgery. *J. Pain* **2013**, *14*, 1694–1702. [CrossRef] [PubMed]
78. Rabbitts, J.A.; Zhou, C.; Groenewald, C.B.; Durkin, L.; Palermo, T.M. Trajectories of postsurgical pain in children: Risk factors and impact of late pain recovery on long-term health outcomes after major surgery. *Pain* **2015**, *156*, 2383–2389. [CrossRef] [PubMed]
79. Friedrichsdorf, S.J. Prevention and treatment of pain in hospitalized infants, children, and teenagers: From myths and morphine to multimodal analgesia. In Proceedings of the Pain 2016: Refresher Courses, 16th World Congress on Pain, Yokohama, Japan, 23–30 September 2016; International Association for the Study of Pain, IASP Press: Washington, DC, USA, 2016; pp. 309–319.

80. World Health Organization. WHO-Principles of Acute Pain Management for Children. Available online: http://apps.who.int/iris/bitstream/10665/44540/1/9789241548120_Guidelines.pdf (accessed on 7 December 2016).

81. Guzman, J.; Esmail, R.; Karjalainen, K.; Malmivaara, A.; Irvin, E.; Bombardier, C. Multidisciplinary bio-psycho-social rehabilitation for chronic low back pain. *Cochrane Database Syst. Rev.* **2002**. [CrossRef]

82. Logan, D.E.; Carpino, E.A.; Chiang, G.; Condon, M.; Firn, E.; Gaughan, V.J.; Hogan, M.; Leslie, D.S.; Olson, K.; Sager, S.; et al. A day-hospital approach to treatment of pediatric complex regional pain syndrome: Initial functional outcomes. *Clin. J. Pain* **2012**, *28*, 766–774. [CrossRef] [PubMed]

83. Hechler, T.; Ruhe, A.K.; Schmidt, P.; Hirsch, J.; Wager, J.; Dobe, M.; Krummenauer, F.; Zernikow, B. Inpatient-based intensive interdisciplinary pain treatment for highly impaired children with severe chronic pain: Randomized controlled trial of efficacy and economic effects. *Pain* **2014**, *155*, 118–128. [CrossRef] [PubMed]

84. Eccleston, C.; Malleson, P.N.; Clinch, J.; Connell, H.; Sourbut, C. Chronic pain in adolescents: Evaluation of a programme of interdisciplinary cognitive behaviour therapy. *Arch. Dis. Child* **2003**, *88*, 881–885. [CrossRef] [PubMed]

85. Maynard, C.S.; Amari, A.; Wieczorek, B.; Christensen, J.R.; Slifer, K.J. Interdisciplinary behavioral rehabilitation of pediatric pain-associated disability: Retrospective review of an inpatient treatment protocol. *J. Pediatr. Psychol.* **2010**, *35*, 128–137. [CrossRef] [PubMed]

86. Palermo, T.M.; Scher, M.S. Treatment of functional impairment in severe somatoform pain disorder: A case example. *J. Pediatr. Psychol.* **2001**, *26*, 429–434. [CrossRef] [PubMed]

87. Lynch, M.E.; Campbell, F.; Clark, A.J.; Dunbar, M.J.; Goldstein, D.; Peng, P.; Stinson, J.; Tupper, H. A systematic review of the effect of waiting for treatment for chronic pain. *Pain* **2008**, *136*, 97–116. [CrossRef] [PubMed]

88. Thompson, L.A.; Knapp, C.A.; Feeg, V.; Madden, V.L.; Shenkman, E.A. Pediatricians' management practices for chronic pain. *J. Palliat. Med.* **2010**, *13*, 171–178. [CrossRef] [PubMed]

89. Simons, L.E.; Smith, A.; Ibagon, C.; Coakley, R.; Logan, D.E.; Schechter, N.; Borsook, D.; Hill, J.C. Pediatric pain screening tool: Rapid identification of risk in youth with pain complaints. *Pain* **2015**, *156*, 1511–1518. [CrossRef] [PubMed]

90. Society, A.P. Pediatric Chronic Pain Programs by State/Province. Available online: http://americanpainsociety.org/uploads/get-involved/PainClinicList_12_2015.pdf (accessed on 7 December 2016).

91. Cormier, S.; Lavigne, G.L.; Choiniere, M.; Rainville, P. Expectations predict chronic pain treatment outcomes. *Pain* **2016**, *157*, 329–338. [CrossRef] [PubMed]

92. Lynch-Jordan, A.M.; Sil, S.; Peugh, J.; Cunningham, N.; Kashikar-Zuck, S.; Goldschneider, K.R. Differential changes in functional disability and pain intensity over the course of psychological treatment for children with chronic pain. *Pain* **2014**, *155*, 1955–1961. [CrossRef] [PubMed]

93. Sherry, D.D.; Wallace, C.A.; Kelley, C.; Kidder, M.; Sapp, L. Short- and long-term outcomes of children with complex regional pain syndrome type I treated with exercise therapy. *Clin. J. Pain* **1999**, *15*, 218–223. [CrossRef] [PubMed]

94. Odell, S.; Logan, D.E. Pediatric pain management: The multidisciplinary approach. *J. Pain Res.* **2013**, *6*, 785–790. [CrossRef] [PubMed]

95. Lee, B.H.; Scharff, L.; Sethna, N.F.; McCarthy, C.F.; Scott-Sutherland, J.; Shea, A.M.; Sullivan, P.; Meier, P.; Zurakowski, D.; Masek, B.J.; et al. Physical therapy and cognitive-behavioral treatment for complex regional pain syndromes. *J. Pediatr.* **2002**, *141*, 135–140. [CrossRef] [PubMed]

96. Wilson, A.C.; Palermo, T.M. Physical activity and function in adolescents with chronic pain: A controlled study using actigraphy. *J. Pain* **2012**, *13*, 121–130. [CrossRef] [PubMed]

97. Jerstad, S.J.; Boutelle, K.N.; Ness, K.K.; Stice, E. Prospective reciprocal relations between physical activity and depression in female adolescents. *J. Consult. Clin. Psychol.* **2010**, *78*, 268–272. [CrossRef] [PubMed]

98. Bowering, K.J.; O'Connell, N.E.; Tabor, A.; Catley, M.J.; Leake, H.B.; Moseley, G.L.; Stanton, T.R. The effects of graded motor imagery and its components on chronic pain: A systematic review and meta-analysis. *J. Pain* **2013**, *14*, 3–13. [CrossRef] [PubMed]

99. Bussing, A.; Ostermann, T.; Ludtke, R.; Michalsen, A. Effects of yoga interventions on pain and pain-associated disability: A meta-analysis. *J. Pain* **2012**, *13*, 1–9. [CrossRef] [PubMed]

100. Evans, S.; Moieni, M.; Taub, R.; Subramanian, S.K.; Tsao, J.C.; Sternlieb, B.; Zeltzer, L.K. Iyengar Yoga for young adults with rheumatoid arthritis: Results from a mixed-methods pilot study. *J. Pain Symptom Manag.* **2010**, *39*, 904–913. [CrossRef] [PubMed]

101. Vas, J.; Santos-Rey, K.; Navarro-Pablo, R.; Modesto, M.; Aguilar, I.; Campos, M.A.; Aguilar-Velasco, J.F.; Romero, M.; Parraga, P.; Hervas, V.; et al. Acupuncture for fibromyalgia in primary care: A randomised controlled trial. *Acupunct. Med.* **2016**, *34*, 257–266. [CrossRef] [PubMed]

102. Verkamp, E.K.; Flowers, S.R.; Lynch-Jordan, A.M.; Taylor, J.; Ting, T.V.; Kashikar-Zuck, S. A survey of conventional and complementary therapies used by youth with juvenile-onset fibromyalgia. *Pain Manag. Nurs.* **2013**, *14*, e244–e250. [CrossRef] [PubMed]

103. Friedrichsdorf, S.; Kuttner, L.; Westendorp, K.; McCarty, R. *Integrative Pediatric Palliative Care*; Oxford University Press: Oxford, UK, 2010.

104. Kuttner, L.; Friedrichsdorf, S.J. Hypnosis and palliative care. In *Therapeutic Hypnosis with Children and Adolescents*, 2nd ed.; Crown House Publishing Limited: Bethel, CT, USA, 2013; pp. 491–509.

105. Hunt, K.; Ernst, E. The evidence-base for complementary medicine in children: A critical overview of systematic reviews. *Arch. Dis. Child.* **2011**, *96*, 769–776. [CrossRef] [PubMed]

106. Evans, S.; Tsao, J.C.; Zeltzer, L.K. Complementary and alternative medicine for acute procedural pain in children. *Altern. Ther. Health Med.* **2008**, *14*, 52–56. [PubMed]

107. Richardson, J.; Smith, J.E.; McCall, G.; Pilkington, K. Hypnosis for procedure-related pain and distress in pediatric cancer patients: A systematic review of effectiveness and methodology related to hypnosis interventions. *J. Pain Symptom Manag.* **2006**, *31*, 70–84. [CrossRef] [PubMed]

108. Hemington, K.S.; Coulombe, M.A. The periaqueductal gray and descending pain modulation: Why should we study them and what role do they play in chronic pain? *J. Neurophysiol.* **2015**, *114*, 2080–2088. [CrossRef] [PubMed]

109. Valet, M.; Sprenger, T.; Boecker, H.; Willoch, F.; Rummeny, E.; Conrad, B.; Erhard, P.; Tolle, T.R. Distraction modulates connectivity of the cingulo-frontal cortex and the midbrain during pain—An FMRI analysis. *Pain* **2004**, *109*, 399–408. [CrossRef] [PubMed]

110. Tracey, I.; Ploghaus, A.; Gati, J.S.; Clare, S.; Smith, S.; Menon, R.S.; Matthews, P.M. Imaging attentional modulation of pain in the periaqueductal gray in humans. *J. Neurosci.* **2002**, *22*, 2748–2752. [PubMed]

111. Derbyshire, S.W.; Osborn, J. Modeling pain circuits: How imaging may modify perception. *Neuroimaging Clin. N. Am.* **2007**, *17*, 485–493. [CrossRef] [PubMed]

112. Bingel, U.; Wanigasekera, V.; Wiech, K.; Ni Mhuircheartaigh, R.; Lee, M.C.; Ploner, M.; Tracey, I. The effect of treatment expectation on drug efficacy: Imaging the analgesic benefit of the opioid remifentanil. *Sci. Transl. Med.* **2011**, *3*, 70ra14. [CrossRef] [PubMed]

113. Yu, R.; Gollub, R.L.; Spaeth, R.; Napadow, V.; Wasan, A.; Kong, J. Disrupted functional connectivity of the periaqueductal gray in chronic low back pain. *Neuroimage Clin.* **2014**, *6*, 100–108. [CrossRef] [PubMed]

114. Giordano, J. The neurobiology of nociceptive and anti-nociceptive systems. *Pain Phys.* **2005**, *8*, 277–290.

115. Tegethoff, M.; Belardi, A.; Stalujanis, E.; Meinlschmidt, G. Comorbidity of mental disorders and chronic pain: Chronology of onset in adolescents of a national representative cohort. *J. Pain* **2015**, *16*, 1054–1064. [CrossRef] [PubMed]

116. Cohen, L.L.; Vowles, K.E.; Eccleston, C. The impact of adolescent chronic pain on functioning: Disentangling the complex role of anxiety. *J. Pain* **2010**, *11*, 1039–1046. [CrossRef] [PubMed]

117. Palermo, T.M.; Eccleston, C.; Lewandowski, A.S.; Williams, A.C.; Morley, S. Randomized controlled trials of psychological therapies for management of chronic pain in children and adolescents: An updated meta-analytic review. *Pain* **2010**, *148*, 387–397. [CrossRef] [PubMed]

118. Eccleston, C.; Palermo, T.M.; Williams, A.C.; Lewandowski Holley, A.; Morley, S.; Fisher, E.; Law, E. Psychological therapies for the management of chronic and recurrent pain in children and adolescents. *Cochrane Database Syst. Rev.* **2014**. [CrossRef]

119. Kashikar-Zuck, S.; Sil, S.; Lynch-Jordan, A.M.; Ting, T.V.; Peugh, J.; Schikler, K.N.; Hashkes, P.J.; Arnold, L.M.; Passo, M.; Richards-Mauze, M.M.; et al. Changes in pain coping, catastrophizing, and coping efficacy after cognitive-behavioral therapy in children and adolescents with juvenile fibromyalgia. *J. Pain* **2013**, *14*, 492–501. [CrossRef] [PubMed]

120. Seminowicz, D.A.; Shpaner, M.; Keaser, M.L.; Krauthamer, G.M.; Mantegna, J.; Dumas, J.A.; Newhouse, P.A.; Filippi, C.G.; Keefe, F.J.; Naylor, M.R. Cognitive-behavioral therapy increases prefrontal cortex gray matter in patients with chronic pain. *J. Pain* **2013**, *14*, 1573–1584. [CrossRef] [PubMed]

121. Forgeron, P.A.; McGrath, P.; Stevens, B.; Evans, J.; Dick, B.; Finley, G.A.; Carlson, T. Social information processing in adolescents with chronic pain: My friends don't really understand me. *Pain* **2011**, *152*, 2773–2780. [CrossRef] [PubMed]

122. Palermo, T.M.; Wilson, A.C.; Lewandowski, A.S.; Toliver-Sokol, M.; Murray, C.B. Behavioral and psychosocial factors associated with insomnia in adolescents with chronic pain. *Pain* **2011**, *152*, 89–94. [CrossRef] [PubMed]

123. Palermo, T.M.; Law, E.; Churchill, S.S.; Walker, A. Longitudinal course and impact of insomnia symptoms in adolescents with and without chronic pain. *J. Pain* **2012**, *13*, 1099–1106. [CrossRef] [PubMed]

124. Letter, H.H. Blue Light Has a Dark Side. Available online: http://www.health.harvard.edu/staying-healthy/blue-light-has-a-dark-side (accessed on 7 December 2016).

125. Gooley, J.J.; Chamberlain, K.; Smith, K.A.; Khalsa, S.B.; Rajaratnam, S.M.; van Reen, E.; Zeitzer, J.M.; Czeisler, C.A.; Lockley, S.W. Exposure to room light before bedtime suppresses melatonin onset and shortens melatonin duration in humans. *J. Clin. Endocrinol. Metab.* **2011**, *96*, E463–E472. [CrossRef] [PubMed]

126. Logan, D.E.; Simons, L.E.; Carpino, E.A. Too sick for school? Parent influences on school functioning among children with chronic pain. *Pain* **2012**, *153*, 437–443. [CrossRef] [PubMed]

127. Bernstein, G.A.; Hektner, J.M.; Borchardt, C.M.; McMillan, M.H. Treatment of school refusal: One-year follow-up. *J. Am. Aca. Child Adolesc. Psychiatry* **2001**, *40*, 206–213. [CrossRef] [PubMed]

128. King, N.J.; Bernstein, G.A. School refusal in children and adolescents: A review of the past 10 years. *J. Am. Aca. Child Adolesc. Psychiatry* **2001**, *40*, 197–205. [CrossRef] [PubMed]

129. Evans, L.D. Functional school refusal subtypes: Anxiety, avoidance, malingering. *Psychol. Sch.* **2000**, *37*, 183–191. [CrossRef]

130. Lewandowski, A.S.; Palermo, T.M.; Stinson, J.; Handley, S.; Chambers, C.T. Systematic review of family functioning in families of children and adolescents with chronic pain. *J. Pain* **2010**, *11*, 1027–1038. [CrossRef] [PubMed]

131. Liossi, C.; White, P.; Croome, N.; Hatira, P. Pain-related bias in the classification of emotionally ambiguous facial expressions in mothers of children with chronic abdominal pain. *Pain* **2012**, *153*, 674–681. [CrossRef] [PubMed]

132. Higgins, K.S.; Birnie, K.A.; Chambers, C.T.; Wilson, A.C.; Caes, L.; Clark, A.J.; Lynch, M.; Stinson, J.; Campbell-Yeo, M. Offspring of parents with chronic pain: A systematic review and meta-analysis of pain, health, psychological, and family outcomes. *Pain* **2015**, *156*, 2256–2266. [CrossRef] [PubMed]

133. Kaasboll, J.; Lydersen, S.; Indredavik, M.S. Psychological symptoms in children of parents with chronic pain-the hunt study. *Pain* **2012**, *153*, 1054–1062. [CrossRef] [PubMed]

134. Peloso, P.M. Faster, higher, stronger: To the gold medal podium? *Pain* **2014**, *155*, 4–5. [CrossRef] [PubMed]

135. Moore, R.A.; Derry, S.; Straube, S.; Ireson-Paine, J.; Wiffen, P.J. Faster, higher, stronger? Evidence for formulation and efficacy for ibuprofen in acute pain. *Pain* **2014**, *155*, 14–21. [CrossRef] [PubMed]

136. Dowell, D.; Haegerich, T.M.; Chou, R. Cdc guideline for prescribing opioids for chronic pain—United States, 2016. *MMWR Recomm. Rep.* **2016**, *65*, 1–49. [CrossRef] [PubMed]

137. Schechter, N.L.; Walco, G.A. The potential impact on children of the CDC guideline for prescribing opioids for chronic pain: Above all, do no harm. *JAMA Pediatr.* **2016**, *170*, 425–426. [CrossRef] [PubMed]

138. Friedrichsdorf, S.J.; Nugent, A.P. Management of neuropathic pain in children with cancer. *Curr. Opin. Support. Palliat. Care* **2013**, *7*, 131–138. [CrossRef] [PubMed]

139. Vidor, L.P.; Torres, I.L.; Custodio de Souza, I.C.; Fregni, F.; Caumo, W. Analgesic and sedative effects of melatonin in temporomandibular disorders: A double-blind, randomized, parallel-group, placebo-controlled study. *J. Pain Symptom Manag.* **2013**, *46*, 422–432. [CrossRef] [PubMed]

140. Schwertner, A.; Conceicao Dos Santos, C.C.; Costa, G.D.; Deitos, A.; de Souza, A.; de Souza, I.C.; Torres, I.L.; da Cunha Filho, J.S.; Caumo, W. Efficacy of melatonin in the treatment of endometriosis: A phase II, randomized, double-blind, placebo-controlled trial. *Pain* **2013**, *154*, 874–881. [CrossRef] [PubMed]

141. Finnerup, N.B.; Attal, N.; Haroutounian, S.; McNicol, E.; Baron, R.; Dworkin, R.H.; Gilron, I.; Haanpaa, M.; Hansson, P.; Jensen, T.S.; et al. Pharmacotherapy for neuropathic pain in adults: A systematic review and meta-analysis. *Lancet Neurol.* **2015**, *14*, 162–173. [CrossRef]

142. Hauer, J.M.; Solodiuk, J.C. Gabapentin for management of recurrent pain in 22 nonverbal children with severe neurological impairment: A retrospective analysis. *J. Palliat. Med.* **2015**, *18*, 453–456. [CrossRef] [PubMed]

143. Edwards, L.; DeMeo, S.; Hornik, C.D.; Cotten, C.M.; Smith, P.B.; Pizoli, C.; Hauer, J.M.; Bidegain, M. Gabapentin use in the neonatal intensive care unit. *J. Pediatr.* **2016**, *169*, 310–312. [CrossRef] [PubMed]

144. Derry, S.; Wiffen, P.J.; Moore, R.A.; Quinlan, J. Topical lidocaine for neuropathic pain in adults. *Cochrane Database Syst. Rev.* **2014**, *7*. [CrossRef]

145. El-Chammas, K.; Keyes, J.; Thompson, N.; Vijayakumar, J.; Becher, D.; Jackson, J.L. Pharmacologic treatment of pediatric headaches: A meta-analysis. *JAMA Pediatr.* **2013**, *167*, 250–258. [CrossRef] [PubMed]

146. Campo, J.V.; Perel, J.; Lucas, A.; Bridge, J.; Ehmann, M.; Kalas, C.; Monk, K.; Axelson, D.; Birmaher, B.; Ryan, N.; et al. Citalopram treatment of pediatric recurrent abdominal pain and comorbid internalizing disorders: An exploratory study. *J. Am. Acad. Child. Adolesc. Psychiatry* **2004**, *43*, 1234–1242. [CrossRef] [PubMed]

147. Caperell, K.; Pitetti, R.; Cross, K.P. Race and acute abdominal pain in a pediatric emergency department. *Pediatrics* **2013**, *131*, 1098–1106. [CrossRef] [PubMed]

148. Friedrichsdorf, S.J.; Drake, R.; Webster, L.M. Gastrointestinal symptoms. In *Textbook of Interdisciplinary Pediatric Palliative Care*; Elsevier/Saunders: Philadelphia, PA, USA, 2011; pp. 311–334.

149. Friedrichsdorf, S.J. Cancer pain management in children. In *Anaesthesia, Intensive Care, and Pain Management for the Cancer Patient*; Farquhar-Smith, P., Wigmore, T., Eds.; Oxford University Press: Oxford, UK; New York, NY, USA, 2011; pp. 215–227.

150. Michelson, J.D.; Addante, R.A.; Charlson, M.D. Multimodal analgesia therapy reduces length of hospitalization in patients undergoing fusions of the ankle and hindfoot. *Foot Ankle Int.* **2013**, *34*, 1526–1534. [CrossRef] [PubMed]

151. Giordano, J. The neuroscience of pain, and the neuroethics of pain care. *Neuroethics* **2009**, *3*, 89–94. [CrossRef]

152. Giordano, J. Pain research: Can paradigmatic revision bridge the demands of medicine, scientific philosophy and ethics? *Pain Phys.* **2004**, *7*, 407–410.

153. Jorgenson, L.A.; Newsome, W.T.; Anderson, D.J.; Bargmann, C.I.; Brown, E.N.; Deisseroth, K.; Donoghue, J.P.; Hudson, K.L.; Ling, G.S.; MacLeish, P.R.; et al. The brain initiative: Developing technology to catalyse neuroscience discovery. *Philos. Trans. R. Soc. Lond. Ser. B Biol. Sci.* **2015**, *370*. [CrossRef] [PubMed]

154. Giordano, J.; Schatman, M.E. Pain medicine from "bench to bedside": Bridging the disconnect(s) between research and clinical care. *J. Humanit. Sci. Healthc.* **2011**, *1*, 22–40.

155. Giordano, J. *Pain: Mind, Meaning, and Medicine*; PPM Press: Glen Falls, PA, USA, 2009; p. 48.

156. Giordano, J. Maldynia: Chronic pain as illness, and the need for complementarity in pain care. *Forsch. Komplement.* **2008**, *15*, 277–281. [CrossRef] [PubMed]

157. Giordano, J. Pain and suffering: Körper and leib, and the telos of pain care. *Philos. Psychiatry Psychol.* **2013**, *19*, 279–283.

158. Giordano, J.; Benedikter, R.; Boswell, M.V. Pain medicine, biotechnology and market effects: Tools, tekne and moral responsibility. *J. Ethics Biol. Eng. Med.* **2010**, *1*, 135–142. [CrossRef]

159. Desai, K.; Daughtree, C.; Friedrichsdorf, S.J. An interdisciplinary pain clinic: A year in review (poster). In Proceedings of the 10th International Forum on Pediatric Pain (IFPP), White Point Beach Resort, Hunts Point, NS, Canada, 1–4 October 2015.

160. Friedrichsdorf, S.J.; Postier, A.; Eull, D.; Gilbert, M.; Desai, K.; Gibbon, C.; Flood, A. Interdisciplinary pediatric outpatient pain clinic: Improvement in pain, function and predictors of successful graduation. Unpublished work. 2016.

161. "Little Stars—Treating Chronic Pain in Children". Available online: https://www.youtube.com/watch?t=13&v=Bb1fHxfjdWI (accessed on 7 December 2016).

162. Pediatric Pain Clinics in USA and Canada (American Pain Society). Available online: http://americanpainsociety.org/uploads/get-involved/PainClinicList_12_2015.pdf (accessed on 7 December 2016).

163. Pain Bytes (Australia). Available online: http://www.aci.health.nsw.gov.au/chronic-pain/painbytes (accessed on 7 December 2016).

164. Persistent (Chronic) Pain 5-min video[164]. Available online: https://www.youtube.com/watch?v=RWMKucuejIs (accessed on 7 December 2016).

165. Kiran Stordalen and Horst Rechelbacher Pediatric Pain, Palliative and Integrative Medicine Clinic Tour. Available online: https://vimeo.com/122654881 (accessed on 7 December 2016).
166. Elliot Krane (TED-Talk) The mystery of chronic pain. Available online: https://www.youtube.com/watch?v=J6--CMhcCfQ (accessed on 7 December 2016).
167. The Department of Pain Medicine, Palliative Care, and Integrative Medicine, Children's Hospitals and Clinics of Minnesota. Available online: https://www.childrensmn.org/painpalliativeintegrativemed (accessed on 7 December 2016).

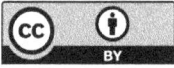

children

MDPI

Review

Evidence-Based Psychological Interventions for the Management of Pediatric Chronic Pain: New Directions in Research and Clinical Practice

Rachael Coakley [1,2,*] and Tessa Wihak [1]

[1]   Division of Pain Medicine, Department of Anesthesiology, Perioperative and Pain Medicine, Boston Children's Hospital, Pain Treatment Service, 333 Longwood Avenue, Boston, MA 02115, USA; tessa.wihak@childrens.harvard.edu

[2]   Department of Psychiatry, Harvard Medical School, 25 Shattuck St, Boston, MA 02115, USA

*   Correspondence: rachael.coakley@childrens.harvard.edu; Tel.: +1-617-3565-7581; Fax: +1-617-730-0199

Academic Editor: Lynn S. Walker
Received: 22 October 2016; Accepted: 13 January 2017; Published: 4 February 2017

Abstract: Over the past 20 years our knowledge about evidence-based psychological interventions for pediatric chronic pain has dramatically increased. Overall, the evidence in support of psychological interventions for pediatric chronic pain is strong, demonstrating positive psychological and behavioral effects for a variety of children with a range of pain conditions. However, wide scale access to effective psychologically-based pain management treatments remains a challenge for many children who suffer with pain. Increasing access to care and reducing persistent biomedical biases that inhibit attainment of psychological services are a central focus of current pain treatment interventions. Additionally, as the number of evidence-based treatments increase, tailoring treatments to a child or family's particular needs is increasingly possible. This article will (1) discuss the theoretical frameworks as well as the specific psychological skills and strategies that currently hold promise as effective agents of change; (2) review and summarize trends in the development of well-researched outpatient interventions over the past ten years; and (3) discuss future directions for intervention research on pediatric chronic pain.

Keywords: chronic pain; pediatric; psychological intervention; parent; child; evidence-based; empirically supported

---

1. Introduction

Current estimates suggest that up to one in four children will have an episode of chronic pain lasting three months or longer [1]. This type of persistent pain is linked to significant physical, psychosocial, and psychological burdens for children and families [2,3]. Chronic pediatric pain also places a significant burden on our healthcare system, ranking among the most expensive pediatric health problems in the United States and costing an estimated $19.5 billion dollars per year [4]. Psychological interventions for pain and pain-related functional deficits (i.e., school impairment, sleep disruption, peer-based challenges, etc.) have been considered an integral part of treatment for the recovery from chronic pain for almost twenty years [5,6]. Taken as a whole, psychological skills and strategies such as cognitive reframing, biobehavioral relaxation, graded in vivo exposure, and mindfulness are demonstrated to decrease pain, improve functioning, increase self-efficacy, and reduce the daily stress that commonly co-occurs in children and adolescents with persistent pain. Moreover, parent-based interventions that reduce maladaptive responses to child pain are demonstrated to further promote a child's recovery [7].

Presently, most psychological interventions for pain are designed with a multi-component structure and are often concerned with evaluating the value-add to standard biomedical approaches to care, the "dose" needed to effect change, the effectiveness of novel delivery methods that can increase access to care, and in many cases assessing how the direct involvement of systems such as parents or families may enhance outcomes. However, the treatment of chronic pain is not a one-size fits all solution and it is unlikely that a single intervention strategy will systematically work for all children with pain. Psychological comorbidities, family-based influences, school environments, developmental factors, functional disability, and underlying pathophysiology of pain all vary by individual. As such, we need to develop various intervention strategies, with the goal of understanding how we can maximally apply these skills and strategies to enhance recovery or coping with pain and to reduce the stress and psychosocial burden for children and parents.

Despite the proven effectiveness of psychologically based strategies for pain, too few pediatric patients referred to psychological services for pain management obtain services due to a lack of available providers, scheduling conflicts, inadequate knowledge of efficacy, and financial or insurance constraints [8,9]. These logistical barriers highlight the need to create models of care that can be flexible in meeting the time, cost, and limited resource barriers that interfere with service acquisition [9]. Additionally, psychological interventions for pediatric pain must also be packaged and administered in a format that is acceptable, attending closely to the common biomedical biases that may inhibit initial engagement in services. For example, when parents perceive their child to have a solely physical problem, they may dismiss or minimize the need for psychological intervention [8,10,11]. Fortunately, gaining a foundational understanding of the biopsychosocial model of pain helps to illuminate how psychological interventions can effectively foster recovery and may increase the likelihood of obtaining targeted psychological services for pain [12].

Helping children and families to effectively manage pain may ultimately be similar to how we help our children succeed in school; all children need to be taught the academic material as well as the skills and strategies that help cement the learning process. How well any individual child succeeds in school, however, is due to a variety of factors such as attentional capacity, intelligence quotient (IQ), motivation, family reinforcement, etc. Children who have poor attention or low motivation, may ultimately be identified as needing additional services such as individual tutoring, small group instruction, or a more structured learning environment to obtain success. Similarly, one of our primary goals in pediatric pain is to identify patient characteristics that may signal the need for more intensive or focused intervention efforts that can help foster recovery [13]. As a corollary, considering that our patients with pain are akin to students in school highlights how first line education and intervention may be necessary, even if not sufficient to produce change for all children. Interventions that provide the building blocks for effective pain management early in a child's experience of pain—for example, before functional deficits occur—may help to change a child's long term trajectory in the same way that obtaining a short course of tutoring *before* a child fails a class may ultimately help a child to stay on pace with peers. Thus, in our current line of research and clinical practice we need to think about generating evidence-based first line interventions, such as targeted pain education and cognitive behavioral coping skills, while at the same time devising specialized or more intensive psychological treatments for those with more entrenched difficulties.

This review includes an overview of pediatric chronic pain intervention research in the past 10 years. Our search terms and findings are presented in Table 1. This is not intended to be an exhaustive list of all interventions tested for all chronic pain conditions, but rather to represent a broad overview of what is being developed and tested for "chronic pediatric pain." Based on a review of this literature, we will present an overview of current theoretical frameworks that are currently guiding the development of interventions in this field and highlight specific ways in which these frameworks map onto pain-management skills and strategies. We will further evaluate current barriers and challenges in clinical application, and discuss future directions for more seamlessly integrating psychological interventions into the clinical management of pediatric pain.

Table 1. Evidence-Based Psychological Interventions for Pediatric Chronic Pain from 2005–2015.

Authors, Year	Target Population [1]	N	Pain Type [2]	Therapy Type [3]	Duration: Session/Weeks (Total Time)	Mode of Delivery	Setting	Outcome
Kashikar-Zuck et al., 2005 [14]	Adol Parent	30	MSK	CST	4 weeks individual/parent-adol + 2 biweekly telehealth (unknown)	Individual + 3 parent-adol sessions + telehealth	Outpt	Reduced functional disability and depressive symptoms in CST group and self-monitoring group at post-treatment. CST showed greater improvement in coping skills and trend towards reduced pain intensity.
Robins et al., 2005 [15]	Child Adol Parent	69	AB	CBT	5 weeks (3–4 h)	Family-based	Outpt	Reduced pain intensity compared to standard medical care alone at post-treatment and 1-year follow-up.
Connelly et al., 2006 [16]	Child Adol	37	HA	CBT	4 weeks (4 h)	CD-ROM + telehealth	Home	Reduced pain intensity, frequency and duration compared to standard medical care waitlist control at 1-, 2- and 3-month follow-up.
Degotardi et al., 2006 [17]	Child Adol Parent	67	MSK	CBT, +SFT + IP	8 weeks (unknown)	Parent-child/ adol group + weekly parent meetings	Outpt	Reduced pain intensity, functional disability, somatic symptoms, anxiety and fatigue at post-treatment.
Duarte et al., 2006 [18]	Child Adol Parent	32	AB	CBT	12 weeks (3–4 h)	Family-based	Outpt	Reduced frequency of pain crises compare to standard medical care at post-treatment.
Hicks et al., 2006 [19]	Child Adol Parent	47	Multi	CBT	7 weeks (unknown)	Internet + telehealth	Home	Reduced pain intensity compared to standard medical care waitlist control at 1 and 3-mo follow-up.
Abram et al., 2007 [20]	Child Adol Parent	81	HA	CBT + ED	1 day (1 h)	Parent-child/ adol group	Outpt	Increased headache knowledge and reduced physician face-to-face time compared to neurological consultation group at 3 and 6months post-treatment. Reduced headache-related disability in both groups.
Vlieger et al., 2007 [21]	Child Adol	53	AB	HT	12 weeks (5 h)	Individual	Outpt	Reduced pain intensity and frequency compared to standard medical care at 1-year follow-up.

Table 1. *Cont.*

Authors, Year	Target Population [1]	N	Pain Type [2]	Therapy Type [3]	Duration: Session/Weeks (Total Time)	Mode of Delivery	Setting	Outcome
Palermo et al., 2009 [22]	Adol Parent	48	Multi	CBT	8 weeks (4 h child + 4 h parent + 1 h therapistcontact)	Internet + telehealth	Home	Reduced pain intensity and functional disability compared to standard medical care wait-list control at post-treatment and 3-month follow-up.
van Tilburg et al., 2009 [23]	Child Adol Parent	34	AB	Guided Imagery	8 weeks (2–3 h)	Portable CD Audio-Recordings	Home	Reduced pain intensity, functional disability and improved QOL for audio exercises compared to standard medical care alone at post-treatment and 6-month follow-up.
Wicksell et al., 2009 [24]	Child Adol Parent	32	Multi	ACT	10 weeks (4.5 h individual + 1.5 h parent-child/adol)	Individual + 1-2 parent-child/ adol sessions	Outpt	Reduced pain intensity, functional disability, pain intensity and pain-related worry compared to MDT group at post-treatment and at 3.5- and 6.5- month follow-up.
Barakat et al., 2010 [25]	Adol Parent	53	SCD	CBT	3 weeks (4–5 h) + 1 booster (1.5 h)	Family-based	Home	Exploratory analyses showed small to medium effects in favor of CBT group on pain frequency, health service use, SCD knowledge, and family cohesion at post-treatment.
Gerber et al., 2010 [26]	Child Adol Parent	34	HA	SCT + SMT + PCST	8 child sessions (12 h) + 4 parent sessions (8 h)	Child group + parent group	Outpt	Reduced headache frequency and duration and improved school and daily functioning in multimodal behavioral education group and BFT group at post-treatment.
Levy et al., 2010 [27]	Adol Parent	200	AB	SLCBT	3 weeks (3 h)	Family-based	Outpt or Home	Reduced pain, gastrointestinal symptom severity and parental solicitous responses to child symptoms compared to educational intervention at post-treatment and 1-week, 1- and 3-month follow-up.
Logan and Simons, 2010 [28]	Adol Parent	40	Multi	CBT	4 weeks or day workshop (4 h adol + 4 h parent-adol)	Adol group + parent-adol group	Outpt	Reduced pain intensity, negative mood/self-esteem and improved school functioning at post-treatment.

Table 1. *Cont.*

Authors, Year	Target Population[1]	N	Pain Type[2]	Therapy Type[3]	Duration: Session/Weeks (Total Time)	Mode of Delivery	Setting	Outcome
Stinson et al., 2010 [29]	Adol Parent	46	MSK	CBT + ED	12 weeks (5 h)	Internet + telehealth	Home	Improved JIA-related knowledge and average weekly pain intensity compared to internet intervention control group at post-treatment.
Trautmann and Kroner-Herwig, 2010 [30]	Child Adol	65	HA	CBT vs. Self-Help/RT	6 weeks (unknown)	Internet + telehealth	Home	Reduced pain frequency, duration and catastrophizing in CBT, AR and educational intervention groups at post-treatment.
Warner et al., 2011 [31]	Child Adol Parent	40	Multi	CBT	10 weeks (9–12 h child + 2 h parent) + 2 booster	Individual + 3 parent meetings	Outpt	Reduced anxiety and somatic symptoms compared to standard medical care waitlist control at post-treatment and 3-month follow-up.
Kashikar-Zuck et al., 2012 [32]	Child Adol Parent	114	MSK	CBT	8 sessions (6 h child + 2–3 h parent-child/adol) + 2 boosters (1.5 h)	Individual + 3 parent-child/adol sessions	Outpt	Reduced pain intensity, functional disability and depressive symptoms in CBT group and Fibromyalgia Education group at post-treatment. CBT showed greater reduction in functional disability compared to fibromyalgia education.
Law et al., 2012 [33]	Adol Parent	26	Multi	CBT	17–27 weeks (unknown)	Internet + telehealth	Home + Outpt	Sending messages to online coach was associated with reduced pain intensity and functional disability at post-treatment.
Myrvik et al., 2012 [34]	Child Adol Parent	10	SCD	BFT + RT	1 day (1 h)	Parent-child/adol + telehealth	Home + Outpt	Reduced pain frequency at post-treatment and 6-week follow-up.
Vlieger et al. 2012 [35]	Child Adol	52	AB	HT	12 weeks (5 h)	Individual	Outpt	Reduced pain, pain frequency and somatic symptoms at mean follow-up of 4.8 years.
Kashikar-Zuck et al., 2013 [36]	Adol Parent	114	MSK	CBT	9 weeks (unknown)	Individual + 3 parent-adol sessions	Home	Improved functional disability at post-treatment.

Table 1. *Cont.*

Authors, Year	Target Population [1]	N	Pain Type [2]	Therapy Type [3]	Duration: Session/Weeks (*Total Time*)	Mode of Delivery	Setting	Outcome
Levy et al., 2013 [37]	Child Parent	200	AB	SLBT	3 weeks (*3 h*)	Family-based	Outpt or Home	Reduced pain and improved coping skills at 1-year follow-up compared to education group. Similarly, SLCBT group exhibited decreased parental solicitousness and maladaptive pain-related beliefs.
Shiri et al., 2013 [38]	Child Adol	10	HA	BFT	10 sessions (*5 h*)	Individual virtual reality	Outpt	Reduced pain and improved QOL and daily functioning at 1 and 3 months post-treatment.
Stern et al., 2014 [39]	Child Adol	27	AB	BFT	8 sessions (*4 h*)	Individual	Outpt	Reduced pain frequency and severity at post-treatment and 2-week follow-up.
Armbrust et al., 2015 [40]	Child Adol Parent Sibling	64	MSK	CBT+ ED	14 weeks (*14 h*)	Internet + 4 group with parent + 1 group with sibling/friend	Outpt	Program commitment similar to internet-based JIA self-help program via phone support and higher commitment compared to other internet interventions for youth.
Hesse et al., 2015 [41]	Adol	20	HA	MBI	8 weeks (*16 h*)	Group	Outpt + Home	Adolescents report improved depressive symptoms and pain-related acceptance at post-treatment. Parents report improved QOL and physical functioning.
Law et al., 2015 [42]	Adol Parent	83	HA	CBT	8–10 weeks (*4 h adol + 4 h parent + 1 h online coach*)	Internet + telehealth	Outpt +Home	Reduced headache frequency in Internet CBT group and headache treatment group at post-treatment and 3-month follow-up.

Search Terms: pediatric/child/adolescent chronic pain + intervention; CBT; biobehavioral; cognitive behavioral; education; psychoeducation; parent training; hypnotherapy; pain coping; mindfulness; acceptance; internet; telehealth; group. [1] **Target Population:** Children = ages 7–11, Adolescents (Adol) = ages 12–18. [2] **Pain Type:** MSK = musculoskeletal, HA = headache, AB = abdominal, Multi = multiple pain, SCD = sickle cell disease, Neuro = neuropathic. [3] **Therapy Type:** ACT = Acceptance and Commitment Therapy, BFT = Biofeedback Therapy, CBT = Cognitive Behavioral Therapy, ED = Psychoed CST = Coping Skills Training, HT = Hypnotherapy, IP = Interpersonal Therapy, MBI = Mindfulness-Based Intervention, MDT = Multidisciplinary Treatment, PCST = Pain Coping Skills Training, RT = Relaxation Therapy, SCT = Sensory Coping Training, SFT = Strategic Family Therapy, SLCBT = Social Learning and Cognitive Behavioral Therapy. [4] **Setting:** Outpt = Outpatient.

2. Theoretical Foundations

Pediatric pain interventions are based on the understanding that pain is a complex biopsychosocial experience shaped not only by underlying pathophysiology but also by individuals' thoughts, feelings, and behaviors [43]. Interventions based in the foundational theories of cognitive behavioral, biobehavioral, and acceptance-based models of care currently encompass the majority of psychological interventions for children and adolescents with pain. However, these theoretical approaches are not necessarily mutually exclusive, as many of the current interventions for pediatric pain contain elements of two or more theoretical orientations. Collectively, these theoretical approaches demonstrate promising improvements in self-efficacy, self-management, family functioning, psychosocial well-being, pain severity, school attendance, anxiety, depression and feelings of hopefulness [7,44,45]. The vast majority of evidenced-based interventions for pediatric pain are designed as brief, goal-oriented treatments incorporating learning experiences that help to modify negative cognitions about pain and eliminating dysfunctional behavioral patterns that occur as a result of the pain. Psychological interventions for pain are also commonly designed to help un-link the association between the sensory experience of pain and the cognitive affective evaluation of the pain that triggers a fight or flight response, often referred to as a "pain alarm" [46]. Specifically, most psychological treatments for pain are designed to address the negative or fearful thoughts about pain (e.g., 'it's going to hurt too much', 'I can't do this') that produce physiological changes (e.g., racing heart, shortness of breath, increased discomfort) and resultant behavioral changes (e.g., withdrawal from activity, poor sleep). Interventions may also use strategies such as graded exposure to anxiety producing stimuli and reinforcement for adaptive behaviors.

As pediatric pain is conceptualized as a biopsychosocial process, intervention efforts are ideally targeted towards a systems framework inclusive of parents, families and schools. It has been well documented that the way parents respond to their child's pain is associated with pain severity, functional disability and other somatic complaints [3,7,47]. Moreover, without targeted parent support at home and school, it is more challenging for children and adolescents to make steady gains. Parents can be collaborators in treatment when they are involved in the planning and reinforcement of their child's psychological intervention plan [48]. For example, parents may be taught how to use relaxation techniques to help reinforce the use of these strategies at home, or may collaborate by consistent provision of rewards or consequences for a child's established behavior plan [17]. But perhaps more importantly, parents can be co-treated along with their child. For example, it's common for parents to become highly focused on their child's pain. This attention to pain is known to inadvertently reinforce a child's focus on his or her own pain increasing disability [49,50]. In contrast, when parents are taught how to reduce their focus on a child's pain, a child's pain and function may improve [27]. Research also suggests that parent-focused treatments such as Problem Solving Therapy (PST) may directly improve parent behaviour and parent psychological functioning [51], an important outcome given that parents are known to experience significant stress in the context of their child's pain [52].

School performance has also been an identified target for intervention because functional impairment in schools—including poor grades, absenteeism, and peer victimization—is a well-documented problem for children with pain [53–55]. It's easy to understand why pain can reduce a child's ability to cope with school demands and contribute to poorer grades. However, for some children school pressures and peer victimization may also be a contributory factor to the onset of pain, thus requiring intervention to reduce the underlying psychosocial stress.

3. Intervention Components

Psychologists typically teach a broad complement of cognitive, behavioral, and biobehavioral strategies, often in the context of multidisciplinary treatments that might also incorporate physical therapy and non-opioid medications. The literature includes many reports of effective multicomponent Cognitive Behavioral Therapy (CBT) treatments for pediatric chronic pain (see Table 1). However, with some notable exceptions for conditions such as headache pain, [5] there is little conclusive evidence about which component parts of psychological intervention are most effective for which population of children with pain. Many investigations have tried narrowing down this area of research by investigating interventions via defined primary pain (e.g., abdominal, musculoskeletal, neuropathic), developmental level (children vs. adolescents), pain severity, psychological comorbidities (e.g., anxiety, depression) and other factors. Yet, in clinical practice, where the majority of children with chronic pain have more than one pain condition and an array of psychological and psychosocial stressors [1], these research-defined classifications may be less salient.

While randomized controlled trials (RCTs), both individually and collectively evaluated in meta analyses, provide our best evidence that psychological strategies offer benefit to pediatric patients with pain, a broader examination of the current research in this field may help us to better conceptualize new directions in this field. Specifically, we can learn how evidenced-based psychological interventions are being implemented across pediatric pain conditions, in various settings, using novel delivery methods and unique combinations of skills and strategies.

Below we briefly review the most common outpatient intervention frameworks cited in the last ten years (2005–2015), highlighting how a variety of skills and strategies may be applied in helping children, adolescents, and parents in the management of pediatric pain.

3.1. Pain Education

Psychoeducation is a fundamental component of most interventions for pediatric pain. Educational interventions provide a rationale for how and why psychological strategies can effectively reduce pain and pain-related stress and improve daily function. The type of psychoeducation that is empirically shown to improve chronic pain outcomes has been termed "Neuroscience Education (NE)." NE is described as an educational intervention that clearly explains "the neurobiology and neurophysiology of pain and pain processing in the nervous system" [56]. The goal of NE is to teach patients about the basic neuroscience of pain—for example, nerve hypersensitivity, central sensitization, neuroplasticity, and brain modulation of pain signals—to enhance a patient's understanding that pain experience does not necessarily represent ongoing harm to the body. Research suggests that thinking about pain in this way can produce immediate and long term improvement in pain severity, physical activity, fear, and catastrophic thinking [57–59]. Additionally, NE can provide clear evidence regarding the bi-directional relationship between stress and pain and a rationale for how and why cognitive-behavioural strategies can effectively reduce pain and restore function. NE has been well studied in adults with chronic pain [56], but to date no pediatric pain investigations have examined an exclusive NE approach.

3.2. Cognitive Reframing/Positive Self-Statements

Cognitive reframing refers to modifying one's thoughts about a distressing situation so that they are less focused on negative aspects of the situation. Typically, children are taught first to *identify* their negative thoughts or 'self-talk' about pain, then to *challenge* these thoughts, for example, by listing out evidence in support of the thought and evidence against it, and finally to *modify* these thoughts to produce less negative emotional responses. A related technique, positive self-statements, focuses on developing a set of statements that emphasize one's ability to cope positively with a challenging situation. These techniques are widely applied, as persistent negative thinking, referred to as 'catastrophizing', is commonly associated with chronic pain [50,60–62] and can contribute to increased pain and disability [63,64]. Modifying catastrophic thinking—for children with pain and their parents—can help to foster adaptive recovery [51].

3.3. Graded Exposure and Psychological Desensitization

Exposure and psychological desensitization techniques involve gradually increasing exposure to a feared stimulus over time while minimizing associated anxiety. Typically, systematic desensitization entails developing a hierarchy of anxiety-provoking situations ordered from least- to most-feared. The goal is to encounter the situations safely, without the previously experienced distress, to unlink them from associated anxiety. The clinician may teach the child to engage in positive coping strategies (e.g., relaxation) during this desensitization process. Desensitization can also be used to reduce this pain-avoidance pattern, decrease fear of pain, and help children to re-engage in activities, which can in turn help to reduce pain [24,65].

3.4. Biobehavioral Relaxation Techniques

Relaxation is widely used in the treatment of chronic pain. Relaxation strategies focus on acquiring specific skills that can be used to decrease pain perception by promoting a general sense of physical and psychological well-being. The decreased physiological state of arousal that results from the practice of different relaxation based strategies may also serve to diminish pain and its related emotional symptoms. Relaxation approaches include diaphragmatic breathing, progressive muscle relaxation (PMR), and guided imagery techniques. Hypnosis also relies heavily on relaxation and has demonstrated benefit, especially for youth with IBS or functional abdominal pain disorders [21,66]. In a meta-analysis published in 2010, Palermo and colleagues concluded that relaxation asa stand-alone cognitive-behavioural treatment was effective in reducing pain across studies of children and adolescents with a variety of chronic pain conditions including headache, abdominal pain, and fibromyalgia [45]. Typically, however, relaxation strategies are incorporated into multicomponent interventions.

3.5. Biofeedback/Biofeedback-Assisted Relaxation Training (BART)

Biofeedback is a therapeutic intervention that measures and 'feeds back' information about an individual's physiological activity (typically indicators of autonomic arousal) to increase awareness of and control over one's physiological processes. Biofeedback for pain management typically incorporates a focus on respiration (pace and depth of breathing), muscle electromyography, peripheral skin temperature, and blood flow or heart rate variability. The 'feedback' can be visual and/or auditory. Children often find biofeedback engaging and benefit from the concrete, visual aspects of this technique. While biofeedback is shown to have positive effects on pain severity [45], additional well-designed studies are needed to compare biofeedback training to placebo conditions to determine whether there is a potential influence of the novelty of this treatment approach.

3.6. Acceptance-Based Approaches

There is growing evidence that the cognitive practice of acceptance and "staying-in the-moment" combined with the behavioral approach-based practice of actively engaging in valued activities may be an important component of treatment for chronic pain. Research on these strategies demonstrates their effectiveness in adult chronic pain populations [67,68]. At this time, there is a limited but growing body of literature supporting the application of these skills in children with chronic pain [69].

3.7. Other

A few other treatment modalities including techniques from structural family therapy, interpersonal therapy [17], coping skills training [14], social learning [37] and problem solving therapy [70] have been used in the treatment of chronic pain. These have had fewer completed investigations, but suggest that there may be additional interventions that may offer benefit.

4. New Developments in Evidence-Based Research

4.1. Primary Pain

The first generation of pain treatment interventions almost exclusively focused on diagnostic-specific populations (e.g., gastrointestinal pain, headache, complex regional pain syndrome.

Developing interventions that are specific to a presenting pain problem has helped to establish an important foundation in pain management, ,but in some cases this diagnostic specific focus may unintentionally obscure opportunities to more broadly address the psychological challenges that universally impact recovery from chronic pain [71]. In contrast, treating chronic pain as a primary disorder "promotes the conceptualization of chronic pain as a more generalized nociceptive process with common functional limitations (e.g., sleep, school function, activity) and emotional correlates (e.g., fear, worry, hopelessness, helplessness)" [72]. Additionally, a primary pain conceptualization opens the door for the functional treatment of pain even when a clear biomedical etiology is not determinable. From an intervention standpoint, conceptualizing pain as a primary disorder means that interventions have the potential to serve a wide population base, inclusive of various pain disorders. In the research reviewed, about 30% of the studies included multiple pain populations, suggesting that viewing pain as a primary disorder may be a viable way to design and evaluate intervention efficacy. For patients with more entrenched psychological or functional deficits, more comprehensive interventions may be most effective when they specifically target psychological symptoms—for example depression, anxiety, avoidance behaviors, family factors, or fear of pain—as opposed to pain-specific etiologies [71].

4.2. Evaluating Intervention Delivery

With a growing evidence base demonstrating short and long-term benefits for psychological intervention for pain, developing effective methods for disseminating these skills and interventions to the millions of children and parents who need them most is part of the new frontier for this line of research. The historical model of providing 1:1 individualized psychological intervention may not be the most efficient model of care for pediatric pain for several reasons. First, as chronic pain is a relatively new area of practice in pediatric psychology, there are too few pediatric psychologists to meet the demand for intervention. In urban areas, this deficit can contribute to lengthy wait lists for services and in rural areas there may not be any psychologists available to provide this relatively specialized area of treatment. Second, while biomedical biases may continue to inhibit engagement in traditional psychotherapy interventions, novel delivery methods that frame psychological intervention as a component part of pain treatment or as a way to attain skills or support for a challenging problem, may help to reduce this bias and increase patients' view of the intervention as an integrated part of their care. Third, traditional models of psychotherapeutic intervention commonly require weekly or bi-weekly in-person visits. Chronic pain treatment can often be very costly and demanding on a family's schedule requiring frequent appointments such as physical therapy, occupational therapy, tutoring, and physician visits. Developing psychological intervention platforms that can effectively deliver evidence-based treatment in cost, time and resource efficient ways may enhance patient engagement and outcomes.

4.2.1. Internet and Telehealth

There has been a recent emergence of Internet-based CBT interventions for pediatric pain [73]. Internet-delivered CBT for chronic pain has a number of advantages to traditional treatment delivery models. It reduces waiting lists and scheduling conflicts, can be self-paced, and minimizes stigma [74,75]. Moreover, while time-intensive and costly to develop, web-based programs can be extremely cost and time efficient from a patient care perspective. Web-based protocols have been found to be a promising way to introduce pain education, thought restructuring, relaxation training, and other CBT skills. Additionally, some programs can teach parent-based strategies to reinforce positive coping and improve parent-child communications [22]. Findings of a RCT demonstrate significant reductions in pain and activity limitations post-treatment, with gains maintained at a 3-month follow-up. Several Internet-based CBT interventions for children with headaches have also demonstrated reductions in pain and in pain-related negative thinking [19,30].

Limitations to internet delivery methods include the automated aspects of this approach, requirement of access to appropriate technology, and in the case of unguided approaches, a lack of immediate response to individual needs [75]. Moreover, while some interventions have shown benefit [76,77], other studies have high attrition rates suggesting it can be challenging to engage children and adolescents via a home-based, self-administered program [19].

Telehealth treatments that can be personalized and delivered into a patient's home via face-to-face software programs (e.g., skype), personalized email or individualized phone contacts, has also received increased attention in the pediatric pain research over the past 10 years. In most cases, the telehealth portion of an intervention was designed to reinforce skills that were previously taught via other modalities and to problem solve new situations. As intervention dissemination continues to expand, additional telehealth, eHealth and mHealth technologies will likely become more available. Whether these interventions will be sufficient as stand-alone treatments or will alternatively become a valued adjunct to in-person therapies may also be a focus of future research.

4.2.2. Group Interventions

Group-based CBT interventions have been shown to be cost- and time-efficient and as effective as individual treatment in numerous studies [28,78]. The group format also promotes psychosocial support, a particularly salient factor for children with chronic pain who often feel alienated by their condition [79]. Group therapy programs can also incorporate other family members in treatment sessions to help modify pain responses within the family environment [40,80]. In the pediatric literature, group CBT has already demonstrated effectiveness for a variety of pain-related problems such as irritable bowel syndrome [15], headache [26] and pain-related school absenteeism [28]. The most common limitations to group treatments include the possibility of missing sessions and therefore only attaining a partial dose of the interventions. Relatedly, all of the group treatments in this review were administered in person. Thus, access to group treatment may be a logistical barrier.

4.3. Inclusion of Psychosocial Systems

Overwhelmingly, the research on pediatric pain in the past ten years has incorporated parents into treatment. This is an excellent example of how the foundation of our evidence- based research has informed current practice. With strong evidence finding that for all psychological interventions in pediatric pain, inclusion of parents in the treatment fosters better outcomes, it's encouraging to see that the vast majority of newly designed interventions are focused on treating parents. Though almost 70% of the studies we reviewed included parents in their target population, there was tremendous variability in how parents were integrated into treatment. For example, some studies provided only a session or partial session of treatment to parents [17], while other studies fully incorporated parents into all aspects of the treatment [14].

Despite our understanding that other psychosocial systems such as family environments [51,52,81,82] and schools [55,83–85] can influence a child's pain and recovery, there remain few interventions designed to address these broader systems. In our current review, only a single study included siblings, parents, and peers [40] and no studies directly targeted schools. Part of the challenge may be that these more contextual environments require more comprehensive models of care that may be considered too logistically challenging or costly for wider scale clinical implementation. However, given that chronic pain is among the most common and costly problems for children, evaluating whether or not targeted modification of these systems may provide significant benefit may ultimately offer cost benefit.

5. Future Directions

Over the last ten years, our increased knowledge of the neurobiology of pain in combination with a promising research foundation demonstrating that evidenced-based psychological intervention can offer immediate and long-term benefit to children with chronic pain, has led to more nuanced questions regarding the dose, application and dissemination of these interventions. For example, the majority of interventions have been designed as brief models of care (<8 h), increasing our confidence that positive outcomes are possible within a relatively short duration and enhancing opportunities to treat more patients. Effective group treatments similarly enhance opportunities to treat larger numbers of patients while simultaneously providing social support. Moreover, new models of care including internet and telehealth assisted delivery, suggest that our current technology affords opportunities to bring these evidence-based skills and strategies into patients' homes, eliminating many of the logistical barriers to treatment.

Even with these advances, intervention research for pediatric chronic pain is still in its relative infancy and there remain several gaps in our intervention research. For example, our review finds that many interventions did not clearly specify the duration of treatment, leaving out important details such as the number of sessions or the length of each session. Without this "dose" information, it can be difficult to compare efficacy across interventions and challenging to determine how much treatment might be needed for any particular child or family. The use of a tiered care approach to treatment, whereby various levels of intervention intensity are recommended based on a child's particular profile, may emerge as a useful way to direct care. Thus, the availability of various "doses" of intervention is highly relevant. In some cases, patients may first be directed through lower levels of intervention with non-responders proceeding to more intensive interventions, though the use of rapid screening tools (e.g., Pediatric Pain Screening Tool [86]) may also allow providers to identify patients who, according to identified risk factors (i.e., functional disability, depression) need to be fast-tracked to higher levels of intervention (e.g., Intensive Interdisciplinary Rehabilitation Therapy).

Within the current model of care there still remain too many patients who do not seek or attain any psychological interventions for pain due to biomedical biases [8]. Continuing efforts to disseminate basic neuro-science education and to arm children and parents with the necessary skills and strategies early in a child's experience of chronic pain, or even *preventively*, remains a goal for intervention research. Interventions that use non-diagnostic titles such as "The Comfort Ability" [80], "Web-Map" [76], "Teens Taking Charge" [77] or "Headstrong" [16] may help to reduce patient bias [87,88]. Additionally, including psychological interventions as an integrated part of an interdisciplinary treatment program can enhance acceptability. Recent success with social media efforts to shift public opinion about the management of acute pain in children [89] suggests that beyond our focus on patient bias, pediatric psychologists may also have a role to play in shifting general public awareness towards a broader understanding of psychological intervention for managing pediatric chronic pain.

When patients do demonstrate a willingness to engage in psychological intervention for chronic pain, we still have too few options available for clinical use. To date, even with the proliferation of research-based internet programs, there are no web-based protocols available for public use. Moreover, only a handful of the interventions reviewed over the past ten years are maintained outside the research arena as ongoing clinical services. Thus, we need to continue to focus efforts on how to effectively share our knowledge and integrate evidence-based interventions into our current healthcare systems. Programs such as The Comfort Ability, a one-day CBT workshop for children with pain and their parents, is one such example. This program, inclusive of leaders' manuals and patient and parents' workbooks, is designed as a first-line intervention for pediatric pain. Now actively running at eight healthcare institutions, it has demonstrated feasibility for transfer to other sites.

While evidence in the field suggests that many patients and parents benefit from first-line education and intervention, there is also a need to become more specialized in our approach to intervention for those who have high levels of disability or complex comorbidities. There is a need to more fully establish a personalized medicine approach, enabling the identification of patient-specific mood, cognitive, developmental and behavioral patterns that may map onto specialized or tailored interventions leading to improved long-term pain-related outcomes. Without such efforts, patients may become frustrated with trial and error approach or even become treatment resistant [71]. One such example of a specialized approach to care is the "GET Living" intervention, designed to target pain-related fear [90]. With past research demonstrating that patients with high pain-related fear may only partially respond to general CBT [91], more tailored or specialized treatment is warranted for this patient subgroup. Graded in vivo exposure, a specific cognitive–behavioral technique that is effective at improving function for individuals with pain-related fear is being evaluated as the hallmark treatment of GET Living. Though this more intensive treatment is not needed for all pediatric patients with pain, the specialization of this intervention may provide an important path forward for patients with pain and high levels of associated fear.

6. Conclusions

In conclusion, pediatric chronic pain intervention research in the past ten years has made tremendous gains. Collectively there is compelling research demonstrating meaningful gains in reducing pain severity and improving functional outcomes for many brief, outpatient interventions. Nevertheless, there remains a continued need to develop interventions that help to diminish biomedical biases and reduce logistical barriers to care. Moreover, we need sustained efforts in identifying and developing first-line interventions that have wide-scale applicability as well as more nuanced and targeted treatment for patients with more psychophysiological complexities. Psychologists must also consider how to translate our current research initiatives into routine practice for children with chronic pain. Beyond developing interventions, we must continue to educate patients, providers and the general public toward a comprehensive understanding of how and why these interventions can foster adaptive recovery. As our knowledge of the neurobiology of pain continues to expand and we continue to gain confidence in our intervention research, it will be increasingly possible to effectively implement and facilitate the adoption of our evidence-based research.

Acknowledgments: Boston Children's Hospital, Department of Anesthesiology & Perioperative Medicine and the Sara Page Mayo Endowment for Pediatric Pain Research and Education.

Conflicts of Interest: The Comfort Ability is a licensed program registered to Boston Children's Hospital. A portion of Dr. Coakley's activities are funded from the licensure fees associated with this program.

References

1. King, S.; Chambers, C.T.; Huguet, A.; MacNevin, R.C.; McGrath, P.J.; Parker, L.; MacDonald, A.J. The epidemiology of chronic pain in children and adolescents revisited: A systematic review. *Pain* **2011**, *152*, 2729–2738. [CrossRef] [PubMed]
2. Palermo, T.M. Impact of recurrent and chronic pain on child and family daily functioning: A critical review of the literature. *J. Dev. Behav. Pediatr.* **2000**, *21*, 58–69. [CrossRef] [PubMed]
3. Eccleston, C.; Crombez, G.; Scotford, A.; Clinch, J.; Connell, H. Adolescent chronic pain: Patterns and predictors of emotional distress in adolescents with chronic pain and their parents. *Pain* **2004**, *108*, 221–229. [CrossRef] [PubMed]
4. Groenewald, C.B.; Essner, B.S.; Wright, D.; Fesinmeyer, M.D.; Palermo, T.M. The economic costs of chronic pain among a cohort of treatment-seeking adolescents in the United States. *J. Pain* **2014**, *15*, 925–933. [CrossRef] [PubMed]
5. Fisher, E. Systematic review and meta-analysis: Psychological therapies for children with chronic pain. *J. Pediatr. Psychol.* **2014**. [CrossRef] [PubMed]
6. Palermo, T.M. Evidence-based interventions in pediatric psychology: Progress over the decades. *J. Pediatr. Psychol.* **2014**, *39*, 753–762. [CrossRef] [PubMed]
7. Eccleston, C.; Palermo, T.M.; Fisher, E.; Law, E. Psychological interventions for parents of children and adolescents with chronic illness. *Cochrane Database Syst. Rev.* **2015**, *51*, 1036–1038.
8. Simons, L.E.; Logan, D.E.; Chastain, L.; Cerullo, M. Engagement in multidisciplinary interventions for pediatric chronic pain: Parental expectations, barriers, and child outcomes. *Clin. J. Pain* **2010**, *26*, 291–299. [CrossRef] [PubMed]

9. Darnall, B.D.; Scheman, J.; Davin, S.; Burns, J.W.; Murphy, J.L.; Wilson, A.C.; Kerns, R.D.; Mackey, S.C. Pain psychology: A global needs assessment and national call to action. *Pain Med.* **2016**, *17*, 250–263. [CrossRef] [PubMed]

10. Guite, J.W.; Kim, S.; Chen, C.P.; Sherker, J.L.; Sherry, D.D.; Rose, J.B.; Hwang, W.T. Pain beliefs and readiness to change among adolescents with chronic musculoskeletal pain and their parents before an initial pain clinic evaluation. *Clin. J. Pain* **2014**, *30*, 27–35. [CrossRef] [PubMed]

11. Pescosolido, B.A.; Jensen, P.S.; Martin, J.K.; Perry, B.L.; Olafsdottir, S.; Fettes, D. Public knowledge and assessment of child mental health problems: Findings from the national stigma study-children. *J. Am. Acad. Child Adolesc. Psychiatry* **2008**, *47*, 339–349. [CrossRef] [PubMed]

12. Moseley, G.L.; Butler, D.S. Fifteen years of explaining pain: The past, present, and future. *J. Pain* **2015**, *16*, 807–813. [CrossRef] [PubMed]

13. Simons, L.E. Pediatric pain screening tool: Rapid identification of risk in youth with pain complaints. *Pain* **2015**, *156*, 1511–1518. [CrossRef] [PubMed]

14. Kashikar-Zuck, S.; Swain, N.F.; Jones, B.A.; Graham, T.B. Efficacy of cognitive-behavioral intervention for juvenile primary fibromyalgia syndrome. *J. Rheumatol.* **2005**, *32*, 1594–1602. [PubMed]

15. Robins, P.M.; Smith, S.M.; Glutting, J.J.; Bishop, C.T. A randomized controlled trial of a cognitive-behavioral family intervention for pediatric recurrent abdominal pain. *J. Pediatr. Psychol.* **2005**, *30*, 397–408. [CrossRef] [PubMed]

16. Connelly, M.; Rapoff, M.A.; Thompson, N.; Connelly, W. Headstrong: A pilot study of a CD-ROM intervention for recurrent pediatric headache. *J. Pediatr. Psychol.* **2006**, *7*, 737–747. [CrossRef] [PubMed]

17. Degotardi, P.J.; Klass, E.S.; Rosenberg, B.S.; Fox, D.G.; Gallelli, K.A.; Gottlieb, B.S. Development and evaluation of a cognitive-behavioral intervention for juvenile fibromyalgia. *J. Pediatr. Psychol.* **2006**, *31*, 714–723. [CrossRef] [PubMed]

18. Duarte, M.A.; Penna, F.J.; Andrade, E.M.; Cancela, C.S.; Neto, J.C. Treatment of nonorganic recurrent abdominal pain: Cognitive-behavioral family intervention. *J. Pediatr. Gastroenterol. Nutr.* **2006**, *43*, 59–64. [CrossRef] [PubMed]

19. Hicks, C.L.; Von Baeyer, C.L.; McGrath, P.J. Online psychological treatment for pediatric recurrent pain: A randomized evaluation. *J. Pediatr. Psychol.* **2006**, *31*, 724–736. [CrossRef] [PubMed]

20. Abram, H.S.; Buckloh, L.M.; Schilling, L.M.; Wiltrout, S.A.; Ramírez-Garnica, G. A randomized, controlled trial of a neurological and psychoeducational group appointment model for pediatric headaches. *Children's Health Care* **2007**, *36*, 249–265. [CrossRef]

21. Vlieger, A.M.; Menko-Frankenhuis, C.; Wolfkamp, S.; Tromp, E.; Benninga, M.A. Hypnotherapy for children with functional abdominal pain or irritable bowel syndrome: A randomized controlled trial. *Gastroenterology* **2007**, *133*, 1430–1436. [CrossRef] [PubMed]

22. Palermo, T.M.; Wilson, A.C.; Peters, M.; Lewandowski, A.; Somhegyi, H. Randomized controlled trial of an Internet-delivered family cognitive–behavioral therapy intervention for children and adolescents with chronic pain. *Pain* **2009**, *146*, 205–213. [CrossRef] [PubMed]

23. Van Tilburg, M.A.; Chitkara, D.K.; Palsson, O.S.; Turner, M.; Bloismartin, N. Audio-recorded guided imagery treatment reduces functional abdominal pain in children: A pilot study. *Pediatrics* **2009**, *124*, e890–e897. [CrossRef] [PubMed]

24. Wicksell, R.K.; Melin, L.; Lekander, M.; Olsson, G.L. Evaluating the effectiveness of exposure and acceptance strategies to improve functioning and quality of life in longstanding pediatric pain–a randomized controlled trial. *Pain* **2009**, *141*, 248–257. [CrossRef] [PubMed]

25. Barakat, L.P.; Schwartz, L.A.; Salamon, K.S.; Radcliffe, J. A family-based randomized controlled trial of pain intervention for adolescents with sickle cell disease. *J. Pediatr. Hematol. Oncol.* **2010**, *32*, 540. [CrossRef] [PubMed]

26. Gerber, W.D.; Petermann, F.; Gerber-von Müller, G.; Dollwet, M.; Darabaneanu, S.; Niederberger, U.; Schulte, I.E.; Stephani, U.; Andrasik, F. MIPAS-Family-evaluation of a new multi-modal behavioral training program for pediatric headaches: Clinical effects and the impact on quality of life. *J. Headache Pain* **2010**, *11*, 215–225. [CrossRef] [PubMed]

27. Levy, R.L.; Langer, S.L.; Walker, L.S.; Romano, J.M.; Christie, D.L.; Youssef, N.; DuPen, M.M.; Feld, A.D.; Ballard, S.A.; Welsh, E.M.; et al. Cognitive-behavioral therapy for children with functional abdominal pain and their parents decreases pain and other symptoms. *Am. J. Gastroenterol.* **2010**, *105*, 946–956. [CrossRef] [PubMed]

28. Logan, D.E.; Simons, L.E. Development of a group intervention to improve school functioning in adolescents with chronic pain and depressive symptoms: A study of feasibility and preliminary efficacy. *J. Pediatr. Psychol.* **2010**, *35*, 823–836. [CrossRef] [PubMed]

29. Stinson, J.; Mcgrath, P.; Hodnett, E.; Feldman, B.; Duffy, C. Usability testing of an online self-management program for adolescents with juvenile idiopathic arthritis. *J. Med. Internet Res.* **2010**, *12*, e30. [CrossRef] [PubMed]

30. Trautmann, E.; Kroner-Herwig, B. A randomized controlled trial of Internet-based self-help training for recurrent headache in childhood and adolescence. *Behav. Res. Ther.* **2010**, *48*, 28–37. [CrossRef] [PubMed]

31. Warner, C.M.; Colognori, D.; Kim, R.E.; Reigada, L.C.; Klein, R.G. Cognitive-behavioral treatment of persistent functional somatic complaints and pediatric anxiety: An initial controlled trial. *Depress Anxiety* **2011**, *28*, 551–559. [CrossRef] [PubMed]

32. Kashikar-Zuck, S.; Ting, T.V.; Arnold, L.M.; Bean, J.; Powers, S.W. Cognitive behavioral therapy for the treatment of juvenile fibromyalgia: A multisite, single-blind, randomized, controlled clinical trial. *Arthritis Rheum.* **2012**, *64*, 297–305. [CrossRef] [PubMed]

33. Law, E.F.; Murphy, L.K.; Palermo, T.M. Evaluating treatment participation in an internet-based behavioral intervention for pediatric chronic pain. *J. Pediatr. Psychol.* **2012**, *37*, 893–903. [CrossRef] [PubMed]

34. Myrvik, M.P.; Campbell, A.D.; Butcher, J.L. Single-session biofeedback-assisted relaxation training in children with sickle cell disease. *J. Pediatr. Hematol. Oncol.* **2012**, *34*, 340–343. [CrossRef] [PubMed]

35. Vlieger, A.M.; Rutten, J.M.; Govers, A.M.; Frankenhuis, C.; Benninga, M.A. Long-term follow-up of gut-directed hypnotherapy vs. standard care in children with functional abdominal pain or irritable bowel syndrome. *Am. J. Gastroenterol.* **2012**, *107*, 627–631. [CrossRef] [PubMed]

36. Kashikar-Zuck, S.; Flowers, S.R.; Strotman, D.; Sil, S.; Ting, T.V. Physical activity monitoring in adolescents with juvenile fibromyalgia: Findings from a clinical trial of cognitive-behavioral therapy. *Arthritis Care Res. (Hoboken)* **2013**, *65*, 398–405. [CrossRef] [PubMed]

37. Levy, R.L.; Langer, S.L.; Walker, L.S.; Romano, J.M.; Christie, D.L. Twelve-month follow-up of cognitive behavioral therapy for children with functional abdominal pain. *JAMA Pediatri.* **2013**, *167*, 178–184. [CrossRef] [PubMed]

38. Shiri, S.; Feintuch, U.; Weiss, N.; Pustilnik, A.; Geffen, T.; Kay, B.; Meiner, Z.; Berger, I. A virtual reality system combined with biofeedback for treating pediatric chronic headache–A pilot study. *Pain Med.* **2013**, *14*, 621–627. [CrossRef] [PubMed]

39. Stern, M.J.; Guiles, R.A.; Gevirtz, R. HRV biofeedback for pediatric irritable bowel syndrome and functional abdominal pain: A clinical replication series. *Appl. Psychophysiol. Biofeedback* **2014**, *39*, 287–291. [CrossRef] [PubMed]

40. Armbrust, W.; Bos, J.J.F.J.; Cappon, J.; van Rossum, M.A.J.J.; Sauer, P.J.J.; Wulffraat, N.; van Wijnen, V.K.; Lelieveld, O.T.H.M. Design and acceptance of Rheumates@Work, a combined internet-based and in person instruction model, an interactive, educational, and cognitive behavioral program for children with juvenile idiopathic arthritis. *Pediatr. Rheumatol. Online J.* **2015**, *13*, 31. [CrossRef] [PubMed]

41. Hesse, T.; Holmes, L.G.; Kennedyoverfelt, V.; Kerr, L.M.; Giles, L.L. Mindfulness-based intervention for adolescents with recurrent headaches: A pilot feasibility study. *Evid. Based Complement. Alternat. Med.* **2015**, *2015*, 1–9. [CrossRef] [PubMed]

42. Law, E.F.; Bealserickson, S.E.; Noel, M.; Claar, R.; Palermo, T.M. Pilot randomized controlled trial of internet-delivered cognitive-behavioral treatment for pediatric headache. *Headache* **2015**, *55*, 1410–1425. [CrossRef] [PubMed]

43. Yazdani, S.; Zeltzer, L. Treatment of chronic pain in children and adolescents. *Pain Manag.* **2013**, *3*, 303–314. [CrossRef] [PubMed]

44. Barlow, J.H.; Ellard, D.R. Psycho-educational interventions for children with chronic disease, parents and siblings: An overview of the research evidence base. *Child Care Health Dev.* **2004**, *30*, 637–645. [CrossRef] [PubMed]

45. Palermo, T.M.; Eccleston, C.; Lewandowski, A.S.; Williams, A.C.d.C.; Morley, S. Randomized controlled trials of psychological therapies for management of chronic pain in children and adolescents: An updated meta-analytic review. *Pain* **2010**, *148*, 387–397. [CrossRef] [PubMed]
46. Coakley, R.M.; Schechter, N.L. Chronic Pain is Like...The clinical use of analogy and metaphor in the treatment of chronic pain in children. *Pediatr. Pain Lett.* **2013**, *15*, 1–8.
47. Claar, R.L.; Simons, L.E.; Logan, D.E. Parental response to children's pain: The moderating impact of children's emotional distress on symptoms and disability. *Pain* **2008**, *138*, 172–179. [CrossRef] [PubMed]
48. Kendall, P.C. Guiding theory for therapy with children and adolescents. In *Child and Adolescent Therapy: Cognitive-Behavioral Procedures*; Kendall, P.C., Ed.; Guilford Press: New York, NY, USA, 2012; pp. 3–24.
49. Sieberg, C.B.; Williams, S.; Simons, L.E. Do parent protective responses mediate the relation between parent distress and child functional disability among children with chronic pain? *J. Pediatr. Psychol.* **2011**, *36*, 1043–1051. [CrossRef] [PubMed]
50. Langer, S.L.; Romano, J.M.; Levy, R.L.; Walker, L.S.; Whitehead, W.E. Catastrophizing and Parental Response to Child Symptom Complaints. *Child Health Care* **2009**, *38*, 169–184. [CrossRef] [PubMed]
51. Law, E.F.; Fisher, E.; Fales, J.; Noel, M.; Eccleston, C. Systematic review and meta-analysis: Parent and family-based interventions for children and adolescents with chronic medical conditions. *J. Pediatr. Psychol.* **2014**, *39*, 866–886. [CrossRef] [PubMed]
52. Lewandowski, A.S.; Palermo, T.M.; Stinson, J.; Handley, S.; Chambers, C.T. Systematic review of family functioning in families of children and adolescents with chronic pain. *J. Pain* **2010**, *11*, 1027–1038. [CrossRef] [PubMed]
53. Logan, D.E.; Simons, L.E.; Stein, M.J.; Chastain, L. School impairment in adolescents with chronic pain. *J. Pain* **2008**, *9*, 407–416. [CrossRef] [PubMed]
54. Logan, D.E.; Simons, L.E.; Carpino, E.A. Too sick for school? Parent influences on school functioning among children with chronic pain. *Pain* **2012**, *153*, 437–443. [CrossRef] [PubMed]
55. Vervoort, T.; Logan, D.E.; Goubert, L.; De, C.B.; Hublet, A. Severity of pediatric pain in relation to school-related functioning and teacher support: An epidemiological study among school-aged children and adolescents. *Pain* **2014**, *155*, 1118–1127. [CrossRef] [PubMed]
56. Louw, A.; Diener, I.; Butler, D.S.; Puentedura, E.J. The effect of neuroscience education on pain, disability, anxiety, and stress in chronic musculoskeletal pain. *Arch. Phys. Med. Rehabil.* **2011**, *92*, 2041–2056. [CrossRef] [PubMed]
57. Lee, H.; Mcauley, J.H.; Hübscher, M.; Kamper, S.J.; Traeger, A.C. Does changing pain-related knowledge reduce pain and improve function through changes in catastrophizing? *Pain* **2016**, *157*, 922–930. [CrossRef] [PubMed]
58. Moseley, G.L.; Nicholas, M.K.; Hodges, P.W. A randomized controlled trial of intensive neurophysiology education in chronic low back pain. *Clin. J. Pain* **2004**, *20*, 324–330. [CrossRef] [PubMed]
59. Moseley, G.L. Evidence for a direct relationship between cognitive and physical change during an education intervention in people with chronic low back pain. *Eur. J. Pain* **2004**, *8*, 39–45. [CrossRef]
60. Birnie, K.A.; Chambers, C.T.; Chorney, J.; Fernandez, C.V.; McGrath, P.J. Dyadic analysis of child and parent trait and state pain catastrophizing in the process of children's pain communication. *Pain* **2016**, *157*, 938–948. [CrossRef] [PubMed]
61. Crombez, G.; Bijttebier, P.; Eccleston, C.; Mascagni, T.; Mertens, G. The child version of the pain catastrophizing scale (PCS-C): A preliminary validation. *Pain* **2003**, *104*, 639–646. [CrossRef]
62. Leung, L. Pain catastrophizing: An updated review. *Indian J. Psychol. Med.* **2012**, *34*, 204–217. [CrossRef] [PubMed]
63. Liesbet, G.; Eccleston, C.; Vervoort, T.; Jordan, A.; Crombez, G. Parental catastrophizing about their child's pain. The parent version of the Pain Catastrophizing Scale (PCS-P): A preliminary validation. *Pain* **2006**, *123*, 254–263.
64. Wojtowicz, A.A.; Greenley, R.N.; Gumidyala, A.P.; Rosen, A.; Williams, S.E. Pain severity and pain catastrophizing predict functional disability in youth with inflammatory bowel disease. *J. Crohns Colitis* **2014**, *8*, 1118–1124. [CrossRef] [PubMed]
65. Simons, L.E.; Kaczynski, K.J. The Fear Avoidance model of chronic pain: Examination for pediatric application. *J. Pain* **2012**, *13*, 827–835. [CrossRef] [PubMed]

66. Szigethy, E. Hypnotherapy for inflammatory bowel disease across the lifespan. *Am. J. Clin. Hypn.* **2015**, *58*, 81–99. [CrossRef] [PubMed]

67. McCracken, L.M.; Eccleston, C. Coping or acceptance: What to do about chronic pain? *Pain* **2003**, *105*, 197–204. [CrossRef]

68. Vowles, K.E.; McCracken, L.M. Acceptance and values-based action in chronic pain: A study of treatment effectiveness and process. *J. Consult Clin. Psychol.* **2008**, *76*, 397–407. [CrossRef] [PubMed]

69. Martin, S.; Wolters, P.L.; Toledo-Tamula, M.A.; Schmitt, S.N.; Baldwin, A. Acceptance and commitment therapy in youth with neurofibromatosis type 1 (NF1) and chronic pain and their parents: A pilot study of feasibility and preliminary efficacy. *Am. J. Med. Genet.* **2016**, *170*, 1462–1470. [CrossRef] [PubMed]

70. Palermo, T.M.; Law, E.F.; Essner, B.; Jessen-Fiddick, T.; Eccleston, C. Adaptation of problem-solving skills training (PSST) for parent caregivers of youth with chronic pain. *Clin. Pract. Pediatr. Psychol.* **2014**, *2*, 212–223. [CrossRef] [PubMed]

71. Simons, L.E.; Sieberg, C.B.; Coakley, R.M. Patients with pain are not all the same: Considering fear of pain and other individual factors in treatment outcomes. *Pain Manag.* **2013**, *3*, 87–89. [CrossRef] [PubMed]

72. Schechter, N.L. Functional pain: Time for a new name. *JAMA Pediatr.* **2014**, *168*, 693–694. [CrossRef] [PubMed]

73. Voerman, J.S.; Remerie, S.; Westendorp, T.; Timman, R.; Busschbach, J.J.; Passchier, J.; de Klerk, C. Effects of a guided internet-delivered self-help intervention for adolescents with chronic pain. *J. Pain* **2015**, *16*, 1115–1126. [CrossRef] [PubMed]

74. Baer, L.; Greist, J.; Marks, I.M. Computer-aided cognitive behaviour therapy. *Psychother. Psychosom.* **2007**, *76*, 193–195. [CrossRef] [PubMed]

75. Cuypers, M.; Lamers, R.E.D.; Kil, P.J.M.; Poll-Franse, L.V.V.D.; Vries, M.D. Impact of a web-based treatment decision aid for early-stage prostate cancer on shared decision-making and health outcomes: Study protocol for a randomized controlled trial. *Trials* **2015**, *16*, 231. [CrossRef] [PubMed]

76. Palermo, T.M.; Law, E.F.; Fales, J.; Bromberg, M.H.; Jessen-Fiddick, T. Internet-delivered cognitive-behavioral treatment for adolescents with chronic pain and their parents: A randomized controlled multicenter trial. *Pain* **2016**, *157*, 174–185. [CrossRef] [PubMed]

77. Stinson, J. A systematic review of internet-based self-management interventions for youth with health conditions. *J. Pediatr. Psychol.* **2009**, *34*, 495–510. [CrossRef] [PubMed]

78. Morrison, N. Group cognitive therapy: Treatment of choice or sub-optimal option? *Behav. Cognit. Psychother.* **2001**, *29*, 311–332. [CrossRef]

79. Forgeron, P.A.; King, S.; Stinson, J.N.; Mcgrath, P.J.; Macdonald, A.J. Social functioning and peer relationships in children and adolescents with chronic pain: A systematic review. *Pain Res. Manag.* **2010**, *15*, 27–41. [CrossRef] [PubMed]

80. Coakley, R.M.; Barber, B. Overcoming common barriers to engagement in psychological services for chronic pain: A one-day intensive pain management workshop for youth and parents. *Pediatr. Pain Lett.* **2012**, *14*, 10–15.

81. Palermo, T.M.; Valrie, C.R.; Karlson, C.W. Family and parent influences on pediatric chronic pain: A developmental perspective. *Am. Psychol.* **2014**, *69*, 142–152. [CrossRef] [PubMed]

82. Sieberg, C.B.; Manganella, J. Family beliefs and interventions in pediatric pain management. *Child Adolesc. Psychiatr. Clin. N. Am.* **2015**, *24*, 631–645. [CrossRef] [PubMed]

83. Boutilier, J.; King, S. Missed opportunities: School as an undervalued site for effective pain management. *Pediatr. Pain Lett.* **2013**, *15*, 9–16.

84. Dick, B.D.; Pillai Riddell, R. Cognitive and school functioning in children and adolescents with chronic pain: A critical review. *Pain Res. Manag.* **2010**, *15*, 238–244. [CrossRef] [PubMed]

85. Logan, D.E.; Coakley, R.M.; Scharff, L. Teachers' perceptions of and responses to adolescents with chronic pain syndromes. *J. Pediatr. Psychol.* **2007**, *32*, 139–149. [CrossRef] [PubMed]

86. Simons, L.E.; Smith, A.; Ibagon, C.; Coakley, R.; Logan, D.E. Pediatric Pain Screening Tool: Rapid identification of risk in youth with pain complaints. *Pain* **2015**, *156*, 1511–1518. [CrossRef] [PubMed]

87. Brown, J.S.L.; Elliott, S.A.; Boardman, J.; Ferns, J.; Morrison, J. Meeting the unmet need for depression services with psycho-educational self-confidence workshops: A preliminary report. *Br. J. Psychiatry* **2004**, *185*, 511–515. [CrossRef] [PubMed]

88. Brown, J.S.L.; Cochrane, R.; Cardone, D. Large-scale health promotion stress workshops: Promotion, programme content and client response. *J. Mental Health* **1999**, *8*, 391–402.

89. Chambers, C.T. *It Doesn't Have to Hurt*; YouTube: YouTube, 2014; Available online: https://www.youtube.com/watch?v=ge6RY7L2vVo (accessed on 22 October 2016).

90. Simons, L.E. Fear of pain in children and adolescents with neuropathic pain and complex regional pain syndrome. *Pain* **2016**, *157*, S90–S97. [CrossRef] [PubMed]

91. Simons, L.E.; Kaczynski, K.J.; Conroy, C.; Logan, D.E. Fear of pain in the context of intensive pain rehabilitation among children and adolescents with neuropathic pain: Associations with treatment response. *J. Pain* **2012**, *13*, 1151–1161. [CrossRef] [PubMed]

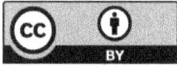

Article

Psychological Neuromodulatory Treatments for Young People with Chronic Pain

Jordi Miró [1,2,3,*], **Elena Castarlenas** [1,2,3], **Rocío de la Vega** [1,4], **Rubén Roy** [1,2,3], **Ester Solé** [1,2,3], **Catarina Tomé-Pires** [1,2,3] **and Mark P. Jensen** [4]

[1]   Chair in Pediatric Pain URV-Fundación Grünenthal, Unit for the Study and Treatment of Pain, ALGOS, 43007 Tarragona, Catalonia, Spain; elenateresa.castarlenas@urv.cat (E.C.); rocio.delavega@urv.cat (R.d.l.V.); ruben.roy@urv.cat (R.R.); ester.sole@urv.cat (E.S.); catarina.tome-pires@urv.cat (C.T.-P.)
[2]   Research Center for Behavior Assessment (CRAMC), Department of Psychology, 43007 Tarragona, Catalonia, Spain
[3]   Institut d'Investigació Sanitària Pere Virgili, Reus 43202, Catalonia, Spain
[4]   Department of Rehabilitation Medicine, University of Washington, Seattle, WA 98105, USA; mjensen@uw.edu
*   Correspondence: jordi.miro@urv.cat; Tel.: +34-977-55-81-79

Academic Editor: Lynn S. Walker
Received: 28 September 2016; Accepted: 30 November 2016; Published: 6 December 2016

Abstract: The treatment of young people with chronic pain is a complex endeavor. Many of these youth do not obtain adequate relief from available interventions. Psychological neuromodulatory treatments have been shown to have potential benefit for adults with chronic pain. Here, we review and summarize the available information about the efficacy of three promising psychological neuromodulatory treatments—neurofeedback, meditation and hypnosis—when provided to young people with chronic pain. A total of 16 articles were identified and reviewed. The findings from these studies show that hypnotic treatments are effective in reducing pain intensity for a variety of pediatric chronic pain problems, although research suggests variability in outcomes as a function of the specific pain problem treated. There are too few studies evaluating the efficacy of neurofeedback or meditation training in young people with chronic pain to draw firm conclusions regarding their efficacy. However, preliminary data indicate that these treatments could potentially have positive effects on a variety of outcomes (e.g., pain intensity, frequency of pain episodes, physical and psychological function), at least in the short term. Clinical trials are needed to evaluate the effects of neurofeedback and meditation training, and research is needed to identify the moderators of treatment benefits as well as better understand the mechanisms underlying the efficacy of all three of these treatments. The findings from such research could enhance overall treatment efficacy by: (1) providing an empirical basis for better patient-treatment matching; and (2) identifying specific mechanisms that could be targeted with treatment.

Keywords: pediatric chronic pain; psychological neuromodulatory treatments; hypnosis; meditation; mindfulness; neurofeedback; efficacy

1. Introduction

Pediatric chronic pain is a common problem worldwide. Although the reported prevalence rates vary as a function of how chronic pain is defined and the reporting period used, the available evidence indicates that pediatric chronic pain is a serious public health problem: prevalence rates range from 6% to 37% [1–3]. The most common pediatric chronic pain problems are headaches, abdominal pain and musculoskeletal pain.

Chronic pain has been defined as "pain without apparent biological value that has persisted beyond normal tissue healing time" [3]. It is a complex experience resulting from the interaction of biological, cognitive, emotional, behavioral, and cultural factors. Chronic pain is known to have significant negative effects on the lives of children and adolescents. For example, research has shown that young people with chronic pain have more cognitive and emotional problems and pain-related worries than their peers without pain [4,5]. Young people with chronic pain also experience more sleep problems [6,7], disability [8,9], impaired social relations [10,11], problems in school function [12,13] and, in general, poorer perceived quality of life [14,15] than their otherwise healthy peers. Moreover, the negative effects of chronic pain also extend to others who live with these youth. For example, family members of children with chronic pain experience more emotional distress, limitations in daily functioning, and problems in marital and social relationships [16,17] than family members of children without chronic pain. Chronic pain also has a significant financial cost, including both direct (e.g., cost of analgesics) and indirect costs (e.g., loss of productivity because one of the parents must stay at home to care for the youth with chronic pain) [18].

Biomedical treatments, consisting primarily of analgesics, are the most common therapeutic strategy used to manage pediatric chronic pain. However, even with the most sophisticated biomedical interventions, many youths continue to experience significant chronic pain and its negative effects [19]. In fact, many of the compounds used in the treatment of pediatric populations with chronic pain have not been licensed for that particular purpose or for the specific pain indication for which they are used with youth [20].

Non-pharmacological treatment options are also sometimes offered to children with chronic pain, although such treatments have traditionally been used as a secondary option (i.e., secondary to the biomedical approach) or as a "last resort" when biomedical treatments are not found to be effective [21]. However, the understanding that chronic pain results from the interaction of biological, emotional, cognitive, behavioral and social factors has led to the promotion of biopsychosocial interventions that address each of these factors [20,22–24]. Furthermore, with the conceptualization of pain as a multidimensional and biopsychosocial phenomenon, and the recognition that pain is ultimately created by the brain (i.e., it is the result of the cortical processing of sensory information in combination with an individual's learning history and evaluations of those sensations), there has been an increased interest in interventions that target brain activity directly to reduce pain and pain-related suffering—so-called psychological neuromodulatory interventions.

There are a number of psychological neuromodulatory treatments that have demonstrated efficacy in adults with chronic pain, and there is a growing number of clinical trials evaluating their efficacy in pediatric populations [25]. The objective of this review paper is to summarize the state of knowledge about the efficacy of three of these psychological neuromodulatory treatments when used with youth with chronic pain: neurofeedback, meditation, and hypnosis. In the sections that follow, and for each of these treatments, we provide a definition and description of the treatment, and then a review of the available evidence regarding its efficacy in youth with chronic pain. The paper ends with a discussion of the clinical implications of the findings and potential avenues for future research.

In order to identify the research studies in this area, we searched the PsycINFO, MEDLINE, PsycARTICLES, Health and Psychosocial Instruments, CINAHL, Scopus and ProQuest Dissertations and Theses databases from their inception to July 2016, using the search terms "((neurofeedback OR meditation OR hypnosis) AND chronic pain AND (child* OR adolescent OR infant OR pediatric OR paediatric OR young OR youth) AND (treatment OR management))". We focused on empirical articles that dealt with chronic non-cancer pain. We also identified systematic reviews which would help to provide the most updated and comprehensive information possible on the topic, both through the original electronic search and through the reference lists of the identified articles. Studies with participants up to 21 years of age are included in this review.

2. Neurofeedback

2.1. Definition and Procedures

Neurofeedback (NF) is a type of biofeedback treatment that provides real-time information to the patient about his or her brain activity, allowing patients to learn how to directly change this activity in ways that are thought to be healthier, more efficient, or provide comfort. As stated by the International Society for Neurofeedback and Research [26], what distinguishes NF from other forms of biofeedback is its focus on the central nervous system; in particular the brain. The assessment of brain activity is performed either through Electroencephalography (EEG) or functional Magnetic Resonance Imaging (fMRI) [25]. The EEG alternative is used much more often because of practical and economic reasons [25]. No studies have examined the efficacy of fMRI-based biofeedback in youth with chronic pain. Therefore, in this review, all references to NF are references to EEG biofeedback.

Although there are a variety of NF protocols, they share the same basic procedures, which are based on operant learning principles [27]. All NF procedures use a Brain Computer Interface; that is, a communication system between the brain and some external device [28]. Briefly, with NF, one or more electrodes is/are placed on the patient's scalp to assess his or her electrical brain activity. The raw electrical signal (which represents the collective activity of hundreds of thousands of neurons in the cortex just below the electrode) is digitalized and the amplitudes of activity in specific frequency bandwidths (e.g., alpha activity, in the 8–12 Hz range) are displayed on the therapist's monitor. Depending on the bandwidths that are the target of treatment—usually bandwidths thought to represent dysfunctional activity—a specific treatment protocol is developed. This protocol is designed to enhance (or inhibit, as appropriate) the power or amount of specific oscillations in order to achieve the therapeutic goals (e.g., increase alpha activity to facilitate perceived relaxation, increase beta or gamma bandwidth activity over the motor cortex to facilitate the inhibition of sensory signals, increase theta or alpha activity over the sensory cortex to inhibit the processing of sensory information, etc.).

Activity in the targeted bandwidth is then "fed back" to the patient, along with instructions to increase or decrease that activity. In children, the feedback is often presented as a game. For example, they are instructed to "fly the rocket" and the software is written to provide the patient with an image of a flying rocket if and when the brain activity changes or maintains in the direction of the training criteria established by the therapist. This feedback enables the patient to influence and progressively change brainwave patterns via operant conditioning [27,29,30]. There are a variety of treatment protocols that are usually named based on the frequencies they intend to alter (e.g., a "Beta protocol" would be one aimed at modifying beta oscillations). It can take a relatively long time for brain activity changes to occur with NF treatment; a full course of NF treatment is normally comprised by 15 to 50 sessions of 20–40 min each [29–31].

Individuals with chronic pain show patterns of EEG activity that differ from those without chronic pain. For example, Pinheiro and colleagues [32] found that individuals with chronic pain display increased alpha and theta frequencies at rest, relative to those without chronic pain [32]. NF treatment for pain usually targets these and other bandwidths in order to: (1) decrease the processing of sensory information; (2) increase activity in areas of the brain that operate to inhibit sensory information; and/or (3) increase perceived relaxation [25]. The electrode placement sites used in the treatment of pain vary, and depend on the specific brain activity patterns thought to underlie a patient's unique pain problem. Electrode placement sites often include central and temporal areas of the cortex [33], but can include as many as 19 different sites in the course of a patient's treatment program [34].

The typical NF session begins with a 2–3 min resting condition to assess baseline EEG activity, which is then followed by several training trials spaced by small breaks. During the training trials, the parameters are set such that one (or more) oscillation bandwidth is reinforced and/or one (or more) oscillation bandwidth is "inhibited" (i.e., the patient needs to demonstrate a decrease in activity in that bandwidth in order to receive the reinforcement). For example, in one recent study evaluating the efficacy of NF to treat chronic neuropathic pain in adults, the investigators reinforced alpha frequency bandwidth (8–12 Hz) activity, and inhibited theta (4–8 Hz) and higher beta (20–30 Hz) bandwidth activity [33]. Reward thresholds are progressively adjusted so that the visual and/or auditory feedback reward is provided to the patient 60%–70% of the time [29].

2.2. Effects

To the best of our knowledge, only two studies have reported on the effects of NF when used for the treatment of youth with chronic pain. Although there are a number of studies that have included adolescents in their samples (e.g., [35,36]), the way in which the data are reported in these studies does not allow us to evaluate the results separately for the children versus adults. Therefore, they were not included in this review.

Siniatchkin and colleagues [37] examined the efficacy of Slow Cortical Potentials NF in a very small sample ($n = 10$) randomized controlled trial of children with migraine without aura. Participants in this trial (which included two control groups; see Table 1) were provided visual feedback in the form of a bar. The protocol was established so that the bar became longer with brain activity thought associated with increased autonomic muscular tension, and shorter with brain activity thought associated with increased relaxation (i.e., soothing thoughts and a restful state). The participants in this study were also asked to pay attention to the thoughts or body sensations that helped them to perform the task. After 10 sessions provided over an eight-week period, the treatment group showed significant reductions in the number of days with migraine per month and the duration of migraine episodes; effects that were not found in the control groups. However, no statistically significant improvements were found in the treatment group on measures assessing the intensity of the migraine headaches, the use of headache medications or other migraine-related symptoms.

In a case series (uncontrolled) study, Stokes and Lappin [38] treated 37 patients with migraine with a combination of NF, passive infrared hemo-encephalography (pIR-HEG), and thermal biofeedback. Thirteen of the study participants were up to 21 years of age, and here we report the results from this subset of patients. The treatment consisted of an average of 40 sessions and included an average of 30 frequency-based NF sessions and an average of 10 pIR-HEG or hand-warming biofeedback session provided over the course of six months. NF training aimed to reduce the amplitude of the frequencies which were assessed at baseline and determined to be "excessive"; that is, treatment was tailored to each participant and was not standardized. The use of a combination of treatments as well as the lack of a control condition does not allow us to determine how much of this benefit was due to the specific effects of NF treatment, how much was due to the specific effects of the other treatment components, and how much was due to non-specific effects (e.g., time, outcome expectancies, therapist attention, etc.).

2.3. Conclusions

NF is an intervention still under development and evaluation for chronic pain. Despite some preliminary encouraging results in adults [25], the lack of controlled trials does not allow us to conclude that NF is an effective treatment for chronic pain in adolescents and children with chronic pain. Nevertheless, the two studies identified do provide preliminary evidence indicating the possibility that NF may benefit young people with chronic pain. Controlled trials are needed to evaluate this possibility. If found to be effective, research is also needed to: (1) understand which NF treatment protocols (number of sessions, electrode training sites, oscillations to reinforce and inhibit, necessity of "booster" treatment sessions, etc.) produce the best results; (2) understand the mechanisms that explain treatment benefits; and (3) identify the patient factors that predict positive treatment responses.

3. Meditation

3.1. Definition and Procedures

Meditation has been defined as "a family of complex emotional and attentional regulatory strategies developed for various ends, including the cultivation of well-being and emotional balance" [39]. Traditionally, meditation procedures have been classified into two types: focused attention meditation and open monitoring meditation [39]. Focused attention meditation includes focusing and sustaining the attention on a specific object (e.g., a flame) or an internally generated image or sound (e.g., image of a flame or mantra), noting when attention begins to wander from that object, and then refocusing attention back onto the object. Open monitoring meditation promotes focusing on and being aware of and accepting without judgment all elements of one's "present experience" without purposefully focusing on any one image or object.

Mindfulness, which is a type of monitoring meditation, is the strategy that has been studied the most in relation to the management of chronic pain in both youths and adults [25]. This procedure has been defined by Kabat-Zinn [40] as "the awareness that emerges through paying attention on purpose, in the present moment, and non-judgmentally to the unfolding of experience, moment by moment". Three common standardized interventions that include mindfulness practice are: (1) Mindfulness–Based Stress Reduction (MBSR) [41]; (2) Mindfulness-based Cognitive Therapy (MBCT) [42]; and (3) Acceptance and Commitment Therapy (ACT) [43].

Mindfulness-based interventions have been described as effective approaches to manage chronic health conditions in young people [44,45], such as in cancer [46] or depression [47]. There are fewer studies evaluating the efficacy of mindfulness in pediatric populations with chronic pain than in adult populations [48,49], although the number of studies using youth samples is growing. In the section that follows, we focus in the results from studies of mindfulness related interventions when used to manage chronic pain in pediatric populations.

3.2. Effects

Mindfulness approaches have been recently used with adolescents with chronic pain, either by using an adaptation of the MBSR program that was original developed for adults [50–52] or as a part of ACT treatment (although mindfulness training is just one of several treatment components of ACT) [53,54]. These interventions have all been implemented in a group format. The available studies have mostly sought to examine the feasibility and acceptability of these treatments; preliminary efficacy data are only reported in a few cases.

It is difficult to compare the results of the available studies due to methodological differences, such as the type of study design (case series versus randomized clinical trial), the content of the mindfulness treatment component, the inclusion of non-mindfulness-based treatment components, the number of treatment sessions provided, and the amount of time of recommended home meditation practice (see Table 1 for a detailed description of the studies reviewed here). Generally speaking, these interventions that include training in mindfulness meditation are well accepted by adolescents with chronic pain, as reflected by the high attendance rates to sessions and high compliance with home practice recommendations. For example, 81% of the participants in one study [52] and 75% in another [50] completed the interventions.

Preliminary results suggest that the MBSR program has significant potential for efficacy (see Table 1). To the best of our knowledge, the first randomized controlled trial using MBSR with pediatric populations with chronic pain was conducted by Jastrowski and colleagues [51]. This study included a very small sample of participants, with four children in a MBSR condition and two in a psychoeducation group. They found that all six participants, regardless of treatment condition, reported increases in mindfulness self-efficacy, but they found inconsistent results regarding the other outcome variables. For example, only three of the participants (two in the mindfulness condition and one in the psychoeducation condition) reported improvements on the total score of a measure assessing physical, emotional, social, and school function.

Two additional studies have adapted the MBSR to be used with adolescents. In one of these studies, Hesse and colleagues [50] conducted a case series study with 20 adolescents with recurrent headache. After eight weeks of treatment, the participants reported a reduction in depressive symptoms and an increase in "pain willingness"; that is, an increase in the belief that pain control is not as important as other life goals. However, no significant pre- to post-treatment differences were found in the other outcome domains, including disability, or anxiety or physical, emotional, social, and school function.

Ruskin and colleagues [52] also adapted MBRS treatment for adolescents with chronic pain and implemented it in a sample of 16 adolescents with a variety of chronic pain conditions (e.g., musculoskeletal pain, abdominal pain). At the end of the treatment, the study participants reported that the treatment helped them to cope better with their pain and to manage their emotions. These results were based on qualitative interviews with the small number of participants who completed the whole program and the assessment at follow-up (see Table 1 for additional details).

Mindfulness techniques have also been used with adolescents with chronic pain as a component of an ACT program [53,54]. Gauntlett-Gilbert and colleagues [53] used a case series study to evaluate changes that occurred following an ACT residential pain management program in a sample of 98 adolescents with chronic pain. The results showed pre- to post-treatment improvements in most of the outcome variables, such as, physical and social disability, pain-related anxiety or pain acceptance, which were maintained for the most part, at the three-month follow-up (see Table 1 for detailed information).

In a more recent study, Martin and colleagues [54] examined changes in outcomes following three two-hour sessions over two days of ACT treatment, which included a number of mindful procedures such as mindful breathing, in a sample of 10 adolescents with neurofibromatosis type 1 and chronic pain. After completion of treatment, the study participants reported significant reductions in pain intensity and pain interference, which maintained at the three-month follow-up assessment point. However, no significant pre- to post-treatment improvements were observed in other outcomes such as pain acceptance, anxiety, and depression.

3.3. Conclusions

Taken as a whole, the findings from research on meditation approaches when used with young people with chronic pain support their feasibility and acceptability. However, data regarding the efficacy of this treatment approach are almost non-existent. The preliminary uncontrolled findings suggest the possibility that mindfulness may help adolescents with chronic pain to improve some (but not all) quality of life domains, including functional status. However, there remain significant methodological limitations that should be addressed in future research. One noteworthy limitation, common for most of the studies, is the small sample sizes. Another related limitation is the quality of the study design. Only one randomized controlled trial has been published [51], but this study was conducted with an extremely small sample, severely limiting the conclusions that can be drawn from the findings. In addition, in many of the studies performed to date, mindfulness training is just one component of a multi-component treatment "package" (e.g., ACT). While it might be argued that the MBSR is at its core a mindfulness training program, we were only able to identify three studies that examined the effects of MBSR (see Table 1). Two of these were case series studies and one was a randomized trial with very few ($n = 6$) subjects. Thus, there is a need for more studies to examine the specific effects of training in mindfulness practice. Furthermore, studies using other meditation procedures, like focused attention meditation, are also needed.

Moreover, the field still needs to reach a consensus regarding how best to adapt mindfulness-based interventions for young people with chronic pain. For example, it would be important to establish the number of sessions needed to maximize any benefits, as well as the number of home-practice hours needed in order to assimilate and integrate the meditation practice into the lives of these youth. In addition, research is also needed to identify the person variables, both internal and external personal characteristics, that facilitate the acquisition of knowledge and skills required in meditation practice. Furthermore, the current research is also limited by the use of participants who are 10 years old or older; future research is needed to evaluate the feasibility and efficacy of meditation practices in children younger than 10 years old.

4. Hypnosis

4.1. Definition and Procedures

Division 30 of the American Psychological Association (APA) defines hypnosis as a "State of consciousness involving focused attention and reduced peripheral awareness characterized by an enhanced capacity for response to suggestion" [55]. Hypnotic procedures usually start with a hypnotic "induction" (thought to increase the patient's response to suggestions), followed by specific suggestions that target the presenting problem. A hypnotic induction can include a number of strategies (e.g., suggestions for relaxation, counting methods) [56,57]. In pediatric chronic pain it is common to use relaxation and/or imagery as induction techniques [58].

In the context of pain management, a typical hypnotic protocol can include suggestions for greater comfort or for coping more adequately with pain, ranging, for example, from direct instructions (e.g., "*You are noticing where in the body you feel the greatest comfort, and can allow this sense of comfort to expand . . . ")* to metaphors (e.g., "*You might visualize any uncomfortable sensations as an image or object, such as a fire or tightly knotted rope,... and now notice how that object changes and as you notice these changes, your experience changes... becoming more and more comfortable"),* to general comfort images (e.g., " . . . *floating* like a big comfortable cloud") or specific suggestions for the problem that is being addressed (e.g., for abdominal pain it can be suggested to patients to "*Feel your hands as warm and place both hands on your abdomen, imagining the warmth spreading into and throughout the abdomen . . . ")* [25,58,59]. Treatment also often includes post-hypnotic suggestions given at the end of the hypnotic sessions which are designed to maintain and extend the therapeutic benefits achieved during the sessions into the patient's daily life. Often, patients are given an audio recording of the sessions to facilitate home practice [58,60].

4.2. Effects

Previous reviews summarizing the findings from randomized controlled trials (RCTs) [58,59], and case studies and non-controlled studies [61], have shown the positive effects of hypnosis when used in the treatment of youth with chronic pain. Most studies for chronic non-cancer related pain have been conducted in samples if children with headache or functional abdominal pain. The results are generally positive, either as presented in uncontrolled case series studies using hypnosis only [62–64] or in combination with other treatments such as acupuncture [65]. The most consistent beneficial effects are found for pain intensity [66–68] and pain frequency [67–69] in samples of children with abdominal pain. These benefits maintain at up to five-year follow-up (see a description of reviewed studies in Table 1) [68].

However, the findings are not as consistently positive in samples of young people with headache. For example, Olness and colleagues [70] found that a hypnotic protocol consisting of standard progressive relaxation exercise, imagery and hypnotic suggestions (e.g., hand anesthesia) significantly reduced the number of headaches but did not decrease headache pain intensity. Positive effects in controlled studies have been also found in samples of children with abdominal pain, in the reduction of disability [66] and school absenteeism [69], although not all studies have reported significant effects on absenteeism [66–68].

Table 1. Summary of reviewed studies.

Author(s) Country	Neuromodulatory Treatment/Study Design	Group and Intervention Description	Sample Description	Assessment Points and Outcome/Process Variables	Summary of Key Findings
		Groups			50% of the treatment group presented a 50% or greater reduction in the number of migraines a month after treatment. Migraine duration reductions were observed in treatment and waiting list groups. No significant changes in the waiting list group in accompanying symptoms (nausea, vomiting, intensity of migraine, or medication intake). No significant differences between the treatment group and the waiting list group in medication intake and migraine intensity. Successful suppression of SCPs' amplitude in the treatment group.
		G1: NF treatment G2: Healthy controls G3: Waiting list		*Assessment points*	
		Session details	G1: *n* = 10 80% male Mean age = 10.5 years Dx.: Migraine without aura	- Baseline - Post-treatment - 6-month follow-up	
		Number of sessions: 1 introductory session + 10 training sessions over 8 weeks.		*Outcome variables*	
Siniatchkin et al. [37]	NF	*Session content:* - 20 trials of baseline CNV recordings (reaction time paradigm).	G2: *n* = 10 70% male Mean age = 11.6 years Dx.: Healthy children	- Average number of days with migraine - Duration of migraine episodes - Headache intensity	
Germany	Non-randomized pilot study	10′ training/5′ break - 30 trials of increasing SCP negativity, 15′ training/5′ break - 30 trials of suppressing SCP negativity 15′ training/5′ break - 15 transfer trials of increasing SCP negativity 7′ training/3′ break - 15 transfer trials of suppressing SCP negativity 7′ training/3′ break	G3: *n* = 10 80% male Mean age = 9.9 years Dx.: Migraine without aura	- Accompanying symptoms (i.e., nausea/vomiting) - Medication intake - Amplitude of the SCPs	

Table 1. Cont.

Author(s) Country	Neuromodulatory Treatment/Study Design	Group and Intervention Description	Sample Description	Assessment Points and Outcome/Process Variables	Summary of Key Findings
Stokes & Lappin [38] USA	NF Case series	*One group only* NF + pirHEG + medication *Session details* Number of sessions: 40 sessions (30 NF + 10 pirHEG; thermal feedback) Session content: – 2 channels NF – Individualized protocols – 5 electrode placement: T3 I T4, C3 I C4, F3 I F4, FP1 I FP2, P3 I P4 – Auditory or visual feedback	*n* = 13 70% female Mean age = 13.4 years Age range = 9–21 years Dx.: Migraine	*Assessment points* – Baseline – Follow-up (variable: from 3 months to 2 years) *Outcome variable* – Average number of days with migraine	Significant decreases observed in the average number of migraine days from pre-treatment to follow-up.
Gauntlett-Gilbert et al. [53] United Kingdom	Meditation Case series	*One group only* ACT residential pain management program *Session details* Sessions duration: 90 h over 3 weeks Session content: – Three components: physical conditioning, activity management, and psychology – Psychology topics included: – Acceptance – Defusion – Present moment contact – Values – Committed action – Self-as-context	*n* = 98 75% female Mean age = 15.6 years Age range = 10.8–19.0 years Dx.: Idiopathic pain, complex regional pain syndrome, back pain, abdominal pain, pain associated with hypermobility	*Assessment points* – Pre-treatment – Post-treatment – 3-month follow-up *Outcome variables* – Physical disability – Social disability – Walk distance – Sit to stand – Pain intensity – Depression – Pain-specific anxiety – Perceived psychosocial development – Pain catastrophizing – Acceptance of pain – School attendance – Number of medications – Health care use	Significant pre- to post-treatment improvements observed in physical and social disability, walking distance, pain anxiety, pain catastrophizing, pain acceptance, school attendance and medication use that were maintained at follow-up. Significant pre- to post-treatment improvements in depression and perceived psychosocial development were observed, but these improvements were not maintained at follow-up. Significant pre- to follow up decrease in health care use. No significant differences in pain intensity at post-treatment and follow-up.

Table 1. *Cont.*

Author(s) Country	Neuromodulatory Treatment/Study Design	Group and Intervention Description	Sample Description	Assessment Points and Outcome/Process Variables	Summary of Key Findings
		One group only		*Assessment points*	Average number of sessions attended: 6.10 of 8 total sessions.
		MBSR		- Pre-treatment	Average of adherence to daily meditation practice: 4.69 of 6 practices per week.
		Session details		- Post-treatment	Number (%) who completed treatment: 15 (75%).
		Number of sessions:		*Process variables*	53% reported the treatment was helpful in coping with stress, relaxing and controlling their
		8 weekly sessions		- Average number of sessions attended	emotions and pain; 40% reported that it was helpful in specific
		Session duration: 2 h		- Average of adherence to daily meditation	ways (i.e., pain reduction);
		Session content:		- Completion rate	13% reported the intervention was not as helpful as expected.
		- Homework and incentives		- Helpfulness of the intervention	33% reported the intervention not affect their headache, 20%
		- Welcoming and centering practice: awareness and mindfulness sound	$n = 20$	- Perceived effect of the intervention to headache	reported having fewer headaches, 13.3% reported having less severe headache, and 7% the headache got better.
Hesse et al. [50]	Meditation	- "Food for thought": relations of quotes or poems with their experiences	100% female	*Outcome variables*	Significant pre- to post-treatment improvements were observed in depressive symptoms and
USA	Case series	- Didactic lessons: awareness of breath, heartfulness, and body scan guided meditations	Mean age = 14.15 years Age range = 11–16 years Dx.: Headache	- Frequency and severity of headache	pain willingness.
		- Learned mindful listening, eating, and walking		- Pain interference	No significant pre- to post-treatment differences were
		- Discussion of home practice		- Headache disability	observed in frequency and severity of headache, disability,
		- Closing mindfulness practice		- Quality of life (physical, emotional, social, and school function)	quality of life, anxiety, or activity engagement.
		- Journaling prompts		- Pain acceptance: activity engagement and pain willingness	
		- Home practice		- Depression	
		- Guided meditation once per day		- Anxiety	
		- Daily diaries			

Table 1. *Cont.*

Author(s) Country	Neuromodulatory Treatment/Study Design	Group and Intervention Description	Sample Description	Assessment Points and Outcome/Process Variables	Summary of Key Findings
		Groups		*Assessment points*	Average number of sessions attended:
		G1: MBSR		- Pre-treatment	G1: 4/6 sessions
		G2: Psycho-educational group		- Post-treatment	G2: 3/6 sessions
				- 4-week follow-up	In general, participants had
		Session details		- 12-week follow-up	positive expectations of the
		Number of sessions:		*Process variables*	proposed interventions.
		6 weekly sessions			75% of the participants in G1
		Session duration: 90	G1:	- Group attendance	reported expecting that MBSR
		Session content:	N = 4	- Participants' expectations	would be "somewhat" to
			75% female	about the benefits of MBSR	"completely helpful" at
		G1:	Mean age = 15.0 years	- Helpfulness of the	pre-treatment. At 12-week
		- Body awareness	Age range = 12–17 year.	treatments components	follow-up one participant
Jastrowski et al. [51]	Meditation	- Basic yoga	Dx.: Chest pain, extremity		reported that MBSR was
		- Relaxation techniques	pain, headache pain, back pain	*Outcome variables*	"completely helpful" and another
USA	Randomized pilot (i.e., very	- Body-scan meditation		- Number of days with pain	that it was "not at all helpful".
	small sample size) study	- Walking meditation	G2:	prior 2 weeks	Qualitative individual analyses
		- Appreciation of the self and	N = 2	- Pain intensity	for outcome variables (data are
		respect for uniqueness	100% female	- Pain duration	missing for several participants
		- Non-judgment of thoughts	Mean age = 12.5 years	- State and Trait Anxiety	and for different assessment
		- Gratitude meditation	Age range = 12–13 years	- Mindfulness self-efficacy	points) indicate that:
		- 30 min homework	Dx.: Abdominal pain	- Quality of life (physical,	- Mindfulness self-efficacy
		6 days/week.		emotional, social, and	increased for all participants
				school functional domains)	in both groups.
		G2:		- Catastrophic thoughts	- Inconsistent results on the
		- Cognitive-behavioral model		- Functional disability	other outcomes measures.
		of chronic pain			
		(anatomy-physiology and			
		misconceptions about pain)			
		- Stress management			
		- Communications skills			

Table 1. *Cont.*

Author(s) Country	Neuromodulatory Treatment/Study Design	Group and Intervention Description	Sample Description	Assessment Points and Outcome/Process Variables	Summary of Key Findings
Martin et al. [54] USA	Meditation Case series	*One group only* ACT *Session details* Number of sessions: 3 Session duration: 2 h over 2 days Session content: - Mindfulness techniques such as mindful breathing - Home practice: ACT exercises to practice between sessions	$n = 10$ 50% girls Mean age = 16.9 years Age range = 12–20 years Dx.: Neurofibromatosis type 1	*Assessment points* - Baseline - 3-month follow-up *Process variables* - Treatment adherence - Satisfaction with treatment (adolescent and parents) *Outcomes variables* *Adolescents:* - Pain interference - Pain intensity - Functional disability - Pain acceptance - Pain-related anxiety - Depression - Health-related quality of life (daily, emotional and cognitive functioning, medical/physical status) - Pharmacological and non-pharmacological techniques used by to manage pain - Disease severity (completed by a nurse practitioner) *Parents* - Child pain interference - Acceptance of child's pain - Health-related quality of life (daily, emotional and cognitive functioning, medical/physical status) - Psychological distress (e.g., anxiety, depression, and somatization)	60% of the participants used mindfulness techniques at least once a week at follow-up. Average participant satisfaction with study was 3.9 on a 0–5 scale. Average parent satisfaction with treatment was 4.6 on a 0–5 scale. Significant pre-treatment to follow-up improvements in pain intensity and pain interference were observed. 60% of the participants reported a decrease of medication at follow-up, relative to pre-treatment. Parents reported a significant pre-treatment to follow-up reduction in pain interference. No significant pre-treatment to follow-up improvements were reported in functional ability, anxiety, depression, quality of life by patient or parent reports, and acceptance of child's pain.

Table 1. *Cont.*

Author(s) Country	Neuromodulatory Treatment/Study Design	Group and Intervention Description	Sample Description	Assessment Points and Outcome/Process Variables	Summary of Key Findings
		One group only		*Assessment points*	Completion rate: 81%
				- Baseline	Average sessions attendance was 6.4 out of 8 sessions.
		MBSR		- Post-treatment	All participants would recommend the intervention.
		Session details		*Process variables*	Average importance of learning and practice mindfulness rated as 4.17 out of 5.
		Number sessions: 8 Session duration: 2 h Session content (meditation exercises):	*n* = 16 100% girls Mean age = 5.75 years	- Completion rate - Sessions attendance - Recommendation of treatment to others	Average confidence in use mindfulness rated as 4 out of 5. MBSR rated as being useful to cope with pain and negative emotions and for being more kind with themselves (average rating = 3.67 out of 5).
Ruskin et al. [52]	Meditation	- Bringing comfort to pain	Age range = 13–17 years Dx: Neurophatic pain,	- Importance of learning and practice mindfulness	
Canada	Pilot uncontrolled clinical study	- Kindness to pain - Body scan	musculoskeletal pain, abdominal pain, mixed pain, headache	- Confidence in using mindfulness	Favorite activities of the treatment included: experiential exercises, meeting others with similar life
		- Mindful eating - Breathing meditation - Mountain meditation		- Helplessness of the intervention (i.e., to cope with pain, negative	experiences, group discussions, and learning new techniques to cope with pain.
		- Loving kindness - Gratitude - Home practice: 5 min daily		emotions and to be more kind with themselves) - Favorite activities of the treatment	Areas of improvement noted: need of more specific and immediate techniques for managing pain flare-ups, need of more time to share pain stories with other participant, and difficulties with getting to the hospital after a school day.

Table 1. *Cont.*

Author(s) Country	Neuromodulatory Treatment/Study Design	Group and Intervention Description	Sample Description	Assessment Points and Outcome/Process Variables	Summary of Key Findings
Anbar &Zoughbi [64] USA	Hypnosis Case series	*One group only* Hypnosis *Session details* Number of sessions: Mean of 2 sessions of hypnosis in clinic with a mean of 3.8 sessions (range 1–16)	*n* = 30 56.6% female Mean age = 15 years Age range: 10–18 years Dx.: Headache	*Assessment points* - Baseline - Post-treatment - Follow-up (time not specified) *Outcome variables* - Headache frequency - Headache pain intensity	96% of the participants reported pre- to post-treatment decreases in headache frequency and intensity. Pre- to post-treatment improvements were maintained at follow-up for 65% of the sample.
Galini, Shaoul & Mogilner [62] Israel	Hypnosis Case series	*One group only* Hypnosis *Session details* Number of sessions: 1	*n* = 20 75% female Age range = 11–18 years Dx.: Chronic recurrent functional abdominal pain	*Assessment points* - Baseline - Post-treatment *Outcome variables* - Pain intensity - Pain frequency	70% of the participants reported pre- to post-treatment improvements in pain intensity and pain frequency.
Kohen & Zajac [63] USA	Hypnosis Case series	*One group only* Hypnosis *Session details* Number of sessions: 3 to 4	*n* = 144 66% female Mean age = 11.0 years Age range = 5–15 years Dx.: Headache	*Assessment points* - Baseline - Post-treatment *Outcome variables* - Headache frequency - Headache pain intensity - Headache duration	88% of the participants reported a decrease in headache frequency (from 4.5 to 1.4/week), 87% a decrease in headache pain intensity (10.3 to 4.7 in a 12-point scale), and 26% experienced a resolution in their headache. Headache duration decreased from 23.6 to 3.0 h, on average.

Table 1. *Cont.*

Author(s) Country	Neuromodulatory Treatment/Study Design	Group and Intervention Description	Sample Description	Assessment Points and Outcome/Process Variables	Summary of Key Findings
Olness et al. [70] USA	Hypnosis Randomized controlled trial	*Groups* G1: Placebo-placebo-hypnosis G2: Propranolol-place-bo-hypnosis G3: Placebo-propranolol-hypnosis *Session details* Number of sessions: 3 during 12 weeks, 10-week placebo or drug treatment period.	G1: $n = 9$ 44.4% female Mean age = 8.4 years Age range = 6–12 years Dx.: Migraine G2: $n = 11$ 18.2% female Mean age = 9.6 years Age range = 6–12 years Dx.: Migraine G3: $n = 8$ 62.5% female/male Mean age = 9.6 years Age range = 6–12 years Dx.: Migraine	*Assessment points* - Baseline - Post-treatment *Outcome variables* - Headache frequency - Headache pain intensity	Participants in the hypnosis group reported a significantly greater pre- to post-treatment decrease in headache frequency relative to control group, but no significant differences were found regarding pain intensity.
Van Tilburg et al. [66] USA	Hypnosis Randomized controlled trial	*Groups* G1: Standard medical care + listening to recorded hypnotic sessions G2: Standard medical care *Session details (G1)* Number of sessions: 3 biweekly sessions, including 1 booster session + 3 daily sessions. Treatment period: 2 months Session content: Listen to tape with self-exercises ≥5 days/week.	G1: $n = 19$ G2: $n = 15$ 71% female Age range = 6–16 years Dx.: Functional Abdominal Pain	*Assessment points* - Baseline - Post-treatment *Outcome variables* - Pain intensity - Composite score of quality of life (physical, emotional, social, and school functional domains) - School absenteeism - Medication use	Participants in the hypnosis group reported significantly greater pre- to post-treatment improvements in pain intensity and perceived "health related quality of life" than participants in the control group. No significant differences between the hypnosis and control groups were observed in school absenteeism or medication use.

Table 1. *Cont.*

Author(s) Country	Neuromodulatory Treatment/Study Design	Group and Intervention Description	Sample Description	Assessment Points and Outcome/Process Variables	Summary of Key Findings
Vlieger et al. [67] Vlieger et al. [68] * Netherlands	Hypnosis Randomized controlled trial	*Groups* G1: Hypnosis G2: Standard medical care + supportive therapy *Session details* Number of sessions: 6 Session duration: 50' over a 3-month period for the G1. Six 30' session over a 3-month period for the G2.	G1: *n* = 27 67% female G2: *n* = 22 86% female Mean age = 13.2 years Age range = 8–18 years Dx.: Irritable bowel syndrome, functional abdominal pain	*Assessment points* - Pre-treatment - Post-treatment - 1-year follow-up - 5-year follow-up *Outcome variables* - Pain intensity - Pain frequency (days per month) - General improvement - School absenteeism	Participants in the hypnosis group reported significantly greater pre- to post-treatment improvements in pain intensity and frequency. Participants in the hypnosis group reported significantly greater general pain improvement at 1-year and 5-year follow up. No significant differences between the hypnosis and control groups were observed in school absenteeism at a 5-year follow-up.
Weydert et al. [69] USA	Hypnosis Randomized controlled trial	*Groups* G1: Standard medical care + 4 hypnosis sessions G2: Standard medical care + breathing techniques *Session details* Number of sessions: 4 weekly sessions Session content: G1: Progressive relaxation + guided imagery. Listen to tape with self-exercises twice a day. G2: Learning three breathing techniques.	G1: *n* = 14 77% female Mean age = 11.0 years Dx.: Abdominal pain G2: *n* = 8 50% female Mean age = 11.1 years Dx.: Abdominal pain	*Assessment points* - Pre-treatment - Post-treatment - 1-month follow up *Outcome variables* - Pain frequency - School absenteeism	Participants in the hypnosis group reported significantly greater pre- to post-treatment improvements in pain frequency that were maintained at 1-month follow up. Participants in the hypnosis group reported significantly greater pre- to post-treatment improvements in school absenteeism that were maintained at 1-month follow up.

Table 1. *Cont.*

Author(s) Country	Neuromodulatory Treatment/Study Design	Group and Intervention Description	Sample Description	Assessment Points and Outcome/Process Variables	Summary of Key Findings
Zeltzer et al. [65] USA	Hypnosis Case series	*One group only* Hypnosis *Session details* Number of sessions: 6 weekly sessions Session content: acupuncture combined with 20′ of hypnotic sessions.	*n* = 31 61% female Mean age = 13 years Age range = 6–18 years Dx.: Headache, abdominal pain associated with irritable bowel syndrome, fibromyalgia, complex regional pain syndrome, juvenile rheumatoid arthritis, myofascial back and chest pain	*Assessment points* - Pre-treatment - Post-treatment *Outcome variables* - Average pain intensity - Current pain intensity - Pain interference in functioning - Anxiety - Depression	Children: Participants reported significantly greater pre- to post-treatment improvements in current and average pain intensity; 42.5% of children reported a decrease in current pain. Participants reported significantly greater pre- to post-treatment improvements in pain interference in functioning. Participants reported significantly greater pre- to post-treatment improvements in anxiety (50% of children reported decrease). No significant changes were reported in depression. Parents: Parents reported significantly greater pre- to post-treatment improvements in current and average pain intensity as well as pain interference in functioning.

* This publication reports on the five-year follow-up of the sample. Data from there participants of the control group are missing; NF: Neurofeedback; SCP: Slow Cortical Potentials; pirHEG: passive infrared hemoencephalography; CNV: Contingent Negative Variation; ACT: Acceptance and Commitment Therapy; MBSR: Mindfulness-based stress reduction; T: temporal area; C: central area; F: frontal area; FP: prefrontal area; P: parietal area; G: group; *n*: number of participants; Dx.: Diagnosis.

4.3. Conclusions

On the basis of the available research, summarized here, it appears that the use of hypnosis for the management of pediatric chronic pain is promising, although its efficacy also appears to vary as a function of the pain condition studied. For example, the efficacy of hypnosis as a treatment for youth with chronic abdominal pain has strong research support whereas its use in the management of headaches only has modest support (based on the criteria proposed by the Society of Clinical Psychology, Division 12 of the American Psychological Association [71], recently updated, see https://www.div12.org/faq/). There are a variety of hypnotic strategies available which can target a variety of outcomes and mechanisms. However, there is not yet any evidence regarding which protocols are most effective for whom and under what circumstances. There is a general belief, however, that treatment should be tailored to the age of the patient for best results [72].

Future research is needed to identify which hypnosis treatment protocols are most effective, and if the efficacy of protocols are moderated by type of pain and age of the patient or other factors. In addition, many investigators and clinicians have expressed the belief that hypnotic suggestions should target the multidimensional experience and effects of pain, including pain intensity, psychological distress (e.g., anxiety), maladaptive thoughts (e.g., catastrophizing), as well as other domains known to be influenced by pain, such as analgesic intake and sleep quality [73–75]. Research is needed to evaluate this assumption, and to identify which outcome domains are most responsive to hypnotic treatment.

5. Conclusions and General Discussion

The results from this review indicate that psychological neuromodulatory treatments are promising treatments for young people with chronic pain. However, there are more findings supporting the efficacy of hypnosis—in particular for chronic abdominal pain—than for either neurofeedback or meditation. In this review, we limited our focus to non-cancer chronic pain-related problems. However, the conclusions from this review—at least those conclusions with respect to the efficacy of hypnosis—are consistent with those from reviews of studies in youth with cancer-related pain (e.g., [58,76]), providing even more support for the efficacy of hypnosis. An additional finding supporting the use of hypnosis for chronic pain in youth—even as a potential "first line treatment"—is its side effect profile; that is, the benefits noted appear to occur in the absence of any significant negative side effects, other than perhaps the effort and time it takes to learn the self-hypnosis skills taught [58].

Not all patients benefit from hypnotic treatment, however. For example, the rates of children who benefited from hypnosis as reported in the studies reviewed here ranged from 67% to 96% (see Table 1). Moreover, we still do not understand the factors that predict outcome. We still do not know for whom hypnotic treatment works best, and which of the many possible hypnotic protocols produce the most benefit. There is a belief among those who are not familiar with hypnosis research that trait hypnotizability predicts response to hypnosis treatment. However, while the association between measures of hypnotizability and hypnosis treatment in adults tends to be positive, the strength of those associations also tends to be weak [77]; high levels of trait hypnotizability do not appear to be necessary to obtain benefits from hypnotic treatments. On the other hand, there is some evidence that adult patients with neuropathic pain may respond better to hypnosis treatment than patients with non-neuropathic chronic pain conditions [25]. However, the generalizability of this finding to children is not known. In short, even as the field continues to evaluate the efficacy of hypnosis for chronic pain conditions in youth, there is also a need to better understand the mechanisms and moderators of the treatment benefits that are found.

With respect to mindfulness meditation and NF in pediatric populations with chronic pain, there are too few clinical trials to be able to draw firm conclusions regarding efficacy. Preliminary data indicate that these treatments are well tolerated, and may be associated with improvements in some important pain outcome variables (e.g., pain intensity, frequency of pain episodes, well-being, physical function) in some populations. However, the long-term benefits of these treatments are not known. Critically, there is a lack of adequately designed randomized clinical trials evaluating the specific effects of these treatments. On the other hand, the side effect profiles of these treatments are positive; studies about meditation and NF do not report many (if any) significant negative effects associated to these treatments.

An additional important advantage of all of these psychological neuromodulatory treatments is that they promote and reinforce self-efficacy and encourage self-care. However, these advantages need to be weighed against the fact that these treatments require the involvement and motivation of the patient. Another disadvantage of NF treatment specifically is that it requires many sessions (as many as 40 or more) and special equipment, both of which increase the cost of this intervention.

We are far from having an adequate level of evidence to provide strong recommendations that hypnosis, NF, and training in meditation should be offered to all youth with chronic pain. However, the preliminary evidence reviewed here is promising, and supports the idea that additional studies about the efficacy of psychological neuromodulatory treatments are warranted. These future studies should include larger samples, use more robust methodologies (i.e., randomized controlled trials), and use manualized (i.e., standardized) interventions to develop an empirical foundation from which to make informed decisions about which treatment(s) should be offered to which patient(s). Ideally, these studies would be conducted in samples of children with a variety of chronic pain problems. For example, although we can conclude based on the available evidence that hypnotic treatment is efficacious for the management of chronic abdominal pain and has moderate evidence in relation to chronic headaches, studies in other chronic pain problems are needed.

Moreover, future research is needed to expand the criteria used to assess the efficacy of these treatments from a focus on pain-related domains (intensity, frequency or duration) to measures of function. The Initiative on Methods, Measurement, and Pain Assessment in Clinical Trials (PedIMMPACT; [78]) recommended a group of common outcome domains and measures for clinical trials, and it would be useful if all those future trials include as many as these domains as possible (i.e., pain intensity, global judgment of satisfaction with treatment, symptoms and adverse events, physical functioning, emotional functioning, role functioning, sleep, and economic factors).

As research in this area expands, and more is known regarding the efficacy and mechanisms of hypnosis, NF, and meditation training and practice in youths with chronic pain, we anticipate that it will provide the necessarily empirical basis for making treatment decisions and recommendations. This should increase the treatment options available to children, which will ultimately result in an improvement in the comfort and overall quality of life of these individuals.

Acknowledgments: Support for this work was provided by grants from Obra Social de La Caixa, Universitat Rovira i Virgili (PFR program), the Spanish Ministry of Innovation (MINECO; PSI2015-70966-P), and the European Regional Development Fund (ERDF). E.C.'s work is supported by grant PSI2014-60180-JIN of the Spanish Ministry of Economy and Competitiveness. R.V.'s work is supported by a Beatriu de Pinós Postdoctoral Fellowship (2014 BP-A 00009) granted by the Agency for Administration of University and Research Grants (AGAUR). J.M.'s work is also supported by the Institució Catalana de Recerca i Estudis Avançats (ICREA-Acadèmia), and Fundación Grünenthal.

Conflicts of Interest: The authors declare no conflict of interest.

References

1. Van Dijk, A.; McGrath, P.A.; Pickett, W.; VanDenKerkhof, E.G. Pain prevalence in nine- to 13-year-old school children. *Pain Res. Manag.* **2006**, *11*, 234–240. [CrossRef] [PubMed]
2. Huguet, A.; Miró, J. The severity of chronic pediatric pain: An epidemiological study. *J. Pain* **2008**, *9*, 226–236. [CrossRef] [PubMed]
3. Stevens, B.J.; Zempsky, W.T. Prevalence and distribution of pain in children. In *Oxfor Textbook of Paediatric Pain*; McGrath, P.J., Stevens, B.J., Walker, S.M., Zempsky, W.T., Eds.; Oxford University Press: Oxford, UK, 2014; pp. 12–19.

4. Huguet, A.; Eccleston, C.; Miró, J.; Gauntlett-Gilbert, J. Young people making sense of pain: Cognitive appraisal, function, and pain in 8–16 year old children. *Eur. J. Pain* **2009**, *13*, 751–759. [CrossRef] [PubMed]

5. Solé, E.; Castarlenas, E.; Miró, J. A Catalan adaptation and validation of the Pain Catastrophizing Scale for Children. *Psychol. Assess.* **2016**, *28*, e119–e126. [CrossRef] [PubMed]

6. De la Vega, R.; Racine, M.; Sánchez-Rodríguez, E.; Tomé-Pires, C.; Castarlenas, E.; Jensen, M.P.; Miró, J. Pain Extent, Pain Intensity, and Sleep Quality in Adolescents and Young Adults. *Pain Med.* **2016**, *17*, 1971–1977. [CrossRef] [PubMed]

7. De la Vega, R.; Miró, J. The assessment of sleep in pediatric chronic pain sufferers. *Sleep Med. Rev.* **2013**, *17*, 185–192. [CrossRef] [PubMed]

8. Miró, J.; Huguet, A.; Jensen, M.P. Pain beliefs predict pain intensity and pain status in children: Usefulness of the pediatric version of the survey of pain attitudes. *Pain Med.* **2014**, *15*, 887–897. [CrossRef] [PubMed]

9. Miró, J.; Huguet, A.; Nieto, R. Predictive factors of chronic pediatric pain and disability: A Delphi poll. *J. Pain* **2007**, *8*, 774–792. [CrossRef] [PubMed]

10. Castarlenas, E.; de la Vega, R.; Tomé-Pires, C.; Solé, E.; Racine, M.; Jensen, M.P.; Miró, J. Student Expectations of Peer and Teacher Reactions to Students With Chronic Pain: Implications for Improving Pain-related Functioning. *Clin. J. Pain* **2015**, *31*, 992–997. [CrossRef] [PubMed]

11. Forgeron, P.A.; King, S.; Stinson, J.N.; McGrath, P.J.; MacDonald, A.J.; Chambers, C.T. Social functioning and peer relationships in children and adolescents with chronic pain: A systematic review. *Pain Res. Manag.* **2010**, *15*, 27–41. [CrossRef] [PubMed]

12. Logan, D.E.; Simons, L.E.; Carpino, E.A. Too sick for school? Parent influences on school functioning among children with chronic pain. *Pain* **2012**, *153*, 437–443. [CrossRef] [PubMed]

13. Roth-Isigkeit, A.; Thyen, U.; Stoven, H.; Schwarzenberger, J.; Schmucker, P. Pain among children and adolescents: Restrictions in daily living and triggering factors. *Pediatrics* **2005**, *115*, e152–e162. [CrossRef] [PubMed]

14. Huguet, A.; Miró, J. Development and psychometric evaluation of a Catalan self- and interviewer-administered version of the Pediatric Quality of Life Inventory version 4.0. *J. Pediatr. Psychol.* **2008**, *33*, 63–79. [CrossRef] [PubMed]

15. Rabbitts, J.A.; Holley, A.L.; Groenewald, C.B.; Palermo, T.M. Association Between Widespread Pain Scores and Functional Impairment and Health-Related Quality of Life in Clinical Samples of Children. *J. Pain* **2016**, *17*, 678–684. [CrossRef] [PubMed]

16. Vowles, K.E.; Cohen, L.L.; McCracken, L.M.; Eccleston, C. Disentangling the complex relations among caregiver and adolescent responses to adolescent chronic pain. *Pain* **2010**, *151*, 680–686. [CrossRef] [PubMed]

17. Hunfeld, J.A.; Perquin, C.W.; Duivenvoorden, H.J.; Hazebroek-Kampschreur, A.A.; Passchier, J.; van Suijlekom-Smit, L.W.; van der Wouden, J.C. Chronic pain and its impact on quality of life in adolescents and their families. *J. Pediatr. Psychol.* **2001**, *26*, 145–153. [CrossRef] [PubMed]

18. Groenewald, C.B.; Wright, D.R.; Palermo, T.M. Health care expenditures associated with pediatric pain-related conditions in the United States. *Pain* **2015**, *156*, 951–957. [CrossRef] [PubMed]

19. Stinson, J.; Bruce, E. Chronic pain in children. In *Managing Pain in Children. A Clinical Guide*; Twycross, A., Dowden, S., Bruce, E., Eds.; Wiley-Blackwell: Chichester, UK, 2009; pp. 145–170.

20. Gregoiré, M.C.; Finley, G.A. Drugs for chronic pain in children: A commentary on clinical practice and the absence of evidence. *Pain Res. Manag.* **2013**, *18*, 47–51.

21. Unruh, A.; McGrath, P.J. History of pain in children. In *Oxford Textbook of Paediatric Pain*; McGrath, P.J., Stevens, B.J., Walker, S.M., Zempski, W.T., Eds.; Oxford University Press: Oxford, UK, 2014; pp. 3–11.

22. Carter, B.D.; Threlkeld, B.M. Psychosocial perspectives in the treatment of pediatric chronic pain. *Pediatr. Rheumatol. Online J.* **2012**, *10*, 15. [CrossRef] [PubMed]

23. McGrath, P.; Stevens, B.; Walker, S.; Zempsky, W. *Oxford Textbook of Paediatric Pain*; Oxford University Press: London, UK, 2013.

24. American pain Society Assessment and Management of Children with Chronic Pain. *A Position Statement Am. Pain Soc.* **2012**.

25. Jensen, M.P.; Day, M.A.; Miró, J. Neuromodulatory treatments for chronic pain: Efficacy and mechanisms. *Nat. Rev. Neurol.* **2014**, *10*, 167–178. [CrossRef] [PubMed]

26. International Society for Neurofeedback and Research Definition of Neurofeedback. Definition of ISNR Board of Directors. Available online: http://www.isnr.org/neurofeedback-introduction (accessed on 10 June 2016).

27. Sherlin, L.H.; Arns, M.; Lubar, J.; Heinrich, H.; Kerson, C.; Strehl, U.; Sterman, M.B. Neurofeedback and Basic Learning Theory: Implications for Research and Practice. *J. Neurother.* **2011**, *15*, 292–304. [CrossRef]
28. Teplan, M. Fundamentals of EGG measurement. *Rev. Meas. Sci.* **2002**, *2*, 1–11.
29. Heinrich, H.; Gevensleben, H.; Strehl, U. Annotation: Neurofeedback—Train your brain to train behaviour. *J. Child Psychol. Psychiatry* **2007**, *1*, 3–16. [CrossRef] [PubMed]
30. Hammond, D.C. What is neurofeedback: An update. *J. Neurother.* **2011**, *15*, 305–336. [CrossRef]
31. Hammond, D.C. What Is Neurofeedback? *J. Neurother. Investig. Neuromodulation Neurofeedback Appl. Neurosci.* **2007**, *10*, 25–36. [CrossRef]
32. Pinheiro, E.S.; Queirós, F.C.; Montoya, P.; Santos, C.L.; do Nascimento, M.A.; Ito, C.H.; Silva, M.; Nunes Santos, D.B.; Benevides, S.; Miranda, J.G.; et al. Electroencephalographic Patterns in Chronic Pain: A Systematic Review of the Literature. *PLoS ONE* **2016**, *11*, e0149085. [CrossRef] [PubMed]
33. Hassan, M.A.; Fraser, M.; Conway, B.A.; Allan, D.B.; Vuckovic, A. The mechanism of neurofeedback training for treatment of central neuropathic pain in paraplegia: A pilot study. *BMC Neurol.* **2015**, 1–13. [CrossRef] [PubMed]
34. Koberda, J.L.; Koberda, P.; Bienkiewicz, A.A.; Moses, A.; Koberda, L. Pain Management Using 19-Electrode Z-Score LORETA Neurofeedback. *J. Neurother.* **2013**, *17*, 179–190. [CrossRef]
35. Santoro, M.M.; Cronan, T.A. Systematic Review of Neurofeedback as a Treatment for Fibromyalgia Syndrome Symptoms. *J. Musculoskelet. Pain* **2014**, *22*, 286–300. [CrossRef]
36. Kayiran, S.; Dursun, E.; Dursun, N.; Ermutlu, N.; Karamürsel, S. Neurofeedback Intervention in Fibromyalgia Syndrome; a Randomized, Controlled, Rater Blind Clinical Trial. *Appl. Psychophysiol. Biofeedback* **2010**, *35*, 293–302. [CrossRef] [PubMed]
37. Siniatchkin, M.; Hierundar, A.; Kropp, P.; Kuhnert, R.; Gerber, W.D.; Stephani, U. Self-regulation of slow cortical potentials in children with migraine: An exploratory study. *Appl. Psychophysiol. Biofeedback* **2000**, *25*, 13–32. [CrossRef] [PubMed]
38. Stokes, D.A.; Lappin, M.S. Neurofeedback and biofeedback with 37 migraineurs: A clinical outcome study. *Behav. Brain Funct.* **2010**, *6*, 9. [CrossRef] [PubMed]
39. Lutz, A.; Slagter, H.A.; Dunne, J.D.; Davidson, R.J. Attention regulation and monitoring in meditation. *Trends Cogn. Sci.* **2008**, *12*, 163–169. [CrossRef] [PubMed]
40. Kabat-Zinn, J. Mindfulness-Based Interventions in Context: Past, Present, and Future. *Clin. Psychol. Sci. Pract.* **2003**, *10*, 144–156. [CrossRef]
41. Kabat-Zinn, J. *Wherever You Go, There You Are: Mindfulness Meditation in Everyday Life*; Hyperion: New York, NY, USA, 1994.
42. Segal, Z.V.; Williams, J.M.G.; Teasdale, J.D. *Mindfulness-Based Cognitive Therapy for Depression: A New Approach to Preventing Relapse*; Guilford Press: London, UK, 2002.
43. Hayes, S.C.; Strosahl, K.D.; Wilson, K.G. *Acceptance and Commitment Therapy: An Experiential Approach to Behavior Change*; The Guilford Press: New York, NY, USA, 1999.
44. Burke, C.A. Mindfulness-based approaches with children and adolescents: A preliminary review of current research in an emergent field. *J. Child Fam. Stud.* **2010**, *19*, 133–144. [CrossRef]
45. Kallapiran, K.; Koo, S.; Kirubakaran, R.; Hancock, K. Review: Effectiveness of mindfulness in improving mental health symptoms of children and adolescents: A meta-analysis. *Child Adolesc. Ment. Health* **2015**, *20*, 182–194. [CrossRef]
46. Jones, P.; Blunda, M.; Biegel, G.; Carlson, L.E.; Biel, M.; Wiener, L. Can mindfulness based interventions help adolescents with cancer? *Psychooncology* **2013**, *22*, 2148–2151. [CrossRef] [PubMed]
47. Ames, C.S.; Richardson, J.; Payne, S.; Smith, P.; Leigh, E. Mindfulness-based cognitive therapy for depression in adolescents. *Child Adolesc. Ment. Health* **2014**, *19*, 74–78. [CrossRef]
48. Rosenzweig, S.; Greeson, J.M.; Reibel, D.K.; Green, J.S.; Jasser, S.A.; Beasley, D. Mindfulness-based stress reduction for chronic pain conditions: Variation in treatment outcomes and role of home meditation practice. *J. Psychosom. Res.* **2010**, *68*, 29–36. [CrossRef] [PubMed]
49. Chiesa, A.; Serretti, A. Mindfulness-based interventions for chronic pain: A systematic review of the evidence. *J. Altern. Complement. Med.* **2011**, *17*, 83–93. [CrossRef] [PubMed]
50. Hesse, T.; Holmes, L.G.; Kennedy-Overfelt, V.; Kerr, L.M.; Giles, L.L. Mindfulness-Based Intervention for Adolescents with Recurrent Headaches: A Pilot Feasibility Study. *Evid.-Based Complement. Altern. Med.* **2015**, *2015*, 1–9. [CrossRef] [PubMed]

51. Jastrowski, K.E.; Salamon, K.S.; Hainsworth, K.R.; Anderson Khan, K.J.; Ladwig, R.J.; Davies, W.H.; Weisman, S.J. A randomized, controlled pilot study of mindfulness-based stress reduction for pediatric chronic pain. *Altern. Ther. Health Med.* **2013**, *19*, 8–14.

52. Ruskin, D.; Ahola Kohut, S.; Stinson, J. The development of a mindfulness-based stress reduction group for adolescents with chronic pain. *J. Pain Manag.* **2015**, *7*, 301–312.

53. Gauntlett-Gilbert, J.; Connell, H.; Clinch, J.; McCracken, L.M. Acceptance and values-based treatment of adolescents with chronic pain: Outcomes and their relationship to acceptance. *J. Pediatr. Psychol.* **2013**, *38*, 72–81. [CrossRef] [PubMed]

54. Martin, S.; Wolters, P.L.; Toledo-Tamula, M.A.; Schmitt, S.N.; Baldwin, A.; Starosta, A.; Gillespie, A.; Widemann, B. Acceptance and commitment therapy in youth with neurofibromatosis type 1 (NF1) and chronic pain and their parents: A pilot study of feasibility and preliminary efficacy. *Am. J. Med. Genet. A* **2016**, *170*, 1462–1470. [CrossRef] [PubMed]

55. Elkins, G.R.; Barabasz, A.F.; Council, J.R.; Spiegel, D. Advancing Research and Practice: The Revised APA Division 30 Definition of Hypnosis. *Am. J. Clin. Hypn.* **2015**, *57*, 378–385. [CrossRef] [PubMed]

56. Weitzenhoffer, A.M. *The Practice of Hypnotism*, 2nd ed.; John Wiley & Sons: New York, NY, USA, 1989.

57. Derbyshire, S.W.; Whalley, M.G.; Oakley, D.A. Fibromyalgia pain and its modulation by hypnotic and non-hypnotic suggestion: An fMRI analysis. *Eur. J. Pain* **2009**, *13*, 542–550. [CrossRef] [PubMed]

58. Tomé-Pires, C.; Miró, J. Hypnosis for the management of chronic and cancer procedure-related pain in children. *Int. J. Clin. Exp. Hypn.* **2012**, *60*, 432–457. [CrossRef] [PubMed]

59. Rutten, J.M.; Reitsma, J.B.; Vlieger, A.M.; Benninga, M.A. Gut-directed hypnotherapy for functional abdominal pain or irritable bowel syndrome in children: A systematic review. *Arch. Dis. Child.* **2013**, *98*, 252–257. [CrossRef] [PubMed]

60. Jensen, M.P.; Patterson, D.R. Hypnotic approaches for chronic pain management: Clinical implications of recent research findings. *Am. Psychol.* **2014**, *69*, 167–177. [CrossRef] [PubMed]

61. Hawkins, R.M. A systematic meta-review of hypnosis as an empirically supported treatment for pain. *Pain Rev.* **2001**, *8*, 47–73. [CrossRef]

62. Galili, O.; Shaoul, R.; Mogilner, J. Treatment of chronic recurrent abdominal pain: Laparoscopy or hypnosis? *J. Laparoendosc. Adv. Surg. Tech. A* **2009**, *19*, 93–96. [CrossRef] [PubMed]

63. Kohen, D.P.; Zajac, R. Self-Hypnosis Training for Headaches in Children and Adolescents. *J. Pediatr.* **2007**, *150*, 635–639. [CrossRef] [PubMed]

64. Anbar, R.D.; Zoughbi, G.G. Relationship of headache-associated stressors and hypnosis therapy outcome in children: A retrospective chart review. *Am. J. Clin. Hypn.* **2008**, *50*, 335–341. [CrossRef] [PubMed]

65. Zeltzer, L.K.; Tsao, J.C.; Stelling, C.; Powers, M.; Levy, S.; Waterhouse, M. A Phase I Study on the Feasibility and Acceptability of an Acupuncture/Hypnosis Intervention for Chronic Pediatric Pain. *J. Pain Symptom Manag.* **2002**, *24*, 437–446. [CrossRef]

66. Van Tilburg, M.A.; Chitkara, D.K.; Palsson, O.S.; Turner, M.; Blois-Martin, N.; Ulshen, M.; Whitehead, W.E. Audio-recorded guided imagery treatment reduces functional abdominal pain in children: A pilot study. *Pediatrics* **2009**, *124*, e890–e897. [CrossRef] [PubMed]

67. Vlieger, A.M.; Menko-Frankenhuis, C.; Wolfkamp, S.C.; Tromp, E.; Benninga, M.A. Hypnotherapy for Children With Functional Abdominal Pain or Irritable Bowel Syndrome: A Randomized Controlled Trial. *Gastroenterology* **2007**, *133*, 1430–1436. [CrossRef] [PubMed]

68. Vlieger, A.M.; Rutten, J.M.; Govers, A.M.; Frankenhuis, C.; Benninga, M.A. Long-term follow-up of gut-directed hypnotherapy vs. standard care in children with functional abdominal pain or irritable bowel syndrome. *Am. J. Gastroenterol.* **2012**, *107*, 627–631. [CrossRef] [PubMed]

69. Weydert, J.A.; Shapiro, D.E.; Acra, S.A.; Monheim, C.J.; Chambers, A.S.; Ball, T.M. Evaluation of guided imagery as treatment for recurrent abdominal pain in children: A randomized controlled trial. *BMC Pediatr.* **2006**, *6*, 29. [CrossRef] [PubMed]

70. Olness, K.; MacDonald, J.T.; Uden, D.L. Comparison of self-hypnosis and propranolol in the treatment of juvenile classic migraine. *Pediatrics* **1987**, *79*, 593–597. [PubMed]

71. Chambless, D.L.; Baker, M.J.; Baucom, D.H.; Beutler, L.E.; Calhoun, K.S.; Crits-christoph, P.; Daiuto, A.; Derubeis, R.; Detweiler, J.; Haaga, D.A.F.; et al. Update on Empirically Validated Therapies, II. *Clin. Psychol.* **1998**, *51*, 3–16.

72. Tomé-Pires, C.; Solé, E.; Racine, M.; de la Vega, R.; Castarlenas, E.; Jensen, M.; Miró, J. Use of hypnotic techniques in children and adolescents with chronic pain: Do age of patients, and years of practice and theoretical orientation of clinicians matter? *Int. J. Clin. Exp. Hypn.* **2016**, *64*, 1–16. [CrossRef] [PubMed]

73. Lang, E.V.; Benotsch, E.G.; Fick, L.J.; Lutgendorf, S.; Berbaum, M.L.; Berbaum, K.S.; Logan, H.; Spiegel, D. Adjunctive non-pharmacological analgesia for invasive medical procedures: A randomised trial. *Lancet (Lond. Engl.)* **2000**, *355*, 1486–1490. [CrossRef]

74. Jensen, M.P. *Hypnosis for Chronic Pain Management: Therapist Guide;* Oxford University Press: Oxford, UK, 2011.

75. Jensen, M.P.; Patterson, D.R. Hypnotic approaches for chronic pain management: Clinical implications of recent research findings. *Am. Psychol.* **2014**, *69*, 167–177. [CrossRef] [PubMed]

76. Richardson, J.; Smith, J.E.; McCall, G.; Pilkington, K. Hypnosis for procedure-related pain and distress in pediatric cancer patients: A systematic review of effectiveness and methodology related to hypnosis interventions. *J. Pain Symptom Manag.* **2006**, *31*, 70–84. [CrossRef] [PubMed]

77. Jensen, M.P.; Adachi, T.; Tomé-Pires, C.; Lee, J.; Osman, Z.J.; Miró, J. Mechanisms of hypnosis: Toward the development of a biopsychosocial model. *Int. J. Clin. Exp. Hypn.* **2015**, *63*, 34–75. [CrossRef] [PubMed]

78. McGrath, P.J.; Walco, G.A.; Turk, D.C.; Dworkin, R.H.; Brown, M.T.; Davidson, K.; Eccleston, C.; Finley, G.A.; Goldschneider, K.; Haverkos, L.; et al. Core Outcome Domains and Measures for Pediatric Acute and Chronic/Recurrent Pain Clinical Trials: PedIMMPACT Recommendations. *J. Pain* **2008**, *9*, 771–783. [CrossRef] [PubMed]

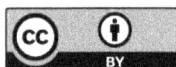

Review

Specialized Rehabilitation Programs for Children and Adolescents with Severe Disabling Chronic Pain: Indications, Treatment and Outcomes

Lorin Stahlschmidt [1,2], Boris Zernikow [1,2] and Julia Wager [1,2,]*

[1] German Paediatric Pain Centre, Children's and Adolescents' Hospital, 45711 Datteln, Germany
[2] Department of Children's Pain Therapy and Paediatric Palliative Care, Faculty of Health,
     School of Medicine, Witten/Herdecke University, 58448 Witten, Germany;
     l.stahlschmidt@deutsches-kinderschmerzzentrum.de (L.S.); b.zernikow@kinderklinik-datteln.de (B.Z.)
*   Correspondence: j.wager@deutsches-kinderschmerzzentrum.de; Tel.: +49-2363-975-184

Academic Editor: Carl L. von Baeyer
Received: 25 October 2016; Accepted: 10 November 2016; Published: 21 November 2016

Abstract: Children and adolescents with highly disabling chronic pain of high intensity and frequency are admitted to specialized pain rehabilitation programs. Some barriers to obtaining this specialized care include a lack of availability of treatment centers, a perceived social stigma and individual barriers such as socioeconomic status. Specialized rehabilitation programs for severe disabling chronic pain worldwide have similarities regarding admission criteria, structure and therapeutic orientation. They differ, however, regarding their exclusion criteria and program descriptions. The short- and long-term effectiveness of some rehabilitation programs is well documented. All countries should promote the establishment of future pediatric pain centers to improve the health care of children and adolescents suffering from severe chronic pain. Standardized reporting guidelines should be developed to describe treatments and outcomes to enable comparability across treatment centers.

Keywords: chronic pain; indication; rehabilitation programs; specialized pain treatment; pediatric; effectiveness

1. Introduction

Approximately 3% to 5% of children and adolescents experience strong negative consequences of chronic pain [1]. They miss a significant amount of school and experience a decline in their grades, a considerable reduction in their quality of life and psychological distress [1–5]. The long-term prognosis of these children and adolescents is poor. Without effective treatment, their chronic pain is likely to continue into adulthood [6–8]. This process of chronification can potentially be interrupted with specialized pain treatments. However, not all children and adolescents seek treatment when they suffer recurrent pain [9,10]. One important and very robust predictor of health care utilization is high pain-related disability [1,10–12]. Additional factors associated with health care utilization include pain characteristics, such as high pain frequency or high pain intensity [1,10–12].

In many health care systems, the first point of contact is typically primary care, with subsequent referrals to secondary or tertiary care [13,14]. However, some health care systems, e.g., those in the USA, do not follow this structured approach; in these types of settings, patients may self-refer and enter the system at any level [13]. Some of the children and adolescents who visit a primary care physician for recurrent or constant functional pain are referred to specialized pain treatment centers, while many patients are (mistakenly) referred to other specialists such as rheumatologists, neurologists, gastroenterologists or orthopedic surgeons [11,15–17]. Before presenting to specialized pediatric pain treatment centers, patients undergo a substantial number of medical visits and pain-related hospital stays [2,11,17,18]. Furthermore, other barriers to accessing specialized pain care exist, such as availability of care [19–21] and socioeconomic status [19,20]. A lack of understanding in society and among friends, family or even primary care physicians due to the invisible nature of pain may also present a barrier to specialized care [22]. In addition, the perceived stigma associated with psychological therapy can prevent patients from seeking specialized care with a psychological focus [22,23], especially if the patients believe that their problem is a physical one [23]. Pain location can represent a barrier to accessing specialized care as well, as not all pediatric pain programs treat all types of pain.

Specialized pain care provides treatment options with different levels of intensity. For patients with a moderate level of functional and emotional impairment, outpatient chronic pain treatment with limited intensity may be sufficient [24–27]. For severely disabled children and adolescents with chronic pain, an intensive specialized rehabilitation program is indicated. Figure 1 displays the usual course of health care utilization due to chronic pain.

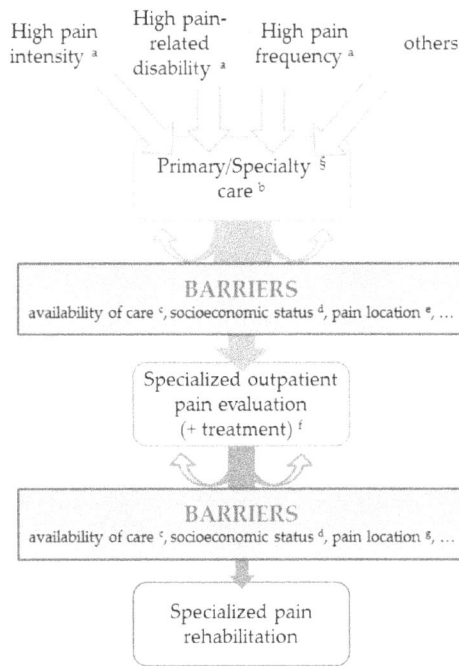

Figure 1. Usual course of health care utilization due to chronic pain. § e.g., rheumatologists, neurologists, gastroenterologists, orthopedic surgeon. [a] e.g., [1,10–12]; [b] e.g., [11,15–17]; [c] e.g., [19–21]; [d] e.g., [19,20]; [e] e.g., [26]; [f] e.g., [25–27]; [g] e.g., [28].

Currently, there are specialized pediatric pain centers in many countries around the world. According to the International Association for the Study of Pain [29], specialized pain clinics are characterized by the concurrent efforts of an interdisciplinary clinical team that is able to treat any type of pain disorder. The patient-centered treatment provided in these clinics is based on the best available evidence, and these clinics implement quality improvement efforts, for example, by routinely monitoring patient characteristics and outcomes (see [30] for an example of a successful implementation of such methods). Specialized pain centers also engage in research and academic teaching. According to the bio-psycho-social model of chronic pain, chronic pain treatment should always include medical, psychological and social treatment methods. There are pain clinics that specialize in only one pain disorder but fulfill all of the other criteria defined by the IASP. The American Pain Society additionally defined parent inclusion and school reintegration as particular requirements of specialized pediatric pain treatment [31]. The overall goal of pediatric chronic pain treatment is to assume an active self-management approach in coping with pain [32,33] and to enable age-appropriate daily activities despite pain [33–35].

In this review, we focus on specialized pain rehabilitation programs in particular and do not address specialized outpatient treatment. A recent systematic review showed strong positive results regarding the short-term effectiveness of specialized pain rehabilitation programs [36]. Here, we aim to provide a comprehensive overview of existing pain rehabilitation programs, their structure and their short- and long-term effectiveness. First, we present the criteria that suggest that intensive pain treatment is indicated. Second, we take an international perspective on the structure and the components of different pain rehabilitation programs worldwide to note their differences and similarities. Third, we provide a summary of the results regarding short- and long-term outcomes of pain rehabilitation programs. With the results presented in this review, we aim to promote the development of further specialized pain programs, to place single programs within a larger context and to advance global networking.

2. Method

We conducted a literature search based on a recent systematic review of intensive interdisciplinary pain treatment [36] initiated by our research group. This published systematic review integrated results from ten studies and had a strong focus on the outcomes of chronic pain treatment. In this review, we concentrated more on providing a comprehensive description of existing specialized rehabilitation programs and therefore further included referenced studies that were excluded from the systematic review, for example due to overlapping samples [25,37–42]. Additionally, we identified five more recent studies on this topic through a nonsystematic search in Medical Literature Analysis and Retrieval System Online (MEDLINE) and by conducting a manual search [16,28,34,43–45]. Overall, information about nine different rehabilitation programs from the USA, the UK, Australia and Germany was available. We extracted information from the included studies concerning the admission criteria of the rehabilitation programs and their structure, therapeutic orientation and treatment components. We further extracted information regarding outcomes according to the core outcome domains listed in the Pediatric Initiative on Methods, Measurement, and Pain Assessment in Clinical Trials (PedIMMPACT) recommendations [46].

3. Results

3.1. Indications for Specialized Rehabilitation Programs

The criteria for admission to specialized rehabilitation centers vary slightly between the rehabilitation programs worldwide. The inclusion criteria showed considerable similarities. Most programs agree that the most important criteria is for the pain to be persistent with a high intensity for at least three months [33,35,47] and for children and adolescents to be severely impaired by the pain in daily activities such as school attendance, sports or leisure activities [32,33,35,47–49]. As family environment may be an important factor in the development or maintenance of pain, patients' and their parents' motivation for and compliance with treatments are important requirements [35,47–49]. In addition, failure of prior outpatient treatment is often mentioned as a necessary admission criterion [32,47,49]. This factor is important for avoiding overtreatment. The exclusion criteria vary widely between the rehabilitation programs. Patients with specific psychiatric needs requiring further treatment are often excluded [32,35,49], as are patients requiring further medical assessments [33,35] and patients with a medical pathology/underlying disease [32,48] or a malignant disease [47,48]. If other effective medical options are available, this can also be an exclusion criteria [48]. Table 1 provides an overview of the criteria for the different rehabilitation programs introduced in the literature.

Table 1. Admission criteria for specialized rehabilitation programs.

Criteria	Specialized Rehabilitation Programs								
Inclusion	AUS	UK	UK	GER	USA	USA	USA	USA	USA
	1	2	3	4	5	6	7	8	9
Pain for more than 3 months		x		x			x		
High pain-related disability		x	x	x	x	x	x		
Patient and parent motivation		x	x	x			x		
Failure of outpatient treatment				x	x	x			
Exclusion	1	2	3	4	5	6	7	8	9
Psychiatric needs		x				x	x		
Further assessment required		x					x		
Medical pathology/underlying disease			x			x			
Active malignant disease			x	x					
Effective medical options			x						

Only criteria explicitly reported in the literature are included for each rehabilitation program, i.e., a missing "x" does not mean that this criterion does not apply to this rehabilitation program, but that it is not reported in the literature; 1: Melbourne, AUS [50]; 2: Bath, UK [35]; 3: Bath, UK [48]; 4: Datteln, GER [41,45,47]; 5: Boston, MA, USA [32,51]; 6: Baltimore, MD, USA [49]; 7: Rochester, MN, USA [33]; 8: Cleveland, OH, USA [34,43]; 9: Philadelphia, PA, USA [28].

3.2. Treatment Components of Specialized Rehabilitation Programs

Specialized rehabilitation includes inpatient chronic pain treatment and intensive day-hospital approaches [36]. Most of these programs treat all types of pain disorders, although some specialize only in musculoskeletal pain [28,32]. Similar to the admission criteria described above, the rehabilitation programs vary slightly around the world; however, they agree on a number of core contents and structures. These programs mainly include operant and cognitive behavioral techniques, as well as some acceptance and commitment therapy-based approaches, and they consist of a number of different medical, psychological and social modules delivered by interdisciplinary teams [28,32–35,41,48–50]. The psychotherapy contents are mainly delivered in one-on-one sessions, but they are also delivered in group or family sessions [28,32–34,41]. Treatment typically lasts three weeks, with approximately eight hours of treatment per day, whether in inpatient or day-hospital treatment settings [32–34,41,48].

One important rehabilitation module is chronic pain education [16,35,41,49], i.e., informing patients about the bio-psycho-social model of chronic pain, the possible etiological causes and factors associated with the maintenance of pain, the consequences of inactivity and the benefit of activity despite pain. Regarding pain management, various strategies are taught, such as relaxation techniques [32–34,41,49,50], attention defocusing techniques [33,41,49], imagery [32,41,43,49], active daily structures [28,32–35,41,48–50], stress management [32,33,45,49] and problem-solving activities [32,43,49]. Physical therapy [28,32–35,41,48–50], biofeedback [32,33,45,49] and therapy for psychological comorbidities [33,41] such as depression or anxiety are also included in rehabilitation. In family sessions, parents actively participate in the treatment [28,32–35,41,48,49]; they are informed about how to support their children or adolescents in active pain management and how to avoid reinforcing inappropriate pain behavior. In addition, familial stress factors can be identified and worked on with the parents. Some programs also incorporate parent-only sessions [28,33,35,48]. Medical interventions include providing medical examinations [32,34,41,49] and tapering off or changing medications [28,33,41,49,50] if necessary and appropriate. Further treatment components incorporated by some of the programs address occupational therapy [28,32–35,41,49], recreational therapy [16,33,49], acupuncture/acupressure [34,49,50], diet [33,34], sleep hygiene [33,44,49], music therapy [28,41,43] and art therapy [16,28,41]. In some programs, the patients also attend some type of hospital school program [32,34,47]. To consolidate treatment strategies, the treatment plans incorporate therapeutic homework and practice [32,35,47]. Relapse prevention is an important part of therapy [32,34,41,49]. This stage is composed of stress tests, reintegration into the patient's home and school routine, and arrangement of outpatient psychotherapy.

Some of the rehabilitation programs offer follow-up care, in which the patient's status and goal attainment are evaluated and treatment is resumed if necessary [24,49,51]. Table 2 provides an overview of the different rehabilitation programs and their specific components. Only components reported by two or more programs in the literature are included.

Table 2. Structural and therapeutic components of the specialized rehabilitation programs.

Components	Specialized Rehabilitation Programs								
	AUS	UK	UK	GER	USA	USA	USA	USA	USA
Structure	1	2	3	4	5	6	7	8	9
Inpatient	x			x		x		x	x
Day-hospital		x	x		x		x	x	x
Interdisciplinary team	x	x	x	x	x	x	x	x	x
Psychotherapy Approach	1	2	3	4	5	6	7	8	9
Operant and cognitive behavioral therapy	x	x	x	x	x	x	x	x	x
Acceptance and commitment therapy			x	x	x				
Medical Interventions	1	2	3	4	5	6	7	8	9
Medication	x			x		x	x		x
Medical examination				x	x	x		x	
Physical therapy	x	x	x	x	x	x	x	x	x
Biofeedback				x	x	x	x		
Psychological Interventions	1	2	3	4	5	6	7	8	9
Education		x		x		x		x	
Relaxation techniques	x			x	x	x	x	x	
Attention defocusing				x		x	x		
Imagery				x	x	x		x	
Active daily structure	x	x	x	x	x	x	x	x	x
Stress management				x	x	x	x		
Problem-solving					x	x		x	
Addressing psychological comorbidities				x			x		
Social Interventions	1	2	3	4	5	6	7	8	9
Family sessions		x	x	x	x	x	x	x	x
Parent-only sessions		x	x		x		x		x
School reintegration	x			x	x	x		x	
Patient group sessions				x	x		x	x	x
Other	1	2	3	4	5	6	7	8	9
Occupational therapy		x		x	x	x	x	x	x
Recreational therapy						x	x	x	
Hospital school program				x	x			x	
Acupressure/acupuncture	x					x		x	
Diet							x	x	
Sleep hygiene					x	x	x		
Music therapy				x				x	x
Art therapy				x				x	x
Therapeutic homework and practicing			x	x	x				
Relapse prevention				x	x	x		x	
Follow-up care				x	x	x			

Only components explicitly reported in the literature for two or more rehabilitation programs are included in this table, i.e., a missing "x" does not mean that this component is not included in this rehabilitation program, but that it is not reported in the literature; 1: Melbourne, AUS [50]; 2: Bath, UK [35]; 3: Bath, UK [48]; 4: Datteln, GER [41,45,47]; 5: Boston, MA, USA [32,44,51]; 6: Baltimore, MD, USA [49]; 7: Rochester, MN, USA [33]; 8: Cleveland, OH, USA [16,34,43]; 9: Philadelphia, PA, USA [28].

3.3. Outcomes of Specialized Rehabilitation Programs

A recent systematic review of rehabilitation programs integrated the results of ten studies regarding the short-term effectiveness two to six months after treatment [36]. We complement these results with more recent studies and with long-term outcomes. The results are presented according to the core outcome domains from the PedIMMPACT recommendations [46].

- **Pain intensity.** The systematic review showed large short-term reductions in pain intensity [36]. More recent studies confirm these short-term reductions in pain intensity [28,34,43]. Several studies also provide evidence for long-term reductions (12 to 24–42 months after treatment) of pain intensity [16,28,34,47,52,53].
- **Satisfaction with treatment, symptoms and adverse events.** None of the studies investigated satisfaction with treatment or treatment-emergent symptoms and adverse events as outcome measures.
- **Physical functioning.** There was a large effect for the reduction of pain-related disability described in the systematic review [36]. Significant short-term effects were also found in more recent studies [28,43]. Studies also reported positive long-term effects (12 months after treatment) of rehabilitation programs on pain-related disability [28,47,52,53].
- **Emotional functioning.** The systematic review revealed a moderate effect for reduction in general anxiety, a large effect for reduction in pain-specific fear and a small to moderate effect for the reduction in depressive symptoms [36]. Benore et al. [43] replicated the short-term effects of specialized rehabilitation programs on general anxiety and on pain-specific anxiety. Sherry et al. [28] found positive short-term effects on emotional functioning that remained stable up to one year after treatment. Two more studies reported significant long-term reductions (12 months after treatment) in anxiety and depression [52,53].
- **Role functioning.** According to the systematic review, school attendance as the recommended measure of role functioning [46] was significantly improved by intensive treatment with moderate to large effect sizes [36]. Recent studies replicated these short-term effects [28,34,43]. Several studies further supported the long-term effectiveness (12 to 24–42 months after treatment) of intensive pain treatment on reducing school absence [28,34,47,52,53].
- **Sleep.** Only three studies used sleep as an outcome measure. All reported improvements in sleep disturbances [44,49,50]. One study further found stable short-term improvements in sleep onset delay, sleep duration, night waking and daytime sleepiness and an overall reduction in the use of sleep medication [44]. However, these results were based on self-report and not on validated objective measures such as actigraphy or sleep recording [46].
- **Economic factors.** A small number of studies investigated the economic effects of intensive pain treatment in terms of health care utilization and indirect costs. Significant reductions were found for health care utilization, in both the short and long term (12 to 24–42 month after treatment) [16,34,48,52]. Indirect costs, such as lost work days [16,34,52] and parental subjective financial burden [52], also showed significant reductions. Evans et al. [16] concluded that chronic pain rehabilitation is a cost-effective treatment for pediatric chronic pain.
- Regarding **moderators of treatment outcome**, the results indicated that sex [38,47], fear of pain [51], pretreatment functional impairment [53], psychological comorbidities [43,53], sleep habits [44] and patients' readiness to self-manage pain [37] were associated with treatment outcomes. Poorer treatment outcomes were associated with female sex [38,47], high levels of fear of pain [51], low levels of school absence before treatment [53] and high levels of anxiety and depression [53]. Furthermore, decreases in anxiety [43], increases in readiness to self-manage pain [37] and improvements in sleep habits, such as sleep duration, night-waking or sleep onset, showed associations with better treatment outcomes [44].

4. Discussion

In this review, we aimed to provide a summary of the published specialized rehabilitation programs around the world regarding their admission criteria, treatment components and outcomes. Specialized rehabilitation programs for chronic pain in children and adolescents seem to have certain similarities around the world and have proven to be effective in treating disabling chronic pain disorders. There are many similarities regarding the admission criteria for specialized rehabilitation programs, of which pain-related disability and patient and parent motivation seem to be the most important. The different programs around the world also showed substantial similarities in structure, therapeutic orientation and individual components. All programs consist of an interdisciplinary team and include operant and cognitive-behavioral therapy, physical therapy and an active daily structure. Most of the programs address medications, use relaxation techniques and occupation therapy and have family sessions as an integral component of the treatment. The results for most of the outcome domains are comparable across all studies and indicate high short- and long-term effectiveness of specialized rehabilitation programs in pain intensity and physical, school and emotional functioning. There are, however, outcome domains, such as sleep and economic factors, for which the conclusions are rather preliminary. None of the studies investigated satisfaction with treatment or symptoms and adverse events.

4.1. Indications for Specialized Rehabilitation Programs

Three rehabilitation programs did not provide admission criteria. The other rehabilitation programs differed mainly in their exclusion criteria. There are large differences regarding medical issues, for example, whether patients with an underlying or active malignant disease are excluded. Furthermore, some programs include children and adolescents with psychiatric comorbidities, while others do not. This difference accounts for certain differences in treatment components. Programs that include children and adolescents with comorbidities need to be more intensive, especially concerning psychological interventions and the need to treat these comorbidities. These different exclusion criteria may further impede the comparability of the rehabilitation program outcomes, since psychological comorbidities are a risk factor for treatment failure [53]. Programs that exclude patients with comorbidities may achieve larger effects in pain-related outcome domains. Therefore, it is important that all specialized rehabilitation programs report their admission criteria to ensure that the outcomes can be interpreted accordingly.

4.2. Treatment Components of Specialized Rehabilitation Programs

Despite the considerable similarities between the program components, it is difficult to compare the rehabilitation programs due to the way they are described in the literature. Some programs are described in abundant detail, while others lack basic information. The descriptions of many programs are not comprehensive. Therefore, the overview of structural and therapeutic components in this review may not be considered absolute, and more similarities or even further components could arise from a more detailed and standardized description of the programs. The medical components, for example, may be considered obvious by most authors, which may be one reason why not all programs reported ongoing medical examinations. In addition, physicians are responsible for a large part of the education process to reduce the somatic fixation of the patients, and although this was not reported, it is likely an important module of most rehabilitation programs. A standardized method of reporting treatments and treatment components is desirable for investigating the similarities and differences between programs. We recommend including a detailed description in at least one publication per rehabilitation program of the characteristics outlined in Table 2, i.e., the structure, psychotherapy approach and the medical, psychological, social and other interventions. For the medical, psychological, social and other interventions, components that are essential and usually implemented should be reported.

In addition to the differences in the components, differences between the programs could arise from the interdisciplinary team (e.g., composition, professional qualifications) or from the standardization of therapy. This information is essential and needs to be reported because a description of the components alone may not capture the core aspects of treatment. Although the rehabilitation programs can be disassembled into separate components, these components are not meant to be simply checked off to create an effective treatment. The effectiveness may instead arise from non-linear effects resulting from the strong interactions within the interdisciplinary team and from interactions between the team, the parents and the patients. These mechanisms need to be studied to precisely understand the drivers of program effectiveness to improve and strengthen existing pain centers and establish new ones.

4.3. Outcomes of Specialized Rehabilitation Programs

Though the short-term effectiveness of specialized rehabilitation programs has largely been demonstrated, reliable evidence regarding the long-term effectiveness over several years is lacking. One problem that arises in longitudinal clinical studies of complex interventions involves the inclusion of an appropriate control group. It is not ethically acceptable to deny severely disabled pediatric patients an effective treatment for such a long time or to provide a treatment that is clearly less effective. Randomized controlled trials (RCTs) have been conducted on psychological interventions, i.e., a subset of components of the rehabilitation programs [54,55], and one RCT has even been conducted on an entire program using a waiting-list control design [52]. However, this design only allows for short-term conclusions regarding efficacy. These RCTs have certainly contributed to good progress in the field, but there remains a need for more and stronger evidence, especially concerning long-term outcomes. One Dutch study conducted a ten-year follow-up of young adults who had received inpatient rehabilitation for chronic pain or fatigue at one of five rehabilitation centers and found that the majority of these former pediatric patients had a paid job and a moderate to good health-related quality of life [56]. However, their quality of life was somewhat lower than that of the normal population. Further long-term studies similar to the Dutch analysis are needed. Additionally, reliable evidence regarding the moderators of treatment is also needed. The existing results should be interpreted with caution due to the comparatively small sample sizes. Hirschfeld et al. [12] showed, that in regression analyses, reliable results can only be achieved with samples of several hundred patients. Such large samples require an extremely long recruitment period or a multicenter data collection process. Collaborative multicenter data collection for complex data analyses and the comparability of effectiveness of different rehabilitation programs are important areas for future research. Multicenter studies also require that comparable treatments be used at each center. Currently, this cannot be assumed, despite a certain overlap across treatment sites.

Regarding the comparability of effectiveness, an important issue concerns the outcome measures used to indicate effectiveness. In 2008, McGrath et al. defined the PedIMMPACT recommendations for the core outcome domains and measures for pediatric acute and chronic/recurrent pain clinical trials [46]. The aim of these recommendations was to standardize the outcome domains and measures assessed in studies to facilitate their comparability and interpretation. However, not all studies adhere to these recommendations. There are, for example, huge differences in assessing pain intensity in the studies mentioned above. Although it is one of the core outcome domains, some studies do not report pain intensity [25,49]. Furthermore, some studies report pain intensity in the present moment [28,32,33], while others report pain intensity in the last 24 h [34], the last seven days [35,47,48], or the last four weeks [24]. Thus, the time period varies greatly between studies. For chronic pain, short time periods are not appropriate because chronic pain is not necessarily persistent or present each day. Thus, the time period should be long enough to also account for pediatric migraine patients, who sometimes experience attacks only once a month. Using a measure of pain intensity of less than one month may lead to distorted results. In addition, the different time periods impede the comparability of study outcomes and thereby of the effectiveness of different rehabilitation programs. The different studies also vary greatly in terms of how many outcome domains they cover. Furthermore, there are outcome domains that have not yet been investigated, despite being recommended as core outcome domains [46], such as satisfaction with treatment and symptoms and adverse events. However, to date, no validated measures exist for these domains.

Another important issue in effectiveness studies of chronic pain patients concerns the definition of what is considered effective. Is a treatment effective if the patients show statistically significant or clinically relevant changes or if the patients return to a normal functional level after treatment? In other words, what is more important: the degree of change or the status of the patient after treatment? Most studies to date have focused on the change from pre- to post-treatment or to follow-up, but what use is a significant or clinically relevant change when the patient is still severely impaired and far from normal? We may need to rethink and redefine the criteria that have to be fulfilled for the treatment to be considered effective or a success.

4.4. Recommendations for Future Research and Patient Care

Several areas of research need to be emphasized according to the results of this review. First, we need to devote more effort into standardizing the reporting of rehabilitation programs and outcomes to enable global comparisons of programs and their effectiveness. This review provides a set of important criteria for reporting. Furthermore, efforts should be made to report outcomes according to the PedIMMPACT recommendations in order to increase comparability. This also requires the development of valid outcome measures for different languages. Reporting a wide range of outcomes over a long follow-up gives proper consideration to the complexity of chronic pain, e.g., in some patients, certain pain symptoms may remain while pain-related disability may be substantially reduced in the long term. Additionally, we need further progress regarding long-term effectiveness, moderators of treatment outcome and mechanisms of change. Therefore, collaborative multicenter data collection may play an important role in advancing research in this field and in improving worldwide networking. Improved collaborations between pain centers and the establishment of new centers are similarly important to overcome barriers to health care utilization. The limited availability of pediatric pain clinics and centers bears the risk of additional barriers to health care. Thus, nationwide availability of appropriate health care for children and adolescents with different chronic pain conditions is one, if not the most important, goal for all countries to address pediatric chronic pain. Recently developed internet-delivered or phone-based treatment approaches may be an alternative for patients with long travel distances [57,58]. However, these programs only consist of a few of the components of specialized rehabilitation programs such as cognitive-behavioral techniques and do not replace the complexity of intensive rehabilitation programs. Thus, the establishment of new pain centers remains essential. However, training primary care providers or nurses in psychoeducation or coping skills to initiate some form of treatment before referral to specialized rehabilitation may be a good possibility to bridge the long waiting times for treatment. Comparable evaluation research is needed for quality assurance and for further development of treatment options.

4.5. Limitations

The results of this review should be interpreted in light of the following limitations. This review was restricted to descriptions of the structure and outcomes of specialized pain treatment programs that have been published, i.e., the programs of specialized pain centers. However, a considerable number of specialized pain clinics do not necessarily engage in research and thus do not conduct or publish studies on their programs. There may be differences in the structure or outcomes between published and unpublished specialized treatment programs. In addition, we did not conduct a systematic literature search. However, we assume that the included articles are nearly exhaustive because our review is based on a systematic review [36].

Author Contributions: Lorin Stahlschmidt contributed to the writing and editing of the manuscript. Boris Zernikow contributed to the writing and editing of the manuscript. Julia Wager contributed to the writing and editing of the manuscript.

Conflicts of Interest: The authors declare no conflict of interest.

References

1. Huguet, A.; Miro, J. The severity of chronic paediatric pain: An epidemiological study. *J. Pain* **2008**, *9*, 226–236. [CrossRef] [PubMed]
2. Zernikow, B.; Wager, J.; Hechler, T.; Hasan, C.; Rohr, U.; Dobe, M.; Meyer, A.; Hübner-Möhler, B.; Wamsler, C.; Blankenburg, M. Characteristics of highly impaired children with severe chronic pain: A 5-year retrospective study on 2249 pediatric pain patients. *BMC Pediatr.* **2012**, *12*, 54. [CrossRef] [PubMed]
3. Logan, D.E.; Simsons, L.E.; Stein, M.J.; Chastain, L. School impairment in adolescents with chronic pain. *J. Pain* **2008**, *9*, 407–416. [CrossRef] [PubMed]
4. Wager, J.; Hechler, T.; Darlington, A.S.; Hirschfeld, G.; Vocks, S.; Zernikow, B. Classifying the severity of paediatric chronic pain—An application of the chronic pain grading. *Eur. J. Pain* **2013**, *17*, 1393–1402. [CrossRef] [PubMed]
5. Voerman, J.S.; de Klerk, C.; Vander Heyden, K.M.; Passchier, J.; Idema, W.; Timman, R.; Jolles, J. Pain is associated with poorer grades, reduced emotional well-being, and attention problems in adolescents. *Clin J. Pain* **2016**. [CrossRef] [PubMed]
6. Brna, P.; Dooley, J.; Gordon, K.; Dewan, T. The prognosis of childhood headache: A 20-year follow-up. *Arch. Pediatr. Adolesc. Med.* **2005**, *159*, 1157–1160. [CrossRef] [PubMed]
7. Hestbaek, L.; Leboeuf-Yde, C.; Kyvik, K.O.; Manniche, C. The course of low back pain from adolescence to adulthood: Eight-year follow-up of 9600 twins. *Spine (Phila Pa 1976)* **2006**, *31*, 468–472. [CrossRef] [PubMed]
8. Walker, L.S.; Dengler-Crish, C.M.; Rippel, S.; Bruehl, S. Functional abdominal pain in childhood and adolescence increases risk for chronic pain in adulthood. *Pain* **2010**, *150*, 568–572. [CrossRef] [PubMed]
9. Ellert, U.; Neuhauser, H.; Roth-Isigkeit, A. [pain in children and adolescents in Germany: The prevalence and usage of medical services. Results of the german health interview and examination survey for children and adolescents (KiGGs)]. *Bundesgesundheitsblatt Gesundheitsforschung Gesundheitsschutz* **2007**, *50*, 711–717. [CrossRef] [PubMed]
10. Perquin, C.W.; Hunfeld, J.A.; Hazebroek-Kampschreur, A.A.; van Suijlekom-Smit, L.W.; Passchier, J.; Koes, B.W.; van der Wouden, J.C. Insights in the use of health care services in chronic benign pain in childhood and adolescence. *Pain* **2001**, *94*, 205–213. [CrossRef]
11. Toliver-Sokol, M.; Murray, C.B.; Wilson, A.C.; Lewandowski, A.; Palermo, T.M. Patterns and predictors of health service utilization in adolescents with pain: Comparison between a community and a clinical pain sample. *J. Pain* **2011**, *12*, 747–755. [CrossRef] [PubMed]
12. Hirschfeld, G.; Wager, J.; Zernikow, B. Physician consultation in young children with recurrent pain—A population-based study. *PeerJ* **2015**, *3*, e916. [CrossRef] [PubMed]
13. Grumbach, K.; Bodenheimer, T. The organization of health care. *JAMA* **1995**, *273*, 160–167. [CrossRef] [PubMed]
14. Mossialos, E.; Wenzl, M.; Osborn, R.; Anderson, C. *International Profiles of Health Care Systems, 2015*; The Commonwealth Fund: New York, NY, USA, 2016.
15. Groenewald, C.B.; Essner, B.S.; Wright, D.; Fesinmeyer, M.D.; Palermo, T.M. The economic costs of chronic pain among a cohort of treatment-seeking adolescents in the united states. *J. Pain* **2014**, *15*, 925–933. [CrossRef] [PubMed]
16. Evans, J.R.; Benore, E.; Banez, G.A. The cost-effectiveness of intensive interdisciplinary pediatric chronic pain rehabilitation. *J. Pediatr. Psychol.* **2016**, *41*, 849–856. [CrossRef] [PubMed]
17. Kaufman, E.L.; Tress, J.; Sherry, D.D. Trends in medicalization of children with amplified musculoskeletal pain syndrome. *Pain Med.* **2016**. [CrossRef] [PubMed]
18. Ho, I.K.; Goldschneider, K.R.; Kashikar-Zuck, S.; Kotagal, U.; Tessman, C.; Jones, B. Healthcare utilization and indirect burden among families of pediatric patients with chronic pain. *J. Musculoskelet. Pain* **2008**, *16*, 155–164. [CrossRef]

19. Ruhe, A.; Wager, J.; Hirschfeld, G.; Zernikow, B. Household income determines access to specialized pediatric chronic pain treatment in Germany. *BMC Health Serv. Res.* **2016**, *16*, 140. [CrossRef] [PubMed]
20. Wager, J.; Ruhe, A.; Hirschfeld, G.; Wamsler, C.; Dobe, M.; Hechler, T.; Zernikow, B. Influence of parental occupation on access to specialised treatment for paediatric chronic pain: A retrospective study. *Schmerz* **2013**, *27*, 305–311. [CrossRef] [PubMed]
21. Peng, P.; Choiniere, M.; Dion, D.; Intrater, H.; LeFort, S.; Lynch, M.; Ong, M.; Rashiq, S.; Tkachuk, G.; Veillette, Y.; et al. Challenges in accessing multidisciplinary pain treatment facilities in Canada. *Can. J. Anaesth.* **2007**, *54*, 985–991. [CrossRef] [PubMed]
22. Stinson, J.; White, M.; Isaac, L.; Campbell, F.; Brown, S.; Ruskin, D.; Gordon, A.; Galonski, M.; Pink, L.; Buckley, N. Understanding the information and service needs of young adults with chronic pain: Perspectives of young adults and their providers. *Clin. J. Pain* **2013**, *29*, 600–612. [CrossRef] [PubMed]
23. Stinson, J.N.; Lalloo, C.; Harris, L.; Isaac, L.; Campbell, F.; Brown, S.; Ruskin, D.; Gordon, A.; Galonski, M.; Pink, L.R. iCanCope with Pain™: User-centred design of a web-and mobile-based self-management program for youth with chronic pain based on identified health care needs. *Pain Res. Manag.* **2014**, *19*, 257–265. [CrossRef] [PubMed]
24. Hechler, T.; Wager, J.; Zernikow, B. Chronic pain treatment in children and adolescents: Less is good, more is sometimes better. *BMC Pediatr.* **2014**, *14*, 262. [CrossRef] [PubMed]
25. Simons, L.E.; Sieberg, C.B.; Pielech, M.; Conroy, C.; Logan, D.E. What does it take? Comparing intensive rehabilitation to outpatient treatment for children with significant pain-related disability. *J. Pediatr. Psychol.* **2013**, *38*, 213–223. [CrossRef] [PubMed]
26. Claar, R.L.; Kaczynski, K.J.; Minster, A.; Donald-Nolan, L.; LeBel, A.A. School functioning and chronic tension headaches in adolescents: Improvement only after multidisciplinary evaluation. *J. Child. Neurol.* **2013**, *28*, 719–724. [CrossRef] [PubMed]
27. Hechler, T.; Martin, A.; Blankenburg, M.; Schroeder, S.; Kosfelder, J.; Hölscher, L.; Denecke, H.; Zernikow, B. Specialized multimodal outpatient treatment for children with chronic pain: Treatment pathways and long-term outcome. *Eur. J. Pain* **2011**, *15*, 976–984. [CrossRef] [PubMed]
28. Sherry, D.D.; Brake, L.; Tress, J.L.; Sherker, J.; Fash, K.; Ferry, K.; Weiss, P.F. The treatment of juvenile fibromyalgia with an intensive physical and psychosocial program. *J. Pediatr.* **2015**, *167*, 731–737. [CrossRef] [PubMed]
29. International Association for the Study of Pain. *Pain Treatment Services*; 2009. Available online: http://www.iasp-pain.org/Education/Content.aspx?ItemNumber=1381 (accessed on 1 August 2016).
30. Lynch-Jordan, A.M.; Kashikar-Zuck, S.; Crosby, L.E.; Lopez, W.L.; Smolyansky, B.H.; Parkins, I.S.; Luzader, C.P.; Hartman, A.; Guilfoyle, S.M.; Powers, S.W. Applying quality improvement methods to implement a measurement system for chronic pain-related disability. *J. Pediatr. Psychol.* **2009**, *35*, 32–41. [CrossRef] [PubMed]
31. American Pain Society—Pediatric Chronic Pain Task Force. *Assessment and Management of Children with Chronic Pain—A Position Statement from the American Pain Society*; 2012.
32. Logan, D.E.; Carpino, E.A.; Chiang, G.; Condon, M.; Firn, E.; Gaughan, V.J.; Hogan, M.; Leslie, D.S.; Olson, K.; Sager, S. A day-hospital approach to treatment of pediatric complex regional pain syndrome: Initial functional outcomes. *Clin. J. Pain* **2012**, *28*, 766–774. [CrossRef] [PubMed]
33. Weiss, K.E.; Hahn, A.; Wallace, D.P.; Biggs, B.; Bruce, B.K.; Harrison, T.E. Acceptance of pain: Associations with depression, catastrophizing, and functional disability among children and adolescents in an interdisciplinary chronic pain rehabilitation program. *J. Pediatr. Psychol.* **2013**, *38*, 756–765. [CrossRef] [PubMed]
34. Banez, G.A.; Frazier, T.W.; Wojtowicz, A.A.; Buchannan, K.; Henry, D.E.; Benore, E. Chronic pain in children and adolescents: 24–42 month outcomes of an inpatient/day hospital interdisciplinary pain rehabilitation program. *J. Pediatr. Rehabil. Med. Inderdiscip. Approach* **2014**, *7*, 197–206.
35. Eccleston, C.; Malleson, P.; Clinch, J.; Connell, H.; Sourbut, C. Chronic pain in adolescents: Evaluation of a programme of interdisciplinary cognitive behaviour therapy. *Arch. Dis. Child.* **2003**, *88*, 881–885. [CrossRef] [PubMed]
36. Hechler, T.; Kanstrup, M.; Holley, A.L.; Simons, L.E.; Wicksell, R.; Hirschfeld, G.; Zernikow, B. Systematic review on intensive interdisciplinary pain treatment of children with chronic pain. *Pediatrics* **2015**, *136*, 115–127. [CrossRef] [PubMed]

37. Logan, D.E.; Conroy, C.; Sieberg, C.B.; Simons, L.E. Changes in willingness to self-manage pain among children and adolescents and their parents enrolled in an intensive interdisciplinary pediatric pain treatment program. *Pain* **2012**, *153*, 1863–1870. [CrossRef] [PubMed]

38. Hechler, T.; Kosfelder, J.; Vocks, S.; Mönninger, T.; Blankenburg, M.; Dobe, M.; Gerlach, A.L.; Denecke, H.; Zernikow, B. Changes in pain-related coping strategies and their importance for treatment outcome following multimodal inpatient treatment: Does sex matter? *J. Pain* **2010**, *11*, 472–483. [CrossRef] [PubMed]

39. Hechler, T.; Dobe, M.; Damschen, U.; Blankenburg, M.; Schroeder, S.; Kosfelder, J.; Zernikow, B. The pain provocation technique for adolescents with chronic pain: Preliminary evidence for its effectiveness. *Pain Med.* **2010**, *11*, 897–910. [CrossRef] [PubMed]

40. Hechler, T.; Dobe, M.; Kosfelder, J.; Damschen, U.; Hübner, B.; Blankenburg, M.; Sauer, C.; Zernikow, B. Effectiveness of a three-week multimodal inpatient pain treatment for adolescents suffering from chronic pain: Statistical and clinical significance. *Clin. J. Pain* **2009**, *25*, 156–166. [CrossRef] [PubMed]

41. Dobe, M.; Damschen, U.; Reiffer-Wiesel, B.; Sauer, C.; Zernikow, B. [Multimodal inpatient pain treatment in children—Results of a three-week program]. *Schmerz* **2006**, *20*, 51–60. [CrossRef] [PubMed]

42. Dobe, M.; Hechler, T.; Behlert, J.; Kosfelder, J. [Pain therapy with children and adolescents severely disabled due to chronic pain—Long-term outcome after inpatient pain therapy]. *Schmerz* **2011**, *25*, 411–422. [CrossRef] [PubMed]

43. Benore, E.; D'Auria, A.; Banez, G.A.; Worley, S.; Tang, A. The influence of anxiety reduction on clinical response to pediatric chronic pain rehabilitation. *Clin. J. Pain* **2015**, *31*, 375–383. [CrossRef] [PubMed]

44. Logan, D.E.; Sieberg, C.B.; Conroy, C.; Smith, K.; Odell, S.; Sethna, N. Changes in sleep habits in adolescents during intensive interdisciplinary pediatric pain rehabilitation. *J. Youth Adolesc.* **2015**, *44*, 543–555. [CrossRef] [PubMed]

45. Dobe, M.; Zernikow, B. *Practical Treatment Options for Chronic Pain in Children and Adolescents: An Interdisciplinary Therapy Manual*; Springer: Berlin/Heidelberg, Germany, 2013; Volume 1, pp. 1–268.

46. McGrath, P.J.; Walco, G.A.; Turk, D.C.; Dworkin, R.H.; Brown, M.T.; Davidson, K.; Eccleston, C.; Finley, A.G.; Goldschneider, K.; Haverkos, L.; et al. Core outcome domains and measures for pediatric acute and chronic/recurrent pain clinical trials: Pedimmpact recommendations. *J. Pain* **2008**, *9*, 771–783. [CrossRef] [PubMed]

47. Hechler, T.; Blankenburg, M.; Dobe, M.; Kosfelder, J.; Hübner, B.; Zernikow, B. Effectiveness of a multimodal inpatient treatment for pediatric chronic pain: A comparison between children and adolescents. *Eur. J. Pain* **2010**, *14*, 97.e1–97.e9. [CrossRef] [PubMed]

48. Gauntlett-Gilbert, J.; Connell, H.; Clinch, J.; McCracken, L.M. Acceptance and values-based treatment of adolescents with chronic pain: Outcomes and their relationship to acceptance. *J. Pediatr. Psychol.* **2013**, *38*, 72–81. [CrossRef] [PubMed]

49. Maynard, C.S.; Amari, A.; Wieczorek, B.; Christensen, J.R.; Slifer, K.J. Interdisciplinary behavioral rehabilitation of pediatric pain-associated disability: Retrospective review of an inpatient treatment protocol. *J. Pediatr. Psychol.* **2010**, *35*, 128–137. [CrossRef] [PubMed]

50. Chalkiadis, G.A. Management of chronic pain in children. *Med. J. Aust.* **2001**, *175*, 476–479. [PubMed]

51. Simons, L.E.; Kaczynski, K.J.; Conroy, C.; Logan, D.E. Fear of pain in the context of intensive pain rehabilitation among children and adolescents with neuropathic pain: Associations with treatment response. *J. Pain* **2012**, *13*, 1151–1161. [CrossRef] [PubMed]

52. Hechler, T.; Ruhe, A.; Schmidt, P.; Hirsch, J.; Wager, J.; Dobe, M.; Krummenauer, F.; Zernikow, B. Inpatient-based intensive interdisciplinary pain treatment for highly impaired children with severe chronic pain: Randomized controlled trial of efficacy and economic effects. *Pain* **2014**, *155*, 118–128. [CrossRef] [PubMed]

53. Hirschfeld, G.; Hechler, T.; Dobe, M.; Wager, J.; Blankenburg, M.; Kosfelder, J.; Zernikow, B. Maintaining lasting improvements: One-year follow-up of children with severe chronic pain undergoing multimodal inpatient treatment. *J. Pediatr. Psychol.* **2013**, *38*, 224–236. [CrossRef] [PubMed]

54. Eccleston, C.; Palermo, T.M.; De C Williams, A.C.; Lewandowski, A.; Morley, S.; Fisher, E.; Law, E. Psychological therapies for the management of chronic and recurrent pain in children and adolescents. *Cochrane Database of Syst. Rev.* **2012**, *12*, CD003968.

55. Fisher, E.; Heathcote, L.; Palermo, T.M.; de, C.W.; Lau, J.; Eccleston, C. Systematic review and meta-analysis: Psychological therapies for children with chronic pain. *J. Pediatr. Psychol.* **2014**, *39*, 753–762. [CrossRef] [PubMed]

56. Westendorp, T.; Verbunt, J.; Remerie, S.; Blécourt, A.; Baalen, B.; Smeets, R. Social functioning in adulthood: Understanding long-term outcomes of adolescents with chronic pain/fatigue treated at inpatient rehabilitation programs. *Eur. J. Pain* **2016**, *20*, 1121–1130. [CrossRef] [PubMed]

57. Palermo, T.M.; Wilson, A.C.; Peters, M.; Lewandowski, A.; Somhegyi, H. Randomized controlled trial of an internet-delivered family cognitive-behavioral therapy intervention for children and adolescents with chronic pain. *Pain* **2009**, *146*, 205–213. [CrossRef] [PubMed]

58. Palermo, T.M.; Law, E.F.; Fales, J.; Bromberg, M.H.; Jessen-Fiddick, T.; Tai, G. Internet-delivered cognitive-behavioral treatment for adolescents with chronic pain and their parents: A randomized controlled multicenter trial. *Pain* **2016**, *157*, 174–185. [CrossRef] [PubMed]

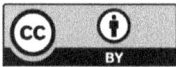

children

MDPI

Review

Acceptance and Commitment Therapy for Pediatric Chronic Pain: Theory and Application

Melissa Pielech [1],*, Kevin E. Vowles [1],* and Rikard Wicksell [2]

[1] Department of Psychology, University of New Mexico, Albuquerque, NM 87131, USA
[2] Department of Clinical Neuroscience, Karolinska Institutet, SE-171 76 Stockholm, Sweden; rikard.wicksell@karolinska.se
* Correspondence: melissapielech@gmail.com (M.P.); k.e.vowles@gmail.com (K.E.V.); Tel.: +1-505-277-1394 (K.E.V.)

Academic Editor: Lynn S. Walker
Received: 4 October 2016; Accepted: 25 January 2017; Published: 30 January 2017

Abstract: Acceptance and Commitment Therapy (ACT) is a third wave behavior therapy approach which aims to increase engagement in activities that bring meaning, vitality, and value to the lives of individuals experiencing persistent pain, discomfort, or distress. This goal is particularly relevant when these aversive experiences cannot be effectively avoided or when avoidance efforts risk their exacerbation, all of which may be common experiences in children and adolescents with chronic pain conditions. The primary aim of the present paper is to review and summarize the extant literature on the application, utility, and evidence for using ACT with pediatric chronic pain populations by: (1) defining the theoretical assumptions of the ACT model; (2) summarizing research study findings and relevant measures from the published literature; and (3) critically discussing the strengths, limitations and areas in need of further development.

Keywords: Acceptance and Commitment Therapy; ACT; children; adolescents; pediatric; chronic pain; pain acceptance

1. Introduction

A significant percentage of young people experience chronic pain, generally defined as pain that persists for three months or longer [1]. A subset of these patients report marked deficits in healthy functioning [2] and commonly experience comorbid mental health difficulties that can persist into adulthood [3]. Treatment efforts for chronic pain often highlight the primacy of pain reduction or elimination. Such efforts to minimize current pain and avoid it in the future are perfectly natural. In acute cases, efficient pain escape and avoidance behaviors can have genuine adaptive value, as they minimize risk of morbidity and mortality by allowing for efficient detection and response to painful or potentially painful situations [4–6].

In the case of chronic pain, however, these perfectly natural responses may not be the most adaptive. In fact, when persistent, avoidance behaviors can be reliably associated with significant disruptions in physical, social, and emotional functioning across the lifespan, often without any corresponding decrease in pain. A prime and well-established example of these findings is the fear-avoidance model, which consistently indicates that more persistent and widespread efforts to avoid pain are associated with worse current and future functioning in both pediatric and adult settings [7–11]. In youth, the role of caregiver responses to pain is also highly relevant, as high fear-avoidance in parents or responses to the child's pain that reinforce avoidance are related to greater levels of child distress and disability [12–14]. Thus, when pain avoidance is a primary goal in youth and their caregivers, there appears to be a heightened risk that pain will be more disruptive in important areas of physical and psychosocial functioning [15,16].

Youth with chronic pain and their family systems are therefore likely in need of treatments that emphasize effective responding to pain, with less reliance on pain control. It is possible that effective responding to chronic pain requires somewhat paradoxical responses to pain. Such paradoxical responses might include, for instance, decreasing pain avoidance attempts, particularly when they are ineffective at avoiding pain over the longer term or when they negatively impact important functioning. Further, effective responding to pain may actually include "approach" behaviors, such as participation in meaningful activities even when pain is present. Importantly, adoption of such strategies requires careful consideration regarding whether one is willing to experience pain in the service of engagement in meaningful activities. Acceptance and Commitment Therapy [17] aims to improve the ability to act in alignment with personal values while in the presence of potentially interfering pain and distress, a response pattern defined as psychological (or behavioral) flexibility. As part of this process, the individual is encouraged to explore and challenge the utility of avoidance, as well as acceptance-oriented strategies, in managing chronic pain. The primary aim of the present paper is to provide a narrative review and summary of the extant literature on the application and utility of ACT specifically for pediatric chronic pain. First, we review the primary goals and theoretical assumptions of the ACT model. Second, we summarize treatment outcomes and relevant measures from the published literature. Finally, we discuss strengths, limitations, and areas in need of development.

1.1. The ACT Model

While a full review of the theoretical and philosophical assumptions of the ACT model is beyond the scope of the present review (see Hayes et al. [17] for more information), it is important to highlight a few key points. The first is to emphasize the overarching goal of ACT, which is to increase successful engagement in activities that bring meaning, vitality, and importance to the lives of individuals experiencing persistent pain, discomfort, or distress. This goal is particularly relevant when these aversive experiences cannot be effectively avoided or when avoidance efforts risk their exacerbation, as is often the case with persistent pain. Each of the following conceptual assertions circle back to this overarching goal.

ACT is based on the philosophical positions of both pragmatism and functional contextualism [18]. Its pragmatic goal is "effective action," meaning it aims to facilitate the effectiveness of behavior in achieving adaptive and functional goals over the longer term. At the level of actual clinical interaction, this goal is described in terms of greater engagement in valued actions. The functional contextual orientation of ACT allows one to define two primary aims: (1) accurate prediction and (2) useful influence on behavior [19]. The pursuit of these aims requires one to attend to the relevant contextual events in any analysis of behavior, including historical events giving rise to the behavior as well as relevant ongoing events in the person's environment. Practically, ACT seeks to undermine the influence of key current and historical stimuli that contribute to ineffective responses to pain, such as persistent avoidance, and bolster the influence of those that contribute to more effective responses, such as the specification and pursuit of desired valued outcomes. These aims of "accurate prediction" and "useful influence on behavior" are concordant with the operant behavioral roots of both ACT and Cognitive-Behavioral Therapy (CBT; [18,19]).

Much discussion has occurred regarding the similarities and differences amongst ACT and other forms of psychotherapy, principally Cognitive Behavioral Therapy (CBT; for information regarding applications of CBT for pediatric chronic pain, please refer to [20,21]). We suggest that there are two key differences between these approaches. The first is the central focus on the facilitation of values-based actions in ACT. While such a focus is both fully compatible and at times apparent within CBT (e.g., [18,19]), its centrality in ACT is distinctive. The second key difference pertains to working with human language and cognition. In brief, ACT seeks not to directly alter the occurrence of certain instances of human cognition (e.g., catastrophic thinking) and sensation (e.g., pain intensity), but to increase the repertoire of responses to these cognitions and sensations, as well as the flexible use of them, to facilitate actions more in line with valued activities over the longer term.

The experimental pain literature provides several examples regarding the utility of altered responding to human cognition and sensation in adults. One of the earliest experimental trials of acceptance involved an acute pain induction task, where participants were asked to submerge a hand into an ice water bath and were randomized to a pain control (e.g., keep your pain under control; don't let it increase) or pain acceptance (e.g., let your pain be; don't let it control your responses) set of instructions [22]. Results indicated that tolerance time for participants in the latter condition were significantly longer than the former. Importantly, participants in the pain acceptance condition viewed pain and thoughts about pain as less influential than those in the pain control condition. This pattern of results has been replicated several times in studies with experimentally induced pain and healthy controls [23–27], as well as in adults with low back pain [28]. Furthermore, laboratory studies suggest that the inclusion of values in experimental pain settings is important. For example, when a pain task is paired with a personally important reason for experiencing the pain, tolerance times tend to be increase and the experience of pain is viewed as a less important determinant of behavior [27,29].

The clinical model of ACT specifies several related treatment processes, each of which is intended to help facilitate more effective responding to difficult or aversive experiences. For example, the central overarching process has been termed "psychological flexibility," which can be simply defined as effectively and flexibly responding to aversives such that engagement in important areas of living is maintained at a level that is sufficient for the needs of the individual [17,30]. Thus, an instance of psychological flexibility in an adolescent with chronic pain may be maintenance of social and scholastic engagement even with the ongoing experience of chronic pain and including times when pain is low as well as when it is high (see Wicksell et al. [31], summarized below, for description of a case example).

Underlying this overarching process of psychological flexibility are three pairs of "sub" processes [17]. These three pairs include (1) acceptance and defusion; (2) moment-to-moment awareness and a transcendent sense of self; and (3) clarity and committed action in pursuit of valued activities (e.g., see [17] for details, as well as [32] for an empirical evaluation of this model in chronic pain). Acceptance and defusion refer to patterns of responding to pain that involve acknowledgement that pain and suffering are a normal part of life many times and choosing to work with these experiences rather than try to avoid or control them [33–35]. Moment-to-moment awareness and a transcendent sense of self refer to aspects of mindfulness that seek to increase consistent, nonjudgmental attention to the present moment, less struggling with present experiences, and the facilitation of a stable sense of self as a person having experiences, rather then an unstable sense of self as a person who is defined by the experiences themselves (see [36,37]). Finally, clarity and committed action in relation to values includes a definition of useful, valued directions to help guide behavior while in the midst of difficult circumstances, as well as a flexible commitment to these values such that behavior can be adjusted over time to facilitate consistent movement towards them [38].

Thus, treatment success in ACT for pediatric chronic pain could be defined as the occurrence of effective responding to the natural variations in pain intensity that occur, such that personal needs and goals are being met or progressed. Furthermore, the model assumes that such treatment success is most likely to occur when one is (1) aware of pain when it is occurring, but is not consumed by that experience to the exclusion of other things happening; (2) aware of present experiences as they are occurring and able to let these experiences come and go; and (3) clear on valued areas and engaged in a flexibly persistent pattern of behaviors to pursue these areas. Overall, the relevance of these processes in adult chronic pain is reasonably well-established in that measures of these processes are reliably and significantly related with pain-related distress, disability, and healthcare use [39–41].

In the case of pediatric pain treatment specifically, this model applies to both caregiver and child. Much like caregiver responses are important in the fear-avoidance model, greater caregiver acceptance of pain and discomfort is associated with less restricted functioning in children [42,43]. Thus, it can be hypothesized that parental support of the child's engagement in valued activities in the presence of pain via operant approaches may be helpful to the child's overall success in adapting effectively to a chronic condition.

1.2. Developmental Considerations

ACT has been successfully adapted and implemented for use with a wide range of pediatric populations including youth with chronic pain (e.g., [44]), cystic fibrosis [45], and anxiety disorders [46], as well as medical conditions that involve pain as a primary symptom [47]. For a review of the application of ACT more broadly with pediatric populations with physical health conditions, please refer to [48]. Given the inherent level of abstraction in some ACT concepts, developmentally sensitive modifications in the language and delivery of treatment may be necessary. Adaptations should be made based on clinical judgment and awareness of the patient's level of cognitive, social, and psychological functioning, as well as abstraction abilities (refer to [49] for a discussion of adapting ACT interventions for adolescent populations). Briefly, adaptations may include age-appropriate simplification of language of complex concepts, such as referring to distressing, pain-related thoughts as coming from a "pain monster" whose advice may serve to restrict functioning and effective engagement in valued activities [31]. Concrete strategies can be used for teaching abstract concepts, like facilitation of values identification by using a heart shaped box that is filled with slips of paper describing patient values or teaching mindfulness via a walking exercise [50]. There are also numerous ACT metaphors that are developmentally relevant for use with adolescents, though it is recommended that use of metaphors be chosen with consideration to the patient's social context and interests. It can also be helpful to reiterate and repeat important topics to reinforce understanding. Additionally, the importance of family factors and inclusion of parents/caregivers in pediatric pain treatment is of clear importance [14,31,51]. From an ACT perspective, more traditional behavioral strategies such as contingency management may favorably be combined with interventions aimed at improving the parent's ability to self-manage distress, which otherwise may interfere with effective coaching [33].

2. The Evidence-Base for ACT with Youth with Chronic Pain

2.1. Search Criteria

Relevant treatment outcome papers using ACT published through December 2016 were identified through searches on PubMed and PsychInfo using search terms such as 'Acceptance and Commitment Therapy' or 'ACT' and 'children,' 'adolescents,' 'youth,' or 'pediatric' and 'chronic pain.' The evidence base for using ACT with youth for chronic pain is modest, and includes one case study, one case series, two randomized controlled trials, and three prospective cohort studies. Each of these studies is reviewed below. In addition, a fourth cohort study is also reviewed. While the study described a CBT-based intervention, mediation analyses were done using a measure of pain acceptance, thus the outcomes seem relevant to include.

2.2. Case Study and Case Series

The first study in the field of ACT for pediatric chronic pain is a case study by Wicksell et al. [33] that facilitated development of ACT treatments for youth with chronic pain and was helpful in distinguishing between ACT and CBT in the context of chronic pain rehabilitation. The patient was a 14-year-old female, who had been experiencing persistent pain for three years. Her array of symptoms were conceptualized as "musculoskeletal pain syndrome" and included generalized joint and body pain, persistent headaches, and features of panic attacks with subsequent school absence, social isolation from friends, and withdrawal from valued activities. Treatment was rehabilitative in nature and primarily consisted of exposure to stimuli related to pain and distress, including avoided activities and places, as well as significant values clarification exercises. Treatment comprised a total of 13 sessions over a six-month period, with three of the 13 sessions including both patient and parents. At discharge, improvements were noted in functional disability, engagement with valued activities, scholastic involvement, and avoidance of emotions. Importantly, these improvements were sustained during a six-month follow up period.

In 2007, a follow-up case series was published describing findings from an individual ACT-based treatment approach used with 14 adolescents (11 females, mean age = 17 years, standard deviation (SD = 2.1) with chronic pain and high levels of pain-related disability [52]. Primary outcome variables were disability and school attendance. Treatment emphasized exposure to private events and previously avoided activities, values clarification and use of values as guiding principles for engagement in exposure, as well as acceptance of distressing and negative feelings. Treatment length varied from 5–29 weekly sessions and included individual sessions with parents, as needed. Significant improvements were observed in the primary outcomes variables, which were maintained through 3 and 6-month follow-ups. Significant improvements were also observed in levels of pain catastrophizing, pain intensity, and pain interference.

2.3. Randomized Controlled Trials (RCT)

Following the case study and pilot case series, Wicksell et al. [44] published the first RCT evaluating the effectiveness of an ACT-based treatment for children and adolescents with chronic pain. ACT was compared to a multidisciplinary treatment (MDT) including amitriptyline medication. The primary components of the 10-week ACT-oriented treatment group were acceptance strategies and exposure, with sessions occurring weekly. A total of 32 youth participated (mean age = 14.8 years, SD = 2.4) with 16 patients randomized to each condition. Patients in the ACT condition improved significantly in multiple domains (e.g., functional disability, health related quality of life) and changes were sustained through follow up, as evidenced by multiple large effect sizes. Patients in the MDT group improved in many domains, as well, but across conditions, patients who received ACT improved significantly more in levels of pain-related fear, overall quality of life, pain intensity, and pain interference. A prolonged treatment period in the MDT condition complicated comparisons at follow up, but results demonstrated the relative utility of ACT in comparison to a multidisciplinary treatment.

In a planned set of post-hoc analyses, Wicksell et al. used data from this same RCT to identify mediators of treatment outcome [41]. Tested mediators were pain intensity, as well as both CBT- and ACT-consistent variables, including self-efficacy, catastrophizing, kinesiophobia, pain-impairment beliefs, and pain reactivity. Only these last two variables, which were argued to be representative of a more flexible and willing pain response style, were shown to be significant mediators of change. Furthermore, in subsequent analyses these same two mediators were independent predictors of outcomes at follow-up for the ACT condition only. Although tentative, the pattern of results suggests that variables consistent with psychological flexibility mediate the effects of ACT-based interventions to improve functioning in patients with chronic debilitating pain.

In a more recent study, Ghomian and Shairi [53] compared an ACT based treatment (*n* = 10) with a control condition (*n* = 10) in children ages 7 to 12 with chronic pain. Details regarding treatment components or the control condition were not provided (Note. the study authors were emailed a request asking for further details regarding treatment and control conditions and no response was received). Data was collected at four time points: pre-treatment, discharge, and 3.5 and 6.5 months post-treatment. Regarding results, patients in the ACT condition reportedly demonstrated significantly greater improvements in functional disability at the end of treatment and through the follow up time points.

2.4. Prospective Cohort Studies

Gauntlett-Gilbert et al. [54] evaluated outcomes from a 3-week residential, interdisciplinary ACT-based program (~90 h of treatment) for adolescents (*n* = 98) with chronic pain. The program, comprised of physical conditioning, activity management, and psychology, also included parent involvement in most sessions, with the exception of a four-day period where parents received therapy separately from their child. Data on self-reported functioning (e.g., depressive and anxious symptoms, levels of pain acceptance) and objective physical ability was collected from child and parent across three time points: baseline, three weeks after discharge from treatment, and at a three-month follow up time point. Patients improved across all domains of functioning in a manner that was theoretically consistent with ACT whereby improvements occurred without efforts to control pain or manipulate cognitions. Additionally, improvements in pain-related acceptance were associated with better treatment outcomes, suggesting a key role of acceptance in pediatric pain rehabilitation.

Martin et al. [55] published outcomes of a feasibility trail of ACT for adolescents with chronic pain and Neurofibromatosis type 1 (NF1), an autosomal disorder. The sample included 10 adolescents, who averaged 17 years of age and seven parents, who participated in a two day group intervention provided in a "workshop" format. At a three-month follow-up, significant declines in pain interference were reported by both patients and parents, while patients only reported decreased pain intensity. The authors suggested that the obtained data supported the feasibility of ACT in young people diagnosed with NF1.

Prospective Studies with Parents

Recently, Wallace et al. [56] published the first pilot study examining the application of an eight-week, ACT-based group intervention with parents (*n* = 8; 6 completed the study) of youth with chronic pain. The primary treatment target was to increase parental psychological flexibility, specifically for parents to identify areas of ineffective action or stuckness within themselves and their family unit, as well as develop strategies to support pursuit of values-based action. Sessions were delivered once a week, on an outpatient basis, and were 75 min long (session by session content is detailed by the authors in the manuscript [56]). Measures of parent psychological flexibility, responses to child pain symptoms, and levels of pain interference were collected during treatment and at three follow up time points, up to six months post treatment. Overall, parents were highly satisfied with the intervention. Furthermore, parent levels of psychological flexibility increased during treatment, as well as through follow up. During follow up, parent protective responses and adolescent-reported levels of pain interference decreased significantly. The authors hypothesize that the delayed improvements observed in parental responses may indicate a potential mediating effect of psychological flexibility on parental responses.

A final study examined changes in pain-acceptance following CBT for chronic pain. While this study was not strictly an application of ACT, the treatment description suggests that there were some goals that were concordant. For example, the authors of the study noted that participants and their parents were told that the goal of treatment was not decrease pain, but to "increase coping skills, functioning, and quality of life" [34]. Thus, it seemed appropriate to include this study within the present review, particularly because it examined how changes in acceptance over the course of the treatment were related to changes in distress and disability. A total of 112 youth, aged 11–18, participated in the treatment program, which included daily relaxation training, physical therapy, occupational therapy, recreation therapy, family therapy, and psychotherapy groups. Levels of acceptance significantly increased during treatment, while levels of depression, pain catastrophizing, and functional disability significantly decreased. Importantly, changes in acceptance significantly predicted changes in all psychosocial variables and functional disability.

3. Measures of ACT Processes in Youth with Chronic Pain and Their Families

Table 1 describes self-report measures for youth and their caregivers that assess constructs relevant to ACT processes and their relation with other psychosocial measures of pain-related functioning. In brief, to date there are four measures that explicitly measure ACT processes in children and adolescents, and three questionnaires developed for use with caregivers either as a proxy report (*n* = 1) or a report of the caregiver's own experience and behaviors (*n* = 3). Three measures not specifically validated with pediatric chronic pain populations were included due to their utility in assessing ACT processes [57–59]. Further research and evaluation on all of the measures is warranted, as the statistical properties have only been preliminarily validated. Notably, however, findings from the published cross-sectional studies with pediatric samples are consistent with similar studies in adults and illustrate that ACT-relevant processes are related to functioning in a manner consistent with the underlying theory of ACT (e.g., greater pain acceptance is associated with better emotional and physical status).

Table 1. Measures of Acceptance and Commitment Therapy (ACT) processes in pediatric chronic pain.

Measures	Description	Relations
Child Specific		
Chronic Pain Acceptance Questionnaire: Adolescent version (CPAQ-A; [60,61])	20 item self-report measure, adapted from the adult version [33]. Assesses two aspects of pain acceptance: (1) Activity Engagement and (2) Pain Willingness. Response options range from (0) *never true* to (4) *always true*.	Correlated with disability, depression, anxiety, self-efficacy. Not correlated with pain-specific variables (e.g., pain duration).
Child and Adolescent Mindfulness Measure (CAMM; [58]) *	10 item measure of mindfulness skills. Normed on four samples of school age children and adolescents. Response options range from (0) *never true* to (4) *always true*.	Correlated with quality of life, school and social functioning and mindfulness-inconsistent processes (e.g., externalizing behavior).
Avoidance and Fusion Questionnaire for Youth (AFQ-Y; [57]) *	17 item measure of psychological inflexibility for youth. There is also a validated eight-item short form of the AFQ-Y.	Scores for both versions correlated with child anxiety, somatic complaints, mindfulness, quality of life, and scholastic functioning.
Parent specific		
Parent psychological flexibility measure (PPFQ; [43,62])	24 item measure to assess parental levels of psychological flexibility in responses to child's pain symptoms. Items range from (0) *never true* to (6) *always true*.	Scores correlated with child disability, depression, and pain acceptance, as well as with parental response behaviors, as assessed by the Adult Responses to Child Symptoms (ARCS) measure [63].
Chronic Pain Acceptance Questionnaire: Parent report (CPAQ-P; [64])	16 item self-report measure of parent perceptions of child's acceptance of pain, adapted from the adult CPAQ [33]. Same two subscales as the CPAQ-A. Response options range from (0) *never true* to (6) *always true*.	Scores correlated with child pain intensity and disability, as well as parent pain catastrophizing, pain-related fear, and maladaptive protective responses.
Parent Pain Acceptance Questionnaire (PPAQ; [42])	15 item self-report measure of parent's own levels of acceptance towards their child's pain. Adapted from the CPAQ-P [64]. Two sub-scales: (1) Activity Engagement and (2) Pain-related Thoughts and Feelings.	Scores correlated with child pain acceptance, pain-related fear, and pain catastrophizing, as well as parental maladaptive responses to pain and pain catastrophizing
Parental Acceptance and Action Questionnaire (PAAQ [59]) *	15 item self-report measure of experiential avoidance in relation to parenting. Two subscales: (1) Inaction and (2) Unwillingness	In preliminary validation, the PAAQ correlated with symptoms of child psychopathology and measures of controlling parental behaviors and affective expression. Predicted significant amounts of variance in parent and clinician ratings of child anxiety symptoms.

* Not a pain specific ACT measure.

4. Strengths, Limitations, and Future Directions

ACT takes a pragmatic and flexible approach to the treatment of pediatric pain. The overarching goal of ACT is to decrease ineffective struggles for control of pain or distressing emotions and increase adaptive responses to pain and facilitate consistent re-engagement with valued activities. Theoretically, the probability of this occurring is assumed to be more likely when one approaches aversive experiences with more openness and fewer struggles for control, and when one is more aware of both one's personal values and currently available opportunities to engage in valued activities.

Although preliminary, the growing body of evidence regarding ACT for pediatric pain is promising and results from existing studies are consistent, offering some support regarding validity and utility. Notably, and unfortunately, the number of studies on ACT for pediatric pain patients is considerably smaller than the body of research and strong evidence for using ACT for adult chronic pain [65]. Furthermore, beyond a small number of studies, the literature on ACT for children and adolescents suffers from either an absence of or poorly defined control conditions, and small sample sizes. Thus, there is a need for more studies and those of higher quality in terms of study design, evaluation across settings (e.g., outpatient, day hospital, individual vs. group), and further identification and replication of the mechanisms by which improvements in functioning occur during treatment. Formal inclusion of parents in treatment and assessment of parent pain-related functioning is also needed to illuminate and optimize their role in their child's pain rehabilitation.

At present, there is also a need for precise measurement of ACT treatment processes in youth with chronic pain. The adult chronic pain literature boasts numerous measures of ACT constructs, such as psychological flexibility [66,67], pain acceptance [33], engagement in valued activities [68–70], and committed action [38], which could potentially be adapted for use with pediatric populations. While there is one measure of pain acceptance for youth, it is curious that no measure of values or assessments related to other aspects of the model have been developed yet for pediatric chronic pain populations. Given the focus within ACT on improvements in values-based actions, the development of a robust measurement method in young people with chronic pain appears highly important. In particular, valued domains in adults may be different than in youth and these differences may require a carefully considered assessment. Furthermore, clinical experience suggests that certain times in one's life, for example, adolescence, are a time of personal determination of what is of personal value. For example, there can be consideration and weighing of socially-constructed values (e.g., be popular) in relation to those that are more personal in nature (e.g., be kind to others). The adult literature on values assessment offers little to no guidance on the assessment of "values formation" (for lack of a better term) and this seems a distinct and important opportunity for those that work in pediatric settings. In addition, further specification of the unique and interactive effects of caregiver and child responses to pain within an ACT framework appears to present an important opportunity for further work. Thus, while some aspects of the ACT model may be appropriate to assess via a process of "downward" extension from adults to youth, there may be particular facets of the pediatric setting that are deserving of careful consideration.

There are several additional considerations in relation to the use of ACT in the treatment of pediatric chronic pain. First, there is little guidance on ages that are appropriate or inappropriate for ACT; notably, only two of the ten studies reviewed explicitly made mention of developmental adaptations or considerations taken into their protocol [31,55]. In particular, it is not currently known if there is a minimum age, or minimum set of developmental milestones that must have been met, for successful treatment participation. The authors' clinical experience suggests somewhere in the 8–10 range may be a lower age limit, but this intuition is in need of empirical examination. Second, there is little guidance on the selection of type of psychological treatment, for example, use of ACT instead of CBT. Given the overlap between approaches, it may be that firm data-based rubrics are unlikely in the near future. Furthermore, given the distinctions between ACT and CBT, as detailed in the first major section of this paper, perhaps ACT is more relevant for use in individuals with significant deficits in values clarity and pursuit of values-based directions, or in those who are so paralyzed by pain and associated cognitions that cognitive methods are unlikely to work in an efficient manner. Third, while caregiver involvement in treatment is important and there is evidence demonstrating that caregiver responses and functioning impact child outcomes, the exact type or duration of such involvement is not clear. For example, is it sufficient to simply have caregivers sit in on some or all treatment sessions, or is it necessary for caregivers to receive treatment specific to their particular needs? Again, clinical experience suggests that the latter is more likely to be of use, but, to our knowledge, there are no data to use for guidance. It seems fair to note that these three issues are important for psychological interventions for pediatric chronic pain writ large and seem necessary to address for the field to move forward to firmer empirical ground.

5. Conclusions

To conclude, a primary goal of ACT for pediatric chronic pain is to support youth in healthy functioning and aid them in the process of re-engagement in valued activities so that their focus may shift back to age- appropriate activities, rather than predominantly on pain control or pain avoidance. The theoretical principles of ACT provide a framework for the structure of such treatment. While the extant data is promising, much more work needs to be done to augment the evidence base for the application of ACT with pediatric pain populations and to ensure that clinical practice is consistent with the hypothesized theoretical principles of ACT.

Acknowledgments: This work was supported by funding from the National Institutes of Health (R34AT008398; PI: Kevin E. Vowles) and the National School of Research in Health Care Science (PI: Rikard Wicksell).

Author Contributions: M.P. and K.E.V. conceived of the idea for this topical review and outlined the paper. M.P. performed the literature search, summarized findings for studies and measures, and put together an initial draft of the paper. K.E.V. wrote and finalized the introduction, provided edits and feedback. R.W. contributed to the conceptual organization of the paper, wrote up summaries on processes of change related studies, and provided valuable edits and feedback to finalize the paper.

Conflicts of Interest: The authors declare no conflict of interest.

References

1. King, S.; Chambers, C.T.; Huguet, A.; MacNevin, R.C.; McGrath, P.J.; Parker, L.; MacDonald, A.J. The epidemiology of chronic pain in children and adolescents revisited: A systematic review. *Pain* **2011**, *152*, 2729–2738. [CrossRef] [PubMed]
2. Huguet, A.; Miró, J. The severity of chronic pediatric pain: An epidemiological study. *J. Pain* **2008**, *9*, 226–236. [CrossRef] [PubMed]
3. Noel, M.; Groenewald, C.B.; Beals-Erickson, S.E.; Gebert, J.T.; Palermo, T.M. Chronic pain in adolescence and internalizing mental health disorders: A nationally representative study. *Pain* **2016**, *157*, 1333–1338. [CrossRef] [PubMed]
4. Loeser, J.D.; Melzack, R.; Melzack, R.; Wall, P.; Levine, J.; Taiwo, Y.; Dubner, R.; Ruda, M.; Gracely, R.; Lynch, S.; et al. Pain: An overview. *Lancet* **1999**, *353*, 1607–1609. [CrossRef]
5. van Damme, S.; Crombez, G.; Eccleston, C. Coping with pain: A motivational perspective. *Pain* **2008**, *139*, 1–4. [CrossRef] [PubMed]
6. Woolf, C.J.; Bennett, G.J.; Doherty, M.; Dubner, R.; Kidd, B.; Koltzenburg, M.; Lipton, R.; Loeser, J.D.; Payne, R.; Torebjork, E. Towards a mechanism-based classification of pain? *Pain* **1998**, *77*, 227–229. [CrossRef]
7. Simons, L.E.; Kaczynski, K.J. The Fear Avoidance model of chronic pain: Examination for pediatric application. *J. Pain* **2012**, *13*, 827–835. [CrossRef] [PubMed]
8. Asmundson, G.J.G.; Noel, M.; Petter, M.; Parkerson, H.A. Pediatric fear-avoidance model of chronic pain: Foundation, application and future directions. *Pain Res. Manag.* **2012**, *17*, 397–405. [CrossRef] [PubMed]
9. Lethem, J.; Slade, P.D.; Troup, J.D.; Bentley, G. Outline of a Fear-Avoidance Model of exaggerated pain perception—I. *Behav. Res. Ther.* **1983**, *21*, 401–408. [CrossRef]
10. Vlaeyen, J.W.; Linton, S.J. Fear-avoidance and its consequences in chronic musculoskeletal pain: A state of the art. *Pain* **2000**, *85*, 317–332. [CrossRef]

11. Leeuw, M.; Goossens, M.E.J.B.; Linton, S.J.; Crombez, G.; Boersma, K.; Vlaeyen, J.W.S. The fear-avoidance model of musculoskeletal pain: Current state of scientific evidence. *J. Behav. Med.* **2007**, *30*, 77–94. [CrossRef] [PubMed]

12. Guite, J.W.; McCue, R.L.; Sherker, J.L.; Sherry, D.D.; Rose, J.B. Relationships among pain, protective parental responses, and disability for adolescents with chronic musculoskeletal pain: The mediating role of pain catastrophizing. *Clin. J. Pain* **2011**, *27*, 775–781. [CrossRef] [PubMed]

13. Logan, D.E.; Simons, L.E.; Carpino, E.A. Too sick for school? Parent influences on school functioning among children with chronic pain. *Pain* **2012**, *153*, 437–443. [CrossRef] [PubMed]

14. Palermo, T.M.; Valrie, C.R.; Karlson, C.W. Family and parent influences on pediatric chronic pain: A developmental perspective. *Am. Psychol.* **2014**, *69*, 142–152. [CrossRef] [PubMed]

15. Chow, E.T.; Otis, J.D.; Simons, L.E. The longitudinal impact of parent distress and behavior on functional outcomes among youth with chronic pain. *J. Pain* **2016**, *17*, 729–738. [CrossRef] [PubMed]

16. Simons, L.E.; Smith, A.; Kaczynski, K.; Basch, M. Living in fear of your child's pain: The Parent Fear of Pain Questionnaire. *Pain* **2015**, *156*, 694–702. [CrossRef] [PubMed]

17. Hayes, S.C.; Strosahl, K.D.; Wilson, K.G. *Acceptance and Commitment Therapy: The Process and Practice of Mindful Change*, 2nd ed.; Guilford Press: New York, NY, USA, 2012.

18. Zettle, R.D. The Evolution of a Contextual Approach to Therapy: From Comprehensive Distancing to ACT. *Int. J. Behav. Consult. Ther.* **2005**, *1*, 77–89. [CrossRef]

19. Biglan, A.; Hayes, S.C. Should the behavioral sciences become more pragmatic? The case for functional contextualism in research on human behavior. *Appl. Prev. Psychol.* **1996**, *5*, 47–57. [CrossRef]

20. Noel, M.; Petter, M.; Parker, J.A.; Chambers, C.T. Cognitive Behavioral Therapy for Pediatric Chronic Pain: The Problem, Research, and Practice. *J. Cogn. Psychother.* **2012**, *26*, 143–156. [CrossRef]

21. Palermo, T.M.; Law, E.F.; Bromberg, M.; Fales, J.; Eccleston, C.; Wilson, A.C. Problem Solving Skills Training for Parents of Children with Chronic Pain: A Pilot Randomized Controlled Trial. *Pain* **2016**, *157*, 1213–1223. [CrossRef] [PubMed]

22. Hayes, S.C.; Bissett, R.; Korn, Z.; Zettle, R.D.; Rosenfarb, I.; Cooper, L.; Grundt, A. The impact of acceptance versus control rationales on pain tolerance. *Psychol. Rec.* **1999**, *49*, 33–47.

23. Keogh, E.; Bond, F.W.; Hanmer, R.; Tilston, J. Comparing acceptance- and control-based coping instructions on the cold-pressor pain experiences of healthy men and women. *Eur. J. Pain* **2005**, *9*, 591–598. [CrossRef] [PubMed]

24. McMullen, J.; Barnes-Holmes, D.; Barnes-Holmes, Y.; Stewart, I.; Luciano, C.; Cochrane, A. Acceptance versus distraction: Brief instructions, metaphors and exercises in increasing tolerance for self-delivered electric shocks. *Behav. Res. Ther.* **2008**, *46*, 122–129. [CrossRef] [PubMed]

25. Gutiérrez, O.; Luciano, C.; Rodríguez, M.; Fink, B.C. Comparison between an acceptance-based and a cognitive-control-based protocol for coping with pain. *Behav. Ther.* **2004**, *35*, 767–783. [CrossRef]

26. Masedo, A.I.; Esteve, M.R. Effects of suppression, acceptance and spontaneous coping on pain tolerance, pain intensity and distress. *Behav. Res. Ther.* **2007**, *45*, 199–209. [CrossRef] [PubMed]

27. Branstetter-Rost, A.; Cushing, C.; Douleh, T. Personal values and pain tolerance: Does a values intervention add to acceptance? *J. Pain* **2009**, *10*, 887–892. [CrossRef] [PubMed]

28. Vowles, K.E.; McNeil, D.W.; Gross, R.T.; McDaniel, M.L.; Mouse, A.; Bates, M.; Gallimore, P.; McCall, C. Effects of pain acceptance and pain control strategies on physical impairment in individuals with chronic low back pain. *Behav. Ther.* **2007**, *38*, 412–425. [CrossRef] [PubMed]

29. Páez-Blarrina, M.; Luciano, C.; Gutiérrez-Martínez, O.; Valdivia, S.; Ortega, J.; Rodríguez-Valverde, M. The role of values with personal examples in altering the functions of pain: Comparison between acceptance-based and cognitive-control-based protocols. *Behav. Res. Ther.* **2008**, *46*, 84–97. [CrossRef] [PubMed]

30. McCracken, L.M.; Vowles, K.E. Acceptance and Commitment Therapy and mindfulness for chronic pain: Model, process, and progress. *Am. Psychol.* **2014**, *69*, 178–187. [CrossRef] [PubMed]

31. Wicksell, R.K.; Dahl, J.; Magnusson, B.; Olsson, G.L. Using acceptance and commitment therapy in the rehabilitation of an adolescent female with chronic pain: A case example. *Cogn. Behav. Pract.* **2005**, *12*, 415–423. [CrossRef]

32. Vowles, K.E.; Sowden, G.; Ashworth, J. A comprehensive examination of the model underlying acceptance and commitment therapy for chronic pain. *Behav. Ther.* **2014**, *45*, 390–401. [CrossRef] [PubMed]

33. LMcCracken, M.; Vowles, K.E.; Eccleston, C. Acceptance of chronic pain: Component analysis and a revised assessment method. *Pain* **2004**, *107*, 159–166. [CrossRef]
34. Weiss, K.E.; Hahn, A.; Wallace, D.P.; Biggs, B.; Bruce, B.K.; Harrison, T.E. Acceptance of pain: Associations with depression, catastrophizing, and functional disability among children and adolescents in an interdisciplinary chronic pain rehabilitation program. *J. Pediatr. Psychol.* **2013**, *38*, 756–765. [CrossRef] [PubMed]
35. Kalapurakkel, S.; Carpino, E.A.; Lebel, A.; Simons, L.E. 'pain can't stop Me': Examining pain self-efficacy and acceptance as resilience processes among youth with chronic headache. *J. Pediatr. Psychol.* **2014**, *40*, 926–933. [CrossRef] [PubMed]
36. Hayes, S.C.; Shenk, C. Operationalizing Mindfulness Without Unnecessary Attachments. *Clin. Psychol. Sci. Pract.* **2006**, *11*, 249–254. [CrossRef]
37. McCracken, L.M.; Gauntlett-Gilbert, J.; Vowles, K.E. The role of mindfulness in a contextual cognitive-behavioral analysis of chronic pain-related suffering and disability. *Pain* **2007**, *131*, 63–69. [CrossRef] [PubMed]
38. McCracken, L.M. Committed action: An application of the psychological flexibility model to activity patterns in chronic pain. *J. Pain* **2013**, *14*, 828–835. [CrossRef] [PubMed]
39. Vowles, K.; Fink, B.; Cohen, L. Acceptance and Commitment Therapy for chronic pain: A diary study of treatment process in relation to reliable change in disability. *J. Context. Behav. Sci.* **2014**, *3*, 74–80. [CrossRef] [PubMed]
40. Vowles, K.E.; Thompson, M. Acceptance and Commitment Therapy for chronic pain. In *Mindfulness and Acceptance in Behavioral Medicine: Current Theory and Practice*; McCracken, L.M., Ed.; New Harbinger Publications: Oakland, CA, USA, 2011; pp. 31–60.
41. Wicksell, R.K.; Olsson, G.L.; Hayes, S.C. Mediators of change in acceptance and commitment therapy for pediatric chronic pain. *Pain* **2011**, *152*, 2792–2801. [CrossRef] [PubMed]
42. Smith, A.M.; Sieberg, C.B.; Odell, S.; Randall, E.; Simons, L.E. Living Life With My Child's Pain. *Clin. J. Pain* **2015**, *31*, 633–641. [CrossRef] [PubMed]
43. Wallace, D.P.; McCracken, L.M.; Weiss, K.E.; Harbeck-Weber, C. The role of parent psychological flexibility in relation to adolescent chronic pain: Further instrument development. *J. Pain* **2015**, *16*, 235–246. [CrossRef] [PubMed]
44. Wicksell, R.K.; Melin, L.; Lekander, M.; Olsson, G.L. Evaluating the effectiveness of exposure and acceptance strategies to improve functioning and quality of life in longstanding pediatric pain—A randomized controlled trial. *Pain* **2009**, *141*, 248–257. [CrossRef] [PubMed]
45. Casier, A.; Goubert, L.; Theunis, M.; Huse, D.; de Baets, F.; Matthys, D.; Crombez, G. Acceptance and well-being in adolescents and young adults with cystic fibrosis: A prospective study. *J. Pediatr. Psychol.* **2011**, *36*, 476–487. [CrossRef] [PubMed]
46. Arch, J.J.; Craske, M.C. Acceptance and Committment Therapy and Cognitive Behavioral Therapy for anxiety disorders: Different treatments, similar mechanisms? *Clin. Psychol. Sci. Pract.* **2008**, *15*, 263–279. [CrossRef]
47. Kallesøe, K.H.; Schröder, A.; Wicksell, R.K.; Fink, P.; Ørnbøl, E.; Rask, C.U. Comparing group-based acceptance and commitment therapy (ACT) with enhanced usual care for adolescents with functional somatic syndromes: A study protocol for a randomised trial. *BMJ Open* **2016**, *6*, e012743. [CrossRef] [PubMed]
48. Wicksell, R.K.; Kanstrup, M.; Kemani, M.K.; Holmström, L.; Olsson, G.L. Acceptance and Commitment Therapy for children and adolescents with physical health concerns. *Curr. Opin. Psychol.* **2015**, *2*, 1–5. [CrossRef]
49. Halliburton, A.E.; Cooper, L.D. Applications and adaptations of Acceptance and Commitment Therapy (ACT) for adolescents. *J. Context. Behav. Sci.* **2014**, *4*, 1–11. [CrossRef]
50. Murrell, A.R.; Coyne, L.W.; Wilson, K.G. ACT with children, adolescents, and their parents. In *A Practical Guide to Acceptance and Commitment Therapy*; Hayes, S.C., Strosahl, K.D., Eds.; Springer: New York, NY, USA, 2005.
51. Palermo, T.M.; Chambers, C.T. Parent and family factors in pediatric chronic pain and disability: An integrative approach. *Pain* **2005**, *119*, 1–4. [CrossRef] [PubMed]
52. Wicksell, R.K.; Melin, L.; Olsson, G.L. Exposure and acceptance in the rehabilitation of adolescents with idiopathic chronic pain—A pilot study. *Eur. J. Pain* **2007**, *11*, 267–274. [CrossRef] [PubMed]

53. Ghomian, S.; Shairi, M.R. The Effectiveness of Acceptance and Commitment Therapy for Children with Chronic Pain on the Quality of Life on 7 to 12. *Int. J. Pediatr.* **2014**, *2*, 47–56.

54. Gauntlett-Gilbert, J.; Connell, H.; Clinch, J.; Mccracken, L.M. Acceptance and values-based treatment of adolescents with chronic pain: Outcomes and their relationship to acceptance. *J. Pediatr. Psychol.* **2013**, *38*, 72–81. [CrossRef] [PubMed]

55. Martin, S.; Wolters, P.L.; Toledo-Tamula, M.A.; Schmitt, S.N.; Baldwin, A.; Starosta, A.; Gillespie, A.; Widemann, B. Acceptance and commitment therapy in youth with neurofibromatosis type 1 (NF1) and chronic pain and their parents: A pilot study of feasibility and preliminary efficacy. *Am. J. Med. Genet. Part A* **2016**, *170*, 1462–1470. [CrossRef] [PubMed]

56. Wallace, D.P.; Woodford, B.; Connelly, M. Promoting psychological flexibility in parents of adolescents with chronic pain: Pilot study of an 8-week group intervention. *Clin. Pract. Pediatr. Psychol.* **2016**, *4*, 405–416. [CrossRef]

57. Greco, L.A.; Lambert, W.; Baer, R.A. Psychological inflexibility in childhood and adolescence: Development and evaluation of the Avoidance and Fusion Questionnaire for Youth. *Psychol. Assess.* **2008**, *20*, 93–102. [CrossRef] [PubMed]

58. Greco, L.A.; Baer, R.A.; Smith, G.T. Assessing mindfulness in children and adolescents: Development and validation of the Child and Adolescent Mindfulness Measure (CAMM). *Psychol. Assess.* **2011**, *23*, 606–614. [CrossRef] [PubMed]

59. Cheron, D.M.; Ehrenreich, J.T.; Pincus, D.B. Assessment of parental experiential avoidance in a clinical sample of children with anxiety disorders. *Child Psychiatry Hum. Dev.* **2009**, *40*, 383–403. [CrossRef] [PubMed]

60. McCracken, L.M.; Gauntlett-Gilbert, J.; Eccleston, C. Acceptance of pain in adolescents with chronic pain: Validation of an adapted assessment instrument and preliminary correlation analyses. *Eur. J. Pain* **2010**, *14*, 316–320. [CrossRef] [PubMed]

61. Wallace, D.P.; Harbeck-Weber, C.; Whiteside, S.P.H.; Harrison, T.E. Adolescent acceptance of pain: Confirmatory factor analysis and further validation of the chronic pain acceptance Questionnaire, Adolescent version. *J. Pain* **2011**, *12*, 591–599. [CrossRef] [PubMed]

62. McCracken, L.M.; Gauntlett-Gilbert, J. Role of psychological flexibility in parents of adolescents with chronic pain: Development of a measure and preliminary correlation analyses. *Pain* **2011**, *152*, 780–785. [CrossRef] [PubMed]

63. Walker, L.S.; Levy, R.L.; Whitehead, W.E. Validation of a measure of protective parent responses to children's pain. *Clin. J. Pain* **2006**, *22*, 712–716. [CrossRef] [PubMed]

64. Simons, L.E.; Sieberg, C.B.; Kaczynski, K.J. Measuring parent beliefs about child acceptance of pain: A preliminary validation of the Chronic Pain Acceptance Questionnaire, parent report. *Pain* **2011**, *152*, 2294–2300. [CrossRef] [PubMed]

65. Society of Clinical Psychology. *Acceptance and Committment Therapy for Chronic Pain*; American Psychological Association: Washington, DC, USA, 2013; Available online: http://www.div12.org/PsychologicalTreatments/treatments/chronicpain_act.html (accessed on 21 May 2015).

66. Vowles, K.; McCracken, L.; Sowden, G.; Ashworth, J. Psychological flexibility in coping with chronic pain: Further examination of the brief pain coping inventory-2. *Clin. J. Pain* **2014**, *30*, 324–330. [CrossRef] [PubMed]

67. McCracken, L.M.; Vowles, K.E. Psychological flexibility and traditional pain management strategies in relation to patient functioning with chronic pain: An examination of a revised instrument. *J. Pain* **2007**, *8*, 700–707. [CrossRef] [PubMed]

68. McCracken, L.M.; Yang, S. The role of values in a contextual cognitive-behavioral approach to chronic pain. *Pain* **2006**, *123*, 137–145. [CrossRef] [PubMed]

69. Jensen, M.P.; Vowles, K.E.; Johnson, L.E.; Gertz, K.J. Living well with pain: Development and preliminary evaluation of the Valued Living Scale. *Pain Med.* **2015**, *16*, 2109–2120. [CrossRef] [PubMed]

70. Pielech, M.; Bailey, R.W.; McEntee, M.L.; Ashworth, J.; Levell, J.; Sowden, G.; Vowles, K.E. Preliminary evaluation of the values tracker: A two-item measure of engagement in valued activities in those with chronic pain. *Behav. Modif.* **2016**, *40*, 239–256. [CrossRef] [PubMed]

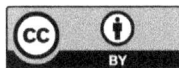

![children logo] *children*

MDPI

Article

A Clinical Pilot Study of Individual and Group Treatment for Adolescents with Chronic Pain and Their Parents: Effects of Acceptance and Commitment Therapy on Functioning

Marie Kanstrup [1,2,*], Rikard K. Wicksell [1,2], Mike Kemani [1,2], Camilla Wiwe Lipsker [1,2], Mats Lekander [2,3] and Linda Holmström [1,4]

1   Functional Area Medical Psychology, Functional Unit Behavioral Medicine, Karolinska University Hospital Solna, P8:01, 171 76 Stockholm, Sweden; Rikard.Wicksell@karolinska.se (R.K.W.); Mike.Kemani@karolinska.se (M.K.); Camilla.Wiwe-Lipsker@karolinska.se (C.W.L.); Linda.Holmstrom@ki.se (L.H.)
2   Department of Clinical Neuroscience, Karolinska Institutet, Nobels väg 9, 171 77 Stockholm, Sweden; Mats.Lekander@ki.se
3   Stress Research Institute, Stockholm University, 106 91 Stockholm, Sweden
4   Department of Women's and Children's health, Karolinska Institutet, H2:00, Karolinska University Hospital Solna, 171 76 Stockholm, Sweden
*   Correspondence: Marie.Kanstrup@ki.se; Tel.: +46-8-517-779-29

Academic Editor: Lynn S. Walker
Received: 9 September 2016; Accepted: 7 November 2016; Published: 16 November 2016

Abstract: Pediatric chronic pain is common and can result in substantial long-term disability. Previous studies on acceptance and commitment therapy (ACT) have shown promising results in improving functioning in affected children, but more research is still urgently needed. In the current clinical pilot study, we evaluated an ACT-based interdisciplinary outpatient intervention (14 sessions), including a parent support program (four sessions). Adolescents were referred to the clinic if they experienced disabling chronic pain. They were then randomized, along with their parents, to receive group ($n = 12$) or individual ($n = 18$) treatment. Adolescent pain interference, pain reactivity, depression, functional disability, pain intensity and psychological flexibility, along with parent anxiety, depression, pain reactivity and psychological flexibility were assessed using self-reported questionnaires. There were no significant differences in outcomes between individual and group treatment. Analyses illustrated significant ($p < 0.01$) improvements (medium to large effects) in pain interference, depression, pain reactivity and psychological flexibility post-treatment. Additionally, analyses showed significant ($p < 0.01$) improvements (large effects) in parent pain reactivity and psychological flexibility post-treatment. On all significant outcomes, clinically-significant changes were observed for 21%–63% of the adolescents across the different outcome measures and in 54%–76% of the parents. These results support previous findings and thus warrant the need for larger, randomized clinical trials evaluating the relative utility of individual and group treatment and the effects of parental interventions.

Keywords: cognitive behavior therapy (CBT); acceptance and commitment therapy (ACT); treatment; intervention; pain disability; persistent pain; adolescent

---

1. Introduction

Chronic pain is common among children and adolescents and is related to disability for up to 80% of those affected, for example negatively affecting leisure or school activities [1,2]. Pediatric chronic pain is related to poorer family functioning and may lead to an economic burden for parents and society [3,4]. Hence, there is a great need for interventions that effectively improve patient and family functioning. Although current medical treatment has often proven to be insufficient in reducing symptoms and improving functioning in pediatric chronic pain patient, systematic review findings support the use of psychological treatments, particularly those based on cognitive behavior therapy (CBT) [5]. CBT commonly includes a broad spectrum of interventions, based on different theoretical perspectives and models, aimed at both reductions in pain and distress, as well as improvement in overall functioning. Although there is evidence for the efficacy of CBT to treat pediatric chronic pain, debilitating symptoms can still remain for a number of patients, and therefore, there is a need to better understand change processes. Furthermore, considering the need for further research of the effects on functioning and mood [5], interventions aimed at decreasing pain interference (i.e., the impact of pain on functioning) and emotional reactivity to the pain experience, are crucial. Acceptance and commitment therapy (ACT) constitutes such a development within CBT [6]. From an ACT perspective, a primary source of disability and reduced quality of life is the inflexible use of avoidance strategies (psychological inflexibility), especially in the presence of pain and distress. Therefore, the key treatment target in ACT is to increase psychological flexibility (i.e., the ability to actively choose and act in line with long-term goals and values, even when in the presence of disturbing symptoms), by undermining the dominance of distressing thoughts, emotions and physical sensations, using various techniques, such as defusion and acceptance [6]. This specific focus on increasing behaviors in the direction of functionality in important life areas despite ongoing pain is consistent with the Pediatric Initiative on Methods, Measurement, and Pain Assessment in Clinical Trials (PedIMMPACT) recommendations [7], which emphasize the importance of targeting pain-related functioning in physical, emotional and social domains for treatments of pediatric chronic pain. Today, the empirical support for ACT for adult, unspecific chronic pain is strong [8]. However, only a few studies so far have been conducted analyzing children and adolescents.

Of these studies, findings from three ACT-based outpatient interventions for pediatric chronic pain by Wicksell et al., include an RCT consistently illustrate improvements in functioning [9–11]. In the RCT it was shown that these improvements in functioning at follow-up were mediated by improvements in pain impairment beliefs and pain reactivity, which are two variables strongly associated with psychological flexibility [12]. Similarly, results from a study evaluating an ACT-based intensive inpatient-program [13] showed that adolescents reported improved functioning along with increased levels of acceptance. A recent study by Ghomian and Shairi [14] on ACT for young children with chronic pain found increased functional ability after treatment compared with the control group. Furthermore, a pilot study on pediatric patients suffering from chronic pain and neurofibromatosis type 1 [15] showed that ACT may decrease pain interference.

Notably, previous interventions for adolescents have been delivered both individually [9–11] and in a group format [13,15], but to date, there is no scientific evaluation comparing the relative utility of these treatment formats. Furthermore, despite the evident relationship between pediatric chronic pain and family functioning, studies evaluating the effects of parental support programs on parent behaviors and distress are scarce [16]. Recent studies suggest the importance of ACT-consistent behaviors in parental management of pediatric chronic pain. For example, parental psychological flexibility has been found to correlate positively with adolescent acceptance and negatively with an adolescent pain-related impact on functioning and dysfunctional parental responses [17]. Therefore, parent psychological flexibility is suggested to be a potentially important target for the treatment of children and adolescents with chronic, debilitating pain [17,18]. In addition, considering the impact of pain on family functioning [3], parent emotional reactivity to child pain should also be explored. To date, one study has explored the utility of ACT for parents of children suffering from chronic pain [15], and the results suggest that interventions may improve parent acceptance.

Thus, there is preliminary support for the use of ACT to treat pediatric chronic pain, but more research is needed to further investigate the effects of ACT interventions in children and adolescents with chronic pain conditions. Furthermore, more studies are needed to evaluate the effects of ACT-based parental support programs. Positive effects have been seen in both individually- and group-delivered ACT interventions although these formats have not been compared using the same protocol. This is an important clinical question, as services might be providing both formats. Hence, the aims of the present clinical pilot study were to preliminarily evaluate the effects of (1) an ACT-based intervention provided in a group or in an individual format to adolescents with disabling chronic pain conditions, on functioning (i.e., pain interference, pain reactivity, depressive symptoms and functional disability), pain intensity and psychological flexibility; and (2) an ACT-based parental support program on parent emotional functioning, pain reactivity and psychological flexibility.

2. Methods

2.1. Study Setting and Design

This pilot study was performed by a team of five psychologists, two pain physicians and one physiotherapist, at a tertiary pain specialist clinic in Stockholm, Sweden. Patients between 12 and 18 years referred to the clinic due to chronic debilitating pain and their parents were considered eligible for inclusion in this study. Participants were randomized to either group ($n = 24$) or individual ($n = 24$) ACT treatment. The randomization sequences were generated via an online randomization service accessible at https://www.random.org/. An administrator who was not involved in treatment delivery randomized the participants, placed the information in coded sealed envelopes and informed the participants about which condition they had been assigned to by opening the envelopes in their presence. Data collection began in 2009 and ended in 2012. Pre-treatment assessments from study participants were included as part of previously-reported cross-sectional studies [19,20]. This clinical pilot trial was not registered.

2.2. Participants

Inclusion and exclusion criteria were assessed in semi-structured clinical interviews during the first visit to the clinic. Patients were included if they (1) were referred to our tertiary care pain clinic; (2) were between 14 and 18 years old (initial criterion 12 and 18 years, see below); (3) had suffered from pain >6 months; (4) reported insufficient effects of previous pain treatments; (5) reported substantial pain-related disability. They were excluded if (1) improvement was expected without treatment (e.g., had improved between referral and assessment); (2) psychiatric co-morbidity was considered the main reason for disability, required immediate intervention or was assumed to interfere with the planned intervention; (3) there was a substantial risk for suicide; (4) they had substantial cognitive dysfunction or reduced proficiency in Swedish; (5) they had other on-going or planned treatments (i.e., within the next 6 months); (6) pain was recurrent rather than continuous (defined as ≥ 4 completely pain-free days per week); and (7) pain was fully explained by a pathophysiological process, e.g., cancer. Adolescents not eligible for the study, who declined participation (e.g., those who did not want to take part in randomization) or who dropped out (e.g., those who changed their mind after being randomized to group treatment), were offered standard treatment at the clinic.

Parents of included adolescents were invited to participate in the parent support program, and all included adolescents had at least one parent who participated in the study. Parents data were collected from the same parent at all time points, although both parents, if applicable, were participating in the parent sessions.

As shown in Figure 1, 48 adolescent-parent dyads were randomized (24 participants randomized to individual treatment and 24 participants to group treatment). Attrition rates were 6 and 12 participants for the individual treatment condition and group treatment condition, respectively. Reasons for attrition are reported in the flow chart (Figure 1). The group condition included four groups, with 2–4 participants per group at post-treatment. At post-treatment assessment, 30 adolescents remained in the study, and these were included in the analyses. Out of all included parents, 28 parents provided data. Six parents were excluded from analysis because ratings were performed by different parents at different time-points (i.e., mother ratings at pre- and mid-, but father ratings at post-assessment). Therefore, data of 22 parents were included in the analyses.

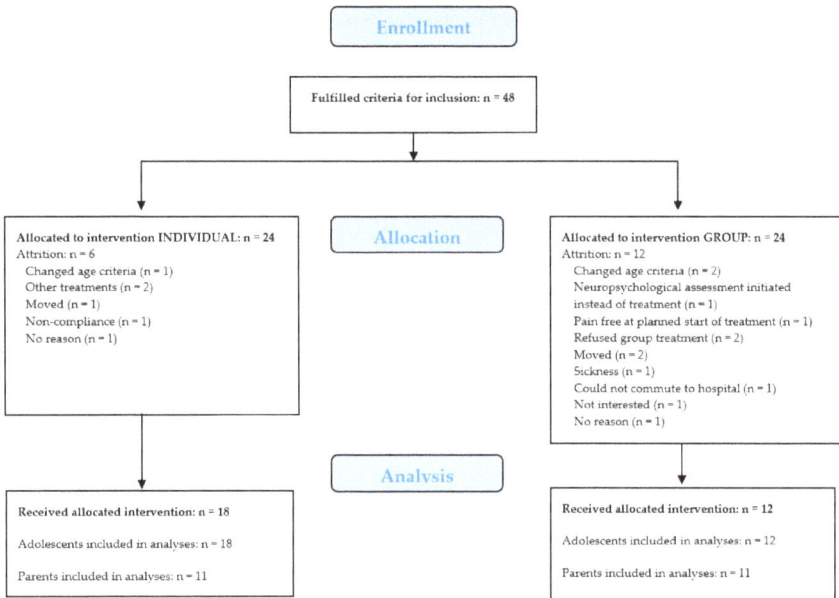

Figure 1. Flow diagram. Changed age criteria: researchers initially aimed to include participants from the age of 12 years, but due to low inflow of younger adolescents, the age range was set to 14–18 years, and three randomized participants were excluded.

2.3. Intervention

The intervention consisted of an interdisciplinary ACT-based outpatient treatment based on a protocol from a previous RCT with 10 adolescent sessions and one to two parent sessions [10]. In the current protocol, we increased the involvement of the pain physician, included two sessions with a physiotherapist to address pain interference in regard to physical activity, and added sessions conducted by the psychologists for both adolescents and parents. This resulted in a total of 18 sessions (Table 1). The majority of sessions were conducted by a psychologist.

The treatment can be divided into four phases with different, although related, treatment objectives: (1) preparing for behavior change (including pain education, conducted separately with parents and adolescents by a pain physician); (2) shifting perspective (i.e., changing the focus from pain reduction to a valued life); (3) acceptance (i.e., willingness to experience symptoms and thoughts without trying to change them) and cognitive defusion (i.e., have a perspective on and step back from thoughts and feelings); and (4) values-oriented behavior activation (i.e., behavior change in the service of living a meaningful life). All phases included the use of age-appropriate metaphors and experiential exercises and an emphasis on functional restoration and behavior activation. Importantly, although two sessions focused specifically on the processes of acceptance and defusion, these behavioral strategies were addressed and practiced continuously during all phases of the treatment. In every session, participants were given individualized home assignments related to the treatment content and to their own specific challenges, and these outcomes were discussed in the beginning of the following session.

The parent support program was embedded in the treatment and comprised of four sessions (Sessions 3, 6, 11 and 12). Session 12 was a joint session, with both adolescents and parents participating in continued pain education and discussion about pain and symptoms, in relation to values-oriented behavioral activation. In short, the objective of the parent support program was to improve the parents' ability to use values- and acceptance-based coaching behaviors, in order to support their child to increase functioning, even in the presence of pain and distress. Parents were given home assignments between Parent Sessions 6 and 11.

Table 1. Interdisciplinary ACT-based outpatient treatment

Prior to treatment: Assessment of pain and pain-related disability through semi-structured screening interviews with psychologist, pain physician and physiotherapist (3 × 1 h) followed by team discussion regarding suitability for treatment; feedback to the patient and a joint decision regarding the initiation of treatment.		
Pre-treatment assessments		
	Adolescent session	Parent session
Sessions 1–3: Preparing for behavior change.	(1) Introduction to behavior analysis of difficult pain-related situations, such as ABC-analysis * with antecedent (2) Pain education with physician directed towards adolescents (e.g., information about the pain system and differences between adaptive avoidance reactions to acute pain and potentially dysfunctional avoidance reactions to long-term pain).	(3) Pain education with physician directed towards parents.
Sessions 4–6: Shifting perspective.	(4) Individual life values: What is important in life? How have previous strategies to avoid pain and distress led away from a valued life? (5) Introduction to the concept of increased functioning also in the presence of persisting pain.	(6) Introduction to ABC-analysis of difficult pain-related parent-child situations. Pain reduction as opposed to valued living. Clarification of parental values. Being an effective coach to your child. Home assignment: practice ABC-analyses on parent-child interactions.
Mid-treatment assessments		
Sessions 7–8: Acceptance and cognitive defusion.	(7) Evaluation of previous strategies and creative hopelessness (i.e., how have previous attempts at symptom reduction prevented a valued living). (8) Acceptance and cognitive defusion.	
Sessions 9–17: Values-oriented behavioral activation.	(9) Goal setting, gradual behavior activation and exposure to previously-avoided situations, in line with life values. (10) Physiotherapist: Goal setting focused on physical activities in line with chosen values. (12) Physician: Joint session. Continued pain education and discussion about symptoms in relation to behavior change. (13) Exposure, continued. (14) Physiotherapist: Evaluation and gradual increase of values oriented physical activities. (15) Exposure, continued. (16) Recruiting family and friends for support. (17) Formulating individual plan for relapse prevention and summary of treatment.	(11) Practice of acceptance and defusion in order to facilitate behaviors in line with long-term goals and values also in the presence of own worry and distress. Follow up on parent-as-coach. (12) Physician: Joint session.
Post-treatment assessments: Concluding team session together with both adolescent and parent.		

* ABC-analysis: (A) antecedent, (B) behavior, (C) short- and long-term consequences.

The intervention was carried out either individually or in a small-group format, with the same treatment content in both conditions. Group sessions were 2 h including a break, and individual sessions were 45 min. Group sessions were longer, in order to allow participation from all group members. Both adolescent and parent sessions were conducted in a parallel format (i.e., parents in the group treatment arm received group-based parent support sessions, and parents in the individual treatment arm received individual parent support sessions). If a participant in either condition missed a session, a short summary was individually given before the start of the next session.

Treatment fidelity was assured via the use of the detailed protocol, and all five psychologists involved in delivering treatment had formal training in CBT and ACT, with varying years of experience working with pediatric chronic pain patients. All psychologists were continuously supervised by a senior researcher with extensive experience using ACT for pediatric chronic pain.

2.4. Assessment

Data collection took place at pre-, mid- and post-assessment. Demographic and medical information (e.g., pain duration, pain location, temporal aspects of pain and pain medication) was collected in semi-structured screening interviews. Parents provided background information regarding educational status and work, through a self-reported questionnaire. Adolescent and parent functioning was assessed through self-reported questionnaires at all time points.

2.4.1. Adolescent Measures

2.4.1.1. Pain Intensity

Current pain intensity for all time points was rated on a numerical rating scale from 0 (no pain at all) to 6 (extreme pain).

2.4.1.2. Pain Interference Index (PII)

The Pain Interference Index (PII) was used to assess the influence of pain on behaviors, or to what extent pain impacts everyday functioning. PII consists of six items, concerning whether pain has made it difficult to do schoolwork, leisure activities, spend time with friends, has affected mood, physical activities or sleep. Items are rated on a scale from 0 (not at all) to 6 (completely), and the maximum score is 36. The Swedish version of PII has shown sensitivity to change [10], along with satisfying reliability and internal consistency [20]. It has also been used in an English version for parents, providing further support for the consistency and validity of the instrument [21]. At pre-treatment assessment, Cronbach's alpha for PII in this sample was 0.82.

2.4.1.3. Pain Reactivity Scale (PRS)

The Pain Reactivity Scale (PRS) measures worry and general emotional reactivity to pain [10]. It contains five items: (1) How often do you worry about your pain? (2) How often are you worried that you will not be able to do things because of your pain? (3) How often are you worried that you will not be able to do things in the future because of your pain? (4) How difficult do you think it is to think about things that are related to your pain? (5) How often are you angry or said because it hurts? PRS is rated on a scale from 0 (never/not at all) to 6 (always/very much), with a maximum total score of 30. The instrument has shown sensitivity to change in ACT-treatment [10]. At pre-treatment assessment, Cronbach's alpha for PRS in this sample was 0.83.

2.4.1.4. Center for Epidemiological Studies Depression Scale Children (CES-DC)

The Center for Epidemiological Studies Depression Scale Children (CES-DC) [22,23] was used to assess depressive symptoms. The scale consists of 20 items concerning feelings and actions relevant for depressive disorder, and they are rated on a scale from 0 (not at all) to 4 (a lot), with four reversed items. The maximum score is 60. CES-DC has shown adequate psychometric properties and the ability to discriminate depressive disorder in a Swedish population of adolescents, where a cut-off of 24 was proposed [24]. At pre-treatment assessment, Cronbach's alpha for CES-DC in this sample was 0.90.

2.4.1.5. Functional Disability Index (FDI)

The Functional Disability Index (FDI) [25] was used to assess child functioning. FDI has been evaluated for pediatric patients with chronic pain, with evidence of reliability and validity [26], and it is recommended by the PedIMMPACT as a core outcome measure of physical functioning [7]. The instrument has 15 items rated on a scale from 0 (no problems) to 4 (impossible), and the maximum score is 60. There are established cut-off scores for the FDI, with 0–12 indicative of no/minimal disability, 13–20 indicative of mild disability, 21–29 indicative of moderate disability and scores of 30 or over indicative of severe disability [27]. In the present study, we used the parent version, which has been found to correlate significantly with child ratings [26]. At pre-treatment assessment, Cronbach's alpha for FDI-P in this sample was 0.93.

2.4.1.6. Psychological Inflexibility in Pain Scale (PIPS)

The Psychological Inflexibility in Pain Scale (PIPS) is a measure of psychological inflexibility (i.e., the inability to carry out behaviors in line with a valued life when pain, unpleasant thoughts or emotions are present) [6]. PIPS consists of 12 items rated on a scale from 1 (never true) to 7 (always true), and the maximum score is 84. Examples of items are: "I would do almost anything to get rid of my pain" and "it's not me that controls my life, it's my pain". Previous research with adults with chronic pain supports the psychometric properties and the use of PIPS as a process measure to assess changes in pain-related disability after ACT-based treatment [28–30]. At pre-treatment assessment, Cronbach's alpha for PIPS in this sample was 0.85.

2.4.2. Parental Measures

2.4.2.1. Hospital Anxiety and Depression Scale (HADS)

The Hospital Anxiety and Depression Scale (HADS) [31] was used to measure parental levels of anxiety and depressive symptoms. The scale consists of 14 items divided into two subscales, HADS-A and HADS-D, with seven items respectively. Agreement is rated on a scale from 0 to 3, for example "I still enjoy the things I used to enjoy" most of the time (0), a lot of the time (1), from time to time, occasionally (2) or not at all (3). A score between 0 and 7 on each subscale respectively indicates non-cases of anxiety or depressive disorder; a score between 8 and 10 indicates possible cases; and scores of 11 and above indicate probable cases (i.e., a score >8 on each scale respectively defines caseness) [32]. HADS has been used extensively across both patient and general populations with results in favor of using the instrument for both identification of caseness and of symptom severity [32], and results from a study in the general population support the validity of the Swedish version used in this sample [33] At pre-treatment assessment, Cronbach's alpha for HADS in this sample was 0.82.

2.4.2.2. Pain Reactivity Scale Parent (PRS-P)

The Pain Reactivity Scale described above was also used for parents (PRS-P) to measure their emotional reactivity to their child's pain. Parents were asked the same questions as in PRS, but in relation to their child, e.g., "How often do you worry about your child's pain". At pre-treatment assessment, Cronbach's alpha for PRS-P in this sample was 0.91.

2.4.2.3. Parent Psychological Flexibility Questionnaire (PPFQ)

The Parent Psychological Flexibility Questionnaire (PPFQ) was developed with the aim of measuring parental psychological flexibility in the context of pediatric chronic pain [17]. Further development of the instrument supported the validity and reliability of a shorter, 17-item version, and the authors suggest its potential for assessment of parent psychological flexibility in treatment interventions for pediatric patients with chronic pain [18]. Items are rated on a scale from 0 (never true) to 6 (always true), and examples of items are: "Even though my child has pain we can continue to do things that are important and enjoyable" and "My child's pain makes it impossible to focus on anything else" (reversed scoring). In this study, we used a 10-item version of the instrument, with seven reversed items and a maximum score of 60, on the basis of a psychometric evaluation and factor analysis of a Swedish version of the instrument [34]. At pre-treatment assessment, Cronbach's alpha for PPFQ in this sample was 0.82.

2.5. Data Management

Throughout the whole dataset, 12 (<1%) items were missing completely at random (MCAR). These were manually imputed via person mean imputation, in order to maximize *n* for all analyses.

2.6. Data Analysis

Due to the fact that the data was non-normally-distributed, a non-parametric approach was applied. For a comparison of non-completers versus completers, and for comparisons of conditions (group versus individual) across all assessments, Mann–Whitney U tests were used. To assess when changes occur (pre–mid-assessment, mid–post assessments and pre–post-assessment), Wilcoxon signed-rank tests were used. Effect sizes were calculated from *z*-scores and the number of total observations by use of *r* [35]. Correlational effect sizes above 0.10 indicate a small effect, above 0.30 a medium effect and above 0.50 a large effect, according to Cohen [36]. Mean-based statistics were used to calculate clinically-significant changes for all significant outcome variables and pain intensity using the 1991 Jacobson–Truax method for reliable change, where a change of two standard deviations (*SD*) in the direction of functionality from the mean of the population under investigation is considered clinically significant [37,38]. Pairwise deletion was chosen for all analyses, and all analyses were conducted with SPSS 23 and Excel 2011 for Mac. The significance level was set at a conservative level of $p < 0.01$ to account for multiple comparisons.

2.7. Ethical Considerations

All participants (parents and children) were given oral and written information about the study and provided signed informed consent. The study was approved by the Ethical Review Board in Stockholm, Sweden (2009:815:31/4, approved 2009/4:6).

3. Results

3.1. Initial Analyses

To assess potential differences between completers and non-completers/exclusions at pre-treatment assessment (*n* = 48), a series of Mann–Whitney U tests was performed. No statistically-significant differences in the pre-treatment assessments were found between children and parents who dropped out or were excluded, and children and parents who completed the study for any of the variables included in further analyses (PII, PRS, CES, FDI-P, PIPS, actual pain intensity and pain duration and parent HADS (total and subscales), PRS-P, PPFQ and parent chronic pain). All further analyses are based on the final sample of completers (*n* = 30).

3.2. Descriptive Statistics

The final sample included 30 adolescent participants (24 girls), with a mean age of 16 years and mean pain duration of more than four years. The majority of adolescents reported continuous pain from multiple sites. The parent sample included 28 parents (24 mothers), with a mean age of 47 years. Demographic and medical information is provided in Table 2.

Table 2. Demographic and medical data for adolescents and parents.

	Total Sample	Group Condition	Individual Condition
Children	30	12	18
Age *m (SD)*	16.0 (1.6)	16.3 (1.5)	15.8 (1.6)
Gender			
Girls *n* (%)	24 (80.0)	11 (91.7)	13 (72.2)
Boys *n* (%)	6 (20.0)	1 (8.3)	5 (27.8)
Pain characteristics			
Head *n* (%)	27 (90.0)	10 (83.0)	17 (94.0)
Abdominal *n* (%)	12 (40.0)	4 (33.0)	8 (44.0)
Back *n* (%)	13 (43.0)	7 (58.0)	6 (33.0)
Joint *n* (%)	5 (17.0)	4 (33.0)	1 (5.5)
Other (e.g., parts of limbs) *n* (%)	18 (60.0)	9 (75.0)	9 (50.0)
CRPS [a] *n*(%)	1 (3.3)	-	1 (5.5)
Widespread *n* (%)	6 (20.0)	4 (33.0)	2 (11.0)
Pain locations > 3 *n* (%)	16 (53.0)	8 (67.0)	8 (44.0)
Pain duration in months *m (SD)*	57.87 (49.5)	43.18 (36.3)	67.35 (55.4)
Pain duration ≥36 months *m (SD)*	17 (60.7)	6 (54.5)	11 (64.7)
Current pain intensity (0–6) *m (SD)*	3.31 (1.4)	3.75 (1.0)	3.00 (1.7)
Continuous pain *n* (%)	22 (73.3)	10 (83.3)	12 (66.7)
Pain every day *n* (%)	5 (16.7)	2 (16.7)	3 (16.7)
Pain every week *n* (%)	3 (10.0)	-	3 (16.7)
Current pain medication *n* (%)	15 (50.0)	6 (50.0)	9 (50.0)
School absence *n* (%)			
None	4 (13.3)	3 (25.0)	1 (5.6)
Moderate	16 (53.3)	4 (33.3)	12 (66.7)
Extensive (>1 day/week)	4 (13.3)	3 (25.0)	1 (5.6)
Total absence	4 (13.3)	1 (8.3)	3 (16.7)
N/A	1 (3.3)	1 (8.3)	1 (5.6)
Parents	28	12	16
Mothers *n* (%)	24 (86.0)	10 (83.3)	14 (87.5)
Age *m (SD)*	47.3 (4.8)	48.42 (4.5)	46.5 (5.0)
Parent pain duration ≥1 year *n* (%)	16 (57.1)	7 (58.3)	9 (56.2)
Marital status *n* (%)			
Married	14 (50.0)	6 (83.0)	8 (50.0)
Co-habiting	6 (21.4)	2 (16.7)	4 (25.0)
In a relationship	2 (7.1)	1 (8.3)	1 (6.3)
Single	6 (21.4)	3 (25.0)	3 (18.8)
Educational status *n* (%)			
Basic/high school	16 (57.1)	5 (41.7)	11 (68.8)
University studies	12 (42.9)	7 (58.3)	5 (31.3)
Occupational status *n* (%)			
Full time work/study	20 (71.4)	9 (75.0)	11 (68.8)
Part time work/study	5 (17.9)	-	5 (31.3)
Not working/studying	3 (10.7)	3 (25.0)	-

[a] CRPS = Complex Regional Pain Syndrome; *m* = mean; *SD* = standard deviation.

3.3. Initial Analyses: Comparison of Group and Individual Treatment

For adolescents, no statistically-significant differences were found between the conditions at baseline regarding pain duration (p = 0.409) or prevalence of parent chronic pain (p = 0.209). Similarly, there were no significant differences between the conditions in any of the outcome variables at any of the time points (pain interference, pain reactivity, depression, functional disability, psychological inflexibility and pain intensity, p = 0.109–1.00). For parents, no statistically-significant differences were found between the conditions for any of the outcome variables at any of the time points (anxiety and depression and parent pain reactivity and psychological flexibility, p = 0.022–0.961). Table 3 shows median and min-max values for the total sample and group and individual conditions, respectively, for each time point. Further evaluations of treatment effects concern the total sample ($n = 30$) if not stated otherwise.

Table 3. Median (Md) and min–max scores for adolescent and parent variables at pre-, mid- and post-treatment assessment.

Outcome Variable		Pre-Md (Min–Max)	Mid-Md (Min–Max)	Post-Md (Min–Max)
		Children		
PII (0–36)	Total	24.5 (5–35)	20.0 (4–35)	12.5 (1–35)
	Group	24.5 (11–35)	22.5 (9–35)	13.5 (6–35)
	Individual	22.5 (5–34)	18.0 (4–30)	11.0 (1–32)
PRS (0–30)	Total	21.5 (13–29)	21.0 (10–30)	13.0 (0–29)
	Group	20.0 (14–27)	21.5 (11–30)	15.0 (8–29)
	Individual	23.0 (13–29)	16.0 (10–29)	10.0 (0–28)
CES-DC (0–60)	Total	28.0 (10–47)	27.0 (15–52)	20.0 (6–47)
	Group	26.0 (10–47)	30.5 (15–52)	22.0 (9–47)
	Individual	28.5 (12–45)	26.0 (16–46)	17.0 (6–46)
FDI-P (0–60)	Total	15.5 (3–57)	10.5 (0–37)	6.0 (0–39)
	Group	19.0 (9–39)	9.5 (6–36)	6.5 (0–34)
	Individual	15.0 (3–57)	11.0 (0–37)	6.0 (0–39)
PIPS (12–84)	Total	54.0 (27–81)	49.5 (33–72)	37.0 (17–75)
	Group	54.0 (27–81)	51.0 (33–72)	40.5 (17–45)
	Individual	55.5 (38–76)	48.0 (35.50–71)	32.5 (22–65)
Pain intensity (0–6)	Total	4.0 (0–6)	4.0 (1–6)	3.0 (0–6)
	Group	4.0 (2–6)	4.0 (3–6)	4.0 (1–5)
	Individual	3.0 (0–6)	3.0 (1–6)	2.0 (0–6)
		Parents		
HADS (0–42)	Total	15.0 (0–31)	17.0 (0–30)	13.5 (0–32)
	Group	13.5 (4–19)	12.5 (0–28)	17.0 (0–23)
	Individual	17.0 (0–31)	20.0 (6–30)	10.5 (0–32)
HADS-A (0–21)	Total	9.0 (0–17)	9.5 (0–18)	7.5 (0–16)
	Group	7.5 (4–13)	6.0 (0–17)	6.5 (0–15)
	Individual	11.0 (0–17)	10.5 (3–18)	7.5 (0–16)
HADS-D (0–21)	Total	5.5 (0–14)	8.5 (0–15)	3.5 (0–16)
	Group	4.5 (0–12)	6.0 (0–11)	7.0 (0–12)
	Individual	5.5 (0–14)	9.0 (0–15)	3.0 (0–16)
PRS-P (0–30)	Total	22.5 (5–30)	20.0 (4–30)	15.0 (1–28)
	Group	22.0 (13–30)	15.0 (5–23)	14.0 (5–28)
	Individual	22.5 (5–30)	24.0 (4–30)	15.0 (1–28)
PPFQ (0–60)	Total	32.0 (9–51)	38.0 (6–48)	42.0 (15–55)
	Group	34.5 (19–51)	40.0 (31–47)	42.0 (23–55)
	Individual	24.5 (9–46)	25.5 (6–48)	41.5 (15–54)

Measurement abbreviations: PII, Pain Interference Index; PRS, Pain Reactivity Scale; CES-DC, Center for Epidemiological Studies Depression Scale Children; FDI-P, Functional Disability Inventory Parent rating; PIPS, Psychological Inflexibility in Pain Scale; HADS, Hospital Anxiety and Depression Scale; HADS-D, depression subscale; HADS-A, anxiety subscale; PRS-P, Pain Reactivity Scale Parent; PPFQ, Parent Psychological Flexibility Questionnaire.

3.4. Effects of ACT-Treatment on Adolescent Functioning, Psychological Flexibility and Pain

Pain interference was significantly higher at pre- than at post-treatment assessment, median (Md) = 24.5 versus Md = 12.5, respectively, $p < 0.001$. The effect size was large ($r = 0.51$). Pain reactivity was significantly higher at pre- than at post-treatment assessment (Md = 21.5 versus Md = 13.0, respectively, $p < 0.001$), with a medium effect size ($r = 0.49$). Depressive symptoms were significantly higher at pre- than at post-treatment assessment (Md = 28.0 versus Md = 20.0, respectively $p = 0.004$), with a medium effect size ($r = 0.37$). FDI-P-scores did not change significantly from pre- to post-treatment assessment (Md = 15.5 versus Md = 6.0, respectively, p = 0.032), but a medium effect size was seen (r = 0.35). Psychological inflexibility was significantly higher at pre- than at post-treatment assessment (Md = 54.0 versus 37.0, respectively, $p < 0.001$), with a large effect size (r = 0.59). As expected, given the treatment objective in ACT, there were no significant changes in pain intensity at any of the time points ($p > 0.608$). Details on median and min–max values are provided in Table 3, and z-scores, p-values and effect sizes are listed in Table 4.

3.5. Effects of ACT-Treatment on Parent Anxiety, Depression, Pain Reactivity and Psychological Flexibility

No significant changes were seen in parent emotional functioning overall or anxiety and depression separately ($p > 0.413$). Improvement was seen in parent pain reactivity, with significantly higher ratings at pre- than at post-treatment assessment (Md = 22.5 versus Md = 15.0, respectively, $p < 0.001$), illustrating a large effect size (r = 0.57). Parent psychological flexibility was significantly increased from pre- to post-treatment assessment (Md = 49.5 versus Md = 67.0, respectively, $p < 0.001$) with a large effect size (r = 0.62).

Table 4. Treatment effects for the total sample, for all time points, including z-scores, p-values, effect sizes and clinically significant changes.

Outcome Variable	Wilcoxon Signed Rank Test Pre–Mid Change	Wilcoxon Signed Rank Test Mid–Post Changes	Wilcoxon Signed Rank Test Pre–Post Changes	Effect Size (r) [a] Pre–Post	Clinically Significant Change [b] Pre–Post	Deterioration [c] Pre–Post
			Children			
PII	$z = -2.203$, p = 0.026	$z = -2.962$, p = 0.002 *	$z = -3.949$, $p < 0.001$ *	$r = -0.51$	14 of 30	-
PRS	$z = -0.930$, p = 0.362	$z = -3.651$, $p < 0.001$ *	$z = -3.765$, $p < 0.001$ *	$r = -0.49$	14 of 29	2 of 29
CES-DC	$z = -1.264$, p = 0.213	$z = -3.597$, $p < 0.001$ *	$z = -2.788$, p = 0.004 *	$r = -0.37$	11 of 28	2 of 28
FDI-P	$z = -2.584$, p = 0.008 *	$z = -0.142$, p = 0.901	$z = -2.134$, p = 0.032	$r = -0.35$	4 of 19	2 of 19
PIPS	$z = -2.199$, p = 0.027	$z = -4.314$, $p < 0.001$ *	$z = -4.607$, $p < 0.001$ *	$r = -0.59$	19 of 30	-
Pain intensity	$z = 0.525$, p = 0.697	$z = -1.206$, p = 0.255	$z = -0.980$, p = 0.346	$r = -0.13$	4 of 26	1 of 26
			Parents			
HADS	$z = -0.299$, p = 0.777	$z = -0.142$, p = 0.899	$z = -0.222$, p = 0.838	-	-	-
HADS-A	$z = -0.916$, p = 0.373	$z = -0.234$, p = 0.836	$z = -0.843$, p = 0.413	-	-	-
HADS-D	$z = -0.643$, p = 0.537	$z = -0.114$, p = 0.933	$z = -0.694$, p = 0.508	-	-	-
PRS-P	$z = -2.138$, p = 0.031	$z = -2.987$, p = 0.001 *	$z = -3.672$, $p < 0.001$ *	$r = -0.57$	16 of 21	-
PPFQ	$z = -2.315$, p = 0.019	$z = -3.144$, p = 0.001 *	$z = -4.117$, $p < 0.001$ *	$r = -0.62$	12 of 22	-

[a] for r, effect sizes >3 are considered of medium size and >5 large; [b] clinically-significant changes are defined as a change of >2 *SD* in the direction of functionality; [c] deterioration is defined as a change of >2 *SD* in the direction of dysfunction; * $p < 0.01$, two-tailed.

3.6. Analyses of Temporal Change Patterns

Significant changes from pre- to mid-treatment assessments were only found for functional disability (pre–mid change p = 0.008). From mid- to post-assessments, however, the changes were significant in all other variables with significant overall treatment effects. Thus, the pattern of results illustrates more significant changes from mid- to post- than from pre- to mid-treatment assessments.

3.7. Clinically Significant Changes

3.7.1. Adolescents

Table 4 shows the number of participants who have a clinically-significant change (≥ 2 *SD*) in the direction of functionality. A clinically-significant change in pain interference from pre- to post-treatment assessments was found for 47% of the participants, and a clinically-significant change in pain reactivity was found for 48%. Clinically-significant reductions of depressive symptoms were reported by 39%. For functional disability, improvement was seen in 21% of participants, and for pain intensity, 15% reported a clinically-significant reduction. Finally, 63% of participants reported a clinically-significant change in psychological flexibility. There were no significant differences between the conditions regarding the number of participants with clinically-significant improvement from pre- to post-treatment assessment for any of the variables (*p* between 0.083 and 1.00), but for depressive symptoms, there was a trend towards a significant difference ($z = -2.41$, $p = 0.028$), with more participants reporting clinically-significant reductions in depressive symptoms in the individual condition.

3.7.2. Parents

Parent reactivity to child's pain changed to a clinically-significant degree in the direction of functionality for 76% of the parents (Table 4). Similarly, 54% of parents reported clinically-significant increases in psychological flexibility. There were no significant differences between the conditions regarding the number of participants with clinically-significant improvement in neither parent pain reactivity nor psychological flexibility (*p* = 0.198).

3.8. Deterioration from Pre- to Post-Treatment Assessment

As seen in Table 4, a few adolescent participants reported deterioration (i.e., a change of ≥ 2 *SD* from pre- to post-treatment assessment). Deterioration in pain reactivity was reported by 7% of participants. In depressive symptoms, 7% also reported deterioration, and in functional disability, deterioration was seen in 11% of the adolescents. Deterioration in pain intensity was reported by 4% of participants. However, deterioration was not reported in parent pain reactivity or psychological flexibility.

4. Discussion

This clinical pilot study aimed to evaluate (1) the effects on functioning of an ACT-based intervention provided in a group or in an individual format to adolescents with disabling chronic pain conditions; and (2) the effects of a parental support program on parent functioning. Results showed improvements in adolescent functioning, as well as in parent psychological flexibility, with clinically-significant changes in the direction of a better functionality for a large portion of both adolescent and parent participants. Taken together, our findings of improved functioning in adolescents are consistent with previously-published studies on ACT for pediatric chronic pain conducted by our research group, as well as by researchers in other settings [9–15]. They are also in line with findings on improved functioning post-treatment in a systematic review on psychological therapies for pediatric chronic pain primarily based on CBT (including 37 studies, but only one ACT study) [5].

In addition to our aims, a preliminary comparison of treatment formats was conducted, which did not show any significant differences in effects between group and individually-delivered ACT treatment. However, as the sample is too small for an adequately-powered study with a non-inferiority design, the results should be seen as highly tentative, and larger studies are warranted in order to investigate the relative utility of these treatment formats. The pattern of changes between assessment points illustrated that changes occurred primarily from mid- to post-assessments. These results are interesting, as they suggest that treatment may be effective also when no or marginal improvements are seen in the first place. However, the design of the present study does not allow for any causal interpretation, and this pattern should merely be seen as indicative of the importance for future studies, including component analyses of treatment content, as well as the dose-response relationship.

In treatment of pediatric chronic pain, an overarching goal should be to decrease the impact of pain on a wide array of functioning outcomes [7,39]. The reported pre- to post-treatment assessment changes in pain interference scores and pain reactivity scores are in line with this goal. Similarly, the decreases in depressive symptoms from high pre-assessment scores in the current study (CES-DC Md = 28, which can be compared to the recommended cut-off of 24 for depressive disorder [24]) fits this pattern. Depression and functional disability commonly co-occur in chronic pain [40,41], and treatments that successfully target depressive symptoms are likely to have an important impact on overall pain-related functioning. Findings from recent systematic reviews on treatment for pediatric chronic pain [5,42] highlight the limited evidence for effects on depression in both psychological therapies overall and in intensive interdisciplinary treatment. Our results support previous findings from our research group regarding improvement in depressive symptoms (medium effect sizes) [10], suggesting that ACT treatment may hold promise in effectively targeting pain-related emotional dysfunction.

In this study, significant changes were only observed from pre- to mid-treatment assessment in functional disability (FDI-P), with baseline scores being relatively low as compared to PII-scores. This is consistent with previous findings [20] and suggests that FDI due to item content (e.g., "difficulties watching TV") does not fully capture pain-specific concerns experienced by many patients. Adolescents in our study also reported significant changes in psychological flexibility, indicating that they were dealing with private events, such as pain and emotional distress in a more efficient way post-treatment. For example, instead of shutting the blinds and taking a rest, an adolescent with headache, fatigue and the thought "I can't do it, I'd better wait until I feel better" (pain, distress and thoughts that dictate avoidance) observes these private events, decides not to act in accordance with short-term symptom relief and instead accepts symptom presence and chooses to pick up the phone and call a friend (exposure to previously-avoided situation and achievement of behavioral goal) because friendship is important (life value) and therefore worth pursuing.

This study provides an important contribution to the existing body of research on ACT-treatment for pediatric chronic pain, through the examination of clinically-significant changes in outcomes. In line with PedIMMPACT recommendations [7], pain intensity was included as a treatment outcome. While our finding for paint intensity, namely that changes in pain were not seen post-treatment, are in contrast to psychological therapies overall [5], they are still consistent with ACT-specific predictions [43]. Additionally, using the literature suggested cut-off of 2 *SD* in the direction of functionality [37], a large proportion of patients reported clinically-significant outcomes. It should be considered, however, that this cut-off is arbitrary and, in light of the severity of functional impairment and high chronicity of the population under investigation, may be seen as conservative. For example, a cut-off set at 1 *SD*, as suggested in adult chronic pain trials [44], would have rendered different results. What constitutes a clinically meaningful improvement in functioning for an adolescent with longstanding, debilitating pain should be further discussed and addressed in future trials.

The inclusion of parents in psychological therapies for pediatric chronic pain is encouraged, both on the basis of related family impact and dysfunction [3,4], and on the basis of existing evidence on child outcomes, but also because there is a need for more research concerning parent mental health and parent behavior outcomes [16,45]. That is, in addition to evaluating the importance of both overt parent behaviors and parent psychological states in relation to child dysfunction, such as observable dysfunctional parent behaviors [46] and self-reported parent behaviors and parent distress that are predictive of child distress and functioning over time [47], more studies are needed that specifically examine parent outcomes after treatment. One recent and important contribution is an Internet-delivered evaluation of family-based CBT for adolescents with chronic pain and their parents, where increased parent mental health and decreased dysfunctional parent behaviors were seen [48]. Similar to psychological therapies overall, there are only a few ACT studies evaluating parent support for parents of children and adolescents with physical health concerns [49], but findings indicate that ACT can be beneficial regarding parental adjustment for parents of children with autism [50] and can improve both child and parent outcomes in families where the child has traumatic brain injury [51] or cerebral palsy [52]. An adapted ACT-parent support program was carried out with parents of children with life-threatening illness, and parents reported decreased distress and increased psychological flexibility and mindfulness after participation [53]. Although parents have been involved in previous trials of ACT for pediatric chronic pain, to our knowledge, only one previous study exists specifically examining the effects of ACT support for parents of pediatric chronic pain patients [15]. Our study, evaluating the effects of a brief and structured ACT-based parent support program on parent mental health, parent pain reactivity and parent psychological flexibility, is therefore an important addition and extends previous findings. A majority of parents in our study reported clinically-significant improvements in dealing with their child's pain post-treatment, indicating that both the novel variable parent pain reactivity and parent psychological flexibility, which have previously been reported on [17,18], in relation to child's pain may be important treatment targets for enhancing effective parent behaviors. Regarding parent mental health, the parents in our study tended to be in the "possible cases" range of HADS at pre-treatment assessment (i.e., possibly suffering from anxiety) [32]. They reported no significant changes over the course of treatment. Future studies could include treatment content more specifically aimed at parent depressive or anxious symptoms, as such problems are commonly reported by parents of children with chronic pain [45,54] and potentially hamper effective parent behaviors for a subset of parents. Furthermore, chronic pain is common in parents of children with chronic pain [55], which is also seen in our sample, and the interference of parent chronic pain on parent behavior [56] and parent mental health should therefore be examined further.

A number of limitations should be considered when interpreting the results from this clinical pilot study. Due to the small sample, there was not enough power to adequately evaluate the relative effects from group versus individual treatment, and we suggest this as a focus for future studies. As in most clinical trials, improvements may partially be due to spontaneous recovery or other unspecific factors. However, spontaneous improvements in functioning for this sample with their long mean pain duration (>4 years) and level of disability would not be expected. Notably, our sample is similar regarding, e.g., pain duration as seen in other studies, which indicates representativeness and generalizability [42]. Furthermore, the adolescents in our study presented with relatively higher scores of depressive symptoms [57]. The representativeness of the sample was also seen in parents, as they appear similar to parent samples in other studies on pediatric chronic pain in tertiary care, regarding age and gender [13], as well as in anxiety and depression [54]. Problems with recruitment and retention in clinical trials have been described in the literature [58] and account also for this study where attrition was very high. In the present study, unexpected difficulties occurred after randomization to individual and group treatment, with two participants changing their mind after being allocated to the group condition and, thus, not initiating treatment. In addition, some parent assessments had to be excluded from the analyses due to different parents completing the questionnaires (i.e., when analyzing data, it was found that the mother conducted the rating at baseline and the father at post-assessment). Apart from following a structured protocol and regular supervision, no fidelity checks were performed in this clinical study, e.g., analyses of videotaped sessions. This is advisable for future studies to ensure protocol adherence and that sessions are performed in accordance with ACT theory. Furthermore, for adolescent pain interference and functional disability, the adolescent version of the PII and the parent version of the FDI were used when ideally both parent and adolescent ratings of both these outcomes should have been included. Finally, instead of measuring current pain intensity, a more expanded assessment, e.g., using a daily pain diary for a shorter period, would have given more detail and thereby also more confidence in regards to findings.

Compared to medical or surgical interventions aimed at pain relief, the potential harms from psychological treatments, such as ACT, are presumably low. However, the treatment objective or other related factors might induce negative feelings and expectations, highlight the fact that pain has had a major negative impact on life, and for some even provoke pain. In the present study, this might be the case for those five participants reporting clinically-significant deterioration for one or two of the variables PRS (two reports) CES-DC (two reports), FDI-P (two reports) and pain intensity (one report). This together with the wide range of values observed in most variables at all assessment points illustrates clinical challenges and a need to identify subgroups of non-responders, as well as the need to develop individually-tailored interventions and conduct careful follow-up. Our findings further support the notion that future research should address the questions of what works for whom [59,60]. As seen in our evaluation of clinically-significant changes, it is evident that some adolescents and parents benefit greatly from the interventions, whereas some do not. In a recent study of pain and functional disability trajectories during Internet-delivered CBT-treatment in an adolescent sample with chronic pain, the authors also note improvements for some participants and worsening or minimal improvements for others [61]. To date, we lack sufficient evidence for which components of treatment are related to change or which characteristics of pediatric patients suffering from chronic pain predict or moderate outcomes of both traditional CBT- and ACT-based interventions. Designing future studies to assess the details regarding change processes, including mediators and moderators of treatment outcome, is important. On a final note, it is crucial to conduct long-term follow-up. Currently, the evidence for the maintenance over time of short-term improvements in pediatric pain and disability is limited for psychological therapies overall [5], and although improvements seen post-treatment have been sustained at follow-up in previous ACT-studies [9–11,13,14], no study including pediatric participants with chronic pain has been conducted following up on ACT-treatment outcomes >1 year.

5. Conclusions

Significant improvements following an ACT-based interdisciplinary outpatient program were seen in adolescent pain interference, pain reactivity, depressive symptoms and psychological flexibility post-treatment. Furthermore, their parents reported decreased pain reactivity and increased psychological flexibility after completing a brief ACT-based parental support program. Clinically significant changes occurred for a large proportion of participants. Similar effects were seen for individual and group formats. Though tentative due to the study design, our findings provide further support for the utility of ACT to improve adolescent and parent functioning in pediatric chronic pain.

Acknowledgments: Funding for Kanstrup was provided from the Doctoral School in Health Care Sciences at Karolinska Institutet and from the Functional Area Medical Psychology at Karolinska University Hospital. Funding for Kemani was provided from the Functional Area Medical Psychology at Karolinska University Hospital. Funding for Wiwe Lipsker was provided from the KID-funding at Karolinska Institutet and from the Functional Area Medical Psychology at Karolinska University Hospital. Lekander was funded by Stockholm University (Stress Research Institute) and Karolinska Institutet (Osher Center for Integrative Medicine). Financial support for Holmström and Wicksell was provided through the regional agreement on medical training and clinical research (ALF) between Stockholm City Council and Karolinska Institutet.

Author Contributions: Wicksell conceived of and designed the study. Kanstrup, Kemani, Wiwe Lipsker and Holmström performed the study by collecting data and being involved in delivering the intervention. Kanstrup was responsible for compiling and analyzing data and wrote the paper. Holmström, Lekander and Wicksell contributed with statistical knowledge. All authors contributed substantially in reviewing and revising the manuscript and approved the final manuscript as submitted.

Conflicts of Interest: The authors declare no conflict of interest.

References

1. Hoftun, G.B.; Romundstad, P.R.; Zwart, J.-A.; Rygg, M. Chronic idiopathic pain in adolescence—High prevalence and disability: The young hunt study 2008. *Pain* **2011**, *152*, 2259–2266. [CrossRef] [PubMed]
2. King, S.; Chambers, C.T.; Huguet, A.; MacNevin, R.C.; McGrath, P.J.; Parker, L.; MacDonald, A.J. The epidemiology of chronic pain in children and adolescents revisited: A systematic review. *Pain* **2011**, *152*, 2729–2738. [CrossRef] [PubMed]

3. Lewandowski, A.S.; Palermo, T.M.; Stinson, J.; Handley, S.; Chambers, C.T. Systematic review of family functioning in families of children and adolescents with chronic pain. *J. Pain* **2010**, *11*, 1027–1038. [CrossRef] [PubMed]
4. Groenewald, C.B.; Essner, B.S.; Wright, D.; Fesinmeyer, M.D.; Palermo, T.M. The economic costs of chronic pain among a cohort of treatment-seeking adolescents in the United States. *J. Pain* **2014**, *15*, 925–933. [CrossRef] [PubMed]
5. Eccleston, C.; Palermo, T.M.; Williams, A.C.; Lewandowski Holley, A.; Morley, S.; Fisher, E.; Law, E. Psychological therapies for the management of chronic and recurrent pain in children and adolescents. *Cochrane Database Syst. Rev.* **2014**. [CrossRef]
6. Hayes, S.C.; Luoma, J.B.; Bond, F.W.; Masuda, A.; Lillis, J. Acceptance and commitment therapy: Model, processes and outcomes. *Behav. Res. Ther.* **2006**, *44*, 1–25. [CrossRef] [PubMed]
7. McGrath, P.J.; Walco, G.A.; Turk, D.C.; Dworkin, R.H.; Brown, M.T.; Davidson, K.; Eccleston, C.; Finley, G.A.; Goldschneider, K.; Haverkos, L.; et al. Core outcome domains and measures for pediatric acute and chronic/recurrent pain clinical trials: Pedimmpact recommendations. *J. Pain* **2008**, *9*, 771–783. [CrossRef] [PubMed]
8. Society of Clinical Psychology, American Psychological Association, division 12. Acceptance and Commitment Therapy for Chronic Pain. 2011. Available online: https://wwwdiv12org/psychological-treatments/disorders/chronic-or-persistent-pain/acceptance-and-commitment-therapy-for-chronic-pain/ (accessed on 1 September 2016).
9. Wicksell, R.K.; Melin, L.; Olsson, G.L. Exposure and acceptance in the rehabilitation of adolescents with idiopathic chronic pain—A pilot study. *Eur. J. Pain* **2007**, *11*, 267–274. [CrossRef] [PubMed]
10. Wicksell, R.K.; Melin, L.; Lekander, M.; Olsson, G.L. Evaluating the effectiveness of exposure and acceptance strategies to improve functioning and quality of life in longstanding pediatric pain—A randomized controlled trial. *Pain* **2009**, *141*, 248–257. [CrossRef] [PubMed]
11. Wicksell, R.K.; Dahl, J.; Magnusson, B.; Olsson, G.L. Using acceptance and commitment therapy in the rehabilitation of an adolescent female with chronic pain: A case example. *Cogn. Behav. Pract.* **2005**, *12*, 415–423. [CrossRef]
12. Wicksell, R.K.; Olsson, G.L.; Hayes, S.C. Mediators of change in acceptance and commitment therapy for pediatric chronic pain. *Pain* **2011**, *152*, 2792–2801. [CrossRef] [PubMed]
13. Gauntlett-Gilbert, J.; Connell, H.; Clinch, J.; McCracken, L.M. Acceptance and values-based treatment of adolescents with chronic pain: Outcomes and their relationship to acceptance. *J. Pediatr. Psychol.* **2013**, *38*, 72–81. [CrossRef] [PubMed]
14. Ghomian, S.; Shairi, M. The effectiveness of acceptance and commitment therapy for children with chronic pain on the function of 7 to 12 year-old. *Int. J. Pediatr.* **2014**, *2*, 47–55.
15. Martin, S.; Wolters, P.L.; Toledo-Tamula, M.A.; Schmitt, S.N.; Baldwin, A.; Starosta, A.; Gillespie, A.; Widemann, B. Acceptance and commitment therapy in youth with neurofibromatosis type 1 (nf1) and chronic pain and their parents: A pilot study of feasibility and preliminary efficacy. *Am. J. Med. Genet. Part A* **2016**, *170*, 1462–1470. [CrossRef] [PubMed]
16. Eccleston, C.; Fisher, E.; Law, E.; Bartlett, J.; Palermo, T.M. Psychological interventions for parents of children and adolescents with chronic illness. *Cochrane Database Syst. Rev.* **2015**. [CrossRef]
17. McCracken, L.M.; Gauntlett-Gilbert, J. Role of psychological flexibility in parents of adolescents with chronic pain: Development of a measure and preliminary correlation analyses. *Pain* **2011**, *152*, 780–785. [CrossRef] [PubMed]
18. Wallace, D.P.; McCracken, L.M.; Weiss, K.E.; Harbeck-Weber, C. The role of parent psychological flexibility in relation to adolescent chronic pain: Further instrument development. *J. Pain* **2015**, *16*, 235–246. [CrossRef] [PubMed]
19. Kanstrup, M.; Holmstrom, L.; Ringstrom, R.; Wicksell, R.K. Insomnia in paediatric chronic pain and its impact on depression and functional disability. *Eur. J. Pain* **2014**, *18*, 1094–1102. [CrossRef] [PubMed]
20. Holmstrom, L.; Kemani, M.K.; Kanstrup, M.; Wicksell, R.K. Evaluating the statistical properties of the pain interference index in children and adolescents with chronic pain. *J. Dev. Behav. Pediatr.* **2015**, *36*, 450–454. [CrossRef] [PubMed]

21. Martin, S.; Nelson Schmitt, S.; Wolters, P.L.; Abel, B.; Toledo-Tamula, M.A.; Baldwin, A.; Wicksell, R.K.; Merchant, M.; Widemann, B. Development and validation of the english pain interference index and pain interference index-parent report. *Pain Med* **2015**, *16*, 367–373. [CrossRef] [PubMed]

22. Faulstich, M.E.; Carey, M.P.; Ruggiero, L.; Enyart, P.; Gresham, F. Assessment of depression in childhood and adolescence: An evaluation of the center for epidemiological studies depression scale for children (CES-DC). *Am. J. Psychiatry* **1986**, *143*, 1024–1027. [PubMed]

23. Weissman, M.M.; Orvaschel, H.; Padian, N. Children's symptom and social functioning self-report scales. Comparison of mothers' and children's reports. *J. Nerv. Ment. Dis.* **1980**, *168*, 736–740. [CrossRef] [PubMed]

24. Olsson, G.; von Knorring, A.L. Depression among swedish adolescents measured by the self-rating scale center for epidemiology studies-depression child (CES-DC). *Eur. Child Adolesc. Psychiatry* **1997**, *6*, 81–87. [CrossRef] [PubMed]

25. Walker, L.S.; Greene, J.W. The functional disability inventory: Measuring a neglected dimension of child health status. *J. Pediatr. Psychol.* **1991**, *16*, 39–58. [CrossRef] [PubMed]

26. Claar, R.L.; Walker, L.S. Functional assessment of pediatric pain patients: Psychometric properties of the functional disability inventory. *Pain* **2006**, *121*, 77–84. [CrossRef] [PubMed]

27. Kashikar-Zuck, S.; Flowers, S.R.; Claar, R.L.; Guite, J.W.; Logan, D.E.; Lynch-Jordan, A.M.; Palermo, T.M.; Wilson, A.C. Clinical utility and validity of the functional disability inventory among a multicenter sample of youth with chronic pain. *Pain* **2011**, *152*, 1600–1607. [CrossRef] [PubMed]

28. Wicksell, R.K.; Renofalt, J.; Olsson, G.L.; Bond, F.W.; Melin, L. Avoidance and cognitive fusion—Central components in pain related disability? Development and preliminary validation of the psychological inflexibility in pain scale (pips). *Eur. J. Pain* **2008**, *12*, 491–500. [CrossRef] [PubMed]

29. Wicksell, R.K.; Olsson, G.L.; Hayes, S.C. Psychological flexibility as a mediator of improvement in acceptance and commitment therapy for patients with chronic pain following whiplash. *Eur. J. Pain* **2010**, *14*, 1059.e1–1059.e11. [CrossRef] [PubMed]

30. Wicksell, R.K.; Lekander, M.; Sorjonen, K.; Olsson, G.L. The psychological inflexibility in pain scale (pips)—Statistical properties and model fit of an instrument to assess change processes in pain related disability. *Eur. J. Pain* **2010**, *14*, 771.e1–771.e14. [CrossRef] [PubMed]

31. Snaith, R.P.; Zigmond, A.S. The hospital anxiety and depression scale. *Br. Med. J. (Clin. Res. Ed.)* **1986**, *292*, 344. [CrossRef]

32. Bjelland, I.; Dahl, A.A.; Haug, T.T.; Neckelmann, D. The validity of the hospital anxiety and depression scale: An updated literature review. *J. Psychosom. Res.* **2002**, *52*, 69–77. [CrossRef]

33. Lisspers, J.; Nygren, A.; Söderman, E. Hospital anxiety and depression scale (had): Some psychometric data for a swedish sample. *Acta Psychiatr. Scand.* **1997**, *96*, 281–286. [CrossRef] [PubMed]

34. Wiwe Lipsker, C.; Kanstrup, M.; Holmström, L.; Kemani, M.; Wicksell, R.K. The parent psychological flexibility questionnaire —Item reduction and validation in a clinical sample of Swedish parents of children with chronic pain. *Children*. accepted.

35. Field, A. *Discovering Statistics Using SPSS*, 3rd ed.; SAGE Publications: London, England, 2009; p. 821.

36. Cohen, J. *Statistical Power Analysis for the Behavioral Sciences*; L. Erlbaum Associates: Hillsdale, NJ, USA, 1988.

37. Jacobson, N.S.; Truax, P. Clinical significance: A statistical approach to defining meaningful change in psychotherapy research. *J. Consult. Clin. Psychol.* **1991**, *59*, 12–19. [CrossRef] [PubMed]

38. Wise, E.A. Methods for analyzing psychotherapy outcomes: A review of clinical significance, reliable change, and recommendations for future directions. *J. Pers. Assess.* **2004**, *82*, 50–59. [CrossRef] [PubMed]

39. Palermo, T.M. Enhancing daily functioning with exposure and acceptance strategies: An important stride in the development of psychological therapies for pediatric chronic pain. *Pain* **2009**, *141*, 189–190. [CrossRef] [PubMed]

40. Zernikow, B.; Wager, J.; Hechler, T.; Hasan, C.; Rohr, U.; Dobe, M.; Meyer, A.; Hoebner-Moehler, B.; Wamsler, C.; Blankenburg, M. Characteristics of highly impaired children with severe chronic pain: A 5-year retrospective study on 2249 pediatric pain patients. *BMC Pediatr.* **2012**, *12*, 54. [CrossRef] [PubMed]

41. Kashikar-Zuck, S.; Goldschneider, K.R.; Powers, S.W.; Vaught, M.H.; Hershey, A.D. Depression and functional disability in chronic pediatric pain. *Clin. J. Pain* **2001**, *17*, 341–349. [CrossRef] [PubMed]

42. Hechler, T.; Kanstrup, M.; Holley, A.L.; Simons, L.E.; Wicksell, R.; Hirschfeld, G.; Zernikow, B. Systematic review on intensive interdisciplinary pain treatment of children with chronic pain. *Pediatrics* **2015**, *136*, 115–127. [CrossRef] [PubMed]

43. Hayes, S.C.; Duckworth, M.P. Acceptance and commitment therapy and traditional cognitive behavior therapy approaches to pain. *Cogn. Behav. Pract.* **2006**, *13*, 185–187. [CrossRef]

44. Kemani, M.K.; Olsson, G.L.; Lekander, M.; Hesser, H.; Andersson, E.; Wicksell, R.K. Efficacy and cost-effectiveness of acceptance and commitment therapy and applied relaxation for longstanding pain: A randomized controlled trial. *Clin. J. Pain* **2015**, *31*, 1004–1016. [CrossRef] [PubMed]

45. Palermo, T.M.; Eccleston, C. Parents of children and adolescents with chronic pain. *Pain* **2009**, *146*, 15–17. [CrossRef] [PubMed]

46. Dunford, E.; Thompson, M.; Gauntlett-Gilbert, J. Parental behaviour in paediatric chronic pain: A qualitative observational study. *Clin. Child Psychol. Psychiatry* **2014**, *19*, 561–575. [CrossRef] [PubMed]

47. Chow, E.T.; Otis, J.D.; Simons, L.E. The longitudinal impact of parent distress and behavior on functional outcomes among youth with chronic pain. *J. Pain* **2016**, *17*, 729–738. [CrossRef] [PubMed]

48. Palermo, T.M.; Law, E.F.; Fales, J.; Bromberg, M.H.; Jessen-Fiddick, T.; Tai, G. Internet-delivered cognitive-behavioral treatment for adolescents with chronic pain and their parents: A randomized controlled multicenter trial. *Pain* **2016**, *157*, 174–185. [CrossRef] [PubMed]

49. Wicksell, R.K.; Kanstrup, M.; Kemani, M.K.; Holmström, L.; Olsson, G.L. Acceptance and commitment therapy for children and adolescents with physical health concerns. *Curr. Opin. Psychol.* **2015**, *2*, 1–5. [CrossRef]

50. Blackledge, J.T.; Hayes, S.C. Using acceptance and commitment training in the support of parents of children diagnosed with autism. *Child Fam. Behav. Ther.* **2006**, *28*, 1–18. [CrossRef]

51. Brown, F.L.; Whittingham, K.; Boyd, R.N.; McKinlay, L.; Sofronoff, K. Improving child and parenting outcomes following paediatric acquired brain injury: A randomised controlled trial of stepping stones triple p plus acceptance and commitment therapy. *J. Child Psychol. Psychiatry Allied Discipl.* **2014**, *55*, 1172–1183. [CrossRef] [PubMed]

52. Whittingham, K.; Sanders, M.; McKinlay, L.; Boyd, R.N. Interventions to reduce behavioral problems in children with cerebral palsy: An RCT. *Pediatrics* **2014**, *133*, e1249–e1257. [CrossRef] [PubMed]

53. Burke, K.; Muscara, F.; McCarthy, M.; Dimovski, A.; Hearps, S.; Anderson, V.; Walser, R. Adapting acceptance and commitment therapy for parents of children with life-threatening illness: Pilot study. *Fam. Syst. Health* **2014**, *32*, 122–127. [CrossRef] [PubMed]

54. Eccleston, C.; Crombez, G.; Scotford, A.; Clinch, J.; Connell, H. Adolescent chronic pain: Patterns and predictors of emotional distress in adolescents with chronic pain and their parents. *Pain* **2004**, *108*, 221–229. [CrossRef] [PubMed]

55. Hoftun, G.B.; Romundstad, P.R.; Rygg, M. Association of parental chronic pain with chronic pain in the adolescent and young adult: Family linkage data from the hunt study. *JAMA Pediatr.* **2013**, *167*, 61–69. [CrossRef] [PubMed]

56. Wilson, A.C.; Fales, J.L. Parenting in the context of chronic pain: A controlled study of parents with chronic pain. *Clin. J. Pain* **2015**, *31*, 689–698. [CrossRef] [PubMed]

57. Holm, S.; Ljungman, G.; Asenlof, P.; Linton, S.J.; Soderlund, A. Treating youth in pain: Comparing tailored behavioural medicine treatment provided by physical therapists in primary care with physical exercises. *Eur. J. Pain* **2015**. [CrossRef] [PubMed]

58. Gul, R.B.; Ali, P.A. Clinical trials: The challenge of recruitment and retention of participants. *J. Clin. Nurs.* **2010**, *19*, 227–233. [CrossRef] [PubMed]

59. Kazdin, A.E. Mediators and mechanisms of change in psychotherapy research. *Annu. Rev. Clin. Psychol.* **2007**, *3*, 1–27. [CrossRef] [PubMed]

60. Vlaeyen, J.W.; Morley, S. Cognitive-behavioral treatments for chronic pain: What works for whom? *Clin. J. Pain* **2005**, *21*, 1–8. [CrossRef] [PubMed]

61. Palermo, T.M.; Law, E.F.; Zhou, C.; Holley, A.L.; Logan, D.; Tai, G. Trajectories of change during a randomized controlled trial of internet-delivered psychological treatment for adolescent chronic pain: How does change in pain and function relate? *Pain* **2015**, *156*, 626–634. [CrossRef] [PubMed]

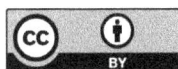

children

Article

The Parent Psychological Flexibility Questionnaire (PPFQ): Item Reduction and Validation in a Clinical Sample of Swedish Parents of Children with Chronic Pain

Camilla Wiwe Lipsker [1,2,*], Marie Kanstrup [1,2], Linda Holmström [1,3], Mike Kemani [1,2] and Rikard K. Wicksell [1,2]

[1] Functional Area Medical Psychology/Functional Unit Behavior Medicine, Uppgång P8:01, Karolinska University Hospital, SE-171 76 Stockholm, Sweden; marie.kanstrup@ki.se (M.K.); linda.holmstrom@ki.se (L.H.); mike.kemani@ki.se (M.K.); rikard.wicksell@ki.se (R.K.W.)
[2] Department of Clinical Neuroscience, Karolinska Institutet, 171 77 Stockholm, Sweden
[3] Department of Women's and Children's Health, Karolinska Institutet, 171 77 Stockholm, Sweden
* Correspondence: camilla.wiwe-lipsker@karolinska.se; Tel.: +46-76-225-6510

Academic Editor: Lynn Walker
Received: 20 September 2016; Accepted: 7 November 2016; Published: 19 November 2016

Abstract: In pediatric chronic pain, research indicates a positive relation between parental psychological flexibility (i.e., the parent's willingness to experience distress related to the child's pain in the service of valued behavior) and level of functioning in the child. This points to the utility of targeting parental psychological flexibility in pediatric chronic pain. The Parent Psychological Flexibility Questionnaire (PPFQ) is currently the only instrument developed for this purpose, and two previous studies have indicated its reliability and validity. The current study sought to validate the Swedish version of the 17-item PPFQ (PPFQ-17) in a sample of parents (n = 263) of children with chronic pain. Factor structure and internal reliability were evaluated by means of principal component analysis (PCA) and Cronbach's alpha. Concurrent criterion validity was examined by hierarchical multiple regression analyses with parental anxiety and depression as outcomes. The PCA supported a three-factor solution with 10 items explaining 69.5% of the total variance. Cronbach's alpha (0.86) indicated good internal consistency. The 10-item PPFQ (PPFQ-10) further explained a significant amount of variance in anxiety (29%), and depression (35.6%), confirming concurrent validity. In conclusion, results support the reliability and validity of the PPFQ-10, and suggest its usefulness in assessing psychological flexibility in parents of children with chronic pain.

Keywords: psychological flexibility; validation; pediatric chronic pain; parents; anxiety; depression; distress; Acceptance and Commitment Therapy (ACT)

1. Introduction

Psychological flexibility, the core treatment target in Acceptance and Commitment Therapy (ACT) [1], is conceptualized as the ability for adaptive, values-oriented behavior in the presence of distressing experiences [2]. Psychological flexibility has also been described as a "fundamental aspect of health", with high relevance to distress, such as anxiety and depression, where there is typically a lack of flexibility [3]. Current research further indicates that parental psychological flexibility may act as a possible moderator in the relationship between parent- and child-distress [4], and also that psychological flexibility within the parenting role is associated with adaptive parenting behavior in non-clinical samples [4,5].

There is emerging evidence for the utility of ACT in pediatric chronic pain [6–9]. In the context of pediatric chronic pain, parental psychological flexibility is defined as the parent's willingness to experience distress related to the child's pain, in the service of long-term values and related behavioral goals for both parent and child [10,11]. Research on parents of children with chronic pain has also shown a positive relationship between parental psychological flexibility and level of functioning in the child, and has pointed to the utility of targeting parental psychological flexibility in treatments with ACT for pediatric chronic pain, in order to potentially improve child treatment effects [10,11]. There is also mounting evidence concerning the association between parental distress, such as anxiety, fear, catastrophizing, and depression, and functional disability in children with chronic pain [12–14], even at subclinical levels of parental distress [15]. For example, research shows that parental distress influences parent behavior toward more protecting and monitoring, which contributes to the child's distress, fear, catastrophizing, and avoidance behaviors; factors with a direct impact on pain related functional disability in the child [16–18].

Psychological flexibility appears to be a context specific construct, in terms of the area of study (e.g., pain, parenting, workplace, or other), and therefore needs to be assessed as such [4,19]. This implies the need for reliable and valid instruments to assess parental psychological flexibility within the context of pediatric chronic pain. To date, only one such instrument has been specifically developed, the Parent Psychological Flexibility Questionnaire (PPFQ) [10,11]. However, the PPFQ has not yet been validated in a Swedish sample. The first study by McCracken and Gauntlett-Gilbert included development of the PPFQ by generating a set of items constructed to reflect aspects related to psychological flexibility (e.g., acceptance, cognitive defusion, and values-based action), of which 24 of the original 31 items were retained for analysis. Results supported internal reliability for the preliminary instrument and suggested concurrent validity through associations with child functioning and parent responses to child pain [11]. The second study by Wallace et al. [10] aimed to further refine and examine the reliability and validity of the 24-item PPFQ (PPFQ-24). This resulted in a 17-item questionnaire (PPFQ-17) with four factors: (1) values-based action (VBA); (2) emotional acceptance (EA); (3) pain acceptance (PA); and (4) pain willingness (PW). The subscales and the full measure generally had adequate internal reliability (though weaker for the three-item PW subscale), and demonstrated adequate correlations with adolescent-reported measures of pain, functioning, pain acceptance, and distress. The authors concluded the PPFQ-17 to be a reasonably reliable and valid measure for clinical use and further research. However, it was also noted that the PA subscale, with few significant correlations and "no unique contributions within the measures included", should be further investigated in future studies designed to test, for example, parental distress, which may result in a briefer measure excluding the PA subscale [10]. Therefore, the objectives of the current study were to (1) explore the factor structure and reliability of the Swedish version of the PPFQ-17 in a sample of parents of children referred to a tertiary pain clinic for chronic pain; and (2) to investigate the concurrent validity of the PPFQ by analyzing its relation to parental distress (anxiety and depression) among parents of children and adolescents with chronic debilitating pain.

2. Materials and Methods

2.1. Procedure and Participants

The study utilized a cross-sectional design including 263 parents of children with chronic pain who had been consecutively referred to a tertiary care pain clinic in Stockholm County, Sweden. Participants were recruited during a period of four years, and were excluded from the study if they were non-Swedish speakers. Mean age for the participating parents was 44.4 years, and the sample consisted of 81% women. A majority of the participating parents (53%) reported having studied at the university level. The regional ethical review board in Stockholm (Regionala etikprovningsnamnden i Stockholm; FE 289; 171 77; Stockholm, Sweden) approved of the study and participants provided written and informed consent. Assessments of the children were also collected, and analyses and results based on these assessments have been previously reported [20,21]. In brief, most children reported multisite pain (76%), the mean pain duration was four years, the majority of the children were girls (72%), and the mean age was 14 years (*SD* = 2.64).

2.2. Assessments

Data was collected by means of self-report questionnaires by the parent accompanying the child to the first visit at the clinic prior to any assessment or intervention.

2.2.1. Demographic Variables

Demographic variables included parental age, parental gender, and parental level of education divided into two categories: basic education/high school and university studies.

2.2.2. Distress (Anxiety and Depression)

The Hospital Anxiety and Depression Scale (HADS) was used to assess anxiety and depression in parents. The two subscales, anxiety (HADS-a) and depression (HADS-d), each consist of seven items rated on a four-point Likert scale (0–3) [22]. The scale has established clinical cutoffs at a score of 8 for each scale [23], and the HADS is one of the most widely used measures of anxiety and depressive symptoms in general medical settings and has been used with a wide variety of medical patients [24]. It has also been used in a number of validation, intervention, and correlational studies concerning acceptance and psychological flexibility, in relation to chronic pain, but also for other conditions as well [25–31]. Furthermore, it has been used with parents of adolescents with chronic illness and, compared with other measures of anxiety or depression, it excludes symptoms that might be somatic aspects of physical illness, such as, for example, insomnia or fatigue [32]. In the current sample, Cronbach's alpha was 0.88 for both subscales (HADS-a and HADS-d).

2.2.3. Parental Psychological Flexibility

The PPFQ aims to assess parents' ability to effectively manage their own distress concerning their adolescent's pain, while keeping actions directed towards goals and values [10,11]. The version used in the current study contained the 17 items as proposed by Wallace et al. [10] and four subscales (factors) as described above, and parents responded to each item using a seven-point scale ranging from 0 = never true to 6 = always true. Items were developed to reflect aspects of relevance to psychological flexibility [2], namely acceptance, cognitive defusion, and values-based action. Cronbach's alpha for the original 24-item scale was 0.91, and this scale was validated by comparison with demographic variables, pain related variables, adolescent functioning, and parent responses to child pain. Initial analyses suggested the reliability and validity of the scale regarding parent behavior, as well as its potential importance in relation to adolescent functioning [11]. Cronbach's alpha for PPFQ-17 was 0.87 in the original study by Wallace et al. [10] and 0.90 in the current sample.

2.3. Translation and Swedish Adaptation

Permission to translate and validate the PPFQ from the English version, originally developed by McCracken et al. [11], to Swedish, was obtained from the authors of the original PPFQ. Based on standards for self-report translation and cross-cultural adaption processes [33], the PPFQ was translated by a clinical psychologist specialized in chronic pain and ACT, with a PhD in clinical psychology, and back-translated by two proficient English speakers. Prior to the study, the pre-final version was administered to a group of parents of children with chronic pain. They provided input on the wording and content of the questionnaire and were asked about possible difficulties related to understanding item-content.

2.4. Analytical Approach

2.4.1. Data and Missing Values Analysis

All analyses were computed using SPSS Statistics (Version 22; IBM: Armonk, NY, USA, 2013). Frequency distributions were analyzed to ascertain multivariate normality of data. Analysis of missing values was performed, and the Expectation-Maximization algorithm (E-M) for imputing missing data was employed.

2.4.2. Factor Structure and Internal Consistency

Initial analyses included inter-item correlations, sampling adequacy, and factorability of the PPFQ-17 [34]. In line with the aim of further exploration, rather than testing the model fit of the existing factor solution, a principal components analysis (PCA) was performed to examine the underlying factor structure of PPFQ items, and to optimize the possibility for data reduction [34]. Both varimax (orthogonal) and direct oblimin (oblique; with delta = 0) rotations of the factor loading matrix were used to achieve the simplest factor structure possible [35], before deciding on a rotation for the final model. The rotated factor structure was examined for items with poorer extraction (communality; lower than 0.4) within the factor structure or cross-loadings (higher than 0.32 on a second factor) to determine the most simple solution with clear and meaningful factors [35]. The internal consistency of the total scale and the respective subscales was calculated using Cronbach's alpha in an iterative process in order to identify items that did not contribute, or had a negative contribution, to the scales' alpha. Items with a negative impact were subsequently removed. The strength of Cronbach's alpha was determined according to the reliability matrix for research in psychology by Ponterotto and Ruchdeschel [36].

2.4.3. Concurrent Criterion Validity

The concurrent criterion validity of the PPFQ (subscales and total scale) was investigated by analyzing the relationship with anxiety (HADS-a) and depression (HADS-d). Pearson product-moment correlation coefficients were calculated between demographic variables, psychological flexibility, anxiety, and depression. A correlation $r = \pm0.00–0.29$ was considered weak, $r = \pm0.30–0.49$, moderate, $r = \pm0.50–0.89$, strong, and $r \geq \pm0.90$, very strong [37]. Following correlations, two hierarchical regression analyses were performed to investigate the variance explained by PPFQ in anxiety and depression respectively. Age, gender, and education were included as control variables in the first step (step 1), followed by the PPFQ (step 2).

3. Results

3.1. Data and Missing Values Analysis

Of the 280 participants recruited, 94% (n = 263) had data on the main variables included (i.e., PPFQ and HADS) and could therefore be used for the analyses. Across all parent forms, 30 data points were missing for the PPFQ (0.8% of possible responses), and 18 data points were missing for HADS (0.5% of possible responses). Missing data was found to be missing completely at random (MCAR) [38]. Visual inspection of histograms, Q-Q plots, and box plots showed that the scores on the main variables were approximately normally distributed.

3.2. Exploratory Factor Analysis

All 17 PPFQ-items correlated at least 0.3 with at least one other item, and no item correlated with another item above 0.8, suggesting reasonable factorability. Communalities were all above 0.3, indicating that items shared some common variance with other items. The Kaiser-Meyer-Olkin measure of sampling adequacy was 0.89, and Bartlett's test of sphericity was significant (χ^2 (136) = 2263.964, $p < 0.000$). The diagonals of the anti-image correlation matrix were all over 0.5.

All 17 PPFQ-items were subjected to a PCA. Three components achieved eigenvalues greater than 1 (the initial five eigenvalues were 6.68, 2.23, 1.38, 0.94, and 0.84), and inspection of the scree plot also suggested a three-factor solution. Based on previous research resulting in four factors, three- and four-factor solutions were examined using both varimax and oblimin rotations of the factor loading matrix. The three-factor solution, which explained 60.5% of the variance in the PPFQ-17, was finally chosen based on eigenvalues and the pattern in the scree plot, and because there were an insufficient number of primary loadings and difficulties in interpreting the fourth factor. We subsequently repeated the analysis with a forced extraction of three factors. Since there was little difference between the varimax and oblimin solutions, we decided on an oblimin rotation for the final solution, assuming that the latent factors would be related [34].

In order to determine as simple a solution as possible, with clear and meaningful factors and best possible internal consistency, items were then sequentially eliminated due to loading on multiple factors, poorer extraction (communality) within the factor structure, or negative contribution to each subscale's alpha, according to the criteria detailed in Section 2.4.2. This process resulted in a 10-item measure (PPFQ-10) with three factors that explained 69.5% of the variance (Table 1). All factor loadings were greater than 0.68, and each subscale had a number of items loading strongly upon it. Three of the four-factor labels proposed by Wallace et al. [10], VBA, PW, and EA, suited the three extracted factors perfectly and were subsequently retained. In line with the previous discussion in Wallace et al. [10], one of the factors, PA, was eliminated in the process. Internal consistency for each of the scales was examined using Cronbach's alpha, taking into account the number of items [36]. The subscales had fair, moderate, and excellent internal consistency (PW, VBA, EA, respectively, α between 0.73 and 0.87), and the full measure had good internal consistency (α = 0.86). The skewness and kurtosis were within a tolerable range for assuming a normal distribution, and examination of the histograms further suggested that the distributions were approximately normal. Alpha values and descriptive statistics are presented in Table 2.

Table 1. Factor loadings and communalities, based on a principle components analysis (PCA) with oblimin rotation, for 10 items from the 17-item version of The Parent Psychological Flexibility Questionnaire (PPFQ-17; *n* = 263).

Item No. [a]	Item [a]	Factor Loadings [b]			Communality (Extraction)
		EA	PW	VBA	
7	Despite my child's pain, we are able to pursue activities that are important to our family.		0.157	0.820	0.721
8	When my child has pain episodes, I am able to remain aware of our goals and other things that are important to us as a family.	0.271	−0.113	0.715	0.696
11	It is possible to live a normal life while my child suffers with pain.			0.814	0.652
9r	I avoid situations where my child will have pain.		0.756	0.124	0.607
13r	Pain control must come first whenever my child does activities.		0.780	−0.138	0.698
24r	My child must avoid activities that lead to pain.		0.826		0.683
22r	I suffer terribly from my child's pain and need to make this suffering stop.	0.830			0.744
26r	My child's pain makes it impossible to focus on anything else.	0.683		0.243	0.717
28r	I am overwhelmed by worry over my child's pain.	0.845			0.753
31r	I struggle with my own thoughts and feelings about my child's pain.	0.853			0.681

[a] From the original PPFQ by McCracken et al. [11]; *r* = reversed scored item. Values are reported from the pattern matrix, sorted by subscale; total variance explained = 69.5%; Factor loadings < 0.1 are suppressed; [b] Extraction method: PCA, with oblimin as the rotation method (kaiser normalized; rotation converged in five iterations); EA, emotional acceptance; PW, pain willingness; VBA, values-based action.

Table 2. Descriptive statistics for the 10-item PPFQ (PPFQ-10) subscales and full scale (*n* = 263).

Scale	No. of Items	Mean (SD)	Skewness	Kurtosis	Alpha
VBA	3	10.41 (4.06)	−0.208	−0.363	0.76
PW	3	7.23 (4.32)	0.269	−0.698	0.73
EA	4	12.48 (5.97)	0.166	−0.741	0.87
Full scale	10	30.12 (11.45)	−0.059	−0.306	0.86

3.3. Concurrent Criterion Validity

3.3.1. Descriptive Analyses and Correlations

Means, standard deviations, and bivariate correlations for all variables are presented in Table 3. Regarding parental distress, as measured by the HADS (with clinical cutoffs of 8 for each scale) [23], 35% of parents reported levels of anxiety symptoms at 8 or above and 21% reported depressive symptoms at 8 or above.

There was a significant positive relationship between the PPFQ-17 and the PPFQ-10 versions ($r = 0.96$, $n = 263$, $p < 0.000$). This correlation was very strong. All three PPFQ-10 subscales had a significant positive and strong correlation with both the PPFQ-10 and PPFQ-17 full scales. Furthermore, results revealed significant negative correlations between psychological flexibility and anxiety (PPFQ-17: $r = -0.48$, $n = 263$, $p < 0.000$; PPFQ-10: $r = -0.52$, $n = 263$, $p < 0.000$), and between psychological flexibility and depression (PPFQ-17: $r = -0.49$, $n = 263$, $p < 0.000$; PPFQ-10: $r = -0.53$, $n = 263$, $p < 0.000$). Lower psychological flexibility was associated with higher levels of anxiety and depression. These correlations were moderate for PPFQ-17 and strong for PPFQ-10. Concerning the three PPFQ-10 subscales; there was a significant strong negative correlation between EA and both anxiety and depression, a significant moderate negative correlation between PW and anxiety, a significant weak negative correlation between PW and depression, and furthermore significant moderate negative correlations between the VBA subscale and both anxiety and depression.

3.3.2. Regression Analyses

Hierarchical regression analyses illustrated that PPFQ-10 contributed significantly to the prediction of both anxiety ($p < 0.000$) and depression ($p < 0.000$). The PPFQ-10 further accounted for 29% of the variation in HADS-a, and 35.6% of the variation in HADS-d when age, gender, and education were controlled for. Concerning the individual contributions of the PPFQ-10 subscales, VBA obtained significant beta coefficients for both anxiety and depression, with a larger unstandardized beta coefficient value for depression; EA obtained significant beta coefficients for both anxiety and depression with equally large unstandardized coefficient values; and PW did not obtain any significant beta coefficients for either criteria variable. The results from the hierarchical regression analyses are presented in Table 4.

Table 3. Descriptive statistics and correlations between controls and variables of sample ($n = 263$).

Variables	Mean (%)	SD	Age	Gender	Education	PPFQ-17 Total	PPFQ-10 Total	PPFQ-10 VBA	PPFQ-10 PW	PPFQ-10 EA	HADS-a
1. Age	44.4	6.5									
2. Gender (F, M)	(81, 19)	N/A	-0.22 **								
3. Education (Hi, Lo)	(53, 47)	N/A	0.24 **	0.05							
4. PPFQ-17 total	47.0	18.0	0.09	0.01	0.19 **						
5. PPFQ-10 total	30.1	11.5	0.08	0.04	0.19 **	0.96 **					
6. PPFQ-10 VBA	10.4	4.0	0.00	0.02	0.11	0.070 **	0.76 **				
7. PPFQ-10 PW	7.2	4.3	0.11	0.10	0.21 **	0.71 **	0.73 **	0.34 **			
8. PPFQ-10 EA	12.5	6.0	0.08	-0.01	0.24 *	0.86 **	0.88 **	0.53 **	0.44 **		
9. HADS-a	6.1	4.5	-0.06	0.11	-0.06	-0.48 **	-0.52 **	0.39 **	-0.30 **	-0.52 **	
10. HADS-d	4.4	4.0	0.03	0.01	-0.04	-0.49 **	-0.53 **	-0.49 **	-0.23 **	-0.53 **	0.72 **

Variables above the line, controls; variables below the line, predictors in the regression analyses; HADS-a, The Hospital Anxiety and Depression Scale—anxiety; HADS-d, The Hospital Anxiety and Depression Scale—depression; * Correlation is significant at the 0.05 level (two-tailed); ** Correlation is significant at the 0.01 level (two-tailed).

Table 4. Hierarchical regression analysis to evaluate the criteria validity of the PPFQ-10.

Criteria	Step	Predictor Variables	R²	R² Change	F Change (df)	Sig. F Change	Unstandardized [a]		Standardized Coefficients Beta [a]		
							B	SE	β	t	Sig.
HADS-a	1	Control variables	0.013	0.013	1.104 (3252)	0.348					
		Age					-0.001	0.038	-0.001	-0.021	0.983
		Gender					1.203	0.626	0.106	1.921	0.056
		Education					0.283	0.493	0.032	0.575	0.566
	2	PPFQ-10	0.303	0.290	34.512 (3249)	0.000					
		VBA					-0.182	0.070	-0.168	-2.621	0.009
		PW					-0.094	0.062	-0.092	-1.505	0.134
		EA					-0.287	0.051	-0.385	-5.685	0.000
HADS-d	1	Control variables	0.002	0.002	0.195 (3252)	0.900					
		Age					0.044	0.034	0.072	1.30	0.20
		Gender					0.489	0.550	0.048	0.889	0.375
		Education					0.478	0.435	0.060	1.098	0.273
	2	PPFQ-10	0.358	0.356	46.003 (3249)	0.000					
		VBA					-0.310	0.060	-0.318	-5.184	0.000
		PW					0.007	0.053	0.008	0.131	0.896
		EA					-0.246	0.043	-0.369	-5.671	0.000

Results show the amount of variance explained by PPFQ-10 in anxiety and depression (criteria variables); [a] Results are displayed from the final model; Sig., significance.

4. Discussion

The present study assessed the adequacy of the Swedish translation of the PPFQ and evaluated the factor structure of the PPFQ-17 in a Swedish sample of 263 parents of children with chronic pain. Exploratory factor analysis with PCA supported a three-factor solution. Seven items were removed in an iterative process due to poorer extraction, significant cross loadings, or negative contributions to the overall reliability of the scale, resulting in a final version with 10 items. Notably, the three factors in the final version matched three of the four labels proposed by Wallace et al. perfectly and were retained. One of the factors, PA, was eliminated in the process, in line with author discussions in the first factor study [10]. The suggested final version of the questionnaire has three theoretically discernible subscales: VBA, PW, and (EA) [10], demonstrating fair to excellent internal consistencies. In addition, the PPFQ-10 correlated very strongly with the PPFQ-17 and was able to explain a significant amount of variance in parental anxiety and depression. Some differences regarding the subscales' individual contributions were seen, where VBA and EA obtained significant beta coefficients, while PW did not. This result is in line with the study by Wallace et al. [10], which described the PW subscale as "the most divergent from the total", in the sense that it had unique correlations with other main variables included in that study which the other subscales did not have. Consequently, the results from the current study are promising in their similarity to the results by Wallace et al. [10], and confirm the construct validity of the instrument when used in a different country and different language. The fact that the construct of parental psychological flexibility displays such consistency across samples and countries, points to the fact that parents' distressing experiences in relation to their child's pain may be of direct clinical importance. However, future studies should evaluate the psychometric properties and utility of the PPFQ-10 in different subgroups, cultures, and languages.

The levels of anxiety and depression were elevated in the current sample compared to Swedish and German normative samples [39,40]. These results are consistent with previous research on parents of children with chronic pain [15,41], and serve as yet another indication of pediatric chronic pain not only being a matter of the child, but also a family concern [42], and further point to the need for targeted parental interventions in the specific context of pediatric chronic pain. For example, earlier studies on parental distress in pediatric chronic pain have reported parents feeling a lack of life control, being caught in a pattern of short-term avoidance behaviors, and unable to change a style of parenting that they know is not appropriate in relation to their child's age [43]. Although the correlation and regression analyses between parental distress and parental psychological flexibility in the current study had the primary objective of concurrent criteria validation, the results nevertheless provide further insight on the interrelation between these variables in parents of children with chronic pain. One possible explanation for the interrelationship seen in this study could be that lower psychological flexibility in a parent of a child with chronic pain potentially increases the risk for less adaptive and values incongruent parental behaviors, which may eventually lead to parental rumination and depression [17,43].

There are, however, a number of limitations that need to be taken into account when interpreting the findings of the current study. With a cross-sectional design, the direction of causality between parental depression and psychological flexibility remains inconclusive. A second potential restriction is that all data are based on self-report and other sources of verification of psychiatric diagnoses of parents are lacking. Further research could, for example, make use of health care records to cross-check results for parental illness. Moreover, the choice of HADS as the sole variable for concurrent criterion validation is not comprehensive, and future validation analyses of the PPFQ-10 could benefit from using a broader set of measures, including parental acceptance, parental reactivity to the child's pain, observational data on relevant parent and child interactions, and possibly also parental cognitive flexibility and executive function. Measures of parental encouragement of the child's illness behavior could also be helpful in establishing discriminant validity. Furthermore, some differences between the subscales' individual contributions were seen, and the relative merits of the subscales could benefit from further examination with other samples, in outcome studies as well as in mediation analyses. Also, longitudinal or experimental designs are required to evaluate the predictive utility of the instrument for child treatment outcomes, and also to establish if treatment interventions specifically targeted at increasing parental psychological flexibility may ultimately benefit both parent and child outcomes.

In conclusion, the factor structure and reliability of this revised and shortened version of the original PPFQ are supported within our results. Results also illustrate the importance of the PPFQ-10 in explaining variance in parental anxiety and depression, supporting criterion validity. Based on the existing data, the PPFQ-10 could serve as a useful tool to assess psychological inflexibility in parents of children with chronic pain, simultaneously reducing the burden of research and assessment.

Acknowledgments: Funding for Wiwe Lipsker was provided from the KID-funding at Karolinska Institutet, and from the Functional Area Medical Psychology at Karolinska University Hospital. Funding for Marie Kanstrup was provided from the Doctoral School in Health Care Sciences at Karolinska Institutet, and from the Functional Area Medical Psychology at Karolinska University Hospital. Financial support for Linda Holmström and Rikard K. Wicksell was provided through the regional agreement on medical training and clinical research (ALF) between Stockholm City Council and Karolinska Institutet. Funding for Mike Kemani was provided from the Functional Area Medical Psychology at Karolinska University Hospital.

Author Contributions: Rikard K. Wicksell conceived and designed the study. Wiwe Lipsker, Marie Kanstrup, Mike Kemani, and Linda Holmström performed the study by collecting data. Wiwe Lipsker was responsible for compiling and analyzing data, and wrote the paper. Linda Holmström and Rikard K. Wicksell contributed with statistical knowledge. All authors contributed substantially in reviewing and revising the manuscript, and approved the final manuscript as submitted. All authors have read and approved the final manuscript.

Conflicts of Interest: The authors declare no conflict of interest. The founding sponsors had no role in the design of the study; in the collection, analyses, or interpretation of data; in the writing of the manuscript, nor in the decision to publish the results.

References

1. Hayes, S.C. Acceptance and commitment therapy, relational frame theory, and the third wave of behavioral and cognitive therapies. *Behav. Ther.* **2004**, *35*, 639–665. [CrossRef]
2. Hayes, S.C.; Luoma, J.B.; Bond, F.W.; Masuda, A.; Lillis, J. Acceptance and commitment therapy: Model, processes and outcomes. *Behav. Res. Ther.* **2006**, *44*, 1–25. [CrossRef] [PubMed]
3. Kashdan, T.B.; Rottenberg, J. Psychological flexibility as a fundamental aspect of health. *Clin. Psychol. Rev.* **2010**, *30*, 865–878. [CrossRef] [PubMed]
4. Moyer, D.N.; Sandoz, E.K. The role of psychological flexibility in the relationship between parent and adolescent distress. *J. Child Fam. Stud.* **2015**, *24*, 1406–1418. [CrossRef]
5. Brassell, A.A.; Rosenberg, E.; Parent, J.; Rough, J.N.; Fondacaro, K.; Seehuus, M. Parent's psychological flexibility: Associations with parenting and child psychosocial well-being. *J. Context. Behav. Sci.* **2016**, *5*, 111–120. [CrossRef]
6. Wicksell, R.K.; Melin, L.; Lekander, M.; Olsson, G.L. Evaluating the effectiveness of exposure and acceptance strategies to improve functioning and quality of life in longstanding pediatric pain—A randomized controlled trial. *Pain* **2009**, *141*, 248–257. [CrossRef] [PubMed]
7. Wicksell, R.K.; Melin, L.; Olsson, G.L. Exposure and acceptance in the rehabilitation of adolescents with idiopathic chronic pain—A pilot study. *Eur. J. Pain* **2007**, *11*, 267–274. [CrossRef] [PubMed]
8. Wicksell, R.K.; Dahl, J.; Magnusson, B.; Olsson, G.L. Using acceptance and commitment therapy in the rehabilitation of an adolescent female with chronic pain: A case example. *Cogn. Behav. Pract.* **2005**, *12*, 415–423. [CrossRef]
9. Kanstrup, M.; Wicksell, R.K.; Kemani, M.; Lipsker, C.W.; Lekander, M.; Holmström, L. A clinical pilot study of individual and group treatment for adolescents with chronic pain and their Parents: effects of acceptance and commitment therapy on functioning. *Children* **2016**, *3*, 30. [CrossRef]
10. Wallace, D.P.; McCracken, L.M.; Weiss, K.E.; Harbeck-Weber, C. The role of parent psychological flexibility in relation to adolescent chronic pain: Further instrument development. *J. Pain* **2015**, *16*, 235–246. [CrossRef] [PubMed]
11. McCracken, L.M.; Gauntlett-Gilbert, J. Role of psychological flexibility in parents of adolescents with chronic pain: Development of a measure and preliminary correlation analyses. *Pain* **2011**, *152*, 780–785. [CrossRef] [PubMed]

12. Palermo, T.M.; Holley, A.L. The importance of family environment in pediatric chronic pain. *JAMA Pediatr.* **2013**, *167*, 93–94. [CrossRef] [PubMed]

13. Logan, D.E.; Scharff, L. Relationships between family and parent characteristics and functional abilities in children with recurrent pain syndromes: An investigation of moderating effects on the pathway from pain to disability. *J. Pediatr. Psychol.* **2005**, *30*, 698–707. [CrossRef] [PubMed]

14. Smith, A.M.; Sieberg, C.B.; Odell, S.; Randall, E.; Simons, L.E. Living life with my child's pain: The parent pain acceptance questionnaire (ppaq). *Clin. J. Pain* **2015**, *31*, 633–641. [CrossRef] [PubMed]

15. Palermo, T.M.; Eccleston, C. Parents of children and adolescents with chronic pain. *Pain* **2009**, *146*, 15–17. [CrossRef] [PubMed]

16. Simons, L.E.; Smith, A.; Kaczynski, K.; Basch, M. Living in fear of your child's pain: The parent fear of pain questionnaire. *Pain* **2015**, *156*, 694–702. [CrossRef] [PubMed]

17. Jaaniste, T.; Jia, N.; Lang, T.; Goodison-Farnsworth, E.M.; McCormick, M.; Anderson, D. The relationship between parental attitudes and behaviours in the context of paediatric chronic pain. *Child Care Health Dev.* **2016**, *42*, 433–438. [CrossRef] [PubMed]

18. Chow, E.T.; Otis, J.D.; Simons, L.E. The longitudinal impact of parent distress and behavior on functional outcomes among youth with chronic pain. *J. Pain* **2016**, *17*, 729–738. [CrossRef] [PubMed]

19. Bond, F.W.; Lloyd, J.; Guenole, N. The work-related acceptance and action questionnaire: Initial psychometric findings and their implications for measuring psychological flexibility in specific contexts. *J. Occup. Organ. Psychol.* **2013**, *86*, 331–347. [CrossRef]

20. Holmstrom, L.; Kemani, M.K.; Kanstrup, M.; Wicksell, R.K. Evaluating the statistical properties of the pain interference index in children and adolescents with chronic pain. *J. Dev. Behav. Pediatr.* **2015**, *36*, 450–454. [CrossRef] [PubMed]

21. Kanstrup, M.; Holmstrom, L.; Ringstrom, R.; Wicksell, R.K. Insomnia in paediatric chronic pain and its impact on depression and functional disability. *Eur. J. Pain* **2014**, *18*, 1094–1102. [CrossRef] [PubMed]

22. Zigmond, A.S.; Snaith, R.P. The hospital anxiety and depression scale. *Acta Psychiatr. Scand.* **1983**, *67*, 361–370. [CrossRef] [PubMed]

23. Olsson, I.; Mykletun, A.; Dahl, A.A. The hospital anxiety and depression rating scale: A cross-sectional study of psychometrics and case finding abilities in general practice. *BMC Psychiatry* **2005**, *5*, 46. [CrossRef] [PubMed]

24. Jutte, J.E.; Needham, D.M.; Pfoh, E.R.; Bienvenu, O.J. Psychometric evaluation of the hospital anxiety and depression scale 3 months after acute lung injury. *J. Crit. Care* **2015**, *30*, 793–798. [CrossRef] [PubMed]

25. Hulbert-Williams, N.J.; Storey, L. Psychological flexibility correlates with patient-reported outcomes independent of clinical or sociodemographic characteristics. *Support. Care Cancer* **2016**, *24*, 2513–2521. [CrossRef] [PubMed]

26. Bardeen, J.R.; Fergus, T.A. The interactive effect of cognitive fusion and experiential avoidance on anxiety, depression, stress and posttraumatic stress symptoms. *J. Context. Behav. Sci.* **2016**, *5*, 1–6. [CrossRef]

27. Fish, R.A.; McGuire, B.; Hogan, M.; Morrison, T.G.; Stewart, I. Validation of the chronic pain acceptance questionnaire (CPAQ) in an internet sample and development and preliminary validation of the CPAQ-8. *Pain* **2010**, *149*, 435–443. [CrossRef] [PubMed]

28. Bendayan, R.; Esteve, R.; Blanca, M.J. New empirical evidence of the validity of the chronic pain acceptance questionnaire: The differential influence of activity engagement and pain willingness on adjustment to chronic pain. *Br. J. Health Psychol.* **2012**, *17*, 314–326. [CrossRef] [PubMed]

29. Fledderus, M.; Bohlmeijer, E.T.; Fox, J.-P.; Schreurs, K.M.G.; Spinhoven, P. The role of psychological flexibility in a self-help acceptance and commitment therapy intervention for psychological distress in a randomized controlled trial. *Behav. Res. Ther.* **2013**, *51*, 142–151. [CrossRef] [PubMed]

30. Barke, A.; Riecke, J.; Rief, W.; Glombiewski, J.A. The psychological inflexibility in pain scale (PIPS)—Validation, factor structure and comparison to the chronic pain acceptance questionnaire (CPAQ) and other validated measures in german chronic back pain patients. *BMC Musculoskelet. Disord.* **2015**, *16*, 1–10. [CrossRef] [PubMed]

31. Eccleston, C.; Crombez, G.; Scotford, A.; Clinch, J.; Connell, H. Adolescent chronic pain: Patterns and predictors of emotional distress in adolescents with chronic pain and their parents. *Pain* **2004**, *108*, 221–229. [CrossRef] [PubMed]

32. Cohen, L.L.; Vowles, K.E.; Eccleston, C. Parenting an adolescent with chronic pain: An investigation of how a taxonomy of adolescent functioning relates to parent distress. *J. Pediatr. Psychol.* **2010**, *35*, 748–757. [CrossRef] [PubMed]

33. Beaton, D.E.; Bombardier, C.; Guillemin, F.; Ferraz, M.B. Guidelines for the process of cross-cultural adaptation of self-report measures. *Spine* **2000**, *25*, 3186–3191. [CrossRef] [PubMed]

34. Floyd, F.J.; Widaman, K.F. Factor analysis in the development and refinement of clinical assessment instruments. *Psychol. Assess.* **1995**, *7*, 286. [CrossRef]

35. Gorsuch, R.L. *Factor Analysis*, 2nd ed.; Lawrence Erlbaum Associates: Hillsdale, NJ, USA, 1983.

36. Ponterotto, J.G.; Ruckdeschel, D.E. An overview of coefficient alpha and a reliability matrix for estimating adequacy of internal consistency coefficients with psychological research measures. *Percept. Motor Skills* **2007**, *105*, 997–1014. [CrossRef] [PubMed]

37. Field, A. *Discovering Statistics Using IBM Spss Statistics*; Sage Publications Ltd.: London, UK, 2013; p. 952.

38. Little, R.J. A test of missing completely at random for multivariate data with missing values. *J. Am. Stat. Assoc.* **1988**, *83*, 1198–1202. [CrossRef]

39. Lisspers, J.; Nygren, A.; Söderman, E. Hospital anxiety and depression scale (HAD): Some psychometric data for a Swedish sample. *Acta Psychiatr. Scand.* **1997**, *96*, 281–286. [CrossRef] [PubMed]

40. Hinz, A.; Brähler, E. Normative values for the hospital anxiety and depression scale (HADS) in the general german population. *J. Psychosom. Res.* **2011**, *71*, 74–78. [CrossRef] [PubMed]

41. Campo, J.V.; Bridge, J.; Lucas, A.; Savorelli, S.; Walker, L.; Di Lorenzo, C.; Iyengar, S.; Brent, D.A. Physical and emotional health of mothers of youth with functional abdominal pain. *Arch. Pediatr. Adolesc. Med.* **2007**, *161*, 131–137. [CrossRef] [PubMed]

42. Sinclair, C.M.; Meredith, P.; Strong, J.; Feeney, R. Personal and contextual factors affecting the functional ability of children and adolescents with chronic pain: A systematic review. *J. Dev. Behav. Pediatr.* **2016**, *37*, 327–342. [CrossRef] [PubMed]

43. Jordan, A.L.; Eccleston, C.; Osborn, M. Being a parent of the adolescent with complex chronic pain: An interpretative phenomenological analysis. *Eur. J. Pain* **2007**, *11*, 49–56. [CrossRef] [PubMed]

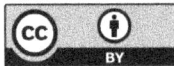

children

MDPI

Article

Supporting Teens with Chronic Pain to Obtain High School Credits: Chronic Pain 35 in Alberta

Kathy Reid [1,2,*], Mark Simmonds [1,2], Michelle Verrier [2] and Bruce Dick [1,2]

[1] Stollery Children's Hospital, Alberta Health Services, Edmonton, AB T6G 2B7, Canada; mark.simmonds@ualberta.ca (M.S.); bruce.dick@ualberta.ca (B.D.)

[2] Department of Anaesthesiology and Pain Medicine, University of Alberta, Edmonton, AB T6G 2R3, Canada; mrheault@ualberta.ca

* Correspondence: Kathy.Reid@ahs.ca; Tel.: +1-780-407-1363

Academic Editor: Carl L. von Baeyer
Received: 16 September 2016; Accepted: 7 November 2016; Published: 19 November 2016

Abstract: Chronic pain is a significant problem in children and teens, and adolescents with chronic pain often struggle to attend school on a regular basis. We present in this article a novel program we developed that integrates attendance at a group cognitive-behavioural chronic pain self-management program with earning high school credits. We collaborated with Alberta Education in the development of this course, Chronic Pain 35. Adolescents who choose to enroll are invited to demonstrate their scientific knowledge related to pain, understanding of and engagement with treatment homework, and demonstrate their creativity by completing a project, which demonstrates at least one concept. Integrating Chronic Pain 35 into an adolescent's academic achievements is a creative strategy that facilitates the engagement of adolescents in learning and adopting pain coping techniques. It also helps teens to advocate for themselves in the school environment and improve their parents' and teachers' understanding of adolescent chronic pain. This is one of the first successful collaborations between a pediatric health program and provincial education leaders, aimed at integrating learning and obtaining school credit for learning about and engaging in health self-management for teens. The authors hope this paper serves as an effective reference model for any future collaborating programs aimed at supporting teens with chronic pain to obtain high school credits.

Keywords: chronic pain; adolescent; school; cognitive-behavioural therapy

1. Introduction

Chronic pain is a significant problem in the pediatric population. Chronic pain is defined as any prolonged pain that lasts longer than the expected healing time or any recurrent pain that occurs at least three times during a three-month period [1,2]. Common pain diagnoses in children and adolescents include headaches, chronic abdominal pain, back pain, and musculoskeletal pain [3]. The pain may result from a disease, injury, a trauma, or surgery. For a significant number of children, there are no identifiable causes for the reported pain. Increasingly, this type of pain is discussed as a result of neurobiological changes that result in pain syndromes including pain centralization and pain amplification [4,5]. Population studies demonstrate that 20%–35% of children and adolescents report symptoms meeting research definitions of chronic pain [1,2,6]. It is estimated that between 5%–8% of children with chronic pain will develop significant pain-related disability [7,8]. This pain-related disability is known to affect children's functioning including their ability to attend school on a regular basis [9]. These children often require an interdisciplinary team to help manage chronic pain and pain-related disability.

Research has demonstrated that adolescents with chronic pain report being less socially developed than their peers [10] and that they may avoid social situations with peers [11]. Lower social functioning can contribute to school impairment, and therefore having children socially connected to their peers can limit the detrimental effects on school functioning [12].

As mentioned, evidence demonstrates that children and adolescents with chronic pain often struggle to attend school on a regular basis [9]. In one study, 44% of students with chronic pain missed at least 25% of school days, and 20% missed more than one half of school days [13]. In addition, 44% of the students reported a decline in grades. A study comparing school absences of children with functional abdominal pain (FAP), inflammatory bowel disease (IBD), and healthy controls found that children with both IBD and FAP missed significantly more school than healthy controls [14]. In the Pediatric Pain Program at the Stollery Children's Hospital (Edmonton, AB, Canada), our records suggest that a majority of individuals presenting with chronic pain miss at least one half to two days per week on average, and approximately 15%–20% of adolescents are either no longer attending school on a regular basis or have stopped attending in person and complete their studies in a correspondence program. In addition, chronic pain is shown to affect children's cognitive function, but more research is required to determine the long-term effects of this cognitive dysfunction on the developmental trajectory of young people with chronic pain [15].

Given the prevalence of chronic pain, and the magnitude of its effects on adolescents' social development and school functioning, it is critical that teens be provided with the opportunity to continue to learn. Additionally, young people in our program report that it is important to their mental health and self-concept to make progress in their educational programming and pursuit of their school and life goals, despite experiencing ongoing pain. It is also important to maintain contact with a peer group, in order to support normal social adolescent development.

2. Managing Chronic Pain: Biopsychosocial Approach

Adolescents with chronic pain benefit from multimodal approaches to improve their function and return to regular activities, including school. Interventions that include the 3Ps—physical, psychological and pharmacological approaches—are more likely to be successful than single interventions. One of the most effective treatments for chronic pain is cognitive-behavioural therapy (CBT), which has been shown to be effective in managing headache, recurrent and functional abdominal pain in children [16], sickle cell disease [17], and juvenile fibromyalgia [18]. CBT strategies for chronic pain management address pain education, and teach active coping strategies such as relaxation and imagery, stress management, cognitive restructuring, goal setting, and relapse prevention [19]. Treatment approaches that enhance self-efficacy, or increase confidence to function despite pain, have been suggested as helpful for youth with headaches [20,21].

A group intervention for adolescents with chronic pain (*n* = 40) and their parents, called "Coping with Pain School" in Boston, MA, USA, by Logan and Simons [22] provided either four sessions of CBT or a day long CBT session aimed at improving school function. The study found the program was feasible, families who participated were satisfied with the program and school attendance improved after completion of the sessions; however, enrollment challenges were a significant problem identified by the authors in the study. They recommended the need to develop treatments focusing on school functioning and involving school personnel in future studies.

3. The Stollery Experience

The Pediatric Chronic Pain Program at the Stollery Children's Hospital opened in 2008, to provide treatment for children and adolescents with chronic, difficult to manage pain. The large geographical catchment area includes northern Alberta, the Northwest Territories, and North Eastern British Columbia. Children from Saskatchewan and Manitoba have also been included. All patients must be referred to the clinic by a physician or nurse practitioner and must meet the clinic's referral criteria (tab:children-03-00031-t001).

Table 1. Stollery Chronic Pain Clinic referral criteria.

Request for Consultation: Referral by Physician/Nurse Practitioner only	The goal of this service is to treat and care for children 17 years and under who are experiencing chronic, difficult-to-manage pain. Children should always have been seen and assessed first by the appropriate pediatric services prior to being referred to the Pediatric Chronic Pain Clinic.
Inclusion criteria	<ul><li>0–17 years, 11 months</li><li>chronic pain of at least three months' duration</li><li>chronic pain as primary complaint</li><li>chronic pain which impacts activities of daily living, school attendance, sleep, quality of life or family functioning</li></ul>

The family attends an intake appointment in person with the full interdisciplinary team to share their pain experience. The team consists of a chronic pain physician, a nurse practitioner, a physiotherapist and a psychologist. The initial appointment takes up to two hours to complete a comprehensive physical and psychosocial history, physical examination and development of a treatment plan with input from the child and family. For many of the children, participation in group cognitive behavioural therapy becomes part of the treatment plan. This program, called Pain 101, consists of 10 sessions, provided jointly by the psychologist and nurse practitioner. Pain 101 is a treatment program provided by our clinic to children 12–18 years old. Although the treatment is offered for a broad range of ages, due to the careful screening process that takes place prior to Pain 101 admission, we have yet to experience significant issues associated with developmental differences in participant responses.

Participants are invited to attend the sessions in person or by telehealth (secure videoconferencing). Given the large catchment area of our program, telehealth is offered to children who reside outside of the city, which makes attending the program much more feasible, especially to children whose school has access to this secure videoconference service. Pain 101 classes take place in the afternoon to best accommodate high school students who can set their schedule to avoid missing core classes. Group sizes for the class range from 5–15 participants for each 10-session block. Teens who participate are expected to attend all sessions and complete the homework as outlined. In addition to the classes for teens, sessions for parents are offered and provided by the nurse practitioner. The purpose of these sessions is to help parents understand the science of chronic pain, factors that exacerbate pain, and self-management techniques aimed at promoting increased function, mental health, coping, self-efficacy, mindfulness, acceptance, and self-compassion. Attendance for these sessions is encouraged but not required for the program, and consequently attendance of the parent session varies. However, since implementing a parallel course, Chronic Pain 35 (see Section 4), we have noted an increase in the number of parents who attend, as well as requests for additional sessions to be held. For parents, sessions aim to teach them appropriate developmental expectations, strategies to facilitate children's self-management and parent coping all with a global aim help their child function despite pain. It is important that parental behaviours, especially protectiveness [23] and parent pain–related fear [24], be addressed in order to facilitate the return to school for the small but significant number of students who miss extensive amounts of school.

3.1. Pain 101 Session Content

3.1.1. Pain Education

The biopsychosocial model of chronic pain is introduced (Figure 1), and this model is reviewed throughout Pain 101. Pain pathways in the body are reviewed, including how pain messages are sent from the periphery and received by the brain. Participants learn how chronic pain differs from acute pain. The Gate Control Theory of Pain is introduced and up-to-date scientific information on our understanding of this theory is discussed. For homework, participants are asked to complete specific questionnaires.

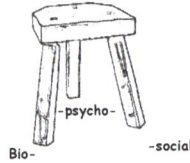

Biopsychosocial model

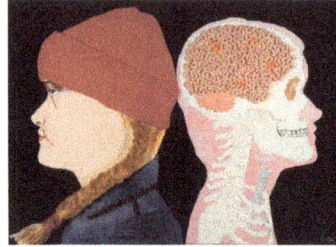

(A)   (B)

Figure 1. (**A**) Biopsychosocial model—the example of a three-legged stool is often used to discuss this topic with the participants, focusing on the concept that all three legs are needed to be able to sit on the stool; (**B**) this image, created by a student of the Pain 101 course entitled "Untitled", is often used to assist in the explanation of the biopsychosocial model, in order to explain pain locations in the brain to participants.

3.1.2. Tension and Relaxation

Participants learn how tension opens pain gates and thereby increases pain and how relaxation strategies have the potential to modify the pain experience. Relaxation exercises including progressive muscle relaxation, guided imagery and diaphragmatic breathing are taught and practiced with the group. For homework, participants are asked to complete relaxation diaries and practice the techniques daily.

3.1.3. Pacing

Participants learn how activity avoidance and activity cycling can open pain gates and lead to disability in chronic pain. Methods to break this downward cycle are reviewed. Participants are expected to complete activity goals for themselves. The goals are broken down from long-term goals to intermediate goals to mini goals. Activity tolerance times are calculated, and then, from this time, baseline activity times are calculated. Participants are then expected to meet their baseline activity goals on a daily basis. For homework, participants are asked to develop a specific, measurable, achievable, relevant and time dependent (S.M.A.R.T.) goal and determine tolerance and baseline for individual activities.

3.1.4. Dealing with Negative Thoughts

Participants learn how living with chronic pain can be associated with negative thoughts and negative moods, including sadness or being overwhelmed, and may even contribute to depression or unhealthy, negative coping behaviours. Methods to challenge these negative thoughts are reviewed including active and positive coping strategies, reframing thoughts, recognition of feelings and challenging unhelpful thoughts. For homework, participants are asked to complete the daily thought diary.

3.1.5. Mindfulness

Participants review the theory of mindfulness-based stress reduction. Practice activities for mindfulness are completed in class. Participants are encouraged to practice various daily activities in a mindful way, such as taking the bus, exercising, and completing chores. For homework, participants are asked to complete one mindfulness activity daily.

3.1.6. Sleep and Nutrition

Participants review the importance of sleep in managing chronic pain and closing pain gates. Healthy sleep practice strategies that support restorative sleep are reviewed, including cognitive, behavioural, and environment modification sleep practices. Dietary habits that affect pain and sleep, including caffeine and energy drinks are also reviewed. For homework, participants are asked to perform a practical application of sleep hygiene strategies and a minimum of one dietary change.

3.1.7. Stress and Anxiety

In this session, we discuss how stress and anxiety lead to biological responses that affect pain gates, mood, and sleep, thereby exacerbating pain. Participants review stressors, such as school, homework, dealing with others, and chores. Fear of pain and how that fear contributes to disability are also reviewed. Recognizing the physical effects of stress and anxiety, including physical reactions (fight or flight response) and emotional reactions are discussed. Additionally, methods to decrease stress and anxiety are reviewed, such as recognition and coping strategies that include relaxation and pacing activities. For homework, participants are asked to recognize personal stressors and find coping strategies.

3.1.8. Communication

Pain behaviours and communication are reviewed. Participants learn about both verbal and non-verbal communication messages and discuss how the messages may be interpreted by others. This session includes a video demonstrating how society sees what they are conditioned to see. Discussion takes place regarding how strategies can be practically applied to teach family, friends, and others about pain. For homework, participants are asked to complete a communication diary.

3.1.9. Setback Planning (Relapse Prevention)

Participants learn how to develop their own personal setback plan to be utilized whenever they have a flare in their pain. This plan includes recognizing the flare early, implementing the various strategies reviewed through the course—relaxation, pacing, thoughts, sleep, stress, and communication. For homework, participants are asked to complete their setback plan worksheet.

3.1.10. Life with Pain

This final session includes strategies to live life to the fullest despite having pain. Concrete methods include simplifying activities of daily living such as school work and activities, chores, work, social activities, and other activities of daily living. We review how strategies that have previously been covered in Pain 101 can be applied to each of these life activities, structuring activities to allow for breaks while still meeting goals. Individual setback plans are reviewed and participants are asked to provide a copy of their set-back plan to the pain clinic staff. For homework, participants are asked to submit the written set-back plan, along with submission of their Chronic Pain 35 project for those who are registered in the parallel course. An example of participant work from this session can be seen in Figure 2.

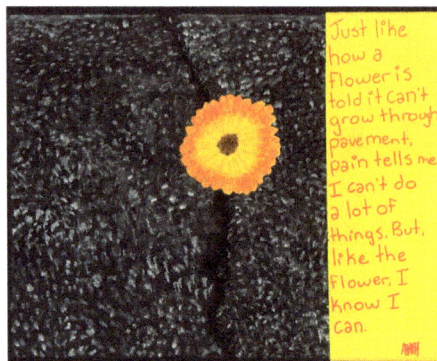

Figure 2. "A flower can grow" created by a Pain 101 participant, A.F.H.

3.2. Participant Measures

All participants who attend Pain 101 are requested to complete questionnaires (tab:children-03-00031-t002) as per the Pediatric Initiative on Methods, Measurement, and Pain Assessment in Clinical Trials (PedIMMPACT) recommendations [25]. These data are used for the establishment of a clinical baseline, monitoring, and, for those who consent, research. The two primary findings from our analyses that have been continually replicated are significant reductions in pain-related disability ($p < 0.001$) and anxiety ($p < 0.005$).

Table 2. Questionnaire measurements.

Pain History and Demographics	Details including age, school grade, gender and school absences are recorded. Additionally, information on pain experience, chronicity, frequency, location and intensity are entered.
Visual Analogue Scale	The child is instructed to illustrate, by drawing a line on a scale from 0–10 (0 = no pain, 10 = worst possible pain), the intensity of pain felt in the past week [26].
Pediatric Quality of Life Inventory	Participants are asked to report how their pain has impacted their quality of life, including their activities, feelings, social interactions and school performance. Parents are asked to fill out the parent version of this scale which includes the same questions, but reporting their observations of their child's quality of life [27].
Children's Sleep Habits Questionnaire	The child is asked 26 questions about own bedtime habits, sleep behaviour and daytime sleepiness. The parent form is constructed of 33 questions on child's bedtime habits, sleep behaviour, waking during the night, morning waking, and daytime sleepiness [28].
Functional Disability Index	Child and parent(s) are asked to report the child's level of physical trouble or difficulty when performing various tasks [29].
Tampa Scale of Kinesiophobia for Children	A self-report form asking the child to identify how they cope with pain. This measure records the child's somatic focus and activity avoidance [30].
Revised Child Anxiety and Depression Scale	This 47-item self-report measure assesses the symptoms of separation anxiety, general anxiety, panic, social phobia, obsession/compulsion, and depression. The child is asked to report the frequency (from 'never' to 'always') of various worrying and sad thoughts [31].
The Children's Chronic Pain Stigma Scale (CCPSS)	This scale is also currently being developed and validated in our program based on the adult Chronic Pain Stigma Scale [32]. This measure explores perceived stigma from physicians, family members and the general public associated with chronic pain.

3.3. Session Completion

The questionnaire measurements are completed prior to the start of Pain 101, at the end of Pain 101 (three months later), and again at the six- and 12-month post-group completion milestones, and then annually at the five-year mark, post-group completion. Additionally, we have begun tracking education outcomes and the number of school days missed in comparison to pre- and post-completion of Pain 101.

4. Chronic Pain 35

In 2010, our healthcare team from the pediatric chronic pain clinic, along with several teens, started to work on ways to consistently obtain high school credits for completing the program and demonstrating their learning. Prior to that point, some students had been granted high school credit for completing Pain 101, but the number of credits granted and the categorization of those credits was highly variable between students. It was up to each student to advocate for themselves at their local school, with support from our team, to obtain credits. Several students were able to obtain between one and three credits, but we lacked consistency at a local or provincial level. In 2014, we approached Alberta Education, which is the provincial government agency responsible for public education in Alberta. We explained the program that we were providing and shared samples of the projects completed by students for successful credits at their local school. Together with educational consultants at Alberta Education and the Alberta Distance Learning program (a provincial online school), we developed the course syllabus. This course syllabus included specific learner outcomes for each of the classes that must be demonstrated for successful completion of the course. Examples of outcomes include: Pain Education—identify two methods by which pain gates in the body are opened; Pacing—develop a S.M.A.R.T. goal for a physical activity and demonstrate following through on that goal; Negative Thoughts—identify at least one cognitive distortion and modify negative thoughts associated with the noted distortion. The course was submitted to the Alberta Education curriculum board, and, in February 2015, it was approved as a locally developed course called Chronic Pain 35. Students who successfully complete the course obtain three credits at the Grade 12 (senior year) level in Alberta. In order to obtain a high school diploma in Alberta, students must complete courses which total 100 credits.

Participants attending Pain 101, enrolled in Grades 10–12 (ages 14–18 years old) are eligible to enroll for the course Chronic Pain 35, in order to earn high school credits. Although junior high school students are allowed to attend Pain 101, there is not a credit program in Alberta for grades 7–9, and therefore the Chronic Pain 35 course is restricted to high school students only. The course is only open to students who are followed in our clinic, as parallel attendance in Pain 101 is required. Not all teens who attend Pain 101 register for Chronic Pain 35, since many teens do not need the credits, live outside of Alberta, or are younger than high school age. Enrollment requires completion of the Alberta Distance Learning (ADL) registration form and written consent of a parent/guardian. Prior to registering, we provide the family with a written outline of the course and completion requirements. Additionally, before registration, teens and their parents choosing to enroll are informed that credits for the course "Chronic Pain 35" will appear on their official transcripts. Any ethical concerns expressed regarding this are discussed with the teen and family directly prior to enrollment. To date, only one student expressed concern over the course name appearing on the transcripts, although the student chose to continue and receive credits.

Students who enroll are required to attend all Pain 101 sessions, submit weekly homework assignments, including completion of relaxation diaries, thought challenging worksheets, development of S.M.A.R.T. goals, and a written setback plan for managing pain flares. Any missed sessions must be made up. Additionally, students must complete a project that demonstrates their learning of at least one concept related to the sessions. Projects have been produced using a variety of media, including written work such as essays, personal reflections and poetry. Other projects have used visual arts, such as collages, story boards, paintings, sculptures, and a host of other genres. A small number of students have composed and produced various forms of music. The course mark is 20% for attendance, participation and homework, and 80% for completion of the project. A certified teacher in the province of Alberta has been assigned to the program and grades all course projects. The teacher attends several sessions to meet the students and answer any questions they may have related to the planned project. She is also available via the online distance learning site to discuss projects with the students.

As of July 2016, 35 students have enrolled in Chronic Pain 35. Of these, 32 students have completed the course and received school credits, since three students completed Pain 101, but chose not to complete the course requirements for Chronic Pain 35. Samples of the participant's work can be found in the Supplementary Material. Feedback from students thus far has been very positive, and attendance and homework completion consistency have markedly risen since the formalization of Chronic Pain 35. To quote one of the 17-year-old student participants: "Without this class I would be short credits to graduate. I used to miss a few days of school each week, but now I barely miss any." In addition to obtaining school credits, several students have discussed the importance of having the opportunity to meet and learn with other students who have chronic pain, and to be with others who understand what it is like to live with chronic pain. These students motivate each other to incorporate the strategies into their own lives and help support each other in achieving goals. These students have reported that one of the most important aspects of the group work is the opportunity to continue to meet with other teens who "get them"; who truly understand what it is like to live with chronic pain. As demonstrated by Forgeron [33], the majority of students who attend group CBT for chronic pain self-management are interested in friendships with their class peers for emotional support.

5. Discussion

This paper highlights our unique program that incorporates attendance at a group CBT program for chronic pain and the provision of high school credits for the completion of a course that is provided in a health care setting. Our CBT program includes many recommendations from previous research studies that have addressed multiple facets of the chronic pain experience while helping young people return to school. School avoidance and absences arise from multiple personal and psychosocial factors. Addressing these factors in a group setting can help youth return to school and thereby improve school performance. In a study of 349 youth treated in a chronic pain clinic, Khan et al. [34] found that anxiety played an important role in both school attendance and function while at school. Addressing anxiety, enhancing self-confidence and self-efficacy, and assisting teens in developing methods to manage anxiety using CBT, are all pillars of practice that are incorporated into our program. Additionally, in a study of 47 adolescents with chronic headache, Claar et al. [35] suggest that having the health care team address methods to return to school can help decrease the frequency and duration of headaches. In several sessions of our program, teens are taught concrete techniques to return to function, such as pacing and goal setting. Additionally, by receiving school credits for completion, the student is increasingly empowered to continue to attend school.

In a study by Logan and Curran [36], 38 teachers were interviewed about their needs when dealing with an adolescent with chronic pain. The study revealed that teachers needed to further understand chronic pain and how to manage pain-related behaviours. In our program, we offer a specific class in which we discuss ways to communicate and how to ask others to help in managing pain, including school personnel. Teachers are further supported by the Alberta Education Chronic Pain 35 curriculum guide, in which teachers can access the relevant information on our program and learn how it can help students succeed. Therefore, the completion of Chronic Pain 35 has opened communication with teachers and school administrators that may not have otherwise occurred. Having a certified teacher involved in the program, who is available to intervene with the teens at a school level, also serves to increase understanding of chronic pain in schools across the province.

As identified by Boutilier and King [37], school sites have been undervalued in helping children with chronic pain management, along with the inherent additional challenges. They recommended increased interdisciplinary collaboration between schools and health care teams. Our program directly meets this recommendation by working with Alberta Education at a local and provincial level to best meet the needs of our students. The program has been endorsed by both the Alberta provincial Education Minister and Health Minister.

Future Directions

Given that up to 50% of adolescents with chronic pain miss several school opportunities, days of classes, and social involvement with peers, it is essential that programs providing services to these children incorporate school functioning efforts into their treatment plans. As recommended by Gorodzinsky et al. [38], measurement of school functioning should include the assessment of absenteeism, academic performance, and cognitive function within a developmental framework. Our program will continue to use outcome measures to determine both short-term and long-term results in adolescents who complete Chronic Pain 35, including tracking school absences and school functioning. We will continue to request permission from the students to share their projects which demonstrate their learning. It is hoped that other jurisdictions can work with their educational boards at a local, provincial (or other) level to develop similar programs. Most importantly, we will continue to advocate for students to be able to return to the classroom and continue with their education, and we encourage other programs to contact us if they are interested in modeling our program or learning more about our work. Children are the future of our societies and children with chronic pain require unique support from teams, including the collaboration of health care providers and teachers, to meet their goals of learning, graduating, gaining fulfilling employment, and contributing to society.

Supplementary Materials: The following figures are available online at http://www.mdpi.com/2227-9067/3/4/31/s1, Figure S1: "Shoes" by B.V.; Figure S2: "Dear Non-Believers" by C.S.; Figure S3: "Pain" by A.S.

Acknowledgments: We would like to thank the students who have granted us permission to share their Chronic Pain 35 projects. We would like to acknowledge Karen Campbell, certified teacher at the Alberta Distance Learning Center, who marked the students' projects for credit. Photo credit Mathew Martin, Alberta Health Services. We received no research funding for this program.

Author Contributions: K.R., M.V., M.S. and B.D. all contributed significantly in the conceptualization, writing, and editing of this article.

Conflicts of Interest: The authors declare no conflict of interest.

References

1. American Pain Society Assessment and Management of Children with Chronic Pain: A Position Statement from the American Pain Society. 2012. Available online: http://americanpainsociety.org/uploads/get-involved/pediatric-chronic-pain-statement.pdf (accessed on 26 July 2016).
2. Van Der Kerkhof, E.; van Dijk, A. Prevalence of Chronic Pain Disorders in Children. In *Encyclopaedia Reference of Pain*; Schmidt, R.F., Willis, W.D., Eds.; Springer: Heidelberg, Germany, 2006; pp. 1972–1974.
3. King, S.; Chambers, C.T.; Huguet, A.; MacNevin, R.C.; McGrath, P.J.; Parker, L.; MacDonald, A.J. The epidemiology of chronic pain in children and adolescents revisited; a systematic review. *Pain* **2011**, *152*, 2729–2738. [CrossRef] [PubMed]
4. Latremoliere, A.; Woolf, C.J. Central Sensitization: A generator of pain hypersensitivity by central neural plasticity. *J. Pain* **2009**, *10*, 895–926. [CrossRef] [PubMed]
5. Woolf, C.J. Cenrtal sensitization: Implications for the diagnosis and treatment of pain. *Pain* **2011**, *152*, S2–S15. [CrossRef] [PubMed]
6. Von Baeyer, C. Interpreting the high prevalence of pediatric chronic pain revealed in community surveys. *Pain* **2011**, *152*, 2683–2684. [CrossRef] [PubMed]
7. Gauntlett-Gilbert, J.; Eccleston, C. Disability in adolescents with chronic pain: Patterns and predictors across different domains of functioning. *Pain* **2007**, *131*, 132–141. [CrossRef] [PubMed]
8. Huguet, A.; Miró, J. The severity of chronic pediatric pain: An epidemiological study. *J. Pain* **2008**, *9*, 226–236. [CrossRef] [PubMed]
9. Logan, D.; Simons, L.; Stein, M.J.; Chastain, L. School impairment in adolescents with chronic pain. *J. Pain* **2008**, *9*, 407–416. [CrossRef] [PubMed]

10. Eccleston, C.; Wastel, S.; Crombez, G.; Jordan, A. Adolescent social development and chronic pain. *Eur. J. Pain* **2007**, *12*, 765–774. [CrossRef] [PubMed]

11. Forgeron, P.; McGrath, P.; Stevens, B.; Evans, J.; Dick, B.; Finley, A.G.; Carlson, T. Social information processing in adolescents with chronic pain; my friends don't really understand me. *Pain* **2011**, *152*, 2773–2780. [CrossRef] [PubMed]

12. Simons, L.; Logan, D.; Chastain, L.; Stein, M. The relation of social functioning to school impairment among adolescents with chronic pain. *Clin. J. Pain* **2009**, *26*, 16–22. [CrossRef] [PubMed]

13. Eccleston, C. Managing chronic pain in children; the challenge of delivering chronic care in a 'modernising' health care system. *Arch. Dis. Child* **2005**, *90*, 332–333. [CrossRef] [PubMed]

14. Assa, A.; Ish-Tov, A.; Rinawi, F.; Shamir, R. School attendance in children with functional abdominal pain and inflammatory bowel diseases. *JPGN* **2015**, *61*, 553–557. [CrossRef] [PubMed]

15. Dick, B.; Pillai-Riddell, R. Cognitive and school functioning in children and adolescents with chronic pain: A critical review. *Pain Res. Manag.* **2010**, *15*, 238–244. [CrossRef] [PubMed]

16. Eccleston, C.; Palermo, T.; de C Williams, A.C.; Lewandowski, A.; Morley, S.; Fisher, E.; Law, E. Psychological therapies for the management of current and chronic pain in children and adolescents (review). *Cochrane Libr.* **2014**. [CrossRef]

17. Anie, K.A.; Green, J. Psychological therapies for sickle cell disease and pain. *Cochrane Database Syst. Rev.* **2015**. [CrossRef]

18. Kashikar-Zuck, S.; Ting, T.V.; Arnold, L.M.; Bean, J.; Powers, S.W.; Graham, T.B.; Passo, M.H.; Schikler, K.N.; Hashkes, P.J.; Spalding, S.; et al. Cognitive-behavioral therapy for the treatment of juvenile fibromyalgia: A multisite, single- blinded, randomized control trial. *Arth. Rheum.* **2012**, *64*, 297–305. [CrossRef] [PubMed]

19. Palermo, T.; Law, E. *Managing Your Child's Chronic Pain*; Oxford University Press: New York, NY, USA, 2015; pp. 1–3, 11–13.

20. Carpino, E.; Segal, S.; Logan, D.; Lebel, A.; Simons, L.E. The interplay of pain-related self-efficacy and fear on functional outcomes among youth with headache. *J. Pain* **2014**, *15*, 527–534. [CrossRef] [PubMed]

21. Kalapurakkel, S.; Carpino, E.; Lebel, A.; Simons, L.E. "Pain can't stop me": Examining pain self-efficacy and acceptance as resilience processes among youth with chronic headache. *J. Pediatr. Psychol.* **2014**, *40*, 926–933. [CrossRef] [PubMed]

22. Logan, D.; Simons, L. Development of a group intervention to improve school functioning in adolescents with chronic pain and depressive symptoms; a study of feasibility and preliminary efficacy. *J. Pediatr. Psychol.* **2010**, *35*, 823–836. [CrossRef] [PubMed]

23. Logan, D.; Simons, S.; Carpino, E.A. Too sick for school? Parent influences on school functioning among children with chronic pain. *Pain* **2012**, *153*, 437–443. [CrossRef] [PubMed]

24. Chow, E.T.; Otis, J.D.; Simons, L.E. The longitudinal impact of parent distress and behavior on functional outcomes among youth with chronic pain. *J. Pain* **2016**, *17*, 729–738. [CrossRef] [PubMed]

25. McGrath, P.J.; Walco, G.A.; Turk, D.C.; Dworkin, R.H.; Brown, M.T.; Davidson, K.; Eccleston, C.; Finley, G.A.; Goldschneider, K.; Haverkos, L.; et al. Core outcome domains and measures for pediatric acute and chronic/recurrent pain clinical trials: PedIMMPACT recommendations. *J. Pain* **2008**, *9*, 771–783. [CrossRef] [PubMed]

26. McGrath, P.A.; Seifert, C.E.; Speechley, K.N.; Booth, J.C.; Stitt, L.; Gibson, M.C. A new analogue scale for assessing children's pain: An initial validation study. *Pain* **1996**, *64*, 435–443. [CrossRef]

27. Varni, J.W.; Seid, M.; Rode, C.A. The PedsQL: Measurement model for the pediatric quality of life inventory. *Med. Care* **1999**, *37*, 126–139. [CrossRef] [PubMed]

28. Owens, J.A.; Spirito, C.E.; McGuinn, M. The childrens' sleep habits questionnaire (CSHQ); psychometric properties of a survey instrument for school-aged children. *Sleep* **2000**, *23*, 1043–1051. [PubMed]

29. Walker, L.S.; Greene, W. The functional disability inventory: Measuring a neglected dimension of child health status. *J. Pediatr. Psychol.* **1991**, *16*, 39–58. [CrossRef] [PubMed]

30. Miller, R.P.; Kori, S.; Todd, D. The Tampa scale; a measure of kinesiophobia. *Clin. J. Pain* **1991**, *7*, 51–52. [CrossRef]

31. Chorpita, B.F.; Moffitt, C.E.; Gray, J. Psychometric properties of the Revised Child Anxiety and Depression Scale in a clinic sample. *Behav. Res. Ther.* **2005**, *43*, 309–322. [CrossRef] [PubMed]

32. Vallab, P.K.; Rashiq, S.; Verrier, M.J.; Baker, G.; Sanderman, B.; Dick, B.D. The effect of a cognitive-behavioral therapy chronic pain management program on perceived stigma: A clinical controlled trial. *J. Pain Manag.* **2015**, *7*, 291–299.

33. Forgeron, P.; Chorney, J.; Carlson, T.E.; Dick, B.D.; Plante, E. To befriend or not; naturally developing friendships amongst a clinical group of adolescents with chronic pain. *Pain Manag. Nurs.* **2015**, *16*, 721–723. [CrossRef] [PubMed]

34. Khan, K.; Tran, S.; Mano, K.E.J.; Simpson, P.M.; Cao, Y.; Hainsworth, K.R. Predicting multiple facets of school functioning in pediatric chronic pain: Examining the direct impact of anxiety. *Clin. J. Pain* **2015**, *31*, 867–875. [CrossRef] [PubMed]

35. Claar, R.; Kaczynski, K.; Minster, A.; McDonald-Nolan, L.; LeBel, A.A. School functioning and chronic tension headaches in adolescents: Improvement only after multidisciplinary evaluation. *JCN* **2012**, *28*, 719–724. [CrossRef] [PubMed]

36. Logan, D.; Curran, J. Adolescent chronic pain problems in the school setting: Exploring the experiences and beliefs of selected school personnel through focus group methodology. *J. Adolesc. Health* **2005**, *37*, 281–288. [CrossRef] [PubMed]

37. Boutilier, J.; King, S. Missed opportunities: School as an undervalued site for effective pain management. *Pediatr. Pain Lett.* **2013**, *15*, 9–15.

38. Gorodzinsky, A.; Hainsworth, K.; Weisman, S.J. School functioning and chronic pain: A review of methods. *J. Pediatr. Psychol.* **2011**, *36*, 991–1002. [CrossRef] [PubMed]

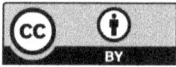

MDPI AG

St. Alban-Anlage 66

4052 Basel, Switzerland

Tel. +41 61 683 77 34

Fax +41 61 302 89 18

http://www.mdpi.com

Children Editorial Office

E-mail: children@mdpi.com

http://www.mdpi.com/journal/children

www.ingramcontent.com/pod-product-compliance
Lightning Source LLC
Chambersburg PA
CBHW051712210326
41597CB00032B/5451